Health Psychology —A Handbook

Theories, Applications, and Challenges
of a Psychological Approach
to the Health Care System

George C. Stone
Frances Cohen
Nancy E. Adler
& Associates

Health Psychology
—A Handbook

Theories, Applications, and Challenges
of a Psychological Approach
to the Health Care System

Jossey-Bass Publishers
San Francisco • Washington • London • 1980

HEALTH PSYCHOLOGY—A HANDBOOK
Theories, Applications, and Challenges of a Psychological Approach to the Health Care System
      by George C. Stone, Frances Cohen, Nancy E. Adler & Associates

Copyright © 1979 by: Jossey-Bass Inc., Publishers
              433 California Street
              San Francisco, California 94104
                    &*
              Jossey-Bass Limited
              28 Banner Street
              London EC1Y 8QE

Library of Congress Catalogue Card Number LC 79-83580

International Standard Book Number ISBN 0-87589-411-9

Manufactured in the United States of America

JACKET DESIGN BY WILLI BAUM

FIRST EDITION
    First printing: May 1979
    Second printing: October 1980

Code 7906

The Jossey-Bass
Social and Behavioral Science Series

Preface

In recent years there has been a growing concern about problems of health and illness and about the state and cost of the current health care delivery system. There has also been increasing awareness of the significance of psychological factors in the etiology, course, and treatment of disease and in the maintenance of health. More and more psychologists have become involved in research and application of psychological knowledge to problems of health and health care, but until now there has been no systematic examination of the contributions of psychology to this critical area. A major purpose of this book is to take stock of these contributions and to consider the state of development of a field that is appropriately called *health psychology*.

This book has been written with a wide range of potential readers in mind. It is, of course, addressed to psychologists, both those who are already at work in the health field and those who are beginning to recognize the challenging opportunities there. *Health Psychology* presents the current state of knowledge and research in the field and identifies issues and tasks that are particularly pressing or have unusual potential for interesting and salient research. The book is designed to inform those who are engaged in health professions and occupations about the potential uses and contributions of psychological theory and research. It is also addressed to our colleagues in the other behavioral sciences who are engaged in research in the health care system. We have found the contributions from other disciplines to be critical to our work and hope that this book will prove useful in defining a psychological approach to health issues: the problems to which psychologists are drawn, the ways in which they formulate and investigate these problems, and the types of interventions they may suggest. Additionally, this book will serve health professionals and students in courses designed to show how psychology can be applied to the health system. Currently, there is no other work that treats a range of psychological topics in sufficient depth to qualify as a survey of health psychology; this book is intended to fill that gap.

Health Psychology is divided into four parts. Part One provides an overview of the health system from the perspective of psychologists and also discusses some of the work of other social and behavioral sciences in the health arena. For psychologists, there is an opening survey of their successes and failures in the health system; for other social and behavioral scientists, there is a description of what psychology is.

Parts Two and Three are concerned with particular aspects of the health system to which psychologists have made significant contributions. Some chapters are overviews; others explore specific issues or topics in depth. Part Two presents topics that focus on the person whose health is at issue. Part Three is concerned with problems of those who undertake to provide health care. (Since the *interactions* between these two groups are crucial, this separation into parts is somewhat arbitrary.) Part Four takes a more prospective viewpoint, outlining theories and approaches from some of the major fields of psychology that might be applied to the health arena in greater measure than has been done so far.

We conclude the book with a discussion of the major themes that emerge in the previous chapters, which, along with other impressions and facts, indicates what form we believe this developing field of health psychology will take. We also consider the training and employment opportunities of future health psychologists.

The concept of this book took shape during a seminar on health psychology led by Gary Schwartz, at the University of California, San Francisco (UCSF). The seminar was an inaugural activity for the newly approved specialization of health psychology, which was to be offered in our doctoral program. Gary Schwartz along with George Stone, who had been planning the health psychology program since 1970, explored questions about the scope and subject matter of this new field and how it might relate to other emerging focuses of scientific and professional activity—behavioral medicine, health care psychology, and medical psychology. Doyle Gentry, Joseph Matarazzo, Peter Suedfeld, Jack Wakely, and Stephen Weiss—guest participants in the seminar—gave us new perspectives on some of the issues, questions, and problems. Their active interest enhanced our excitement about the possibilities for the new field and engendered a determination to explore those prospects more fully. As the core faculty in this new program, we saw the need for a book that would fully investigate what psychologists had done and what they could do to make their expertise more widely available for the resolution of health problems.

In preparing this book we have had the stimulation, support, and assistance of many persons in addition to those already mentioned. We take this opportunity to thank all of you who have, by your interest and suggestions, made it possible for us to complete our task. We would, however, like specifically to acknowledge the help of Pamela Jackson and especially Nancy Snyder, whose work in typing the many drafts of our chapters and in compiling the list of references was invaluable. For their good spirits and calm encouragement throughout we are most grateful.

Finally, we acknowledge the outstanding contributions of our coauthors. Each chapter was written for this book by invitation; however, the contents do not necessarily represent a consensus of opinion. Although we, as editors, reviewed and commented on each chapter, there was no attempt to obtain a consensus of views among authors. Thus this book presents a lively diversity of views and approaches to core issues in health psychology.

San Francisco, California　　　　　　　　　　　　　　　　George C. Stone
April 1979　　　　　　　　　　　　　　　　　　　　　　　Frances Cohen
　　　　　　　　　　　　　　　　　　　　　　　　　　　　Nancy E. Adler

Contents

xiii

Contents

The Authors

George C. Stone is currently professor of psychology at the Langley Porter Institute and director of the graduate academic program in psychology in the Department of Psychiatry, School of Medicine, at the University of California, San Francisco. He received his B.A., M.A., and Ph.D. degrees, all in psychology, from the University of California, Berkeley (1948 to 1954). Before coming to the Langley Porter Institute as research psychologist in 1958, Stone was engaged in research on social perception at the University of Illinois and in the establishment of a psychopharmacology laboratory.

Stone's interests combine social psychology, physiological psychology, and the psychology of information processing. In numerous journal publications, he has reported research on both animal and human subjects, dealing with their learning, perception, and other forms of information-processing under normal conditions and after receiving drugs. Through Stone's leadership the program in health psychology was initiated at the University of California, San Francisco. His present research concerns the use of information in health transactions, with particular emphasis on communication processes.

Stone is a fellow in the American Psychological Association (APA) and the American Association for the Advancement of Science and has played an active role in the development of the new Division of Health

Psychology in the APA, for which he currently chairs the Committee on Education and Training.

Frances Cohen is assistant professor of psychology in the School of Medicine at the University of California, San Francisco, where she is one of the core faculty in the health psychology program. Cohen received her B.S. degree in psychology from the University of Washington, Seattle (1967) and the M.A. and Ph.D. degrees in psychology from the University of California, Berkeley (1970, 1975). She was a postdoctoral fellow in the Department of Psychiatry at the School of Medicine at Stanford University before joining the University of California faculty.

Cohen's research interests focus on theoretical questions concerning stress and coping issues, including psychological factors influencing recovery from surgery, personality factors involved in the etiology of somatic illness, and interventions to aid coping with stressful medical procedures. She also has special interests in the role of social supports in facilitating adjustment in stressful situations and has studied the impact of support on modes of coping and emotional adjustment in women awaiting breast biopsies. She is currently investigating the links between losses, social supports, and childhood emotion and the development of cancer and coronary heart disease.

Cohen is a member of the Division of Personality and Social Psychology and the Division of Health Psychology of the APA.

Nancy E. Adler is associate professor of psychology in the Department of Psychiatry at the University of California, San Francisco. In addition to teaching in the health psychology program, she is an associate of the adolescent health program, an interdisciplinary training program in the Department of Pediatrics. She received her B.A. degree in psychology from Wellesley College (1968) and her M.A. and Ph.D. degrees in social psychology from Harvard University (1971, 1973). From 1972 until 1977, she taught at the University of California, Santa Cruz, where she was a fellow of Kresge College. During that time she was also a visiting research psychologist at the Institute of Personality Assessment and Research, University of California, Berkeley, and at the University of California, San Francisco.

Adler's research interests have focused on social-psychological aspects of reproductive behavior, in particular the use of attitude theories in the study of the creation and resolution of unwanted pregnancies. She has also done research on experimenter effects, group dynamics, and women in graduate education.

Adler is a member of the Society of Experimental Social Psychology, the International Association of Applied Psychology, and the American Psychological Association. She is president elect of the Division of Population and Environmental Psychology of the APA.

Roger Bibace is professor of psychology at Clark University and adjunct professor and director of behavioral sciences, Department of Family and Community Medicine, University of Massachusetts Medical School.

Georges Bordage is a physician and associate professor in the School of Medicine at Laval University, Quebec City, and a doctoral candidate in educational psychology at Michigan State University.

Lillian Kaufman Cartwright is dean of academic affairs at the California School of Professional Psychology, Berkeley.

Rita Y. Cohen is on the faculty at Dennison University.

Arthur S. Elstein is professor and director of the Office of Medical Education Research and Development at Michigan State University.

Norma G. Haan is a research psychologist at the University of California, Berkeley.

Sharon M. Hall is assistant clinical professor of medical psychology at the University of California, San Francisco.

Judith B. Henderson is assistant clinical professor of psychology and a fellow in the Clinical Innovation and Evaluation Program at the University of California, San Francisco.

Earl B. Hunt is professor of psychology at the University of Washington.

Irving L. Janis is professor of psychology at Yale University.

Norman Kagan is professor in the Departments of Counseling Psychology and Psychiatry and in the Office of Medical Education Research and Development at Michigan State University.

John P. Kirscht is professor of health behavior in the School of Public Health at the University of Michigan.

Richard S. Lazarus is professor of psychology at the University of California, Berkeley.

Helene L. Lipton is adjunct associate professor of medical sociology and co-ordinator of technical assistance and dissemination activities, Health Policy Program, University of California, San Francisco.

Colin M. MacLeod is assistant professor of psychology at Scarborough College, University of Toronto.

Norman L. Mages is associate chief of attending staff in the Department of Psychiatry at Mt. Zion Hospital and assistant clinical professor of psychiatry at the University of California, San Francisco.

Gerald A. Mendelsohn is professor of psychology at the University of California, Berkeley and research psychologist at the Institute of Personality Assessment and Research, Berkeley.

Arnold Milstein is director of the Division of Professional Standards Review Organization, Department of Health, Education, and Welfare, Region 9, and clinical instructor in psychiatry at the University of California, San Francisco.

Rudolf H. Moos is professor and director of the Social Ecology Laboratory at the School of Medicine, Stanford University, and the Palo Alto Veterans Administration Hospital.

Judith Rodin is associate professor of psychology at Yale University.

Irwin M. Rosenstock is professor and chairman of the Department of Health Behavior and Health Education in the School of Public Health, University of Michigan.

William Schofield is professor in the Departments of Psychiatry and Psychology at the University of Minnesota.

Gary Schwartz is associate professor of psychology and psychiatry at Yale University.

Lee Sechrest is professor of psychology at the Florida State University, Tallahassee.

Mary E. Walsh is associate professor of psychology at Regis College, adjunct associate professor in the Department of Family and Community Medicine, University of Massachusetts Medical School, and clinical and research associate, Clark University.

Health Psychology — A Handbook

*Theories, Applications, and Challenges
of a Psychological Approach
to the Health Care System*

1

Health and the Health System: A Historical Overview and Conceptual Framework

George C. Stone

The term *health psychology* is a new one. No book before this has borne that name. Until a year or two ago, no school trained health psychologists. In the professional organizations of psychologists, no provision was made for bringing together psychologists who were interested in the study of health, health-seeking behavior, or the health care system. This seeming lack of interest is hard to understand in view of the importance of health to individuals and their societies.

What do we mean by the term *health psychology*? How is it different from *medical psychology*, which has been in use for many years, from *psychological medicine*, which is even more venerable, or from *behavioral medicine*? How does health psychology relate to the other behavioral sciences that concern themselves with the health system? What are the theories, issues, concepts, and methods of health psychology?

Professionals in other behavioral and social sciences have written

1

descriptively and analytically about the health system, or various aspects of it, in books and major articles that date back more than a quarter of a century. So there is a "sociology of medicine" as well as "sociology in medicine," to use Straus' (1957) often-cited distinction. A medical sociology and medical anthropology exist as distinctly identified subfields of their disciplines, and there are books bearing titles like *Health Economics* (Sorkin, 1975) and *The Politics of Health* (Cater and Lee, 1972). Two issues are reflected in these works, both of which will concern us here. One is the matter of self-consciousness of a discipline: Does it reflect on what it is studying? The second has to do with the scope of the field of study: Where are the boundaries drawn? Are inquiries restricted to work within the Western medical tradition; are "alternative forms of treatment" evaluated; is consideration given to the political problems of eliminating major health hazards, such as subsidies to those who grow tobacco?

In this book we will examine the work of psychologists within the health system and of those who have studied its operation. The term *health system* requires specification of the meaning of each component, *health* and *system*, and that specification will require some effort. There is hardly any concept that receives more universal recognition as having positive value than health, but there are many different views as to what should be included in definitions of health and how we can determine when it is present and when it is not. If sufficient agreement can be achieved about what we mean by *health*, and about how its presence can be measured, we can then turn to questions about how it may be secured—what people can do to protect, enhance, and restore health.

One way of approaching these questions, which are fundamental in a health psychology, is to locate health within a *system* of constructs and relationships. Some persons think of systems as rational organizations working effectively to achieve agreed-upon goals. Such persons say—correctly, if we accept their definition of *system*—that there is no health system. Rather, there is chaos and disorder. Later in this chapter a more generally useful definition of the term *system* will be offered, making it possible to outline a conception of the health system that is sufficiently broad to allow us to talk about it freely and to compare and relate different descriptions of the system (Robertson and Heagarty, 1975).

A Brief History of Health Concepts

Before discussing the health system, we need to give some consideration to a working definition of health and some related concepts. The word *health*, like many others related to it semantically—*sickness, illness, ailment, wound*—comes to us from the Germanic roots of our language. The *New English Dictionary on Historical Principles* (1901), known as the Oxford Dictionary, defines *health* as "soundness of body; that condition in which its functions are duly and efficiently discharged." The origin of the word is said to be an Old High German word represented by our modern *hale* and *whole*.

Thus, health is the state of being hale or whole. The concept points to the battlefield. Loss of haleness (wholeness) in early times was usually the result of injury. Attention to health as a desired state to be pursued by means other than skill in battle has not been clearly kept in focus at many points in history. Disease, illness, healing, and hygienic practices are more concretely visible aspects of our lives. While the distinctions among behaviors that foster health, those that prevent disease, and those that cure or ameliorate a pathological condition are actively addressed in contemporary health policy, discussion of these issues is surprisingly absent in previous times. The history of human actions related to such matters reflects a waxing and waning of emphasis on holistic versus highly specialized treatment, paralleling varying conceptions about the causes of illness and disease. Similarly, emphasis on hygienic measures, both public and private, has fluctuated; these measures—sewage systems, for example—do not appear to have been closely bound by theory to the acts of healing.

In this chapter, we trace first the interrelated concepts of health, illness, and healing, and then those of hygiene and public health, in order to convey that our present views represent a very recent convergence of these separate strands, a convergence whose integration may only now be taking place. This historical task cannot be undertaken in any depth here but has fortunately been treated extensively by Sigerist (1941, 1951, 1961) and by Ackerknecht (1968). We discuss the anthropological distinctions between illness and disease and between healing and medical treatment in Chapter Two.

Historical Overview of Health Practices and Beliefs

Paleontological records indicate that bacteria similar to those that cause infections in humans today existed millions of years ago, and that the bones of the earliest humans show signs of morbid processes (Ackerknecht, 1968). Many skulls from Neolithic times have been found in which circular holes, some well healed, give evidence of heroic efforts by early healers. Among the paintings in a cave in southern France is one of an "Ice Age witch doctor wearing an animal mask," which is believed to be more than 17,000 years old (Venzmer, 1972). Thus, human affliction and efforts at healing can be traced as far into antiquity as records go. From our knowledge of the ancients, it appears likely that they construed their afflictions as coming from the gods and that their cures were in the realm of magic.

Even while they still followed magical healing practices, some peoples began to adopt hygienic measures aimed at protecting health. As long as 4,000 years ago, mixtures of sorcery, surgery, pharmacotherapy, and hygiene are found. The Egyptians attributed many illnesses to invasions by worms and practiced hygienic measures of cleanliness that may or may not have had recognized relationships to prevention of such invasions: We know they engaged in rites of cleansing but we do not know the purposes of these rites. The Mesopotamians made soap, built sewage systems, and isolated lepers but, like the Egyptians, intermixed these activities with a hodgepodge of magic and exorcism. The ancient cities of the Indus Valley in India also had highly developed facilities for drainage and baths, but we have no written records from that time to tell us their purpose.

In China, the principle that illness results from alienation from the natural order of the universe dates from about 2600 B.C. Venzmer (1972) describes the chief task of the ancient Chinese doctor as that of restoring a patient's natural balance, which had been disturbed. This formulation, which involves a desired state of health, seems to represent the first record of a concept that is essentially the same as that developed by the Greeks about 2,000 years later. The physician of the Hippocratic school (about 500 B.C.) based treatment "on the fundamental assumption that nature, *physis*, has a strong healing force and tendency of its own, and that the main role of the physician was to assist nature in this healing process, rather than direct it arbitrarily. Health was a state of harmonic mixture of the humors (*eucrasia*), and disease was a state of faulty mixture (*dyscrasia*)" (Ackerknecht, 1968, p. 64). Good diet and the avoidance of excesses were recommended as salutary. Democritus observed that "Men pray to their gods for health; they do not realize that they have control over it themselves."

These holistic conceptions, strangely modern in their tone, gave way to preoccupation once more with local origins of illness, fostered by the pre-eminence of Galen's views, which persisted for more than a thousand years. Galen, who lived and practiced in the second century A.D., was a Greek born in Asia Minor and educated there, in Greece, and in Alexandria. He spent most of his professional life in Rome, where he gained a great reputation as a practitioner, experimenter, lecturer, and writer, and served as physician to Emperor Marcus Aurelius. He left his imprint on medicine as a force of great conservatism, although, for his time, he was an innovator. He was an anatomist who dissected animals of many species (but probably never a human), and made important discoveries about the brain, circulatory system, and kidneys. But his science was mixed with speculation and misinformation, and, because he had written so much that was true, his erroneous ideas were revered for centuries as well. Galen turned away from the Hippocratic holism toward an emphasis on "local pathology," which was based on his belief that "a function is never impaired without the part governing the function being affected" (Ackerknecht, 1968, p. 78). This belief led him to emphasize diagnosis and to focus to a considerable extent on individual diseases like pneumonia, typhoid fever, and malaria, although, in general, he still held to a humoral physiology.

Galen's ideas are said to have overwhelmed and stifled further study, but there was little new learning in any field during the next millennium. With the reemergence of a spirit of inquiry in the Renaissance, attention continued to be focused on individual diseases and the development of new or rediscovered means for their treatment and for the treatment of injuries. A developing knowledge of anatomy and physiology led to an emphasis on their pathological deviations. Tremendous advances in the understanding of the circulatory (Harvey [1628] 1941), respiratory, digestive, and excretory systems, coupled with concurrent advances in physics and, to a lesser extent, chemistry, led to efforts to understand the human body as a machine, subject to localized malfunctions. Even the "British Hippocrates," Thomas Sydenham (1624-1689), who earned that title by following the Hippocratic tradition of very close and careful clinical observation rather than the theoretical rationalism that was predominant at the time, focused much more on individual diseases than on the persons who bore them.

This emphasis on narrowly defined pathological processes led to some vitalistic reactions aimed at restoring a holistic emphasis. Georg Ernst Stahl (1660-1734) proposed that the *anima*, the "sensitive soul," was the force that prevented spontaneous putrefaction of the body. According to William Cullen of Edinburgh (1712-1790), a "nervous force" had to be kept balanced between hazards of overstimulation, leading to *sthenia*, and insufficient response to stimulation, *asthenia*.

The highly individual concepts of global states, or comprehensive views of a person's health, put forward by these two men do not reflect a general attention to an ideal concept of health. Rationalism, science, and analysis were in the ascendancy. Throughout the eighteenth and nineteenth centuries, and continuing into the twentieth, the developing world of science and technology made great progress in overcoming the bodily afflictions that had brought pain and death to humans from their earliest days. At first, these gains were mainly attributable to detailed and meticulous empiricism and to wide sharing of knowledge acquired in such studies. This work further intensified the emphasis on localized changes in organs at the expense of more general considerations. Progress in chemistry, and the development of an experimental physiology, supported by increasingly sophisticated measuring instruments, brought a growing understanding of the actual means by which the bodily functions were accomplished. Great impetus to the understanding of physiology was provided by wide adoption of the theory, pronounced by Schwann in 1838, that the body is formed from individual cells. Major advances in the control of infectious diseases followed the proof, completed by Pasteur and Koch about 1880, that such diseases were transmitted by microorganisms. Developments in the field of surgery followed the adoption of aseptic techniques and the introduction of surgical anesthesia by Thomas Morton in 1846. (Actually, the first use of ether for surgery was made in 1842 by a physician named Long who, because he did not publish, is relegated to a historical parenthesis.)

In reviewing this body of scientific work, Ackerknecht (1968, p. 164) descries an "aversion of the nineteenth-century scientist from any sort of theorizing and larger synthesis." Beginning in the last years of that century, the great theories of biology (evolution), chemistry (valence electrons), and physics (relativity) began to take shape. The speculative rational systems of the eighteenth century had tried in vain to bring large domains of observation under a few relatively simple principles. But now the speculative principles were replaced by principles educed from a century of experiment and careful observation. In the sphere of the human body, this trend may perhaps be exemplified by Sherrington's (1906) *Integrative Actions of the Nervous System* and by Cannon's (1936) theory of homeostasis. Neither of these conceptual frameworks had enough of an impact on medicine during the first half of this century to receive mention in Ackerknecht's *Short History*, although he did take note of empirical work by the same authors. Perhaps these complex conceptions needed the support of accessible mathematical models for complex systems, not developed until World War II, before their influence could be felt. The integrative psychological theories of Freud and Pavlov were better recognized by physicians, and certainly contributed to the "rediscovery" of psychosomatic medicine in the 1930s. Ackerknecht (1968, p. 236) comments on an ironical aspect of this influence: "The fact that bodily diseases or symptoms are profoundly influenced by mental processes, often partially caused by them, was known by all great clinicians from Hippocrates to Charcot [but] the old insights were lost in the shuffle of fascinating objective discoveries with the attendant overmechanization and overspecialization. Doctors became so laboratory-minded, so scientific, and so impersonal, that they forgot, or felt entitled to ignore, the patient as a person. It is a queer reflection on the present age that one of the basic medical functions of all times now had to be reintroduced—as a new specialty." This rediscovery of the influence of mind on body, however, is only now beginning to impress itself on the main body of medicine and on our broad cultural definitions of health (Engel, 1977). The full impact of modern science on our conception of the healthy human being has had to wait upon a widespread dissemination of a sufficiently complex concept of systems that could match the complexity of humans. The models of simple machines, of reflex arcs, and switchboards developed during the first half of this century did not fit us. The systems concepts of the ecologist and the computer scientist provide the basis for incorporating the idea of homeostasis and for recognizing the pervasive working of a brain in control of our bodily functions.

Hygiene and the Public Health Movement

A parallel chronology for the development of a second major aspect of our current understanding of health is required because there has been so little connection between medicine and hygiene over the centuries. Right up until the present, illness has been considered preponderantly a problem of the individual or, at the most, of the patient's immediate community, and healing has been a private matter between physician and patient. Hygienic measures, however, from the beginning of history have been a public concern, unrelated until recently to the treatment of disease. The houses of some cities in India in 2500 B.C. had latrines that drained into sanitary channels, and the *cloaca maxima*, constructed in Rome in the sixth century B.C. and said to be still in use, served not only private homes but 150 public conveniences (Wilcocks, 1965). These early demonstrations of a concern for public hygiene were not accompanied by evidence that they were undertaken with a view to serving public health. In fact, the first recorded history of a governmental body addressing health concerns was in 1348, in Venice, when a "committee of three wise men," chosen from the council of the city, was charged to "consider diligently all possible ways to preserve public health and avoid the corruption of the environment" (Cipolla, 1976, p. 11). This move was taken in response to the horror of the Black Death, which killed a third of the population of Europe in three years, but was not, at that time, accompanied by a restoration of the concern for sanitation that had disappeared with the end of the Roman era. Nor were physicians involved in the "health boards" that grew up in Renaissance Italy until another 180 years had passed. At the beginning, these boards were composed solely of political leaders.

Programs to improve the sanitary conditions of towns and cities gradually reappeared after the Dark Ages. These programs received considerable impetus during the age of the Enlightenment but did not begin to make major inroads into the great scourges like cholera, typhus, malaria, and tuberculosis until the discovery, about 1850, of the bacterial transmission of these diseases. Only then could the concept of combatting epidemics by promoting cleanliness, which the Italians had introduced, give way to a concept of public health, a state in which the epidemics would not arise. Departments and ministries of health began to appear in England and other northern European countries in the middle of the nineteenth century. They represented the institutional core of an emerging field of preventive medicine, which could now envision a time when the impact of all diseases and infections would be greatly reduced, if not eliminated altogether. This trend was and, to a large degree, still is overshadowed by the growth of a highly specialized, highly technologized medicine that has enormously extended the range of conditions from which recovery is possible.

Current Definitions of Health

In the middle of our century, during and immediately following World War II, three major trends culminated in the formulation of a new kind of definition of health. Medical progress made it possible to conceive of the elimination of disease and bodily afflictions. Advances in psychology and psychiatry, coupled with the euphorigenic impact of the ending of the war, enabled us to envision an analogous end to mental illness. And the concept of "One World" opened new horizons in which these social goods would be made available to everyone. Thus, there arose the conception of health in positive terms, rather than as the absence of negative status. "Health is a state of complete physical, mental, and social well-being and is not merely the absence of disease or infirmity." This definition was adopted in 1946 in the original constitution of the World Health Organization (WHO). It draws heavily on the conception given voice a few years earlier by the great historian of medicine, Henry Sigerist (1941, p. 100): "Health is . . . not simply the absence of disease: it is something positive, a joyful attitude toward life, and a cheerful acceptance of the responsibilities that life puts upon the individual." The WHO definition represents, without doubt, the most concerted effort to develop an explicit consensus regarding the meaning of the word *health*, and yet, as we shall see, it has, by no means, been universally accepted as a proper definition. Also, as Crew (1965) points out, this statement leaves us with the task of defining *well-being*. It does, however, purport to establish health as a *state* that can be described, conceptually at least, in positive terms, not merely as the absence of negative elements.

The positive approach was soon criticized as providing an unworkable basis for the guidance of health-seeking behavior. Dubos (1965, p. 346) observed: "The concept of perfect and positive health is an utopian creation of the human mind. It cannot become reality because man will never be so perfectly adapted to his environment that his life will not involve struggle, failures, and sufferings." According to his view, the concept of health as a positive ideal is a creative force, dangerous only if its unattainable character is forgotten. That is, positive definitions of health make of it not a state to be achieved but a *motive*. This kind of definition cannot be used to describe an individual's health status, says Dubos, because the hazards to our health are constantly changing—from microbiological pollution of water to chemical pollution of the atmosphere, from starvation to overindulgence. We strive to remain adapted to our environment, but adaptation can hardly be described using only positive terms because we cannot anticipate what change in the environment may disrupt that adaptation. Primitive people, Dubos points out, are often healthy and vigorous as long as they are isolated and retain their ancestral way of life. But when contact is made with new societies, catastrophic disadaptation often results. In our ever-changing society, we do not have time to reach a state of adaptation. Dubos proposes that: "The nearest approach to health is a physical and mental state fairly free of discomfort and pain which permits the person concerned to function as effectively and as long as possible in the environment where chance or choice has placed him" (1965, p. 351; see also the chapter by Haan in this volume).

Dubos' definition still leaves us with the need to define effective functioning, and also with some ambiguity as to how we should define the health status of those who, like William James and Beethoven, have functioned far more effectively than most of us while afflicted with onerous states that we would ordinarily call ill health. In Dubos' definition we are not advised how we should combine the properties of freedom from pain and discomfort with those of effective functioning. Audy offers a way of retaining the potential values of the positive definition while providing a basis from which a quantitative measure of health status could be developed. He suggests that health be defined as a property of the individual—"a continuing property that can potentially be measured in terms of one's ability to rally from challenges, to adapt to [insults]" (Audy, 1971, p. 140). Audy differentiates four types of health: physiological, immunological, psychological, and social. Although each type of health could be charted separately in an individual, the four types are linked interactively.

In spite of these efforts to recognize the possibility that health can be more than the state that prevails in persons free of injury or disease, working definitions that enter into the design and evaluation of health services are still mostly limited to the use of negative indicators. Rushmer (1975) lists fifteen different categories of illness—for example, "sui-sickness" (self-destructive behavior of all kinds) and "eradic-ailments" (which can be repaired)—in preparation for an analysis of costs and benefits in a humanized health care system. Health indicators and health status indexes (discussed in the chapter by Sechrest in this volume) usually focus on losses from customary levels of function or on experience of distress. A few specific medical tests embody Audy's concept of evaluation by challenge (for example, the tests of organs by their "clearance" of substances such as glucose and creatine, and the skin test for immunological competence against the tuberculosis bacillus). Even though this approach may be appealing because it posits a positive state, it is not clear that ethical considerations would permit the widespread use of tests by "insult."

Perhaps because it is so difficult to arrive at a fully satisfactory definition of health, most contemporary discussions slip quickly from attention to health as a noun to consideration of health as an adjective. We discourse on health care, health services, health facilities, and health behavior. We may find it difficult to agree on what constitutes a state of health, or even whether the term should be considered to represent a state or a motive, but there is much less difficulty in agreeing on whether or not an activity is intended to *improve* someone's health status. Our differences concern the efficacy of the means chosen, how much we should invest, and where we should stop. Mechanic (1972a, pp. 3-4) puts it this way: "The fact that modern societies, however organized, devote such great resources to health attests to its social importance. . . . Since resources are limited, we must make choices. Health care at some point must be weighed against other social preferences and commitments." In other words, in the real world we must inevitably stop short of attaining the ideal of health for all people, however it may be defined. We can devote our attention to considering the ways in which humans go about the business of protecting and improving their health without concluding what such efforts might entail.

Thus, we arrive at a modern definition of health that recognizes it as an unmeasurable state of a complex, continuously adapting organism. Within limits, we can identify changes in health that can be associated with the terms *better* or *worse*. However, the tremendous power of our medical technology to extend life under conditions of reduced capacity to perform normal functions has contributed to a new concern with assessing the quality of life as a whole. At the same time, these medical advances also lead to enormous increases in the costs of medical care and in the amounts that could be effectively invested in public health measures. We have virtually eliminated smallpox from the earth (Boffey, 1977); with sufficient investment, we could surely do the same with malaria, trachoma, malnutrition, and many other conditions.

A Framework for Describing the Health System

This book aims to view the work that has been and is being done by psychologists with respect to health-related behaviors against a framework of the work that needs to be done, and to identify that part of the task for which the psychologist is well fitted by training. The framework required for the attainment of this aim is a comprehensive description of the health system, one that can encompass not only the efforts of psychologists but also of those in all of the disciplines of the behavioral and social sciences. Within this general framework, we can consider how the different disciplines have described and approached the system in their efforts to understand its workings.

Repeated reference has been made to the "health system." Now we must say what we mean by the term and describe that system. Some effort expended at this point in getting a view of the total framework will be repaid by an economy of discussion later on. A good deal of emphasis is placed on the *description* of a system because the first step in the analytic study of a system is a comprehensive description of it. To appraise a description of a system—to know if we have established a sound basis for its study—we must know what are the essential features of the description.

The Concept of a System

A system may be defined as "a purposive collection of interacting entities" (La Patra, 1975, p. 9). It consists of a set of elements that are related to each other in such a way that the actions of one element affect the states of and initiate or modify activity in other elements of the system. The first step in describing a system is to establish its boundaries—setting out principles by which it can be decided whether some particular entity is an element of the system or not. A system is said to be bounded by the relationship of its entities to a purpose, function, or sphere of activity: If the element is relevant to the attainment of the system's objectives, it is an element of the system. If an entity (for example, a knife) impinges on a group of entities (some organs of a body), does it thereby become a part of the system constituted by the organism? That question cannot be answered until we have more completely described the system. Its posing serves to remind us that systems are constructed hierarchically: A heart is a system that forms an element in another system of surgeon, patient, operating theater, and anesthetist; or Aztec priest, victim, and altar; or robber, victim, and assault. If we conceive a system whose purpose is to extend the life of the patient or, for that matter, to terminate it for ritual purposes, then the knife and heart are both elements of the system. In the first case, the knife might even be considered a transient element of the homeostatic system that is the patient —something introduced as a result of the patient's health-seeking behavior. In the case of a thief's assault upon a haphazardly chosen victim, the knife plays a different role: It may be seen as a totally gratuitous insult to the integrity of the person; or, given certain philosophical or religious assumptions, it may still be regarded as an element of a "purposeful collection of interacting entities"—with Fate or God incorporated in the system. The perceived purpose, function, or sphere of activity that bounds the system varies according to who describes the system. Therefore, a statement of the purpose or sphere of activity is a major part of the description of a system, which provides the basis for the enumeration (explicit or implicit) of the system's elements.

Relationships as Rules for Changing Systems

A description of a system also contains a specification of the relationships among those entities. To describe relationships, we first must recognize that every element of a system can exist in multiple states. The heart can be normal, congenitally deformed, enlarged, infarcted, or traumatized. The knife can be in storage, at hand, poised, or cutting. If the change in state of one element is systematically associated with a change in state of another, those elements are said to be related, and a listing of the rules governing these associated changes in state constitutes the description of the relationship. Most elements of a system are related to more than one, usually to many other, elements of the system. The relationship between any two elements is generally conditioned by the state of many, if not all, of the other elements in the system. Thus, each rule—change of element A (knife) from state 1 (at hand) to state 2 (poised) increases the likelihood that element B (heart) will change from state 2 (normal rate of contraction) to state 3 (rapid beating)—must be qualified by specifying the states of all of the other elements in the system (for example, whether the patient is anesthetized or fully conscious). There would be not only one rule but also a whole family of them to describe the relationship of knife to heart.

For any but the most trivial systems, a complete description is an unattainable ideal. For example, if we were concerned with a system of three elements, each capable of taking on only three different states and assuming that the system has no memory of how it got to its present state—a one-stage Markovian system—we would need 648 simple rules to specify all of the relationships. (Starting from each of the $3^3 = 27$ initial states of the system, any one of the three elements could change and in either of two ways. Thus, there are 6 X 27 possible initiating changes. For each, there are two remaining elements that can show altered probabilities of change to each of the two other states it could occupy. If we looked at the matter in a slightly different way, considering that the system was in one of its twenty-seven states at each moment and specifying the probability of its being in each of the twenty-seven states, including the same one, at the next moment we would have to specify $27^2 = 729$ probabilities.) If we had four elements, we would require either 27,648 simple rules or 65,536 probabilities to specify relationships. When we consider the number of different states that can be assumed by the complex entities of the real world (a doctor, a patient), it is clear that our descriptions of real systems must be based on radically limited selections from the set of all relationships. This limitation can be achieved in various ways: by excluding entities from consideration, by selecting from the set of state-change relationships that are considered, and by restricting the number of states of other system entities that are differentiated in describing relationships for any two. For example, the Health Belief Model, a psychological theory described in Chapter Three, focuses on a single change in behavior, usually the taking of a specific action, following a specific kind of state change, the receipt of some health recommendation. By eliminating from consideration all other actions that might have been taken, instead of the one that was recommended, and by averaging over (randomizing) all other types of information input received, a simplification of tenfold to a hundredfold or more can be achieved. Further, the *modifying factors* of this theory, which include such variables as age, sex, ethnic and cultural background, education, and the like, are mentioned but rarely introduced as complex qualifiers on the relationships that are isolated. These various necessary simplifications will be elaborated and exemplified as we proceed to consider various descriptions of the health system.

Simplified and abbreviated descriptions of portions of the health system are usually made in preparation for the proposal of some intervention through which we hope that the system might change from its present distribution of states to one that is deemed preferable. The description may be intended to gain the agreement of others that the change is desirable or to discover how the desired changes may be accomplished. Our purpose in making the description guides our selection of those aspects of the system included in the description, both in terms of the entities we include and our abstraction and organization of the rules listed.

Activities as a Special Type of Relationship

One of the most fruitful approaches to the organization of rules is to group them as "activities." Definition of an activity requires the specification of three subsets of the entities in the system: these may be called the agent, the situation, and the target. Sequenced patterns of state changes in the agent, under specifiable states of the situation (context or environment), give rise to predictable changes in the target. By labeling the activity, we are able to draw bounds around a part of the system, not simply deriving a subsystem made up from a subset of the system elements but also excluding as inconsequential for this activity some of the states of some of the elements that are included. In the system of doctor (agent) and patient (target), if we specify an activity of stethoscopic examination of heart sounds, we know (from prior descriptions of the activity) a good deal about the states of the doctor, patient, and environment. The doctor generally has certain intents (information gathering), certain relationships of responsibility toward this patient, and certain expectations about future aspects of the relationship. Certain spatial relationships between the doctor and patient are obligatory, and so on. Similarly, certain states of the patient are essential, others incompatible, and still others inconsequential to this activity. The environment must be sufficiently free from noise and other physical disturbances that the heart sounds can be heard by the doctor. "Privacy" is usually a desired condition (a condition is a set of states of a set of entities) but is not essential for the activity.

Activities are such potent organizing constructs that many descriptions of the health system are limited to descriptions of and questions about activities that take place within it. However, if we attempt to describe the approach of some discipline to the health system entirely in terms of the collection of activities with which it is concerned, it may be difficult to discern the relationships among the various activities. The overall description is likely to be scattered and incoherent. We will therefore endeavor to generate implicit descriptions of the health system by developing a comprehensive list of the entities that appear in various activities discussed and to abstract an overall purpose or bounding sphere of action from the purposes attributed to individual activities.

Entities of the Health System

The individual descriptions of the health system that emerge from this approach are sufficiently diverse that it is difficult to integrate them without some more comprehensive scheme for categorizing the entities and activities of the health system within a broad statement of its defining purposes. In the broadest definitions, the health system is the system of entities that affect the health of human beings. The defining purpose of the health system is to protect, enhance, and restore the health of humans. This purpose is not necessarily rationally nor efficiently pursued. It is not held as purpose by the system in any self-conscious way since the system has no conscious embodiment. We, as observers, abstract or impute the purpose. Variations in the definition of health lead to variations in the definition of health system. We must be explicit, however, in recognizing that the health system is much broader than the health *care* system, which is that part of the system that deals with activities involving health agents and health targets. This distinction becomes clearer when we consider in more detail the four broad categories of entities that we incorporate within our descriptions: health agents (divided into three subcategories), health targets, health hazards, and health resources.

Health agents. Entities that engage in activities whose explicit purpose is the protection, enhancement, or restoration of health are health agents. There are three subclasses of health agents: people, organizations, and machines.

People act as agents in the health system when they behave deliberately in a way intended to serve some purpose of the health system. When they do so, they become the primary agents in the system. One major class of human agents is that of the health seekers, who include, but are not limited to, those who consume the services and nostrums of health care providers. It may be difficult to determine when a person is acting as a health agent. Sometimes we need to know what is motivating a particular behavior in order to judge. For example, a person who eats nourishing food because it is customary and pleasing to the palate is not behaving as a health seeker, but one who modifies the family diet on recommendation of health experts, or after having taken a course in the physiology of nutrition, is acting as an agent in the health system.

Other classes of people that are entities in the health system are health care providers, family members and other persons who have significant relationships to health seekers, health educators, administrators of health organizations, legislators who promote health legislation, and persons engaged in health-related research. Many other groups could be enumerated here, but need not be, since the principle for their inclusion should be clear.

The category of health *organizations* includes informal groups, collectives, clinics, hospitals, governments, and, in general, all collections of individuals who act together to promote good health. Again the principle of purposive behavior is applied in establishing the definition. An organization that unknowingly pollutes a lake with asbestos fibers is not a health organization, although the fibers are clearly health hazards and organizational activities will affect the amount of the pollutant discharged. If the polluting organization actively resists efforts to document, reduce, or eliminate the hazard, it is still not to be considered a health organization, since it does not further the purposes of the health system. Instead, we would describe it as an "active hazard," discussed later in this chapter. Only if the organization invests some of its resources in the effort to reduce the hazard does it become a health organization.

Although both people and organizations are agents in the health system, and many of their activities may overlap, there are very substantial differences between the ways in which they function. One example of such differences is in the "governing variables" (Argyris and Schön, 1974) which constrain their actions. Preservation of self-esteem figures larger in the actions of humans, while maintenance of organizational integrity is a major factor in the policy choices of organizations. Some of the state variables used to describe organizations and individuals are very different. Emotional states, for example, are important conditions in humans, but not organizations, while accounting principles and distributional structures governing control and the flow of information are used in the characterization of organizations much more effectively than they are with humans.

Increasingly, *machines* such as computers and automated test devices are becoming sufficiently complex in their operation that they must be considered as health agents. Although they, and machinelike bureaucratic procedures, are also listed as tool resources of the health system, both function as agents when no human judgment monitors, and is capable of modifying, their programmed activities. Human agents develop the programs of health machines and they or organizational agents establish policies under which the machines shall operate, but they yield their agency to the machine when they cease observing with the intent to intervene. Unlike an inappropriate bill from a computer, which will usually be detected by the person who has been billed, an inappropriate result from a computerized testing facility may be impossible for the target to detect, and difficult even for the expert agent.

Health targets. Health targets are those persons toward whom health agents direct their activities in order to improve the health states of the target persons. Two major subclasses of targets are patients, who receive restorative care, and persons-at-risk, who are targets of many different kinds of health activities. (The concept of *risk* is used broadly here, to include the risks that people face if they fail to follow the best health-promoting practices of diet, exercise, and the like.)

The separation of the target role (class or entities) from that of health seeker requires some justification. The same individual can be, and usually is, both health seeker and health target. The individual is always the target of his or her own health-seeking behavior, but the same individual may be the target of many other health agents. Furthermore, the person who is unconscious, or incompetent by virtue of age, disability, or other cause, may be target but not agent. The individual who unknowingly takes risks of which others are aware may also be a health target before becoming a health agent, at least with respect to particular hazards. Many of the important issues raised by those who study the health system have to do with relationships between the person-as-agent and person-as-target. How far should the professionals of the health care system go in taking responsibility for those whom they believe to be at risk or to be failing to comply adequately with treatment regimens? When is it appropriate to mandate actions (either by prescription or proscription) that affect only the health of the target and have no effect on other persons? How are the principles that guide our behavior in the previous case affected if the welfare of others is also at stake? In short, the whole issue of coercion and manipulation is involved in the question of whether social agents should address the person-as-agent or the person-as-target: The degree to which social agents acknowledge the autonomy, competence, and responsibility of the other is the degree to which they grant the status of agent.

Health hazards. The agents of the health system engage in activities whose purpose is to reduce the impact of health hazards on the capacity of humans (health targets) to function effectively. Hazards take many forms. Toxins, pathogens, stressors, defects in tools or materials, and attractive nuisances such as crumbling cliffs that offer access to an appealing recreational site are examples. Some hazards are thrust upon persons-at-risk by the activities of other persons or organizations. The person who spreads a contagious disease or the company that resists efforts to clean up its effluents is an active hazard. But the activities of these agents are not considered, in this description, to constitute activities of the health system. They belong conceptually with the metabolic activities of bacteria that generate toxins harmful to the human body. These activities must be understood and modified, as complex states in the health environment, by the activities of health agents. This distinction becomes important when we later confront issues of responsibility. Such issues are relevant to the relationship between health agents and targets, but not to those with active hazards. It is their very refusal to take responsibility that places persons in the category of hazard rather than agent, so the question of *limits* to their responsibility is irrelevant. Coercion is certainly appropriate, and manipulation an option to be considered, in dealing with humans and organizations when they are health hazards.

Health resources. The fourth and last of the major categories of the elements of the health system, health resources, includes all those entities that are used by health agents in the course of their health activities. While one could consider the resources used by agents to be a subsystem of the agents themselves, it is preferable to give them separate status, since many of the activities of health agents are directed toward securing and mobilizing resources. Such activities are qualitatively different from those using the mobilized resources to improve the health status of targets. In fact, some health agents specialize in mobilizing resources for others to use. One of the typical problems of health agents—whether they be voluntary associations like the March of Dimes or researchers in the university laboratory—is that of allocating present resources between health care activities directly oriented to targets and activities whose aim is the garnering of additional resources.

Some of the major subdivisions within the category of health resources are knowledge and technical skills, facilities, tools and machines, therapeutic substances and devices, and commodities for exchange, including money. A very important resource, which cannot be included as a commodity for exchange, is the time of health agents freely committed to health activities: People choose to work as health agents partly out of nonpecuniary motives. This resource is not subject to control by others. Another important category of resources includes regulations, laws, procedures, and other intangible structures that constrain the behavior of humans. This category shares with other resources the property of having been acquired through the expenditure of human effort and ingenuity. The health organization is also a resource. Once it is operational, it functions as an agent, but while it is being formed, the organization is better treated as a resource, because, under the guidance of health agents, other resources are invested in the formation of this entity. A similar situation applies to the training of the health professional, but this has already been taken into account by treating knowledge as a resource.

Health Activities

The classification of health entities can now be used in classifying the activities that occur within the health system. Activities have already been defined as patterns of state changes in one set of entities that give rise predictably to changes in states of other entities. Agents, the entities whose changes of state, or behavior, constitute the activity, have been distinguished from targets, which are the entities whose states are to be changed by the activity. In addition to the human targets of the health system, hazards and resources may also be the targets for change. If the changes that result from activities are labeled outcomes, it is easy to recognize the compatibility of this descriptive framework with the formal model of decision theory (Savage, 1951), which considers how to select among possible activities on the basis of the probabilities of various outcomes associated with each possible action and the values assigned to these outcomes.

All activities of a system consume resources. The allocation of resources among activities is accomplished by many means, some of which are governed by the deliberate actions of health agents. Planning and allocation constitute one of the important classes of health activities. However, frequent calls for a more "rational" health system (better planned and with more equitable allocation of services) do not take sufficient account of the fact that no entity is in a position to guide the total operation of the health system. In most societies, control over allocation of resources is very widely dispersed among parallel, complementary, or competing entities.

Activities can be categorized in terms of the agent who is directing the activity, the target entities, and the kind of change that is sought. Characteristic kinds of change are associated with each agent-target pairing. For example, a health seeker may engage in exercise, dietary practices, or efforts to stop smoking in order to improve his or her own health status. Such activities have been called "health-seeking behavior." A health care provider and a health seeker may jointly engage in behavior designed to diagnose and treat some pathological state of the health seeker. In this *health care* transaction, as in the previous example, the health seeker is simultaneously health target, but in this case another agent is involved as well. The division of responsibility and effort between health care provider and health seeker varies greatly depending on the situation (Stone, in press). Although it is usual for health seekers' activities to be directed toward the immediate improvement of their own health status, some of their activities are directed toward eliminating health hazards (signing a petition to ban smoking in public buildings) and acquiring resources to be used in future activities (purchasing a fever thermometer or enrolling in a health maintenance organization). Other health agents tend to be more specialized in their activities. The health care provider works on the health status of patients, the public health educator on the knowledge of persons-at-risk, the health-oriented politician on the drafting of legislation to reduce hazards or mobilize resources, and the health researcher seeks new knowledge about hazards and the use of resources.

In the chapters that follow, we will examine how many different researchers from various social science disciplines have approached specific problems of the health system. Rarely do they formulate their questions in terms of an abstract system of entities in interrelationships. It may help readers, however, to see the relationships among the topics of the several chapters if they ask themselves which of the groups of entities figure in this discussion and which are absent? Which of the possible activities of health agents are considered and which are not? Thus we may be aided in appreciating not only what has been studied but what has not.

2

Social Science Perspectives on the Health System

Nancy E. Adler

George C. Stone

The bumblebee flew long before there were aeronautical engineers to consider whether its flight was possible, and the health system existed and functioned long before social scientists attempted to describe and understand its working. In Chapter One, we traced, in barest outline, the history of human concerns with health and illness and their efforts to gain control over this sphere of the human condition. We offered, in the most general terms, a framework within which the health system could be described—a framework comprehensive enough to encompass any other more detailed description or analysis within it.

In this chapter, we present a synopsis of the efforts by four social or behavioral science disciplines to comprehend human activities in relation to

Note: We would like to acknowledge our colleagues for their guidance in the disciplines described in this chapter: Richard A. Bailey, Margaret Clark, Marcia Millman, Arnold Milstein, Ann Scitovsky, Richard Suzman, and Irving Zola.

health and illness within the framework of their disciplinary concepts and theories. Our aim is to provide some reference points against which we can appraise the efforts of psychologists to undertake an organized study of the health system. Delving into the history of behavioral and social science studies of health reveals a common pattern: The scientists were present and working in the system for varying lengths of time before they began to reflect on their own activities there and to organize them in some systematic way. Members of each of the four disciplines discussed in this chapter have, however, at one point or another, paused to examine the work their discipline was doing in the health system and its relationship to the theoretical and academic core of the discipline. We draw heavily on those self-examinations here to abstract from them certain generalizations that can guide psychologists as they try to keep their own work on health problems effective and efficient.

We have chosen to concentrate on only four disciplines—sociology, anthropology, economics, and political science—since these have academic traditions that are similar in many ways to those of psychology. Other interdisciplinary fields in which the social sciences are involved—epidemiology, medical geography, human ecology, and systems analysis, for example—are also making significant contributions to the solution of health problems. Health psychologists will need to know about their activities and to participate in them. However, a discussion of these fields is beyond the scope of this chapter.

We present brief descriptions of the work in the health area of the four selected disciplines, beginning with a concise history of the emergence of the specialty or interest group within the discipline that has been concerned with the health system. We then locate these activities within the more general purposes and approaches of the discipline and examine the major health topics studied. Then we consider how the activities of these disciplines relate to the overall framework described in Chapter One. With which of the entities have they concerned themselves? With which activities? What variables do they use to describe the status of health entities? Preliminary answers to these questions provide some sense of how the disciplines relate to the health system and to each other in their work. In this way, we obtain a perspective on the health system that will help us to understand what psychology has done there and what a differentiated health psychology might do.

Medical Sociology

As with the other social science disciplines discussed in this chapter, there was work in the area of medical sociology before there was any organized discipline. In fact, as Rosen (1972) notes, health problems have always been linked to economic, social, and political conditions, and one can find observations as far back as antiquity and medieval times linking social and cultural factors to health. However, despite periodic observations of relationships between the social environment and health and illness, there was no systematic investigation or organized approach to questions that are now addressed by medical sociology.

Medical sociology emerged as an organized field in the 1940s and 1950s (Olesen, 1975), although there was already a great deal of published work before that time. Rosen (1972) traces back an interest in sociology and medicine to 1879, when John Shaw Billings linked the study of hygiene with sociology. As early as 1894, Charles McIntire defined medical sociology in terms that are consistent with certain aspects of current medical sociology. He defined it as: "the science of the social phenomena of the physicians themselves as a class apart and separate; and the science which investigates the laws regulating the relations between the medical profession and human society as a whole; treating of the structure of both, how the present conditions came about, what progress civilization has effected and indeed everything relating to the subject" (pp. 425-426).

Much of the work that immediately preceded medical sociology was in the area of social medicine and social welfare. In contrast to the later, predominantly academic field of medical sociology, work in the first few decades following the turn of the century concerned social policy and social action. In 1910 James Warbasse published *Medical Sociology,* which advocated a variety of reform measures regarding health. Also in 1910 the American Public Health Association formed a section in sociology. Its members were not sociologists but physicians and social workers concerned about social problems and health. Writings on social welfare and medicine remained strong through the early 1940s, reflecting, in part, the New Deal emphasis on programs addressing problems of poverty and disease (Hollingshead, 1973).

In contrast to the applied focus of social medicine, medical sociology was established as an academic discipline and its development was associated with the strengthening of the National Institutes of Health in the late 1940s and the establishment of the National Institute of Mental Health (Hollingshead, 1973). The first medical sociologists were outstanding scholars in the mainstream of general sociology (Bloom, 1976). The key figures included Talcott Parsons, Everett Hughes, Robert Merton, and August Hollingshead. Their interest in medical sociology derived from broader sociological issues. Parsons' work on medicine as a social institution and illness as deviance was an illustration of a larger theory of society; Merton used medicine as an example of a profession in the study of professions; Hughes' work was done within the framework of occupational sociology; and Hollingshead's main focus was on social class (Bloom, 1976). Not surprisingly, centers of training in medical sociology clustered around these leading figures. In the 1940s and 1950s training in medical sociology occurred in four major departments: at Columbia, Harvard, Yale, and the University of Chicago. Each had a somewhat different focus, reflecting the interests of the faculty. For example, training at Harvard under Parsons took a structural-functionalist perspective, while the University of Chicago stressed symbolic interactionism (Olesen, 1975). Yale instituted the first program leading to a Ph.D. in medical sociology in 1954; by 1965 there were fifteen such programs in departments of sociology, and by 1972 there were thirty-nine programs in the United States and Canada (Hollingshead, 1973, pp. 533-534).

In the 1940s and 1950s interest in the field of medical sociology increased, generating a significant body of literature. McCartney (1970) surveyed topical fields in published sociological research. In the period from 1895 to 1904, the sociology of medicine was ranked ninth of all topic fields and accounted for 3.1 percent of all articles. By 1955 this percentage had more than doubled, accounting for 7.5 percent of articles, and by this time it was ranked fourth in frequency of the nineteen fields. Bloom (1976) notes two trends in the 1950s that led to increasing professionalization of medical sociology. One was the collaboration of medical sociologists with medical researchers in large-scale studies. The second was the creation of full-time roles for sociologists in medical institutions rather than exclusively in academic departments of sociology. Rosen (1972) documents the rise in the numbers of sociologists involved in teaching and research in the health field. He cites three reports that show a dramatic increase in the numbers of sociologists with positions in schools of medicine and public health—from 34 sociologists in 1957 (Straus, 1957) to 96 in 1961 (Buck, 1961) to 218 in 1965 (reported in the newsletter of the Medical Sociology Section of the American Sociological Association in 1965). In 1955 an informal committee was established within the American Sociological Association, and a Section on Medical Sociology was created in 1959. In 1960 an official journal was established, the *Journal of Health and Human Behavior*, later changed to the *Journal of Health and Social Behavior*. Freidson (1970a) observes that by the 1960s the Section on Medical Sociology constituted a tenth of the entire membership of the American Sociological Association, and that by 1970 it was one of the largest and most active sections. Interest and involvement in medical sociology has continued to grow, encouraged in part by recent awareness that further improvements in health are less likely to derive from laboratory findings than from changes in people's behavior (Freeman, Levine, and Reeder, 1972).

Focus of Medical Sociology

Medical sociology spans a wide range of topics and theoretical perspectives. This is not surprising since its parent discipline itself lacks any single integrated perspective. However, despite the diversity of approaches, theories, methodologies, and ideologies within sociology, there are some shared assumptions that give coherence to the field. Twaddle and Hessler (1977) identified three basic assumptions. The first is that a social structure does exist and that social behavior is thus ordered to some degree. However, beyond this assumption there is disagreement over the basis of the structure and the manifestation of the structure in social processes. The second shared belief is that the social level (that is, the study of collectivities) is the most useful one for examination and that the study of individuals cannot explain the aggregate-level phenomena. The third assumption is that the social structure imposes constraints on both individuals and groups. Within sociology there is a good deal of debate over the extent of these constraints and whether human behavior is essentially controlled by social processes or is self-determined. There is also disagreement over the ways in which the constraints are conceptualized and studied.

Like general sociology, medical sociology "is concerned with social relationships and social processes, and its theoretical base must of necessity be that of general sociology. The activities of medical sociologists span the various areas of interest to the discipline: social organization, deviant behavior, social control, socialization, and other subjects of generic sociological interest" (Freeman, Levine, and Reeder, 1972, p. 506). Also, like sociology as a whole, medical sociology spans a number of methodological approaches, ranging from large-scale survey research and quantitative analysis to intensive participant-observation focused on a single group of people and qualitative approaches. The diversity of approaches can be seen in the examples given by Mechanic (1978) of the three general approaches to studying deviant responses. One is the positivist approach, which assumes some ideal as a point of reference and then examines deviations from this ideal. The positivist tradition in sociology, as in other disciplines, assumes that events are real and can be defined, and that causal relationships can be studied. In contrast, the idealist tradition asserts that there are no general laws and that one should focus instead on the attributions of meaning associated with social events (Twaddle and Hessler, 1977). This idealist perspective is more consistent with a second approach to deviance that Mechanic defines, the social-reaction approach. This perspective considers how people react to deviant signs in themselves and others, how they come to label them as deviant or not, and how they respond when one or another attribution is made. The third approach to deviance is the statistical one, which simply observes what the most frequent behaviors are. It does not examine the meaning of either moral or deviant behavior but only observes what is actually done.

Given the diversity of issues addressed by medical sociology, it is difficult to present a concise summary of the field. Kendall and Merton (1958) identified four areas: The first area to be established was social etiology and ecology of disease, which borders on epidemiology but considers variations in definitions of health and illness as well as in incidence of disease across social groups. The second area was the sociological study of treatment and recovery, including consideration of social support for illness, which could interfere with health. A third area was the study of the institutional organization of health, its components, and how they are related. The most recent area to emerge while Kendall and Merton wrote was the sociology of medical education, which relates to each of the other three areas.

Twenty years later, in his text on medical sociology, Mechanic (1978) identified twenty-two content areas in the discipline. However, these can roughly be fit within Kendall and Merton's four broad categories. Five of Mechanic's categories relate to the social etiology and ecology of disease: (1)

the distribution and etiology of disease; (2) social influences on patterns of mortality; (3) social epidemiology; (4) sources and effects of social stress with regard to illness; and (5) that aspect of community psychiatry as an area of research that has to do with social correlates of psychiatric problems. Kendall and Merton's second area involved the study of treatment and recovery. Broadened somewhat to consider the range of health behaviors and health care activities, this would encompass another five of the content areas: (1) cultural and social responses to health and illness; (2) utilization of health care services; (3) public health measures to change behavior and the social environment to improve health; (4) new technologies for changing social behavior and improving health-related behaviors; and (5) psychological problems in seeking and responding to medical care and responses of physicians to such problems. The largest number of content areas falls under the study of the institutional organization of health: (1) sociocultural aspects of medical care, focusing on the organization of medical care systems and the influence of the larger social environment; (2) organization of medical practice; (3) organization of the hospital; (4) organization of the healing occupations; (5) organization of the semiprofessions such as the nurse-practitioner area and pharmacy; and (6) organization of community health agencies. In all these categories, different patterns of organization are examined and relationships among agencies, occupations, and organizations are studied. Also included in this grouping is that aspect of studies of community psychiatry that examine it as a movement. The remaining two areas under this category look at health organization at a more macro level and consider the relationship of health institutions to the wider social environment: (7) changes in health care examined in the context of economic and sociocultural changes; and (8) cross-national comparisons of health systems. The last area identified by Kendall and Merton, the study of medical education, is also identified as an area by Mechanic. Finally, three of the content areas named by Mechanic do not fit under any of these four categories. These represent an even broader scope than do earlier categories and have to do with the relationship of sociological concerns to those of other disciplines and professions: (1) legal and ethical issues involved in health care, the introduction of new technologies, and medical research; (2) examination of assumptions of economic models of health care in light of sociological knowledge; and (3) health policy and politics.

In addition to the twenty-two content fields, Mechanic defines three analytic perspectives that are represented in medical sociology. The first is social epidemiology. This perspective views disease in a socioecological context and considers the differential effects of disease agents given varying characteristics of the host and the larger environment. The second is the patient flow perspective, which examines the selective flow of patients into and out of the health system. At each stage of the flow, the question of entry goes beyond a matter of need to questions such as patient characteristics and definitions of illness, physician characteristics, and system characteristics, including availability and accessibility. The third general perspective is the social context of practice. This perspective views the behavior of all participants (patients, doctors, and other health professionals) as being influenced by adaptive needs, social demands, and situational pressures.

One of the first descriptions made of medical sociology and the different approaches represented within it is still one of the most useful. Robert Straus distinguished between sociology *in* medicine and sociology *of* medicine. He suggested that sociology in medicine involves the study of questions in which the medical profession itself is interested. Thus, those who are involved in sociology in medicine are likely to be engaged in collaborative research and/or teaching, working toward the solution of essentially medical problems. In contrast, sociology *of* medicine takes an outside perspective and examines such factors as "the organizational structure, role relationships, value systems, rituals and functions of medicine as a system of behavior" (Straus, 1957, p. 203). The content areas described by Mechanic can be seen to fall roughly into one or the other of these two categories. Areas such as the etiology of disease, responses to health and illness, patterns of mortality, utilization of services, and public health generally represent sociology in medicine since they aim to clarify medical problems. Other content areas involve the study of the sociology of medicine, such as the organization of practice, the sociology of the healing occupations, social change and health care, and medical education.

There is some controversy over which of the two approaches is the more useful and appropriate. Straus noted that the two types of medical sociology are incompatible for a single researcher. Sociology in medicine requires good, collaborative relationships with medical personnel. Sociology of medicine requires an independent perspective. "The sociologist of medicine may lose objectivity if he identifies too closely with medical teaching or clinical research, while the sociologist in medicine risks a good relationship if he tries to study his colleagues" (1957, p. 203).

Much of the research in medical sociology has been in the category of sociology in medicine. Freidson (1970a) states that most studies have been on one of three topics: correlates of illness, utilization of health services, and aspects of behavior of patients and prospective patients. He states further that these share the perspective of the medical profession in defining the problematic aspects of medicine and medical care, and that it is far more likely that the patient and not the practitioner will be chosen for study. Gold (1977, pp. 160-161) reviewed all research presented in the *Journal of Health and Social Behavior* from 1960 to mid 1976. Approximately 60 percent of the articles focused on patient characteristics, and of these, 56 percent showed what Gold termed a "medical bias." Both Gold and Freidson argue for a more independent perspective. Freidson feels that the field needs to develop an understanding that is independent of any single point of view, and that the medical profession should be studied in terms that are independent of the profession's own ideology. Gold identifies two key questions: "How do working relationships within medical organizations constrain sociologists in their freedom of perspective? How can medical sociologists most effectively negotiate working arrangements which allow them greater freedom and autonomy" (1977, p. 166).

Medical Anthropology

In medical anthropology, as in the other disciplines under discussion, there was substantial evolution prior to the self-conscious recognition of the new field of specialization. As most of the major chroniclers of this emergence have pointed out, "Almost every anthropologist since the end of the nineteenth century has included, too often in passing, some reference to medicine or disease in his monographs" (Caudhill, 1953, p. 772). Yet Caudhill's "landmark paper" (Lieban, 1973) on "Applied Anthropology in Medicine" was the first review of its kind. Prior to that, there had been a few significant cross-cultural summaries of ethnographic data related to medicine. Of particular importance was a series of seven papers on "primitive medicine" by Erwin Ackerknecht, historian, physician, and anthropologist, which appeared between 1942 and 1947. These articles had a powerful shaping influence on the framework of medical anthropology and stimulated many other anthropologists to pay greater attention to issues of illness and healing as important aspects of a culture. Caudhill's review cited only about 200 references, of which fewer than half were identifiably anthropological. Polgar (1962) followed Caudhill's lead in the catholicism of his coverage, which was reflected in his title, "Health and Human Behavior: Areas of Interest Common to the Social and Medical Sciences." A year later, Scotch (1963) published the first review explicitly labeled "Medical Anthropology." Polgar cited over 500 publications that had appeared in the decade prior to his review, and Scotch added at least 100 that Polgar had not mentioned, many from fields of ethnopsychiatry, psychosomatics, and other areas to which Polgar had deliberately chosen to give only tangential attention. Another nine years passed before the field was again reviewed comprehensively (Fabrega, 1972). During this interval, the Society for Medical Anthropology was formed, in 1969, and a number of important statements regarding the relationship of anthropology to the health sciences appeared in a book edited by von Mehring and Kasdan (1970). The *Medical Anthropology Newsletter* began publishing in 1968, and in 1977 *Social Science and Medicine* instituted a section devoted to the field.

It is clear that somewhere in the two decades following 1953 this new subspecialty came to recognize itself as partially distinct from its parent discipline. A description of the stages of this emergence has been offered by Weidman (1971, p. 17). According to her view, medical anthropology was successively:

1. A substantive and theoretical area which has developed from an anthropology which looks at health, disease, and medical systems in both evolutionary and cross-cultural perspective.
2. An applied field which involves the introduction of anthropological concepts and methods into our own western medical system.

3. A highly specialized substantive and theoretical field involving the integration of concepts from particular facets of anthropology and a particular branch of medicine.
4. A substantive and theoretical area which draws from medical behavioral science . . . thereby becoming capable of making a unique contribution to general anthropological theory.
5. A substantive and theoretical area resulting from the integration and beginning synthesis of anthropological and medical concepts . . . [It], in this sense, is closely related to and possibly identical to "medical behavioral science."

Although Weidman offers these stages as successive, later ones do not so much supplant the earlier ones as incorporate them into an increasingly coherent and powerful body of theory.

The Anthropological Approach

The nature of this "substantive and theoretical area" to which Weidman refers is revealed in the frameworks that anthropologists have used to structure their reviews of the field. Anthropologists who have worked in the field of health, disease, and medicine are rather sharply divided into two broad subdivisions, corresponding, to some degree, with the division of the major field into sectors of physical and biological anthropology on the one hand and social or cultural anthropology on the other. The field of medical anthropology has been shaped more by the social anthropologists than by those more biological in their orientation. The closely related fields of epidemiology, ecology, and evolutionary biology have tended to draw biological anthropologists into their interdisciplinary endeavors. A good history of the origins and development of the field of anthropology was edited by Brew (1968).

The biological anthropologist studies *etically* (as an outside observer) the adaptive activities of the culture mobilizing its resources of food, work, pharmacotherapy, and so on, to meet these challenges. The social anthropologist takes an *emic* stance in seeking to understand the meaning of the interaction between the health agent and the health target. (The frequently used distinction between *etic* and *emic* corresponds in some ways to that between *behavioral* and *phenomenological* in psychology, or *objective* and *subjective*. Harris, 1976, gives a thorough explication of the terms.)

The focal construct in social anthropology is that of *culture* (Polgar, 1962), and the primary method, *ethnography*. The ethnographic method involves "recording and describing key concepts in the various aspects of culture; the need to understand the thoughts of one's subjects; and the documentation of a legacy of mythological explanation, oral folk-literature, verbal ritual in religion and medicine, oratory and other ceremonial aspects of social and political forms" (Lounsbury, 1968, p. 159). The result of such ethnography is an "ethnology," a detailed history of a people and their customs (Eggan, 1968).

Anthropologists seek a holistic understanding of the patterns of behavior exhibited in a human community. They pay particular attention to the *meanings* that people ascribe to the behavior in which they engage, and to the intricate interrelationships among different aspects of life such as work, religion, procreation, and health. Anthropologists focus on the normative patterns of behavior more than on the range and nature of variation from the norm.

In their long and patient observations, anthropologists establish relationships of deep trust with members of the culture who are their informants. In their contacts with other cultures, they have felt, even more than other social scientists, a profound ethical obligation to keep the impact of their presence in that culture to a minimum, while being acutely aware that they could not fail to influence the data that they were obtaining. Two behavioral tendencies have been noted by self-observing anthropologists to stem from this stance: (1) Medical anthropologists tend to be observers and describers rather than doers; and (2) they tend to identify with the people that they study.

Regarding the first of these tendencies, Polgar (1962) says: "[The anthropologist] may be conscious of his responsibility for the side effects of what he does, but in most instances his socially defined role and the sanctions imposed by his colleagues do not impel him to seek 'practical' results" (p. 179). Of the first third of this century, Foster (1975) says: "In those days, few if any anthropologists routinely collecting data on medical institutions were greatly concerned with the bearing of their findings on health problems of the people being studied" (p. 428). This tendency was greatly reduced when anthropologists began to be drawn into international public health in the years following 1950, and still later as they were called upon to serve as consultants in health care delivery systems, first abroad but then also in our own country (Colson and Selby, 1974). Nevertheless, many anthropologists continue to view their work primarily as an effort "to document and compare the world's curative systems" (Mitchell, 1977), and perhaps to translate "anthropological concepts into clinical language and treatment strategies" (Kleinman, 1977, p. 14).

The second behavioral disposition of medical anthropologists is that of identifying with the people in their traditional cultures. Foster (1976) has traced a sequence of three premises that have guided American-aided health programs in developing countries: First, before the involvement of anthropologists, attempts to help were based on the assumption that American preventive and curative methods would work anywhere and that people everywhere would accept them eagerly. When this assumption proved untenable, the international public health movement adopted the view that their programs would be more successful if they took into account the social, cultural, and psychological characteristics of those whom they sought to assist. Anthropologists, called upon to help provide this understanding of traditional cultures, took issue with what they saw as a pervasive assumption that Western ways were always superior. In fact, Stein (1977, p. 16) remarks that

"Anthropologists have been absolutely phobic in their contempt for Western (read: dehumanizing) medicine." Therefore, the third premise identified by Foster arises from the anthropologists themselves. "The most successful medical and public health programs in developing countries require knowledge about the social, cultural, and psychological factors inherent in the *innovating organizations* and their professional personnel" (Foster, 1976, p. 13). Foster goes on to observe that this assumption, far from being widely accepted, is "stoutly resisted by many." Weidman (1977, p. 26) agrees: "The essence of the Western medical model is its curative (therapeutic) posture. Enormous amounts of money and resources designed to transform it into a responsive, preventive, health maintenance institution as well as a remedial, reparative one have not proved successful. It remains ponderously curative in its orientation." Thus, the ire of the anthropologist is much more often directed at the intruding Western change agent than at the ignorance of the villagers that keeps them subject to "unnecessary" health problems. Most anthropologists, however, do accept the value of bringing Western knowledge to bear on the problems of nutrition, sanitation, inoculation, and other preventive measures to improve the health of those in traditional cultures. They must look, therefore, however reluctantly, at the Western change agents and their activities of organization, education, and the like. But in this examination, anthropologists typically retain their identification with the villager.

Issues in Medical Anthropology

Medical anthropologists are primarily social and cultural anthropologists, whose typical work has been the ethnographic description first of traditional culture systems concerned with health, disease, and curative behavior, and, more recently, of approaches to these matters in our own Western system. Each of six major reviewers of work in medical anthropology has used a somewhat different breakdown of the total field (Caudhill, 1953; Colson and Selby, 1974; Fabrega, 1972; Lieban, 1973; Polgar, 1962; Scotch, 1963). However, by going beneath the first level of classification, one can find a fair degree of agreement on three major groupings of work: ethnomedicine, epidemiology and medical ecology, and culture contact and change.

Ethnomedicine is concerned primarily with the description of the "notions" (Polgar, 1962) people have about health and illness and about the behavior they undertake in search of cures. Examples of this are studies of the relationship between health and harmony in the beliefs of the Navaho (Adair, Deuschle, and McDermott, 1957) and of the moral implications attributed to illness by several cultures (Fabrega, 1972). Ethnomedicine also considers conceptions of specific diseases and the schemes for classifying them. Both biomedically identifiable entities, such as *pinta* (dyschromic spirochetosis), yaws, and worm infestations (Lieban, 1973), and culturally unique disorders like *susto* (Fabrega, 1972) have attracted a good deal of attention. Conceptions of etiology have also been studied extensively. The "hot-cold" theory, prevalent in much of Latin America, Haiti, and West Bengal, is but one of several widely disseminated theories that has attracted considerable attention (Polgar, 1962; Lieban, 1973). This topic is one that provides a point of contact with another major category, the diffusion of Western medicine into nonliterate cultures.

Ethnomedicine has also been much concerned with the behavior of healers and curers in nonliterate cultures, their selection and training, and the efficacy of their treatments. Descriptions are provided of behavior in illness episodes, from labeling of the problem through the seeking of care to the treatment and recovery phases. Fabrega (1972) comments on the rich ore offered by careful case histories of such episodes for increased understanding of a culture's categories of states of health and illness, causes of disease, and appropriate behaviors in response to disordered states. The case method has been applied by Kleinman to illness episodes in our own culture to explicate the relationships between beliefs and behavior. He recounts, for example, the case of a fifty-eight-year-old American machinist whose rehabilitation following an "uncomplicated myocardial infarction" was jeopardized by a traditional familial-cultural belief that heart disease is "caused by stress, especially hard work" (Kleinman, 1975, p. 168). To a much lesser degree, anthropologists have looked at the behavior of the individual that is aimed at maintaining health and preventing illness. Generally, anthropological studies of such health behavior are those in which explicit beliefs play a significant role. In the Guatemala Mayan community, for example, where the belief system stresses the importance of proper balance between "hot" and "cold," great emphasis is placed on measures to prevent chilling (Lieban, 1973). In contrast, dietary practices and other kinds of behavior that are not conceptually related by the culture to health outcomes are usually studied in the context of human ecology.

A third subdivision in ethnomedicine is concerned with the sociocultural matrix within which health practices take place, the interrelationships between health-related behaviors and other cultural concerns, and studies of the mixture and coexistence of competing health care systems— most often, the traditional and the Western. Efforts have been made to apply principles and methods of ethnomedicine to the understanding of our own system of health care. With few exceptions (Caudhill, 1953; Taylor, 1970), most of the work cited under this heading has actually been done by sociologists. More recently, a substantial amount of anthropological work has begun to appear describing such special populations within our society as the aged, the alcoholic, and the drug addict.

Epidemiology and medical ecology is the second major topic treated in all six of the cited reviews. It involves not only the sociocultural specialists of medical anthropology but also physical and biological anthropologists. Social anthropologists see epidemiology primarily as an enterprise of surveying the distribution of illnesses geographically, and cross-culturally, in order to discover or demonstrate the impact of social factors on the health of populations. They are concerned, like many of their colleagues in sociology and psychology, in showing that stress, often arising from the disruption of traditional cultures and from urbanization, is a major factor in the development of various chronic diseases, mental illness, alcoholism, and suicide. They also seek to show how cultural practices in work, ritual, and other aspects of life can affect health.

Biologically oriented anthropologists tend to see epidemiology as the source of information about environmental perturbations and challenges to the adaptive systems of the human community (Haas and Harrison, 1977). Their focus is not on the impact of behavior on health but on the adaptiveness of human systems in responding to problems posed by the environment. Like social anthropologists, biological anthropologists are concerned about the impact of innovations on groups that are in a stable adaptation to their environment. Their emphasis, however, is not on the cultural meanings of change and the resulting psychological stress but rather on the complexly linked system of culture and environment. One of their basic propositions is that human actions are always taken in a context of multiple stresses and causes. For example, the seeking of food in a hunting culture imposes the stresses of work, regulation of body temperature against heat or cold, and exposure to biological hazards ranging from microbes to maneaters. In doing their work, hunters observe ritual taboos and they gain or lose status in the eyes of their peers. Theoretical formulations that treat a population as an adaptive system are summarized by Haas and Harrison (1977). One of the major factors in such systems is nutrition (hence, dietary practices); others are physical stresses such as heat, cold, radiation, and pollution. Recent work has been directed toward "the ecological concept of energy flow in human communities. . . . [This concept] permits biobehavioral interrelationships to be reduced to common caloric units of productivity, consumption, and expenditure" (Haas and Harrison, 1977, p. 82). In this way, the calorie becomes a currency for appraising cultural values.

Medical ecology also considers the effects of health and illness in populations on the development and achievements of their culture. The classic work in this area, Zinsser's *Rats, Lice, and History,* traced the impact of epidemic diseases upon "the fate of nations, indeed, upon the rise, and fall of civilizations" (Zinsser, 1935, p. vii). Polgar (1962) cites a number of more recent works that have investigated both ancient and modern consequences of attacks by bacteria.

In the area of *culture contact and change*, Colson and Selby (1974) point out that the enduring concern of medical anthropologists with the "institutions, personnel, and programs which are available to meet health needs" has traditionally "been focused on the delivery of care across cultural boundaries in a setting of change" (p. 254). This concern has taken several forms: (1) describing and explaining the existence side by side of traditional and Western medical systems, with the same individuals utilizing both; (2) avoiding the "fallacy of the empty vessels" (Polgar, 1962), that is, the assumption that Western medical knowledge can be poured into people without consideration of the knowledge and beliefs they already have; and (3) phrasing recommendations from Western medicine in such a way that they can be incorporated in traditional practices and thus facilitating adoption

(Scotch, 1963). A related topic currently receiving attention is that of finding a role for traditional healers in an integrated health delivery system that
also incorporates Western medicine (Colson, 1976; Foster, 1976).

The Health System as Seen by Medical Anthropologists

Anthropologists have participated significantly in programs to introduce genuinely valuable innovations in health care. At first, they adopted an
"adversary model. . . . It was postulated that scientific and traditional medicine were locked in battle, each trying to win (or hold on to) the allegience
of the community" (Foster, 1976, p. 13). Later many recognized that traditional people were very pragmatic about accepting new ways, adding them to
their customary beliefs and practices, without discarding the old. Caudhill
(1953) early recognized that it is much easier to introduce new therapeutic
techniques than to change underlying beliefs about causation.

In accepting the possibility of a modern health care system existing
side by side with the traditional, planners and administrators must be aware
of cultural practices and social circumstances that will affect the individuals'
access to the new services. Foster (1976, p. 15) presents striking examples of
costs incurred by Indonesian village women using "free" family planning
services, because of customs concerning "outings" and because of transportation costs imposed, in part, by bureaucratic rigidity. Foster sees fully as
many barriers to change in the beliefs and practices of technical bureaucracies as in the folkways of traditional cultures. He urges anthropologists "to
study administrators, planners, and professional specialists as individuals and
as members of professions and bureaucracies, in the same ways and for the
same reasons that we study traditional societies or any other client group"
(p. 15).

A summary characterization of medical anthropology may well re-
emphasize the disposition of anthropologists to describe cultures as they find
them rather than to identify ways in which they may fall short of some
normative culture. Also, more than any of the other disciplines we are examining, anthropology spans the boundary between individual and group because the basic orientation of this science is toward the individual in the
group. Perhaps the most significant aspect of anthropologists' views of the
health system is their tendency to see it not only as a whole but as a whole
embedded inextricably in a larger whole. Rosenstock, a psychologist, saw
that when he wrote, "The central problem in cultural anthropology is the
analysis of entire cultures" (1961, p. 1821). The anthropologist Foster finds
a similar picture today: "A systems approach, a holistic view, the question,
'How do these data fit into the whole picture?' underlies most medical anthropological research" (1975, p. 431).

Health Economics

Economic problems of health care are among the most frequently discussed topics among both lay persons and health professionals today. Surprisingly, the history of health economics as a specialty is quite new. Up

through the mid 1960s, most information on economic aspects of health care was found in proceedings of national commissions and congressional hearings. The sources of the figures were generally individuals or groups who were not specifically trained in economics (Bowen and Jeffers, 1972). The first conference that brought together economists for the express purpose of addressing questions of health economics was held in 1962 in Ann Arbor, Michigan. This "Conference on the Economics of Health Services" was followed by a second conference in 1968. The period between these conferences was an important time of development for health economics. In his introduction to the proceedings of the second conference, Herbert Klarman (1968) identified four changes that had occurred since the initial meeting. By the time of the second conference, there was no longer the need to establish and describe the distinctive economic features of the health care market versus other markets: A body of research had accumulated, there was widespread use of econometrics, and many more economists were working in the area of health. The growing interest of economists in health was documented by Bowen and Jeffers (1972), who noted that 20 health economists attended a special session of health economics at the Annual American Economic Convention in 1967; a similar session in 1970 attracted 120 people. Hauser (1972) credits increased involvement in the area to the rise in the importance of medical care in relation to other national resources, the greater salience of health care as an element of economic growth, and the growing awareness of the need for criteria other than price mechanisms for making decisions about resource allocation in medical care.

Despite the fact that currently "the field of medical economics is active and much outstanding economic talent is devoted to it" (Bowen and Jeffers, 1972, p. 281), most of the research has focused on specific applied problems and the field as a whole remains fragmented (Hauser, 1972). Further, despite the relative burgeoning of the field since its inception, it remains a rather small specialty of economics. Fuchs (1974) noted that, at the time when he wrote, there were only around 100 economists in the United States who devoted all or almost all of their effort to issues of health and medical care. In contrast, despite the fact that health costs account for more of the Gross National Product than agriculture, there were at least five times as many agricultural economists. There is no graduate training program specifically designed to train health economists. In the early 1960s, there was a shift away from teaching programs that were oriented toward specific industries, and graduate programs concentrated more in pure theory and econometric models. Thus, economists are likely to receive general training in economics which they may apply to problems of health (Bailey, 1978). Similarly, there is no journal devoted specifically to health economics. General economists who are testing a hypothesis or applying a theoretical model and choose the area of health for the setting will be likely to publish in regular economics journals. Economists who identify more strongly with the area of health economics per se will be likely to publish in *Inquiry, Medical Care, Milbank Memorial Fund Quarterly,* and *Health Services Research* (Bailey, 1978).

Focus of Health Economics

Victor Fuchs presents three principles on which the general economic perspective rests: in comparison to human wants, resources are inevitably scarce so that some choices in allocation must be made; resources have alternative uses and can fulfill a variety of needs; and people vary from one another in their wants and priorities. The basic economic problem, given these assumptions, is "how to allocate scarce resources so as to best satisfy human wants" (Fuchs, 1974, p. 5). The way that is most frequently applied in our society is the *market mechanism*, which operates under the hypothesis that optimum distribution will occur in a free market. A number of conditions have to be met for a free market to best satisfy human wants. Weisbrod (1961, p. 3), in an early book on the economics of public health, identified three market conditions necessary for optimum production and consumption to occur: "(1) individuals must be able to *determine* the variety and quantities of goods and services upon which to spend their money; (2) means must exist to permit individuals to *transmit* these wants to those who can and will satisfy them; and (3) the consumption and production of these goods and services must occasion no significant external economies or diseconomies" (which means that others should not be affected positively or negatively by this production or consumption). Weisbrod notes that while these conditions are relatively well met for most categories of consumption, they do not hold for the health market. Regarding the first assumption, it is not simple for individuals to decide on the amount of health care to purchase. Further, this assumption includes the further assumption that all participants have full information regarding all relevant factors such as price, effectiveness, and production possibilities (Fuchs, 1974). In many market situations, it is difficult to obtain all relevant information. This is particularly true of the health market, where consumers may not be able to determine for themselves what their actual needs are and must rely on providers for this information. Regarding the second assumption, there are limitations on shopping around for health care, which makes transmission of demand difficult. Finally, there are substantial external economies in health, as in the case of a communicable disease where one person's decision to secure protection by getting a vaccination reduces the chances for others of contracting the disease. Another assumption of the well-functioning free market is that consumption will be determined partly by people's ability to pay and that individuals maximize satisfaction in choosing purchases. However, as Ward (1975) observes, this assumption with regard to health would place a harsh burden on poor individuals, so that some degree of health care costs has been shifted to groups rather than relying fully on individual payment. However, this adjustment introduces some distortion into the market mechanism since incentives to economize at the individual level have been reduced, introducing even more externalities into the system.

Given the general characteristics of the health market and the limitations on its optimal functioning, economists have studied particular problems within it. Questions relating to the operation of this market include: "Who pays for and who receives medical care? How do the cost, quality, and accessibility of medical care vary according to the individual's income, class, sex, and race? Who provides health services and for what compensation? What are the patterns of delivery, and what are the incentives for efficient provision of quality care?" (Harris, 1975, pp. 3-4). Predominant economic concerns about the health care system currently revolve around problems of costs and their rapid increase; access to health care for the population as a whole and for specific groups such as minority, poor, and rural people who may have particularly restricted access; and choices of health care versus other goals (Fuchs, 1974).

Perlman (1974) distinguishes two current approaches to the economics of health and health care. The first, "investment in human capital," emphasizes the costs of disease. In this approach, disease is seen as costly insofar as it interferes with production and thus creates costs for the worker in terms of lost wages or the consumer in terms of added costs of goods. Thus, investment in health is seen as an intermediate product, a means toward lower costs of goods. Research from this approach has generally focused on the costs of particular diseases and cost-benefit analyses of reducing the incidence or curing various diseases. The costs of diseases vary greatly and are determined by variables such as the incidence of death and disability at various age and sex distributions, the average earnings of victims, average duration and severity of the illness, and the extent of permanent disability or increased susceptibility to other diseases (Weisbrod, 1961). The second general approach presented by Perlman is the "production function" perspective. While the first approach looked at health as an intermediate goal, this approach treats it as the end product, a consumption goal. The focus here is on increasing the efficiency of the production system, the health care delivery system. Research has focused on questions such as the substitutability of inputs (for example, the use of paraprofessionals for physician services). This perspective can operate at either the microeconomic level—considering improvements in the practices of specific physicians or in specific hospitals—or at the macro level—considering national health programs.

As noted earlier, research has covered a variety of issues and has been somewhat fragmented. Bowen and Jeffers (1972) summarized seven major areas of research in health economics in the United States. The first is the collection of basic statistics on health service systems. A second area is the study of health manpower to determine current and anticipated future shortages (or excesses) of physicians and health care personnel. Studies of manpower take into account not only supply and demand for services but productivity, since increases in the latter can offset some lack of growth in supply. A third area is the study of economies of scale. These studies focus on hospitals and physician practices to determine the most efficient size. Research has been done on the relationship of size of hospital (within given types of facilities) to average cost, as well as on the relationship of size of physician practices to cost. The fourth area is related to the third and covers the organization of medical practice; this again considers mainly hospitals and physicians and investigates questions such as the effect of the use of nonphysician personnel. A fifth area identified by Bowen and Jeffers concerns financing of health services. Studies have examined the effects of programs such as Medicare on demand for services, quality of care, labor, and costs. With the current debate over national health insurance and other financing plans, this topic of economic research is particularly salient and important. Research involving econometric models is the sixth area. The goal of such research is to develop a model of the entire market for medical care services which could be used to forecast changes due to shifts in economic or other conditions. The seventh area of research is cost-benefit and cost-effectiveness analysis. Bowen and Jeffers point out that since the health market lacks the efficient resource-allocation properties of markets (by failing to fulfill Weisbrod's three assumptions), there is a particularly great need for analytical ways of making decisions about alternative use of resources. The approach of cost-benefit analysis has been picked up by others in the health field as well. Many cost-benefit studies of alternate medical procedures have been done by physicians, administrators, and other noneconomists (Bailey, 1978).

Health economists are well aware of the limits of economic analysis. There are a number of important variables that cannot be translated into economic terms. Weisbrod (1961) notes that in analyses of costs of various diseases, consideration of costs is generally limited to losses to others created by a person's poor health. There is no calculation for nonmonetary costs such as physical discomfort, or psychological pain or loss. Fuchs (1974, p. 29) provides a clear perspective on the limits of the role of economics: "According to one well-known definition, 'economics is the science of means, not of ends': it can explain how market prices are determined, but not how basic values are formed; it can tell us the consequences of various alternatives, but it cannot make the choice for us. These limitations will be with us always, for economics can never replace morals or ethics."

Political Science

Like economics and psychology, which are only beginning to make a formal disciplinary acknowledgment of the work of their members within the health system, political science had neither an organization nor a journal devoted to health issues until 1970. Political scientists do not have a long history of working on health problems: "Even a cursory glance at the basic textbooks on public policy will reveal that health is hardly ever mentioned" (Weller, 1976-1977, p. 466). Lepawsky (1967) noted that in various listings of medically related social sciences, political science tended to be least prominent. As recently as 1968, Kaufman remarked to a meeting of health planners that they would be "fully justified in asking why professional students of politics would attend a meeting of public health specialists" (1969, p. 795). In 1970 the Committee for Health Politics was formed and shortly began to publish the quarterly newsletter "Health Politics Bulletin." In 1976 that periodical gave way to the *Journal of Health Politics, Policy and Law.*

Weller (1976-1977, p. 467) offers several reasons for this relative tardiness in focusing attention on the health system: For one, there may be a "disciplinary boundary problem; that is, political scientists may not be sure whether health policy is really public administration, political science, social administration, or linked to welfare." Also, he suggests, political scientists may only have turned their attention to health when this area became an important focus of government activity. Until the 1960s, governments in the United States and Canada, where most political scientists are to be found (Almond, 1967), had not played a large role in the delivery of health care. Finally, in Weller's view, political scientists have tended to focus too narrowly on the role of pressure groups in developing policy and on the development of health insurance schemes as the only likely outcome of governmental involvement, and have found little to challenge them in these considerations. Whatever the reasons, political scientists have only recently begun to make substantial contributions to the study of the health system.

What is Political Science?

As a background for examining the health problems addressed by political scientists and the approaches they take to these problems, a brief overview of the field of political science is in order. The emergence of this discipline, after 2,500 years of political theory and moral philosophy, is dated by Riker (1977) at the end of the nineteenth century. The first faculty of political science was established at Columbia University in 1880, and the American Political Science Association was organized in 1903 (Lasswell, 1963). Traditionally, political theorists concerned themselves with such questions as the desirability of various forms of government, the nature of representation, the formation of political communities, and the appropriate relation of public officials to partisan politics. They asked: "How can political stability be maintained in the presence of popular participation in government? How can revolution be prevented? How can war be avoided?" (Pool, 1967, p. vi). The very phrasing of these questions reveals the confounding of the descriptive and the normative, the failure to separate discussions of "what is" from "what ought to be." The new discipline of political science began to experiment with the separation of these questions, but found the development of an objective, value-free science to be difficult. The same difficulty has been noted by some members of other social sciences, but there may be in political science a more general and open questioning of the appropriateness of the attempt to be value free.

Although the theoretical posture of political science diverged quite sharply from earlier traditions at its point of inception, its subject matter and methods remained much the same as those of the political theorists— studies of the history of political thought, comparative studies of governments and laws of different nations, and case studies that analyzed closely the impact of specific laws and treaties. These "classical methods" and their associated subject matter have remained an important influence in university departments (Lasswell, 1963; Eulau, 1977).

The major force opposing traditionalism was that of behavioralism. According to Lasswell, Charles Merriam was the leading figure in the development of this new approach, which sought to supplement the traditional library research with new methods, drawing upon the observational, survey, and interviewing techniques being developed in anthropology, psychology, and other social sciences. During the 1920s and 1930s, old theories were shattered, but new theories did not arise to replace them. Easton (1953) saw the need for a systems theory and contributed to its formulation (Easton, 1965). By 1967 Almond (p. 13) could write of "a new paradigm . . . developing in political science" characterized by the systematic use of comparative data drawn from "the total universe of man's experiments with politics." But this seeming convergence of political scientists toward a common conceptual framework is not complete: "Political scientists are still riding off in many directions. . . . Indeed, not even the 48 chapters of the recently published eight-volume *Handbook of Political Science* . . . fully reflect the kaleidoscopic quality of political science" (Eulau, 1977, pp. 5-6). The range is from "an axiomatic science of politics" to a "hermeneutical approach to political knowledge." Yet in spite of this diversity of approach and the diversity of methods to which he points, Eulau perceives a robust (if eclectic) mainstream, with a new methodological sophistication that uses "aggregate statistics, survey studies, intensive personality investigation, content analysis of written documents, historical cases, and other sources" (1977, p. 9) to augment the traditional methods of philosophical and legal analysis and the rigorous methods of axiomatic theory and controlled experiment that are so difficult to apply to intractably complex human events.

Political scientists address themselves to questions about who makes policies and how, for whose benefit, and who pays for their implementation. They concern themselves with the power of different elements of a society in these matters, and the question of how such power is or ought to be acquired and distributed. Politics decides who gets what, when, and how. Political science studies the processes by which these decisions are made.

In their study, however, many political scientists remain concerned not only with describing the processes of decision making but also with prescribing decisions. Easton (1969) said that "To know is to bear the responsibility for acting and to act is to engage in reshaping society" (p. 1052). In a similar vein, Pool (1967, p. 121) says of the luminary authors in a contributed volume on *Contemporary Political Science* that not one had taken a "radically value-free position. All of them have accepted evaluation as a legitimate function for political scientists." Such evaluative tendencies are evident in the analyses of many of those who are now writing on the politics of health. Part of the problem of an outsider in defining the approach of political science to the field of health is that of distinguishing the political scientists from others who write on sociopolitical issues in the health scene.

Involvement of American Government in Health

Lowi (1969) proposes three basic types of public policies in any sphere: distributive, regulatory, and redistributive. Early federal actions with regard to health tended to come from a *distributive policy* of making services available to highly restricted groups, beginning with the Marine Hospital Service in 1798, and adding almost nothing until the establishment of the Children's Bureau in 1912, and the Rehabilitation Services Agency in 1920. Local governments characteristically provided some charity services for the poor, but the overall health policy of our nation, more implicit than explicit, has been characterized by Weller (1976-1977) as one of "benign neglect."

Regulatory actions at a federal level, previously few and scattered, began to be consolidated with the formation of the Food and Drug Administration in 1907. This step reflected another largely implicit policy that the public should be protected from unsafe materials of certain kinds (but not others). A new area of federal action began to develop with the introduction in 1928 of the first bill to appropriate funds ($50 thousand) for the study of cancer. Strickland (1972) details the history that led to the establishment of the National Institute of Health in 1930 and passage of the National Cancer Act in 1937. These acts, he says, signaled the beginnings of a national policy on medical research. Debate continues as to whether research support constitutes a distributive or a regressive redistributive policy.

The Social Security Act of 1935 authorized federal grants-in-aid to states for health programs, an authorization that provided the basis for the first clearly *redistributive policy* of major scope, Medicare, thirty years later (Lee, 1972). During World War II, there was a vast expansion of medical facilities and human resources, and the government adopted a "clear, direct, purposeful medical research policy" (Strickland, 1972, p. 15) of reducing the effects of disease and injury stemming from military action or relating to national defense. Later developments, such as the initiation of Medicare and Medicaid, seem to point to the expansion of this policy to encompass broader sources of insult than the military or defense sectors and to expand services to other segments of our society. However, there is concern among students of national health policy, such as Strickland, that we do not have a well-framed policy to guide this expansion.

Federal expenditures on health, just under $100 million in 1929, constituted only 2.7 percent of the total expenditures on health at that time (Russell and Burke, 1978). The various new programs that were introduced increased the federal share to 9 percent by 1950, a figure that remained stable until 1966. The passage of the Medicare and Medicaid programs, and various smaller programs, led to increases in the proportion of health expenditures coming from the federal government from 9 percent in 1966 to 18 percent in 1967 and 22 percent in 1968. After this time, the rate of increase declined, but by 1976 the proportion stood at 28 percent, which amounted to about $36 billion, and 11 percent of the federal budget.

Political Scientists and the Health System

In reviewing the history of health policies, both here and in other countries, Weller (1976-1977) finds three major eras: benign neglect, health insurance, and governmental regulation. Related to, but not precisely synchronized with these eras of governmental policy, are, according to Weller, three major avenues of approach by political scientists to the politics of health: emphasis on political pressure groups; a modified group approach; and a holistic approach. These approaches also correspond substantially to the evolution of political science during the twentieth century.

Political scientists following Weller's first approach concentrated on analyzing the influence of particular groups, most notably physicians, on policies and on the legislation that was primarily related to the individual groups. A number of analyses of this sort began to appear after 1950 and continued until the later part of the 1960s. At that point, some political scientists began to recognize that they had concentrated on too few groups. Both in concept and in reality, the model of the health system was in the process of shifting from that of a market distributing a commodity, health services, toward that of a political economy regulating access to a public good. The transitional period gave rise to the second approach, which Weller calls a "modified group approach." It views the health system in terms of multiple groups in competition with each other. Alford (1975, p. xiv), for example, describes the system of the present in terms of "a continuing struggle between major structural interests operating within the context of a market society—'professional monopolists' controlling the major health resources, 'corporate rationalizers' challenging their power, and the community population seeking better health via the actions of the equal-health advocates." Cater (1972, p. 4) identifies five elements in what he calls the "subgovernment of health," namely, "political executives, career bureaucrats, key (Congressional) committeemen, legislators, and public interest elites." All of these groups would be among those that Alford called "corporate rationalizers." The era of health insurance is emerging at different rates in different countries out of these struggles, with the era of government regulation still in the offing in the United States.

Weller's third approach is that of the "holists," who "look upon health care as a system" (1976-1977, p. 455). Although, as we have seen, systems analysis is considered by some political scientists as a major theoretical framework for their discipline, none of those who have published holistic analyses of the health system to date is, according to Weller, a political scientist. In his view, such work should have a high place on the agenda of his discipline.

The struggle for power among competing interest groups is only one of eight topics on which political scientists have conducted studies, according to Lieberman and Straetz (1974). Others that they list are: health planning and the restructuring of health delivery programs, public health administration, financing health programs, accountability and governance, health research, professionalism and health manpower development, and mental health. The study of conflict between interest groups, however, may be considered supraordinate to the other topics listed here, for among the crucial issues in planning, administering, financing, and even research are the perennial questions of allocating costs and benefits. For example, Strickland's (1972) book "includes a discussion of the impact of the conflict between scientific research elites and the disease lobbies on the development of federally supported health research programs" (Lieberman and Straetz, 1974, p. 199). The research policy takes shape within the constraints negotiated between these powerful interest groups.

Political scientists pursue these topics by investigating several substantive themes—the proper mix of public and private responsibilities in health, the best means of organizing each, the proper mix of centralization and decentralization of governance and services, and whether one can reduce the difficulty of anticipating the effect of policy-making structures on policy outcomes.

The involvement of political science with the health system has followed a course of sequential focusing on rather specific questions. We can easily understand these selective emphases as we realize that political science concerns itself with the making of policy decisions at the societal level and with the mobilization of power to influence such decisions. Since power resided until recently primarily in the hands of physicians, political scientists interested in health studied physicians. As the government began to become involved in financing and then regulating the delivery of health care, political scientists turned to the study of the emerging conflicts between interest groups. Now the issue of health costs is raising the social question whether we can afford to attempt to meet individual wants as a "right," or whether we will not have to shift to a consideration of societal needs, which may be best met outside of the health care system (Boulding, 1960; Laframboise, 1973). We can anticipate that political scientists will further broaden their perspectives until they do demonstrate the holistic approach, which they have often called for but rarely practiced.

Overview of the Disciplines in Relation to the Health System

Each of the four social science disciplines reviewed in this chapter addresses one or more aspects of the health system. They vary in the number and range of aspects with which they are concerned, in the questions asked about those aspects, and in the methods used to go about answering the questions. One way to compare the disciplines is to view them in light of the description of the health system presented in Chapter One, considering the attributes of the system that each has researched. This will allow us to determine where the approaches are complementary, where there are overlaps, and where gaps exist in the description and examination of the system as a whole.

Sociology

Medical sociology deals with a number of aspects of the health system. Two areas of research in medical sociology—social epidemiology and studies of the etiology of disease—are mainly concerned with *hazards* to health. Studies within these areas examine hazards that are located in the social and cultural environment. To some extent, these studies could also be seen to examine health *targets*, since the determination of social correlates of disease may help to identify those individuals or groups who are more or less likely to be at risk of various diseases and who may thus be more likely to become targets of health activities. Studies involving techniques for changing health-related behaviors and research on the effects of changes in the social environment on health behavior also focus on targets of health care.

Much of the research in medical sociology examines *agents* in the health care system. Sociology of medicine explicitly addresses questions concerning health organizations, such as hospitals, as well as characteristics and activities of health care providers. Research on health behaviors that examines social and cultural differences in definitions of health and illness, responses to symptoms, and utilization of services also deals with agents, since patients or potential patients are seen as directing their own health care activities and thus acting as agents rather than targets. Finally, the study of medical education and the aspect of medical sociology applied to economics focuses on health *resources* and considers how such resources are acquired and distributed.

Anthropology

Medical anthropology also examines several different aspects of the health system. Both social and biological anthropologists study health *hazards*, the biologically oriented scientist attending to their role as stimuli eliciting adaptive responses, and social anthropologists attending to their representations in the symbolic systems of cultures.

In their study of health *agents*, anthropologists have focused, to a large degree, on the curative activities of the traditional healer and on the behavior of individuals as they seek to deal with health problems.

Anthropologists also concern themselves actively with both individuals and communities as health *targets*. They study the meanings of health care activities for the targets who are their recipients, and they may participate in the phrasing of expert messages so that they will mesh with the conceptual frameworks of the targets. Until recently, anthropologists have not considered questions of health resources, but there are increasing signs of their readiness to become involved in recruiting and training health workers, both those who are drawn from indigenous populations and those who are trained in Western schools to work across cultural boundaries.

Economics

In contrast to the two disciplines just described, the focus of health economics has been more circumscribed and has been limited primarily to questions involving tangible *resources* of the health system. Some economic research focuses directly on resource allocation. Cost-benefit studies of the relative impact of resources used for one or another health program would be an example of such research. When other aspects of the health system are examined, the questions that are asked generally involve the relationship of these aspects of the health system to resources. For example, studies of manpower consider health agents as resources in the health system, and studies of economies of scale in the organization of physician practices and hospitals consider the relationship of health organizations to the uses of resources.

Political Science

Political science has a somewhat broader scope. It is concerned with *agents* in regard to the macrolevel interaction between health seekers and health care providers (as in the case where an organization of consumers lobbies for constraint of some behavior of providers by legislative means). Political scientists are concerned with control exercised by professionals. They stress the access of seekers to the commodity, health care, that is dispensed by providers. Effectiveness of agents is evaluated primarily in terms of aggregate statistics on morbidity and mortality. Very little attention has been paid to people as *targets* of health action. A notable exception to this lack is in the radical political critiques of the health system in which the effects of the medical model on individuals are considered (Brown and Margo, 1978).

In their attention to the internal operation of health organizations, by way of their traditional interest in public administration, political scientists have looked at such organizations as agents in the health system. However, they have been much more interested in the *resources* that are used by organizations and in the struggles among organizations for control over social resources. The major import of their study of the health system has concerned the manner in which decisions about the allocations of such resources have been made. There is also a theme, now much in the ascendance, concerning the amount and proportion of our total resources that can be assigned to the health sector. Here the political scientist studies policies for human resources, treating health workers not from the perspective of their agency in combatting health hazards but as resources to be assigned to various problems, populations, and geographical areas.

Until now, political science has devoted surprisingly little attention to the problems of health *hazards*. We do have studies such as Strickland's (1972) which investigate how allocations come to be made to different diseases through the efforts of "disease elites"; and we have the recognition that other social agencies dealing with such matters as public housing for the aged and other kinds of community services do influence health. Largely outside of the academic discipline of political science are the Marxist political theorists, who argue that the health system is not blindly ignoring social options that lie outside of the purview of the health care system—options such as the improvement of nutrition, the curtailment of pollution, and the reduction of occupational hazards—but is rationally pursuing the exploitation of health problems within a profit-oriented, industrial complex (Ehrenreich and Ehrenreich, 1971; Navarro, 1976; Waitzkin and Waterman, 1974).

Comparisons Among the Disciplines

Although each of the disciplines has been examined separately, there is, in fact, a good deal of overlap among them. Both sociology and anthropology focus on a wide range of aspects of the health system. However, while both address questions of hazards, agents, targets, and resources, the questions they ask about these aspects of the system are somewhat different. Olesen (1975) noted a number of substantive differences in the topics of study in the two areas while identifying areas where cooperation between the disciplines would be particularly beneficial: For example, sociologists have done most of the work on socialization of health care professionals, whereas few sociologists, but many anthropologists, have considered alternatives or adjuncts to the traditional health system. In addition to differences in substantive focus, the disciplines differ in the concepts and methods that researchers bring to their work. Sociologists, for example, are far more likely than anthropologists to use survey techniques and quantitative analysis. While both medical anthropologists and some medical sociologists may use field observation as a research tool, they will still differ in their emphasis and final conclusions. Olesen (1975) gives the example of two participant observers in a labor and delivery room. She points out that "the sociological fieldworker might well develop emergent concepts which were influenced by such sociological workhorses as 'role'; Goffman's dramaturgical concepts of 'front and back stage,' 'presentation of self,' 'stress,' 'hierarchy'; while the anthropologist observer might want to entertain concepts of 'kinship,' 'ritual,' 'purity and danger,' 'contagions,' 'mythic properties of birth'" (p. 423).

Similarly, there is overlap among the fields of economics, political science, and sociology in their study of the distribution of resources and the relationship of physicians to the resources. From an outsider's perspective, there does not seem to be a great deal of differentiation among these approaches and, in fact, many of the authors cited in political science are actually sociologists who are engaged in work on the "political economy" of health. In the areas of their overlap, these three descriptions share a focus on behavior of people in the aggregate and tend to use macrolevel statistics descriptive of large systems. To the extent to which they are differentiated, it appears that sociologists tend to focus on the processes by which organizations set and achieve their goals, economists focus on the processes by which resources are allocated and exchanged, and political scientists on the processes by which the power to engage in these activities is acquired.

Understudied Aspects of the System

While there are several aspects of the health system that have received a great deal of attention from one or more of these social science disciplines, there are others that have been mostly overlooked. Within the category of agents, very little attention has been paid to the functioning of machines as health agents. As expanding technology makes direct machine intervention possible in health care, we should examine the possible problems and promise of the functioning of such machines: For example, who will have access to such techniques and to the data that are accumulated? How will patients respond to a diagnosis arrived at by a computer? Will they have greater confidence in it than in the judgment of a fallible human? Will it contribute to feelings of dehumanization? A category of agents that has received some attention, but little in comparison to that given other agents, is that of significant others. Family and friends can play an important role in defining illness and the need for treatment, determining paths to treatment, and coping with illness. With the growing interest in the role of social supports in the etiology and recovery from disease, this should be receiving increasing attention in the future, probably within sociological and anthropological research as well as in psychological studies.

Although targets have been well studied, there has not been a systematic analysis of the nature and needs of a variety of targets. One obvious lack is research on children as health targets (or as health agents). Very little is known about their views on health and openness to health intervention. While much of the research has focused on people as targets of health intervention, more recent trends toward greater responsibility for one's own health and health care suggests that there will be more concern about the relationship of people as targets and as agents. At what point do people receiving information about health problems and preventive possibilities act on the information? What influences whether people will remain as a passive target or will take greater charge over their own information seeking and treatment?

Resources, too, have been well studied, especially from the perspectives of economics and political science. However, several classes of resources have been omitted from analysis. While there have been studies of time as a resource, the questions asked about it have been limited. There have been few studies of freely given time, yet there are many who work in the health system on a volunteer basis or beyond the time for which they are reimbursed. Another aspect of time that has been unexamined is patient time as a potential resource. When waiting times have been included in research, they are generally related to patient satisfaction or to decisions about where to locate facilities. Little attention has been paid to questions such as the scheduling of patient appointments to minimize either physician or patient waiting time. Patients often grumble that their doctor seems to assume that his or her time is more valuable than the patient's in scheduling appointments, since one rarely sees a doctor waiting and often sees long lines of patients. The actual costs and benefits of different schedules, as well as their effects on attitudes and behaviors of patients and providers, have yet to be researched.

The aspect of the health system that has received the least attention is that of hazards. There has been research in both sociology and anthropology on the effects of social hazards on targets. However, almost no work has been done by social scientists on other hazards to health: chemical hazards, such as pollution; physical hazards, such as radiation; and natural hazards, such as weather or earthquakes. Specifically, there has been no research on the relationship of agents to health hazards and how these might be reduced. Writing this chapter in San Francisco, we consider research that could be done about perceptions of hazards—in this case, the San Andreas fault—and of behaviors people take to reduce risks. Do people in San Francisco decide not to live near the fault? Do they choose a house that is on bedrock rather than landfill? Do they have emergency procedures and provisions in case of a quake? It takes little observation to discover that most people are, in fact, coping with the threat by ignoring it. This defensive avoidance may also account for the lack of attention among researchers. If the current trends toward greater awareness of preventive measures and health continue, we may see more individual efforts to deal with hazards and more research on them. In this, as in other areas of the health system, there are many fascinating and important questions for psychologists along with other researchers to investigate.

3 &

Psychology and the Health System

George C. Stone

      "The medical student must be taught that no matter whether he is specializing in surgery, obstetrics, or psychiatry, his subjects are human beings and not merely objects on which he may demonstrate his skill. This shift in his ideas of value will lead him to feel the need of psychologic training and to accept that training."

"It is necessary the student think not in terms of special organs or organs systems but of the whole living organism as a person, reacting physically and mentally to a changing environment primarily social in character.... The conception of a living personality has to be given to students and kept alive in their minds at the same time as they are studying the physical structure and processes of the human body."

These quotations, which express succinctly one of the major premises of the "new" holism that psychologists and others are now seeking to infuse into our patterns of medical care, were not written by members of the current vanguard of health psychologists. They are taken respectively from articles by John B. Watson (1912, p. 917) and E. A. Bott (1928, p. 292). They document emphatically the extended period during which psychologists have given thought to the health care system.

Recent appraisals of psychology's contributions to understanding and improving the health system have emphasized the relative neglect of all aspects except for that of mental health (Schofield, 1969; American Psychological Association, 1976). The impression that one can draw from the flurry of commentary and response in the past decade is that psychologists have just discovered the rest of the health system, after concentrating for many years on mental health, and are thus the most recent of the behavioral and social sciences to turn their attention to it. This is not a true picture. Close examination of the literature reveals that psychologists have been writing, teaching, and doing research on problems of physical (as contrasted to mental) health. There has been a fairly steady growth in the numbers of psychologists involved, in the number of different health topics considered, and in the amount of work devoted to each topic. Growth in health psychology has been slow, however, relative to that of psychology as a whole, biomedical research, and the clinical psychology of mental health. Psychology has not yet attained some of the objectives with respect to the health system that were first identified more than sixty years ago. The present increase in self-consciousness on the part of health psychologists may have initiated a new period of vigorous growth.

Although the rate of growth has seemed insufficient to many of those who have appraised it, much has been accomplished. This chapter cannot review these accomplishments in detail, but will try to discern major patterns and trends. Psychologists, as Leavell (1952) pointed out, were present in medical settings before the other social and behavioral scientists. One reason for this presence is that, to a greater degree than sociology or anthropology, psychology very early developed applied interests and began to offer professional services. Although the first developments of this kind were in education and child guidance clinics, some applications were soon found to have value for the health system. To describe the relationship of psychology to that system it is necessary, therefore, to consider not only the research and theoretical writings of psychologists but also to examine their professional contributions. Also reviewed are discussions of psychology's contributions to medical education. A discipline will propose to teach that which it thinks is important for those engaged in medical care to know. We can thereby learn what psychologists at different points in time considered to be important.

The Discipline and Profession of Psychology

Like the other social and behavioral sciences, psychology is considered to have separated itself from the mother discipline of philosophy during the nineteenth century. Wilhelm Wundt formed the first laboratory of psychology at Leipsig in 1879. William James began teaching psychology at Harvard in 1875; and the first formally designated laboratory of psychology in the United States was established at Johns Hopkins in 1882 by G. Stanley Hall. The American Psychological Association was founded a decade later in 1892. In the first decade of the twentieth century, three lines of work that had major impact on the development of psychology were the reports of Binet's investigations of the intellectual accomplishments of French schoolchildren,

Pavlov's studies of conditioning, and Freud's work with and theories about neurotic patients.

By 1911, when the American Psychological Association sponsored the first symposium on psychology and medical education, a division, largely un-chronicled, into "basic" and "applied" psychology was already taking shape. As in the other behavioral and social sciences, attention to problems of the real world have generally been regarded as somewhat tainted. This division has persisted from that time until the present, although there have always been exceptions to this generalization, and of late there are many voices not-ing that the behavioral sciences, for their future growth, "absolutely require the direction and disciplining effects that come from contact with real world problems" (Glaser, 1973, p. 557; see also Deutsch, 1976).

Academic psychology was dominated during most of this century by six major systems, or "schools." An account of the struggles among them as to which was best able to define the purposes of psychology and account for its data can be found in the systematic history by Marx and Hillix (1973). It is not appropriate to enter into any detailed consideration of these system-atic issues here. However, for the reader who is unfamiliar with psychology's history, it is perhaps worthwhile to note that there are three broad divisions that are reflected in the history of psychology and the health system. These divisions were apparent in 1911, reached their maximum size in the 1930s and 1940s, and persist in much attenuated form into the present. Psychology was divided—into the behaviorists, the psychoanalysts (most of whom were outside of academic psychology), and everybody else—by major cleavages of methodology and, really, of epistemology.

The *Behaviorist* school is dated to a paper by John B. Watson (1913) which urged the discarding of all references to consciousness and to mental states in the development of an objective psychology. Later developments within this school led to widely divergent viewpoints among behaviorists. Most branches of the school adopted a "methodological behaviorism" that acknowledged the importance of inner states but emphasized the necessity of defining them operationally in terms of their relationships to observable behavior. Skinner's *radical behaviorism*, which continues to insist that it is inappropriate for psychologists to posit any variables other than those of contingencies in the environment and observable behavior of subjects, is alone among the behaviorisms of the present in resisting the recent rap-prochement of behavioral psychology with the new cognitive formulations. While there are many contemporary psychologists who seek to combine the *behavior modification* techniques that derived from Skinner's formulations of operant and respondent conditioning with varying numbers of cognitive concepts (Bandura, 1976; Mahoney, 1974a; Meichenbaum, 1977), there also remain a number who hold firmly to Skinner's viewpoint (Azrin, 1977; LeBow, 1975).

Psychoanalysis was a relatively exotic foreign system until mid cen-tury. Aside from a few early experiments that attempted to demonstrate some psychoanalytic phenomena in the laboratory (Sears, 1943), attention was not given by academic psychologists to the ideas of Freud and those who followed him until the great growth of clinical psychology that began during World War II. Its methods of gathering data were too unsystematic and its concepts too loosely tied to observation to satisfy the preponderantly behavioral strictures of psychology.

Although many behaviorists still discount the "explanatory fictions" of psychoanalysis, current students of personality—of the unique patterning of individuals' ways of interacting with the world—are greatly influenced by a number of concepts stressed by the psychoanalysts: the critical importance of interpersonal relations in the earliest years; the presence of deep-lying constraints on behavior, whether these be called *unconscious conflicts* or *conditioned emotional responses*; and the generalization of such constraints along paths of semantic similarity and symbolic association. Recent substantial advances in our methods for representing and investigating verbal memory offer promise of our testing objectively many of the generalizations upon which psychoanalytic theory rests.

The rest of psychology comprised four schools. One of them, Structuralism, disappeared by 1915. The others—Gestalt Psychology, Functionalism, and Associationism—shared an emphasis on the inner processes that lay behind behavior and experience and a commitment to the experiment or some equally objective way of obtaining data, preferably quantitative. Since 1950 the influence of the schools has greatly diminished, and the contributions of these groups has merged with that of much of behaviorism, leading to the emergence of a kind of cognitive behaviorism with many variants but few sharp divisions.

A major new force in the building of psychological theory, the *information-processing approach*, has contributed to this confluence. It began with some of the engineering notions developed during World War II—servomechanisms and control systems, operations research into the effectiveness of complex systems, and mathematical theories of games and of communication—and started to experiment with the application of these models to the behavior of organisms: What if we considered a human a channel to transmit information from stimulus (*source*) to response (*receiver*)? What if we viewed purposive behavior as a system controlled by negative feedback? The early incorporation of digital computers into these efforts led to new metaphors, which have substantially changed the ways in which psychologists conceptualize their venerable topics of perception, learning, and cognition, and have provided a basis for productive investigation of language, problem solving, and adaptive behavior in general. So far, our understanding of motivation has been less affected by this approach, perhaps because computers themselves do not have motives.

A recent development that is important for health psychology is the appearance of what may be a new separatist influence in "Humanistic Psychology." This movement, which has not yet clearly established the scope or direction of its challenge to the main body of psychology, places great emphasis on human values and on the richness and complexity of human experience and of the world in which it takes place. Humanistic psychologists range in their views from those who retain a firm commitment to the objective methods of psychological science to those who completely reject the applicability of scientific method to the understanding of human psychology. The "holistic health movement," with its emphasis on the psychological influences that humans can bring to bear on their own bodies, for better or for worse, has many points of overlap with humanistic psychology.

Growth of the Profession of Psychology

A generic characteristic of psychologists is that they are measurers and manipulators. Their efforts to develop an experimentally based science led them early to a concern with control of variables, quantitative comparisons of behavior displayed under different conditions, and the attempt to *change* behavior to demonstrate the predictive efficacy of their theories. These predilections soon extended themselves beyond the laboratory into much more widespread interventions in the affairs of guidance centers, education, and industry. A child guidance clinic was established by Witmer in 1896; Thorndike began supervising the production of textbooks for elementary schools soon after 1900; and Munsterberg published a textbook on *Psychology and Industrial Efficiency* in 1913.

In spite of these early ventures into application, the applied fields developed largely outside of the purview of academic psychology until after World War II. "Educational psychologists reared their heads but were quite effectively segregated in schools of education amid some profound psychological handwashing. . . . In the twenties and thirties some psychologists became interested in the clinical and industrial areas, but they were treated as sports or even backsliders, and nobody made any effort to train them in their wayward activities" (Bobbitt, 1959, p. 20). These words are from the opening remarks to the first general conference on graduate training in psychology sponsored by the Education and Training Board of the American Psychological Association (APA). This conference, held in 1958, culminated a series of events that ushered in an era of explicit and systematic concern with psychology as a profession. A brief review of this history is relevant because most psychologists in the health system were professional psychologists (Buck, 1961). Some knowledge of their relationships with the rest of the discipline can help us to understand the slow growth of health psychology.

The emergence of applied psychology was not quite as surreptitious as the quotation from Bobbitt suggests. A section on clinical psychology was established in the APA in 1921 (Daniel and Louttit, 1953). By 1937 the number of applied psychologists had grown sufficiently, and the APA was sufficiently unsympathetic to them, that the American Association for Applied Psychology (AAAP) was formed. In 1940 this new organization had over 700 members; of the APA's 2,700 members, 32 percent were in nonteaching positions, mostly working as clinicians, in schools, or in guidance and counseling centers (Daniel and Louttit, 1953). World War II accelerated the shift into applied work and the APA responded. The AAAP merged with the APA in 1945 in conjunction with a major reorganization which introduced a divisional structure. The nineteen original divisions were soon reduced to seventeen. Among these were four that were primarily academic (General, Experimental, Personality and Social, and Esthetics), and eight that were clearly oriented to application (Clinical and Abnormal, Consulting, Industrial and Business, Educational, School, Counseling and Guidance, Public Service, and Military). The other five were somewhat mixed, focusing on a special area of concern and involving both academic and applied aspects (Teaching Psychology, Childhood and Adolescence, Evaluation and Measurement, Psychological Study of Social Issues, and Maturity and Old Age).

Recognizing that psychology had become a profession as well as a science, the APA sponsored a series of conferences to define standards of professional education. The first of these, the Boulder Conference of 1949, established a definition of the clinical psychologist as one who combined the skills of a research scientist and a professional. The *Boulder model* still dominates the training of clinical psychologists, although there have been a number of moves to modify it. A significant number of health psychologists would subscribe to this model as one that is appropriate for the training of future members of this field.

Other conferences in 1951, 1954, 1955, and 1958 dealt with counseling psychology, school psychology, psychology and mental health, and research training, culminating in the Conference on Graduate Education in 1958. Eight days of deliberation did not yield any specified curricula, but did lead to agreement that a defining characteristic of the psychologist is the research training he or she has received. The participants endorsed the idea of accreditation of programs involved in the "synergetic specialties"—"a generic term for the various specialties concerned with a helping relationship with individuals—clinical, school, counseling, etc." (*Graduate Education in Psychology*, 1959, p. 6). The development and support of accrediting and licensing procedures has been a major activity of organized psychology since 1947 (Carlson, 1978).

A recent survey by the APA indicated that about 56 percent of its members report that they provide at least some direct health services (Gottfredson and Dyer, 1978). The number who engage in professional services of all types must be substantially larger.

Psychology in 1978

The history of psychology as an academic discipline has been sketched as passing through a period of theoretical and methodological diversity and into a phase of seeming convergence. From psychobiology to psychodynamics, several common themes are guiding research and the building of theory. Adaptation to the environment, disturbances of adaptation resulting from stressful changes in that environment, particularly as these are cognitively appraised, and the restoration of adaptation through coping mechanisms that depend heavily on human capacities to acquire, encode, store, and retrieve information—these themes will appear in many places in this book as they do throughout psychology. Many psychologists are optimistic that our paradigm is crystallizing—that we may be about to leave the pre-paradigmatic status to which we were consigned by Kuhn (1962).

At the same time, psychology as a profession seems to be stronger than ever before (Dörken, 1977). Psychologists are being accorded independent status as health service providers by law and by agreement. Professionals in the divisions of consulting, counseling, industrial and organizational, and school psychology increase in number and influence. All told, there are now almost 47,000 associates, members, and fellows in the APA, whose interests and specializations are pursued, in part, through the activities of 35 divisions.

Tensions between the basic and the applied, or between the academic and the professional branches of the discipline have not disappeared. Some psychologists see them as posing an imminent threat of a split in organized psychology; others see such a division as desirable. The issue is of grave importance to the prospects of a field of health psychology, if there is to be one; for such a field is located, perhaps more completely than any other area of psychology, directly athwart the fault line between basic theory and application.

Involvement of Psychologists in the Health System

Psychology has been engaged with the health system longer than any other social or behavioral science, but no detailed history of that involvement exists. In this section it can only be sketched. Three major areas of activity can be identified: research into psychological aspects of behavior relevant to the health system; application of psychological concepts and knowledge to problems arising in the health system; and teaching relevant psychological material to the nonpsychologists who work in the health system. Although there is a logical priority to research and theory—one should know before one practices or teaches—in fact, psychologists have emphasized these activities in the reverse order. We began by teaching (or proposing to teach) our general principles to medical students and other health care providers long before we undertook any significant amount of research into the specific problems of health, illness, and health care. We practiced what we had learned in dealing with problems of mental health and in counseling, educational, and even industrial settings before we studied the special aspects of the health system. This brief review will reflect that sequence.

Psychology and Health Professional Education

In December 1911, less than twenty years after its founding, the APA was taking stock of the potential contributions of psychologists participating in medical education. Shephard Ivory Franz, a physiological psychologist, and John B. Watson, soon to proclaim Behaviorism, joined with psychiatrists Adolph Meyer and Morton Prince and a pathologist, E. E. Southard, to consider how psychology could contribute to medical education and practice. By examining their remarks, we can gain considerable insight into their views of the relationships between psychology and medicine at that time.

The physicians on the panel were somewhat skeptical about what the psychology of normal people had to offer to their enterprises. Southard (1912, p. 914) stressed the value of the "pathologic method" for psychology as well as medicine: "The more complex the subject of our study, the less progress do we make by confining our attention to the normal presentment of that object." Prince (1912, p. 918) was even more disparaging: "If by normal psychology is meant that which is taught in the ordinary academic curriculum . . . I am unable to see any particularly close relation between this kind of normal psychology and the problems of medicine." Meyer, one of the important early proponents of the concept of adaptation, saw little use for the laboratory methods of introspection and reaction time measurement, and felt that "psychology will become a much more real issue when it aims to guide students in the correct and critical recording of the plain facts of conduct and behavior" (1912, p. 913). All three, however, agreed that a properly oriented psychology could make essential contributions.

What did the psychologist offer? Franz, after detailing the importance for medicine of mental states, pointed out that a good deal of what was taught in physiology (about sense organs), neurology, psychiatry, and medicine incorporated discussions of mental events. "The physician depends on the mental processes of his patient for the information that will enable him to make a proper diagnosis. At the same time, the accounts of the patients' sensations and feelings help the physician to appreciate or to evaluate the effect of the treatment which is instituted" (Franz, 1912, p. 910). He advocated study of the placebo effect, and the use of psychological methods in pursuing physiological and pharmacological questions. He acknowledged criticisms: "It cannot be doubted . . . that some psychologists have hindered an understanding of and cooperation with medical problems, not only by their aloofness, but also by their 'damn the practical side' " (p. 911). It is more than a little distressing to find us still making the same points (Wexler, 1976; Stone and others, 1977).

Watson took a strong position that psychology (in contrast to psychiatry) had much to offer, but had not been sufficiently appreciated. He outlined a laboratory-based course that would consider such topics as the mixing of spectral colors, demonstrating difference thresholds and the like, laboratory and clinical work with the Binet-Simon tests, experiments with the "curve of work" and the "part that fatigue, disturbances, and emotional factors play in the normal ongoing of mental work" (Watson, 1912, p. 917). Such experiments, he believed, would prepare the medical student to go on to study association, memory, and retention. After such a preparation, "We can safely turn the medical student interested in psychopathology and psychoanalysis over to the psychiatric clinic" (p. 918). The apparent divergence of viewpoints between Franz and Watson was not noted.

Immediately after this symposium, the APA appointed Franz, Southard, and Watson as a committee to survey beliefs and practices of medical
schools with regard to the teaching of psychology. In 71 replies from the
116 medical schools queried, the committee found to be widespread "the
belief that psychology is the equivalent of 'psychoanalysis' or some other
equally restricted part of the whole" (Franz, 1913, p. 557). Of 52 institutions that had some affiliation with academic departments of any kind, only
14 reported that there was any collaboration with psychology departments,
and of these only 7 gave clear indication that psychologists taught medical
students. Most of those who replied, however, felt that students *should* receive instruction in psychology, either during their medical training or prior
to their undertaking it. On the strength of their findings, the committee concluded that courses should be taught by someone with training in both medicine and psychology, "should be practical, and should deal with actual
medical facts as much as possible," but should not be limited to "topics
which have a known practical value at the present time, for it has always
been found that facts apparently incapable of application at the time of, and
immediately after, their discovery are soon applied" (Franz, 1913, p. 566).
The course should be a general course, and should enable the student to "become personally acquainted with the methods and with the general nature of
psychological experimentation, rather than obtain his knowledge from textbooks" (p. 566).

The next major review of teaching in medical schools (Bott, 1928)
commented on, but did not cite, a number of articles on the teaching of
psychology in the medical curriculum in the period from 1912 to the time of
the review. From his reading of these papers, Bott concluded that there was
a wide and growing recognition of the importance of psychological factors in
the life adjustments that are crucial to our health. He found a constant
appeal for preventive as well as remedial measures in improving mental
health and for establishing sound basic mental habits in early childhood.
These mental habits were not limited in their effect to mental health. He
observed a general agreement that "what we require in medicine in order to
do justice to the mental factors that appear in patients or that may tend to
undermine health, is not a few mental specialists but rather more adequately
trained general practitioners able to recognize and deal scientifically with
these situations as they occur in the general run of patients young or old" (p.
291). Bott described a program of instruction at the University of Toronto,
where he taught, that seemed to be modeled closely on the recommendations made by the APA committee in 1913, giving considerable emphasis to
general psychology and experimental methodology. Glover (1934) was the
first to describe a course that was less academic in content. Based upon an
initial assertion that academic psychology is irrelevant to medical education,
the syllabus offered by Glover called for thirty lectures in "medical psychology," which included six lectures on animal psychology, eight on comparative anthropology, ten on child psychology, and six on the psychology of
adolescence and adult life. He recommended emphasizing instincts, the influences of fear and emotional conflict, evolution, and regression.

In these early statements, there is little to indicate that psychologists were giving any thought to making specific application of their knowledge to problems of the health system. Their approach was one of teaching a general course to medical students and expecting that the students would be able to make the adaptations necessary for applying it in their studies and their future practice.

Nearly twenty years went by before psychologists again began to review and consider their potential contributions to medical education. In 1950 the psychology department at the University of Pittsburgh sponsored eight lectures on "The Relation of Psychology to Medicine" (Dennis, 1950). The mood of the contributors was generally optimistic: They spoke in terms of the ending of a period of neglect and of an emerging collaboration of great promise with public health, experimental psychopathology, neurological research, and gerontology, as well as medical education. Carlyle Jacobsen, a psychologist who was then dean for medical education in the State University of New York, emphasized the offering of psychological contributions to medical education in an interdisciplinary context along with the other behavioral and social sciences. This view has gained strong support in the years since it was expressed ("Behavioral Sciences and Medical Education," 1972).

In the interim between the time of these two statements about curricula, there was a continuing slow growth of the number of curriculum hours devoted to psychiatry and behavioral science that continued through the decade of the 1930s (Webster, 1971). It is not easy to tell how much teaching was actually done by psychologists, or what kind. Ambiguous and conflicting reports are the rule. In 1955, appraising data from a survey done by Mensh and others for the Education and Training Board of the APA (Mensh, 1953), Matarazzo (1955) concluded that teaching by psychologists appeared to be minimal, and full responsibility for courses almost nonexistent. Another survey conducted in 1955 led Matarazzo and Daniel (1957) to conclude that growth was occurring in the amount of teaching by psychologists. Buck (1961, pp. 60-61), in replies from 70 medical schools surveyed in 1959, learned of 583 persons identified with psychology, of whom only 36 were described as clinical psychologists. Delivery of formal lectures to medical students was reported for 239 of these psychologists. However, Buck reported that in his visits to 27 of the schools, he found a considerably smaller percentage engaged in formal teaching than his survey results would have indicated. In 1960 the Group for the Advancement of Psychiatry found clinical psychologists participating in teaching of preclinical psychiatry and behavioral science in 51 of 89 medical schools, with other types of psychologists (experimental, developmental, physiological, and others) teaching in only 11 schools. A series of surveys documented the increase in the number of psychologists working in medical schools, although the nature of their activity was not always determined. The most recent of these reports (Lubin, Nathan, and Matarazzo, 1978) traces these numbers: in 1955, 346 psychologists; 1964, 993; 1967-1969, 1,300; and in 1976, 2,336.

This discussion has focused almost entirely on medical education because, until very recently, that is where the attention of psychologists has focused. In the past few years, enough behavioral scientists have found employment on faculties of dental schools (Kleinknecht, Klepac, and Bernstein, 1976) and of schools of pharmacy (Blaug and others, 1975) that interest in and discussion about their tasks is beginning to take form.

Clinical Practice of Psychologists in Health Settings

Whereas nonclinical psychologists who wanted to teach general psychology to medical students succeeded, after half a century, in swelling their numbers in medical schools to at most a few score, clinical psychologists, who began to appear in medical settings in sizable numbers only after World War II, increased their presence tenfold in thirty years. It is difficult from published reports to identify and characterize the work of these clinical psychologists. Although "medical psychology" is recognized as a subspecialty in clinical psychology (American Psychological Association, 1978a), in the older literature the term often referred primarily to the work of medically trained individuals whose involvement with the academic discipline of psychology may have been very slight indeed. "Psychological medicine" has a similar meaning, usually referring to the treatment of those who have mental disorders. While the treatment of mental illness and mental retardation is clearly in the realm of health services (Dörken, 1977), these areas will not be considered here.

Since 1970 there has been a rapid expansion of psychological presence in departments of pediatrics (Drotar, 1977; Routh, 1977), which has developed under the term *pediatric psychology*. Even more recently, many psychologists have been employed in programs teaching the "new" specialty of family practice.

A new term, *Behavioral Medicine*, is being proposed as an overarching rubric to encompass the full range of approaches to health care that derive from psychology and the other behavioral sciences. A number of recent publications have considered how this term ought to relate to the older concept of psychosomatic medicine and to the field that we are attempting to define in this book, health psychology (Schwartz and Weiss, 1977). These terminological issues will be considered again in our last chapter.

Olbrisch (1977) has recently reviewed most of the adequately controlled studies of psychotherapy (broadly defined) applied to medical problems. The studies she cites permit us to discern patterns in the work that has been undertaken. Several general problems have been addressed: (1) Interventions aimed at reducing the burden that "overutilizers" pose to outpatient clinics were first described by Pratt (1934) and Rhoades (1935). These and several other studies during the prewar period reported moderate success, which has been confirmed and extended more recently (Follette and Cummings, 1967; Goldberg, Krantz, and Locke, 1970). (2) Efforts to ameliorate a variety of conditions believed to be related to life stress were undertaken by several groups during the period from 1948 to 1953. Little additional literature appeared until 1968, when a number of different groups began to study the impact of offering psychotherapy in prepaid health plans on the utilization of other services. (3) Early studies by Janis (1958) and Marmer (1959) on the psychological preparation of patients for surgery were once again followed by later work in the same vein. In all three of these areas, there was a marked upsurge of activity beginning in 1968.

Olbrisch also reviews work done with patients of specific diseases: postcardiac patients, and those with headaches, asthma, skin disorders, gastrointestinal illnesses, hypertension, cancer, emphysema, and Parkinsonism. Many of these reports describe psychoanalytic treatment of diseases that were thought to represent symbolic expressions of psychological conflicts. Others have used hypnosis, relaxation training, and various types of supportive and reeducative training.

The overall rate of appearance of the studies reviewed by Olbrisch was quite constant from the mid 1950s through 1970, averaging three per year during that time. A marked shift in rate occurred following the publication in 1969 by Schofield of a significant paper calling attention to psychologists' neglect of both research and service in general medical settings. Whether his statement was a stimulus for change or merely a timely recognition of a condition that had become apparent to many psychologists, it marked a major shift of interest toward the health system at large and resulted in the entry into the system of increasing numbers of clinical psychologists and other service providers. Schofield (1969) tabulated articles in the *Psychological Abstracts* of 1966 and 1967 that were related to twenty-two different categories of health topics. Of these, nine categories that represented the traditional mental health focus of psychology—mental retardation, educational disabilities, alcoholism, psychoneurosis, schizophrenia, psychotherapy (general and research), aging, and suicide—accounted for about 81 percent of the total number of articles. Schofield pointed out expanding opportunities in other areas of the health system.

A number of psychologists responded directly to Schofield's call for action. Weisenberg (1970) indicated the readiness of the National Center for Health Services Research and Development, where he worked, to cooperate with psychologists in exploring better ways to provide health services. Some responded to Schofield's urging that psychology prepare to meet more fully an expanding demand for direct health services (McMillan, 1970; "Psychology and National Health Care," 1971) by developing a model of the psychologist as a "health care professional" to augment the traditional, Boulder model of the scientist-practitioner (Schofield, 1976). Others described new roles that were developing in the health care system. Crary and Steger (1972) discussed the potential value of using diagnostic tests during consultation in medical and rehabilitation clinics. Wiggins (1976) pointed out the special opportunities and hazards posed by new legislation in support of health maintenance organizations. Such legislation threatened to subvert the movement toward gaining full recognition of the psychologist as an independent provider of health services. However, by providing that twenty outpatient mental health visits be made available as a part of the basic health services, the new law encouraged the development of a comprehensive and integrated system offering both physical and mental health services. Such an expansion would foster the emergence of a new definition of the clinical psychologist as one who would be concerned with the psychological aspects of all factors adversely affecting the health of the individual.

Psychologists from various theoretical backgrounds—psychodynamic, existential, and behavioral—are today taking part in the application of behavioral interventions to general health problems. Many recent reports describe adaptations of the paradigms of conditioning to clinical problems. *Behavior modification* is a term applied to a variety of techniques derived from several different branches of psychological learning theory. Behavioral techniques are being applied to a range of problems, including the desensitization of fears of medical and dental treatment, the training of patients with residual deficits after trauma or illness to overcome their physical handicaps and to use prosthetic devices effectively, and the control of vomiting, constipation, torticollis, scratching, chronic pain, asthma, finicky eating, headaches (both tension and migraine), Raynaud's disease, and hypertension, among others (Gambrill, 1977; LeBow, 1975).

The conditioning approaches divide broadly into three categories of intervention: (1) those that attempt to reduce psychologically induced stress by desensitization and by training in relaxation; (2) those that attempt to modify semivolitional behavior such as vomiting, scratching, and jerking by analyzing and modifying contingencies of reinforcement and stimulus control; and (3) those that attempt to bring physiological functions, such as blood pressure or heart rate, under voluntary control through the use of *biofeedback*. Well-controlled studies of clinical biofeedback are still too few, and the results of those that have been done are often equivocal or disappointing (Miller, 1975; Shapiro and others, 1977). Nevertheless, there is a strong sense of optimism among those working in the field (Fuller, 1978; Miller, 1975; Schwartz and Weiss, 1977; Shapiro and Surwit, 1974). Failures are seen as an inevitable part of the process of developing a new domain of therapeutic procedures. Understanding of etiology and treatment will be refined through continued experimentation.

Psychological Research in the Health System

The research literature prior to about ten years ago was small, and there are no comprehensive reviews of early research efforts. This section will not undertake a complete review but will identify some of the areas where considerable effort has been expended and cite some of the specialized reviews. It will not deal with the vast literature in the areas of physiological psychology, psychophysiology, neuropsychology, psychopharmacology, and other such fields at the interface of behavior and the body mechanisms that underlie it. Work of this kind may appear at first sight to have more relevance for health psychology than equally fundamental work in social psychology, cognitive psychology, or personality. We are used to thinking of health issues primarily within the biomedical model—health being the condition in which the body processes are working well, disease the condition in which they are not. Physiological psychologists have been more numerous in medical schools than have most other nonclinical specializations, so we are prone to think that psychologists who study body processes are more closely affiliated with the health system than are those who study perception, learning, or moral development. Part of the purpose in defining a field of health psychology is to correct this biased view about physiological psychology: It is a basic area of specialization, as are social psychology, cognitive psychology, and personality psychology. They are neither parts of health psychology nor supraordinate to it, but basic areas upon which health psychology draws for its solutions to problems and to which it contributes theory in return.

There are also very large bodies of research concerning mental illness, behavior disorders, developmental disabilities, alcoholism, and drug abuse—the domain that has been historically claimed by the National Institute of Mental Health and now by the Alcoholism, Drug Abuse, and Mental Health Administration. This domain, in which the behavior *is* the health problem, is properly a part of health psychology, but no attempt will be made to characterize the research in it because of its sheer quantity and numerous categorical areas. There is too much of it, and it has its own categories. It far overshadows in amount all other psychological research concerned with the health system. Perhaps before too long the mental health area can be viewed as a segment of a thriving field of health psychology, along with rehabilitation psychology, population and fertility, and even environmental psychology. It may well be, as Schwartz and Weiss (1977) and others have suggested, that an integration of the area of mental health with several related areas—population and fertility, environmental psychology, and rehabilitation psychology—can not only facilitate the exchange of knowledge and approaches among various groups but also can foster a holistic attitude and a "biopsychosocial" model (Engel, 1977) that can be applied to all health and disease. Such an integration would lead to a truly comprehensive health psychology.

In the past decade, three publications have reported surveys of the literature in what may be broadly termed health psychology. Schofield (1969), using a "reasonably extensive but not comprehensive list of topics" (p. 567), tabulated from the 1966 and 1967 issues of *Psychological Abstracts* about 4,700 articles. He did not distinguish research-based articles from others but did present the number that were associated with various topics. As reported earlier in this chapter, 81 percent of these articles concerned mental health topics. Schofield categorized the remaining articles as follows: birth and abortion, fertility, and population control (about 3 percent); accidents and highway safety (1 percent); smoking (1 percent); cancer, heart disease, and surgery (about 6 percent); psychosomatics (3 percent); pain (2 percent); and death (2 percent). (The percentages here are rounded, averaged over two years, and approximated from Schofield's tab. 1, p. 568.)

Kahana (1972) obtained a computer search (MEDLARS) of the *Index Medicus* for a period covering "the preceding two to four years" (p. 2), approximately 1967-1970. He focused on "applications of personality concepts in the understanding and managing of physical illness" (p. 2), but defined the variable *personality* very broadly to include references to adaptation, family, physician-patient, stress, and checklists of psychological attitudes, traits, behavior, or symptoms, to name only five of the sixteen rubrics listed in his article. He stopped the "flood of printout" after 5,000 references had been returned, and found about 2,500 of them directly relevant to his topic. Kahana cited only 367 of these references, but intimated that a great many more had to do with psychological elements of physical illness. Kahana grouped his citations according to whether they focused on systems of the body (cardiovascular or hemic and lymphatic, for example), age groups or stages and crises of development, phases of illness (chronic or terminal, for example), special reactions and problems (such as conversion hysteria or severe pain), various settings for medical and surgical treatment (including the effects of hospitalization), and relations of the patient to health care providers or family members. These categories certainly reflect significant attributes of studies; however, in order to get a picture of the research that psychologists have done, we need to know what questions were being asked in the studies. Unfortunately, Kahana did not attempt to classify the research questions.

The most comprehensive effort to characterize contemporary research in health psychology was reported by the American Psychological Association Task Force on Health Research (1976). This group performed a computer search (PASAR) of the *Psychological Abstracts* for the years 1966-1973 on psychological aspects of physical illness, physical disability, and health. From this eight-year period, they retrieved only 3,500 abstracts, compared to Kahana's 5,000 from less than four years. (The reasons for this smaller number can only be guessed at. *Index Medicus* may have a much broader coverage of the relevant journals, and the search terms used in the PASAR search appear to have been narrower.) After all studies that were not direct reports of research and all of those that "dealt primarily with mental health variables or with psychiatric focuses" (1976, p. 270) were eliminated, only about 350 articles remained. These were sorted into three general categories: psychobiological aspects of health, health care delivery, and studies of health-related attitudes. The first of these categories accounted for two thirds of the total number of research papers. Only 56 were devoted to all aspects of health care delivery, including needs and resources, health systems and manpower, improvement of communication, and evaluation of outcomes. The third category, with about 50 papers, included surveys of attitudes held by various populations and studies of attitude change.

The categories that were used to classify the research being done seem less useful than those that would arise from some of the questions posed by the Task Force: Why do many people not follow medical advice? How do constitutional factors or life-styles predispose to illness? What are the primary sources of persisting health care attitudes?

The reviews of reviews, old and new, that were conducted in the preparation of this chapter gave rise to a schema for classifying psychological research in relation to the model of the health system outlined in Chapter One. Table 1 provides an overview of this classification plan. It starts from

Table 1. Classification of Psychological Studies of the Health System

  I. *Studies of the health target*
   A. Psychobiological
    1. Effects of behavior on body processes
    2. Effects of body abnormalities on behavior
   B. Health behavior
    1. Self-destructive behavior
     drug abuse; accident proneness
    2. Preventive health behavior
    3. Illness behavior
     utilization; delay in treatment
    4. Sick role behavior
     adherence; coping with stress of treatment
    5. Adjustment to chronic illness
  II. *Studies of the health care system*
   A. Health care processes
    1. Outreach
    2. Diagnosis
    3. Prescribing; preparing patients for surgery
    4. Provider-patient interactions
   B. Treatment settings and devices
    1. Health care organizations
    2. Human factors
    3. Psychoarchitectural studies
   C. Health care careers
    1. Recruitment; specialty selection
    2. Training
    3. Stresses of health careers
  III. *Planning and resources mobilization*
  IV. *Studies of hazard reduction*

the principle that, since the psychologist studies behavior, it is behavior that should be classified with respect to the health system: Whose behavior was studied? What aspects of their behavior were observed? The various factors that enter into the determination of behavior, such as age, background, and personality of the participants, characteristics of the behavior settings, and physiological influences on behavior, become subsidiary to the functional transactions of the health system. We are not interested primarily in the behavior of old people or of persons with disorders of the liver but in delay in obtaining treatment (by targets) or in capacity to give support (by health care providers), and how this behavior is influenced by age and type of disease. In this system, the specialty areas of psychology are independent of those of the behavior settings of the health system. We can examine a particular aspect of health behavior—the decision to consult a physician, for example—from the vantage point of almost any specialization in psychology. The cognitive psychologist can consider the information that the target individual is using in making the decision; the learning psychologist considers how the information was acquired; the personality psychologist, how the decision is constrained by generalized patterns of coping; the developmental psychologist, how the ways in which these decisions are made differ throughout the life span. Considering the matter in this light immediately raises a question about the relationship between health psychology and the rest of psychology: Since any psychologist can contribute, what is the special contribution of the health psychologist? Consideration of such questions is deferred until the final chapter.

At this point, the classification scheme will be used in organizing a review of work that has been done in the areas of psychological research and theory building. Some estimate will be given in the pages that follow of the amount of work done within each of the categories shown in the table, and reference will be made to appropriate reviews of such work whenever possible.

Research on the behavior of health targets. In the first place, we note that almost all of the research focuses on the first primary category: the behavior of health targets. This category is subdivided into psychobiological research and research on health behavior.

Within the subcategory of research that the Task Force labeled *psychobiological*, there are again two major subdivisions: research into the unintended effects of behavior on body tissues and processes, and the effects of abnormal processes or structures of the body on behavior. In the first of these subdivisions, which includes most of what has been known as psychosomatics, is included the study of the effects of cognitive appraisals and various kinds of symbolic behavior on the physiological systems of arousal and emotion. Also included here is the impact of characteristic patterns of behavior, such as the "Type A" behavior described by Friedman and Rosenman (1974), on the body's functioning. It does not include clinical biofeedback, which falls into the second major subcategory of target behavior—*health behavior*. However, the psychobiology subcategory would include research to discover the possibility of and means for establishing behavioral control over bodily processes.

The second major subdivision of the psychobiological subcategory includes research on the effects of changes in bodily structures or processes induced by disease, trauma, surgery, drugs, stress, or other agents, on the behavioral capacities of the individual. Here we would include those aspects of coping or adapting that are directly demanded by the bodily changes, such as those involved in the use of a prosthetic device, but not the more global kinds of adaptation to changed life opportunities occasioned by health problems and efforts to deal with them. These larger-scale adaptations are also more appropriately grouped with the category *health behavior* because, unlike psychobiological behavior, they are much influenced by sociocultural variables, personality traits, attributions, and so on. The subcategory of psychobiological research as defined here is somewhat smaller than that used by the APA Task Force, but it probably accounts for nearly half of all the research that has been done in health psychology. It will be considered in somewhat more detail shortly. The chapter by Schwartz is also concerned with this topic.

The term *health behavior* is used very broadly here to include all behaviors engaged in by a person that have a significant impact on his or her health. Behaviors with both positive and negative impact on health are included. This area is also one in which a good deal of research and theoretical work has been done. A number of the chapters in this volume are concerned with various aspects of health behavior. To place them in a clearer relationship to each other, a later section of this chapter is also devoted to an explication of the theoretical approaches to health behavior.

Research on the health care system. The second primary category of health psychological research shown in Table 1 is divided into three major subcategories. The first of these, research on health care processes, is closely associated with the treatment phase of health behavior. Research that seeks to determine what the provider should do would fall into this category, but that which focuses on the response of the target would be classified with health behavior. In fact, it may be desirable to recognize a separate category of research that deals specifically with the interactions between target and provider. Many discussions of the doctor-patient relationship have been published over the years, but relatively little research has been reported. Recent reviews in this area are offered by Ley (1976) and Stimson (1976). Research on outreach is reviewed in the chapter by Rosenstock and Kirscht, and different aspects of the diagnostic process are considered by several of the chapters here, especially that of Elstein and Bordage. The presentation of diagnoses, prescribing, and the preparation of patients for stressful treatments are considered in chapters by Haan; Henderson, Hall, and Lipton; Cohen and Lazarus; and Janis and Rodin.

Research on treatment settings has focused more on organizational aspects than on those of the physical environments and devices. Georgopoulos (1975) has presented an extensive review of research on health care organizations. The chapter by Moos in this volume and other publications cited there review much of the work on settings. A book edited by Pickett and Triggs (1975) brings together a number of papers with the perspective of engineering psychology and human factors research. The few psychological studies of architectural features of health settings are scattered widely.

Cartwright's chapter in this volume reviews a good deal of the research that has been done on the careers of health care providers, with regard to the stresses that arise in pursuing such a career. A major review of the psychological research on choosing a career and a specialty is provided by Otis and others (1975). Discussions of the teaching of behavioral science to health professionals have been reviewed earlier. There does not appear to be a comprehensive psychological study of the teaching of health professionals, or of the special learning problems that they face. Hundreds of individual studies have addressed specific teaching-learning problems.

One topic that has attracted a good deal of attention from psychologists is that of teaching communication skills. A recent review by Carroll and Monroe (1978) identified seventy-three reports of efforts to teach communication skills to medical students. A review now in preparation by Tyler and Stone has located about fifty papers that report on at least a quasi-experimental approach to the study of such teaching, almost all of them published within the past ten years. Only one of them, however, has made an evaluation of the impact of the teaching on the actual outcomes of health transactions, and that only on the satisfaction of patients with interviews. Kagan's chapter in this volume offers a review of work on one of the most highly developed approaches to the teaching of interpersonal communications.

Research on health resources. The first two major categories just discussed probably account for more than 90 percent of all psychological research in the health system. Psychological studies of planning and mobilizing resources for the health system are rare. Adler and Milstein's chapter reviews the work on psychological aspects of health planning. Sociologists, political scientists, and economists have concerned themselves with securing resources for the health care system, but we have found no reviews of research that deal with the psychological aspects of decisions or actions in this domain. How do health attitudes and health values affect voting for health facilities or contributions to health organizations? Studies of specific attitudes or intentions with regard to such public health issues as publicly financed abortion or national health insurance are much less common than those that address personal (health behavior) issues such as use of abortion or contraceptive methods or interest in subscribing to a health maintenance organization.

Research on behavior related to health hazards. There is also a disparity of emphasis in research between the health behavior of targets, who are affected by hazards, and the behavior of agents, who attempt to reduce hazards. There is a good deal of psychological research into environmental effects on health and behavior (Hinkle and Loring, 1977) and a smaller amount concerning the health behavior of individuals with respect to such hazards as smoking, drug abuse, improper diets, and the like. (Most of the research here is concerned not with behavior relative to the hazard but with interventions designed to change such behavior.) Individual responses to threats of tornadoes and other natural disasters have attracted a few investigations, which are reviewed by Burton (1972; see also Janis, 1962; Sims and Baumann, 1972). There is almost no examination of individual participation in actions directed toward eliminating or controlling environmental health hazards. Where are the studies of attitudes or behavior with regard to the ozone-depleting fluorocarbons, or asbestos pollution of Lake Superior? Cost-benefit analyses mentioned frequently in the general press strongly suggest that our allocations of resources within the health system are highly irrational in their neglect of these and many other known hazards, but psychologists have not studied this type of irrationality.

At least one community health program in a developing area (Costa Rica) has been taking a broader perspective on the health system than that which focuses on health care delivery and individual health behavior (Ruphuy, 1977). This program has attempted to address the hazards associated with socioeconomic underdevelopment and the attitudes that allow such hazards to persist. As psychologists are drawn into such programs as consultants, we may hope that they will take the opportunity to study the fundamental problems that arise outside of the health care system, where different values, beliefs, and behavior problems are salient.

This brief overview of psychological research in the health system, which will be substantially augmented in the chapters that follow, used the framework of Chapter One in surveying prior work. An effort was made to gain a perspective that not only summarizes what has been done but also shows how the work accomplished to date relates to the overall task of gaining an understanding of the total health system. To obtain a deeper understanding, we will need strong integrative theories that bring together many scattered results. The next section will consider some theories that have been proposed and applied to psychological research in the health system.

Theories in Health Psychology

There are no complete and comprehensive psychological theories of the health system. In fact, it is probably not possible, nor even desirable, to try to create such a theory at this time. What are needed are working theories about various segments of the system which can be linked for special purposes. For example, various theories about the effects of different kinds of hazards on targets might be integrated to good advantage, but there would be little occasion to attempt further integration of such a theory with a theory about the mobilization of resources for new health enterprises. An application of mobilization theory might call, however, for a demonstration of the benefit of the proposed program in terms of reduced impact of hazards. At that point, the two theories would be linked in order to produce the required demonstration. In this review, no attempt is made to analyze any and all applications of psychological theory to the understanding of a health problem. For the most part, it concentrates on work in which a sizable group of researchers has been endeavoring over some period of time to understand a related body of phenomena. There are four major domains of theory that satisfy these criteria. Without claim for the ultimate appropriateness of the labels, these domains are here identified as: adaptation theory, coping theory, psychosomatic theory, and theories of health behavior. Within each of these domains there are contending, specific theories that may differ in minor particulars or in their basic assumptions and approaches.

Two of these domains, adaptation theory and coping theory, discussed in some depth in later chapters, share the characteristic that they have extensive development in relation to phenomena outside of the field of health psychology. They will be given only a brief mention here. A section is devoted to psychosomatic theory, which constitutes a relatively self-contained area that is not described in overview by any of the later chapters. In presenting material on the fourth domain, theories of health behavior, the greatest attention will be given to a single theory, the Health Belief Model (HBM). While numerous individuals and small groups have undertaken to give theoretical accounts of some aspects of health behavior, only the HBM, up to this time, has become a major focal point of work. In order to present it in an adequate context, we will first define more fully what we mean by health behavior and then provide an overview of behavior theories within which the particular theory of the Health Belief Model can be located.

Adaptation theory is represented in this book in the chapter by Schwartz, who presents it in a form that draws very heavily on the *general systems theory* of von Bertalanffy (1968). It starts from the study of the physiological adaptive mechanisms of the body as they respond to challenges or hazards in the form of physical or chemical insults. It then generalizes the principles derived from this study into levels of more complex behavior. The physiological theories fall outside the area of health psychology. Schwartz provides some discussion about the application of these concepts to clinical problems.

Coping theories deal with the ways that people respond to hazards and the threats posed by hazards through complex, learned, and socially modulated patterns of behavior. The domain of coping is clearly much broader than its intersection with health psychology. In health psychology, we are primarily concerned with threats and stresses posed by sickness and health care. A related issue, that of the bodily effects of the coping process, lies at a boundary with psychosomatic theory. Almost any type of behavior may be employed in the course of coping. One of the disagreements within the field has to do with the question of whether defensive behavior that does not reduce the real threat but only the person's awareness of it should be called coping behavior. Two approaches to this issue are reflected in the chapters by Cohen and by Haan in this volume. In the present discussion, the inclusive definition is used. With such a definition, health behavior is almost entirely a subset of coping behavior. It is separated here primarily because there are two separate traditions of research that emphasize different aspects of coping. One, which bears the label *coping*, has been concerned much more with the emotional impact of threats, how this impact contributes to behavior processes, and how the behavior is directed toward keeping emotion and physiological states of arousal within an acceptable range. The other, which is here called *health behavior*, focuses on the factors that influence choice among alternative approaches to dealing with hazards, threats, and bodily insults. The domain of coping theories is addressed by a number of authors in this book: Cartwright, Cohen and Lazarus, Haan, Mages and Mendelsohn, Moos, and, to some extent, by Janis and Rodin. They bring different, sometimes partially conflicting views to the discussion. Among them they offer a good representation of this domain of theory.

The four domains of theory are not sharply differentiated. They tend to share concerns about phenomena more than they share explanatory concepts, but they are sufficiently close to each other that it is possible to conceive of their integration at some point in the foreseeable future. All four domains have to do, in one way or another, with health targets. They are concerned with the impact of hazards upon the target and the responses of the target to those impacts, but they differ in their emphasis on the kinds of hazards and responses.

Psychosomatic theory. Psychosomatic theory originates from a concern with the interaction between biological stressors, symbolic processes, and the body's reactions. In its early years of development, psychosomatic theory made little effort to understand the biological details of the phenomena it studied, but more recently it has come much closer to the domain of adaptation theory. Much of the theoretical writing is to be found in the literature of psychosomatic medicine.

The term *psychosomatic medicine* has found its meaning modified and expanded since it was introduced by Heinroth in 1818 (Wittkower, 1974). The psychosomatic movement began speculatively in the 1920s in Germany and was brought to the United States by Alexander about 1930 and to England in 1933 by Wittkower. Initially, the field was dominated by psychoanalysts who sought to understand bodily symptoms in terms of psychic conflicts. Their concern was directed mainly to diseases in which psychological stress was a prominent feature. Among the conditions first studied in the 1930s were accidents, hypertension, hay fever, hyperemesis of pregnancy (the "hysterical nature" of which was discussed in 1922), menstrual problems, cardiospasm, peptic ulcer, ulcerative colitis, migraine, and skin disorders. Topics first taken up in 1946 or later include allergy, diabetes, disorders of the colon and of the small intestine, and renal and respiratory disorders. In O'Neill's (1955) bibliography of 210 items, almost all references are to medical journals, including *Psychosomatic Medicine* and the *British Journal of Medical Psychology*, which is almost entirely psychiatric (medical) in content, and also to journals of psychoanalysis, psychotherapy, and psychiatry. The contribution of psychologists to the early literature in psychosomatic medicine is undoubtedly greater than these facts would suggest, for there has been noted a tendency for psychologists in medical settings to publish with their medical colleagues in medical journals (American Psychological Association, 1976).

Gradually, patterns of investigation broadened, and psychologists contributed in more identifiable ways to the developing theory. Later reviews of psychosomatic research (Hill, 1970, 1976) included studies of personality characteristics of persons with different types of illnesses (Crowell, 1953; Little and Cohen, 1951; Wishner, 1953); conditioning-based therapies (discussed in an earlier section); biopsychosocial mechanisms (Jenkins and others, 1969); and, particularly, a host of factors associated with stress, adaptation, coping, life change, giving up, and the like (Lipowski, 1976). These matters are reviewed in Chapter Four.

Psychosomatic theory has evolved from a rather narrow attempt to understand particular diseases in relation to psychoanalytic theories about repression and symbolic expression of psychosexual conflicts to a very comprehensive theory. In Lipowski's (1976) formulation, contemporary psychosomatic theory holds that environmental stressors give rise to emotional states through the mediation of cognitive appraisals, which are individualized through the particular cultural, familial, and idiosyncratic learnings of the person. These emotional states, in turn, determine patterns of physiological arousal that serve as information sources but which also may have etiological impact in pathogenesis. Illness and its treatments are stressors themselves, so that both the maintenance of health and the course of a disease involve a dynamic interplay among environmental, social, cognitive, and physiological systems. This formulation is so comprehensive that it may seem to take in every aspect of health and illness. However, we should recognize that its focus is on the mediating impact of the emotions and the responses of the physiological systems to them.

A definition of health behavior. We are now ready to consider theories about behavior that is intended to affect one's health. The term *health behavior* is used here in a more generic sense than it is by proponents of the Health Belief Model, to be discussed shortly. Here it refers to all molar behavior that is guided by health purposes or reinforced by health outcomes. Others have referred to this class of behavior as *health-related behavior*, making of health behavior a subcategory. Readers familiar with that usage will need to take note of this difference.

There is considerable discussion in the literature about meaningful subcategories of health behavior—subcategories that are internally homogeneous and externally heterogeneous with respect to important variables. Reference was made in Chapter Two to the longstanding interest of anthropologists in what people do when they experience symptoms of ill health. The term *illness behavior* is frequently used by anthropologists to describe such behavior. Parsons (1951b) introduced the concept of *sick role behavior* to describe changes in behavior that are sanctioned when an individual is acknowledged to be ill. Much interest has centered on the validation of that concept. The psychological study of behavior directed toward preventing illness or remaining healthy as a distinctive class of behavior was first undertaken by Hochbaum (1958) and by Rosenstock, Derryberry, and Carriger (1959). While specific instances of health-maintaining behavior had been investigated earlier (Cannell and MacDonald, 1956; Herrera and Kiser, 1951), it was Hochbaum and Rosenstock who called attention to the special characteristics of such behavior. The terms *preventive health behavior, illness behavior,* and *sick role behavior* were brought into explicit relationship by Kasl and Cobb (1966) to refer to what a person does to keep from getting sick, how he or she investigates the need for treatment, and how he or she acts after having been designated as sick. Kasl and Cobb's subclasses do not exhaust the realm of health behavior. Suchman (1965), for example, proposed five stages of health-seeking behavior; Baric's (1969) *at-risk* role was accepted by Kasl (1975a) as a worthy addition to his three categories.

Behavior Theories Relevant to Health Behavior

The questions of why people (or other organisms) behave as they do and how they may be induced to behave differently have represented the core of American psychology throughout this century. All psychological theories, therefore, could have offered their particular explanations for health behavior, although few have yet chosen to do so. Most behavior theorists recognize four different levels of determinants that contribute to observed behavior (although the theorists may differ in the level they choose to emphasize and the names they use to denote them): reflex, habit, social custom, and rational choice. Each of these levels will be considered briefly.

In humans, as in other organisms, the level of *reflex* involves relatively inflexible and unmodifiable patterns of response that are characteristic of a species. In the health domain, reflexes play a greater role than in many other spheres of human action—reflexes such as those associated with pain, vomiting, sphincter control, and the physiological systems of arousal and defense. Trauma, illness, and medical treatment are likely to call them into play, and their excessive presence, for whatever reason, is likely to be labeled as a health problem. Mention has already been made of some efforts to develop psychological services directed to the modification of reflex behavior. At the boundaries of physiology, research on reflex behavior concentrates on its modifiability through conditioning methods (Bykov, 1937; Kamiya, 1969; Miller, 1969); in the areas of sociology and anthropology, it is concerned with the influence of cultural patterning on the expression of pain (Zborowski, 1952) and emotion (Ekman, 1972).

Next to the reflex in terms of rigidity and specificity is the *level of the conditioned response* (or *habit*). This level has attracted an enormous amount of attention from psychologists in academic laboratories. In research on health behavior, it has played, until recently, a less significant role. Studies that look at certain of the "psychosomatic" illnesses from the viewpoint of conditioning have been mentioned. Health behaviors that involve the avoidance of harmful substances such as alcohol and tobacco have frequently been studied within a conditioning framework. Occasionally, health-promoting behaviors such as dietary practices and dental prophylaxis (Barnett, 1970) have been treated as conditioned responses or habits maintained by social approval, gustatory or olfactory stimuli, or other positively reinforcing (rewarding) consequences. Surprisingly little attention has been paid to the positively reinforcing contingencies that are operative in those individuals who spontaneously demonstrate effective health behavior. A great deal of attention, however, has been given to the use of fear reduction as a negative reinforcer to build and support health-promoting habits. Generally, these studies go under the label of *fear arousal*, properly reflecting the stress that has been placed on the messages that induce the fear. Major theorists in this field (Janis, 1967; Leventhal, 1973) have stressed that excessive fear may be immobilizing and actually impair existing levels of health behavior and that a means of coping with the fear-inducing messages must be offered if a positive effect on health behavior is to be achieved. The role of fear in causing delay in seeking treatment—discussed in chapters of this volume by Haan, Janis and Rodin, and Kirscht and Rosenstock—cannot properly be located at the level of simple conditioning, however, since complex symbolic appraisals are involved.

Conditioned responses can be organized into complex behavior structures that are nearly as complex as those of the higher levels. In these structures, outcomes of one response serve as cues for later responses. Incorporated in such structures may be behavior that has as its primary function the bridging of gaps in environmental sequences of stimuli—to fill time when there are delays between action and consequence or to provide cues for the next response when environmental consequences do not yield any themselves. In humans, many mediating responses are verbal and much verbal behavior has this function. We name an object or a situation so that we will know what to do with it or about it. One venerable line of psychological research has to do with the impact of labels on what we see (Bruner and Goodman, 1947), what we remember (Wülf, 1922), and the problems we are able to solve (Duncker, 1945). Attribution theory, discussed in the chapter by Janis and Rodin in this volume, is one avenue for studying the impacts of labels on health behavior.

Learning theory merges into cognitive theory when mediating responses become labels. People can label complex patterns of events and then use that label to initiate enormously complex patterns of behavior. A major component of a culture is its set of *customs*. In times past, when people "fell in love," it was appropriate to "have a wedding." If there was a "serious threat to our national interest" (or security or honor), it might be appropriate to "go to war." Study of the impact of social customs, traditions, and rituals on health behavior has been largely left to anthropologists and sociologists, but psychologists clearly have a role to play in the understanding of the interactions between the several levels of determination in the individual. What happens, for example, when traditional values concerning contraception or abortion are in conflict with conclusions drawn from rational appraisal (Swigar, 1976; Zammuner, 1976)?

The level of *rational choice* is the step beyond customary responses and social rituals. In rational behavior, attributes of situations are identified that qualify probabilities above or below some typical value. Various alternative responses are labeled prior to their initiation, and the consequences of each are appraised in light of the particular attributes of the situation. Often, analysis proceeds to postulate a response, examine the possible outcomes of that response, and then consider another and another set of alternative futures. To be fully rational is to be able to describe (convincingly) the elements and steps in such an analysis. Modern decision theory, explained at length in the chapter by Elstein and Bordage in this volume, would allow us to choose the "best" action—the one with the greatest expected value—if we could specify all of the values and probabilities in a situation. Of course, we cannot do this in any real situation. In the view of many theorists, organisms often behave as though they were multiplying the value of each outcome by the probability of its occurrence and choosing the behavior associated with the greatest product. Such theories are frequently labeled *value expectancy* theories. (Expectancy refers to the *subjective probability*—the behaver's estimate—that a particular outcome will materialize in a particular situation.) The differentiation between rational and irrational, or nonrational, behavior lies in the means by which expectancies and values are determined and in the range of alternative actions and environmental possibilities that influence the decision. Verbal descriptions, record keeping, symbolic representations, and study of patterns of outcomes in choice situations can lead to better estimates of probabilities and values and to consideration of more alternatives.

The Health Belief Model

A version of value expectancy theory was adapted by Hochbaum (1958), Rosenstock, Leventhal, and Kegeles (Rosenstock, 1966) to the studies of preventive health behavior they were making for the U.S. Public Health Service. Their theory, which they labeled the Health Belief Model (HBM), was soon applied to a variety of illness and sick role behaviors, and it has guided a substantial amount of research in recent years (Becker, 1974a). In Chapters Seven and Eight in this volume, Rosenstock and Kirscht describe in considerable detail how the HBM has been applied to understand the utilization of health services and the degree to which sick persons adhere to their treatment regimens. A brief outline of the model here will provide the basis for considering some recent critiques of it and alternative models.

The HBM has evolved over the years and should not be considered a finished product. This description is based on a version of it offered by Becker and Maiman (1975). A comparison of that model with a number of other theories of health behavior has been made by a group of associated authors (Becker and others, 1977). According to Rosenstock (1966, p. 98), the HBM was most directly drawn from the theory of Kurt Lewin, which emphasized the subjective world—the perceptions—of the behaver rather than "the objective world of the physician or physicist." (Stone, in press, points out the importance of recognizing that the world of the physician is subjective as well.) In the original version of the model, two major classes of variables were proposed as crucial: *readiness* to take a certain action; and belief that the action would be beneficial, or *perceived benefit*. Readiness was based upon perceived susceptibility to a health threat and on the perceived seriousness of the threat. Belief about the benefits of the proposed action were also assumed to incorporate perceived barriers to taking it. The resultant of these factors was expressed in terms of the likelihood of taking the action. In addition to these factors, it was recognized that there were certain *cues to action* that were necessary to trigger the actual behavior. Pressure toward action could become quite intense without leading to overt action until some internal cue (symptom, pain) or external cue (interpersonal or media message) instigated it. The theory as now presented adds a fourth class of variables, labeled only as *modifying factors*, which are considered to influence all of the others. These factors include "demographic variables" (age, sex, ethnicity), "sociopsychological variables" (personality, social class, reference groups), and "structural variables" (knowledge about the disease, prior contact with it). In essence, the theory says that the likelihood of taking a particular action is a function of perceived threat and perceived benefit. Perceived threat is a function of perceived susceptibility, a subjective probability, and of perceived seriousness, a value. Perceived benefit is the probability that threat will be reduced (by some amount) minus the perceived cost of the action, which must itself be reduced to a set of probabilities times values. The theory does not specify what the functions are that relate these variables, nor how the values of the variables arise and change. Therefore, it does not make quantitative predictions but only relative predictions, such as: If perceived threat is increased (or higher for one group than another), likelihood of action will increase (or be higher for the appropriate group).

Those who work with the HBM have reviewed a great deal of research, most of it cited directly or indirectly in reviews by Becker and Maiman (1975), Becker (1974a), and Rosenstock and Kirscht in Chapters Seven and Eight in this volume. Many of the results are in accord with the predictions of the HBM, but some are not. Most notably, it is clear that people do not always respond to messages about threat by increased adherence to recommendations, and those who know the most about a threat do not always display more appropriate health behavior than those who know less. Proponents of the model admit these difficulties and consider them the subject for further research. Others offer alternative theories that attempt to accommodate such discrepancies in the data.

A Critique of the Health Belief Model

Leventhal and his associates (Safer and others, in press) have criticized the HBM as placing undue emphasis on abstract, conceptual beliefs. These authors stress the importance of the sensory experience of the symptoms and the reactions they elicit—self appraisals, coping responses, emotional reactions, imagined consequences, and situational barriers to care. While acknowledging that these factors could be brought under the rubrics of the HBM, Leventhal believes that in the process the relative independence of conceptual, sensory, imaginal, and emotional systems is obscured, and so are the contributions of these systems to the determination of health behavior.

This developing model, which Leventhal refers to as an information-processing model, is derived from more than a decade of research. The work began with the study, in collaboration with Janis, of the effects of fear-arousing communications on health attitudes and behavior (Janis and Leventhal, 1965). Leventhal is attempting to go beyond the threefold division of health behavior proposed by Kasl and Cobb (1966). He finds, for example, that the stage of illness behavior that intervenes between health and sick role behavior—when the individual is aware of symptoms and is deciding what to do about them—can be further subdivided into three substages. Each of these substages is associated with a period of delay, and these delays are independent of each other in length and associated with different behavioral factors, emotional reactions, negative imagery, and other variables (Safer and others, in press).

Summary: Psychology's Contributions to Date

This chapter has attempted to provide a base from which the psychologist who is relatively unfamiliar with the health system and the health professional who is relatively unfamiliar with psychology can read the chapters that follow with some perspective on their relationships with each other and with the total health system. It has shown psychology beginning its era as an identified behavioral science at the end of the nineteenth century, at about the same time as did the other behavioral and social sciences. It has pointed to an early interest by psychologists in teaching medical students their methods for understanding behavior. Evidence has been presented that psychologists have been present in the health care system longer, and in greater numbers, than sociologists or anthropologists. Psychologists have participated in teaching, research, and practice in the health system, but primarily in collaboration with or under the auspices of psychiatrists. In this collaboration, they have attended mostly to those particular problems of health settings in which emotional and behavioral disturbances perplexed health care providers—physicians and nurses—who never doubted their competence to deal effectively with the normal processes of health care. In their emphasis on patient-as-target, psychologists tended to become just another kind of specialist within a complex of highly specialized experts. They were distinguished from psychiatrists by their training in research methods, experimental techniques, and statistical analyses, but their aim was similar—to understand and control the (bizarre) behavior of patients. In short, they were deeply immersed in the orientation that the sociologist would call *psychology in medicine*, to the almost total exclusion of concern with the *psychology of medicine*. Being participants, they found it difficult to be observers. Having been present for a long time, they were not prompted so much, as were the other behavioral sciences, to examine the conditions of their presence. Anthropologists began by looking at health care systems in other cultures and turned to ours with explicitly comparative concerns. Sociologists examined the system initially as one more realization—another challenging exemplification—of their fundamental principles of social systems. Only later did anthropologists and sociologists begin to participate in the system, and then with much soul searching.

This explanation of the slowness of emergence of a true psychology of health is not fully satisfying. Psychologists were also *in* education almost from the beginning of their existence, but still managed to develop a psychology *of* education—educational psychology—at quite an early date. Perhaps the complex status relationships of the health system, in which even a university professor might be considered a person of limited consequence since he or she lacked the mythic substance of "patient responsibility," was a significant point of difference from educational systems, which often viewed the university professor with an attitude almost of awe.

Whatever the reasons, we have seen that psychologists were slow to begin research in the health system, and that when they did begin, they mostly eschewed research on the process of health care delivery. They largely accepted the medical model of pathology in the target, to be explained and sometimes ameliorated by psychological means. They investigated the irrationality of the patient who sometimes failed to utilize the expertise of the health professional—failed to attend the expert's clinical facilities, and often failed to "comply with" (only recently, "adhere to") his or her advice. Only within the past few years, in response to various forces, have the growing numbers of psychologists in the health system begun to develop a new attitude toward their presence there and toward the work they can do there. Now that they are broadening their attention to include the processes of health care, psychologists do not stand aloof and criticize the failings of those who undertake to provide care to the sick and to alert those who are at risk, as anthropologists and sociologists sometimes do. Rather, they are joining with health care providers in a participative and collegial way, trying to gain a deeper understanding of the human processes of the health system.

4 ❧

Personality, Stress, and the Development of Physical Illness

Frances Cohen

❧ There has recently been increasing interest in the role that psychological factors play, as one part of a multifactorial model, in the precipitation (and prevention) of physical illness. Yet frequently, findings are reported that relate such factors and disease without specification of how such relationships are mediated psychologically and physiologically. This chapter will review various theories and research findings linking psychological factors to the etiology of somatic illness, discuss issues of physiological and psychological mediation, and outline several models that illustrate the basic mechanisms through which such linkages may occur.

There are basically two different ways in which psychological factors are investigated as independent variables in disease. One is via *personality characteristics* thought to predispose to certain emotional states—for example, by affecting appraisals and subsequent emotional reactions to various situations (Lazarus, 1966)—to produce inadequate coping strategies that prolong stressful encounters, to result in behavior (such as smoking or drinking) that is damaging to health, and so on. For example: those with low self-esteem may interpret many situations as stressful and see themselves as

77

unable to cope, resulting in increased anxiety or depression; those who characteristically use repression as a defense may, as a result, not confront threats that can be altered, thereby prolonging the stress; those with oral needs may be more likely to smoke or drink excessively. Another focus has been on *stressful life situations* or events demanding increased coping efforts, resulting in negative emotional states, or creating strain in other areas of life functioning. Although these two focuses have generated separate research approaches, this separation of focus is somewhat artificial. The consequences of having certain personality traits or of undergoing certain stressful life experiences could also be highly interactive. On the one hand, personality characteristics could influence whether stressful life events are encountered or avoided and whether an appraisal of stress is made, and such traits could also affect the outcome of the person-environment transaction. On the other hand, stressful life experiences could influence the development of personality. In addition, it may be useful to look at life experiences and personality characteristics in combination, rather than separately, in trying to predict health outcomes.

There are several different hypotheses about which stress or coping factors are most likely to lead to disease (see also discussions by Lipowski, 1977, and Weiner, 1977). In focusing on stress, different investigators have suggested the following variables as most likely to produce disease outcomes: (1) situations that involve loss, such as bereavement, or events that result in loss of important gratifications (*loss events*), (2) an accumulation of diverse life stresses or events requiring readjustment (*accumulation of life changes*), and (3) the occurrence of life events that the individual appraises as stressful (*stress-appraised events*). The first two approaches focus largely on the occurrence in a person's life of one or many events thought to be stressful or to require adjustment and do not specifically consider whether the individual appraises the events negatively. The third approach emphasizes the individual's perception of events and suggests that if life changes are not perceived as stressful, no disease outcome is likely. In those studies that have focused on personality or coping, the following variables have been suggested by different investigators as most likely to lead to disease: (1) the way the individual copes—for example, by using repression, inhibiting emotional expression, or engaging in agitated interactions with the environment (*mode of coping*), (2) the failure of the individual's coping efforts (*failure of coping*), (3) a generalized emotional state indicating the failure of coping and a sense of giving up (*giving-up*), (4) having particular unconscious psychological conflicts that affect the way events are perceived and coped with (*specific psychological conflicts*), and (5) having personality trait characteristics thought to produce negative emotional states, such as depression and anxiety, or to lead to ineffective coping behaviors (*maladaptive personality traits*).

Although many studies focus specifically on stress—that is, investigate loss events, accumulation of life changes, or stress-appraised events—and others look only at coping or personality—that is, measure mode of coping, failure of coping, giving-up, specific psychological conflicts, or maladaptive personality traits—some studies combine these two perspectives. For example, giving-up is usually studied in connection with loss events, expressions of distress and judgments about the failure of coping are often used as indicators that stress-appraised events have occurred, and personality traits are considered maladaptive when they lead to ineffective coping in response to stress. Although it is important to keep in mind the different ways that stress and coping variables can be conceptualized, it will be necessary to combine categories to describe the research investigating psychological factors in disease.

Major Methodological Problems

There are two major methodological problems present in most of the research in this area. The first involves the indicators of illness used: the dilemma is that of distinguishing between illness and "illness behavior" (Mechanic, 1962b, 1968). It is a major thesis of this chapter that much of the literature cited as support for the idea that psychological factors are related to the development of physical illness may support only the notion that psychological factors influence illness behavior, that is, result in increased treatment seeking or increased reports of illness but not necessarily increased incidence of illness. The second methodological problem is the inadequacy of studying etiological factors in disease through retrospective studies.

Illness Versus Illness Behavior

As will be discussed in detail later, many investigators have reported evidence that illnesses of all kinds increase after stressful life events that require increased coping efforts or during times when individuals' coping efforts fail. The negative emotions that result from the failure of coping or the wear-and-tear that results from the constant readjustment are thought to have negative physiological consequences, resulting in lowered resistance and increased susceptibility to illness. In later sections of this chapter, I shall outline various physiological mechanisms through which such links may occur. However, if some of the research studies investigating these relationships measure illness behavior rather than illness, then psychological rather than physiological mediation may be involved. The illness behavior literature suggests that there may be purely psychological mechanisms that can explain the association between reports of life stresses or failure to cope and increase in illness indicators. It will thus be useful to discuss at some length the distinction between illness and illness behavior and to consider the adequacy of the various outcome measures used (see also Mechanic, 1968; Mechanic and Volkart, 1961).

Illness behavior perspective. The illness behavior literature has investigated factors that influence whether and when physiological activation is interpreted as bodily symptoms requiring medical attention. As defined by Mechanic (1968), illness behavior involves three components: (1) attentiveness to physical symptomatology, (2) processes affecting how symptoms are defined and accorded significance, and (3) the extent to which help is sought, life routine altered, and so on. To the extent that people differ in their sensitivity to physical symptoms, in the likelihood of their defining various symptoms as serious or important, and/or in the likelihood of their seeking treatment when symptoms are present, they will also differ in how frequently they report being sick and in whether they seek treatment. People who are less sensitive or less likely to seek treatment may also have physical symptoms but not report them as such or make appointments to see a physician. Mechanic (1968), Spilken and Jacobs (1971), and others have suggested that the development of illness and the seeking of medical treatment may actually be two distinct phenomena, and that the latter should not be used as a direct measure of the former (Mechanic and Newton, 1965; Mechanic and Volkart, 1961).

Examination of the literature reveals that there are strong individual differences in treatment-seeking behavior for bodily symptoms (Mechanic, 1968; Zola, 1972). Many people have physical symptoms long before they seek treatment (Antonovsky and Hartman, 1974; Cameron and Hinton, 1968; Katz and others, 1970; Olin and Hackett, 1964; von Kugelgen, 1975; see also Chapter Seven in this volume), whereas others do not seek treatment at all, despite symptoms. Indeed, survey data suggest that two out of three individuals do not consult a doctor for an illness episode (White, Williams, and Greenberg, 1961; Zola, 1972; see also Aakster, 1974), and even such serious symptoms as those involved in angina pectoris or myocardial infarction may go unreported in a substantial number of cases (Margolis and others, 1973; Mayou, 1973).

Further, there is evidence of cultural differences in the way bodily symptoms are interpreted and presented. For example, Zola (1966) found that patients of Italian descent described their symptoms vividly and dramatically, in a way that implied illness in their whole body. Patients of Irish descent, however, described their symptoms in a more restrained and calm manner, and localized the specific symptoms. Further, Zola found that more patients of Irish descent denied that pain was a feature of their illness, even if asked directly. Thus, Zola felt that Irish patients limited and understated their difficulties whereas Italian patients spread and generalized theirs. Zborowski (1952) found differences in the way Jewish, Italian, and "Old American" patients interpreted and responded to pain.

Illness indicators. Various indicators of illness have been used in the studies linking psychological factors and disease: subjects' reports of physical symptoms or illness (without confirmation of the existence of organic disease), number of visits to a physician (without confirmation of the existence of organic disease), documented cases of physical illness in subjects who self-select to seek medical treatment, and documented cases of physical illness in all members of a population (that is, physical examinations are carried out on everyone in the population, including those with no complaints of physical symptomatology). The last-mentioned indicator is clearly the most objective measure of illness and can be accomplished only through longitudinal studies that involve regular medical examinations (for example, Hinkle and others, 1961; Margolis and others, 1973; Meyer and Haggerty, 1962). However, because of the expense involved, few studies make such objective assessments, although the importance of using such measures is increasingly being emphasized by researchers in the field (Rahe and Arthur, 1978; Weiner, 1977).

When study is made of subjects with documented cases of illness who self-select for medical treatment, problems of sampling bias are encountered. That is, the disease group under study includes only those people who seek medical treatment for symptoms; others with similar symptoms who do not report to a health care facility are excluded from consideration. As mentioned earlier, there may be important individual or situational differences in whether and when physiological activation is interpreted as bodily symptoms requiring medical attention. Especially in the case of minor illnesses, those who self-select treatment may be those with certain specific personality characteristics (such as a tendency toward chronic anxiety or a need for reassurance). Thus, in comparison with those who do not seek treatment, the diagnosed symptomatic group may score higher on scales measuring these characteristics, not because anxiety or need for reassurance produces illness through physiological mechanisms but because the process of self-selection results in a greater preponderance of patients with these characteristics forming the diagnosed group.

When symptomatic groups are studied, adequate control groups are needed to determine whether there actually are differences in the independent variables for symptomatic and nonsymptomatic subjects. For example, it has been found that evidence of a recent actual, threatened, or symbolic loss with feelings of helplessness or hopelessness can be inferred in 80 percent of patients who are physically ill (Schmale, 1972, p. 23). Whether a similar percentage of healthy people have also experienced actual or symbolic losses cannot be evaluated unless a control group is included. Investigators making such judgments should also be blind to the physical condition of the patient and to the hypotheses under study.

When the number of physician visits is used as the outcome variable and no confirmation is made of the existence of organic disease, the problems are multiplied. Not only is there self-selection for treatment among patients with organic illnesses but the utilization group also includes people with problems-in-living rather than organic disease—those Garfield (1970) has referred to as the "worried well." Such patients in whom physicians can find no organic illness nonetheless show two to three times the utilization of medical facilities as patients without such life difficulties (Harrington, 1978, p. 420). Identical problems exist when questionnaire reports of illness or symptoms are used as the illness outcome measures. In addition, illnesses may be underreported or overreported depending on their social desirability and other characteristics (Brzezinski, 1965; Chambers and others, 1976; Meltzer and Hochstim, 1970). For example, Medalie and his colleagues (1973, p. 590) found that 49 of 256 subjects diagnosed with definite angina pectoris at the beginning of a large-scale study reported that they had never had chest pain (one of the requisite symptoms for the diagnosis of this illness) when reexamined five years later.

All of this suggests that reports of illness or symptoms, number of physician visits, and self-selection into medical treatment are really subjective measures of illness; each involves a self-report aspect that could be highly dependent on the person's psychological state of mind and on characteristic ways of responding to physical symptomatology. When self-report measures of life stresses or personality are used as the independent variable, correlations between variables may merely reflect a reporting tendency. That is, a single personality dimension or process may be manifesting itself in two different assessment situations.

Possible psychological mechanisms. In what specific ways could illness behavior be affected by stress or personality? Two different hypotheses could explain these relationships: (1) Stressful experiences may alter one's appraisal of physical symptoms and the mode utilized in coping with them (*appraisal hypothesis*); or (2) a personality dimension involving either a response tendency to complain about physical symptoms and life difficulties or hypersensitivity to physical symptoms and to negative aspects of one's life situation may affect how symptoms are perceived, reported, and treated (*personality dimension hypotheses*). These two models are outlined in Figure 1, part 1. The other models presented in this figure will be discussed later.

The *appraisal hypothesis* suggests that stressful experiences may affect the individual's appraisals of bodily symptoms and the means of coping with them. That is, processes involved in coping with stressful experiences may increase sensitivity to symptoms, reduce tolerance for symptoms, or encourage adoption of the "sick role." Individuals may become more worried about physical symptoms during times of stress, be less able to ignore minor symptoms (which may interfere with other coping efforts), or be more willing to avoid a work situation that they dislike. Mechanic (1968, 1974b) has suggested that "illness behavior" may be one "method of coping" with an unpleasant or dissatisfying experience. That is, "illness behavior may be seen as part of a coping repertoire, an attempt to make an unstable, challenging situation more manageable for the person who is encountering difficulty" (1968, p. 117). Mechanic further suggests that there may be individual differences in inclination to adopt the "sick role"; stress may enhance this inclination for those high on this trait.

The hypothesis that coping with stressful experiences affects one's appraisal of physical symptoms and the means used to cope with them has not been studied empirically with regard to illness, although the work of Lazarus and his colleagues (Lazarus, 1966; Lazarus, Averill, and Opton, 1970) supports the notion that appraisal and coping modes are dependent on characteristics of the person (including one's physical and mental state) and

Figure 1. Models Linking Stress and Disease

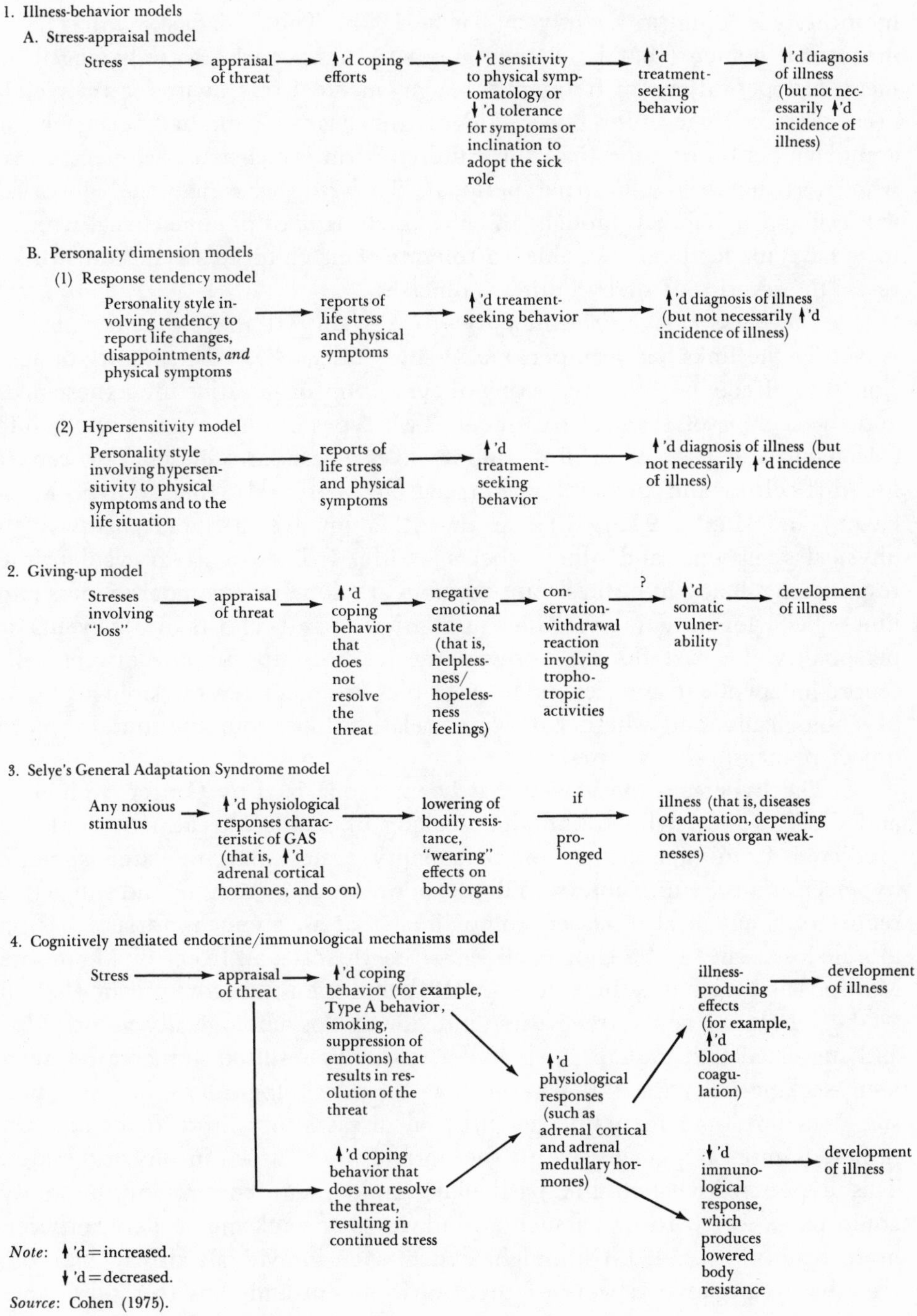

1. Illness-behavior models

   A. Stress-appraisal model

   Stress ⟶ appraisal of threat ⟶ ↑'d coping efforts ⟶ ↑'d sensitivity to physical symptomatology or ↓'d tolerance for symptoms or inclination to adopt the sick role ⟶ ↑'d treatment-seeking behavior ⟶ ↑'d diagnosis of illness (but not necessarily ↑'d incidence of illness)

   B. Personality dimension models

   (1) Response tendency model

   Personality style involving tendency to report life changes, disappointments, *and* physical symptoms ⟶ reports of life stress and physical symptoms ⟶ ↑'d treatment-seeking behavior ⟶ ↑'d diagnosis of illness (but not necessarily ↑'d incidence of illness)

   (2) Hypersensitivity model

   Personality style involving hypersensitivity to physical symptoms and to the life situation ⟶ reports of life stress and physical symptoms ⟶ ↑'d treatment-seeking behavior ⟶ ↑'d diagnosis of illness (but not necessarily ↑'d incidence of illness)

2. Giving-up model

   Stresses involving "loss" ⟶ appraisal of threat ⟶ ↑'d coping behavior that does not resolve the threat ⟶ negative emotional state (that is, helplessness/ hopelessness feelings) ⟶ conservation-withdrawal reaction involving trophotropic activities ⟶[?] ↑'d somatic vulnerability ⟶ development of illness

3. Selye's General Adaptation Syndrome model

   Any noxious stimulus ⟶ ↑'d physiological responses characteristic of GAS (that is, ↑'d adrenal cortical hormones, and so on) ⟶ lowering of bodily resistance, "wearing" effects on body organs ⟶[if prolonged] illness (that is, diseases of adaptation, depending on various organ weaknesses)

4. Cognitively mediated endocrine/immunological mechanisms model

   Stress ⟶ appraisal of threat ⟶ ↑'d coping behavior (for example, Type A behavior, smoking, suppression of emotions) that results in resolution of the threat

   ↑'d coping behavior that does not resolve the threat, resulting in continued stress ⟶ ↑'d physiological responses (such as adrenal cortical and adrenal medullary hormones) ⟶ illness-producing effects (for example, ↑'d blood coagulation) ⟶ development of illness

   ↓'d immunological response, which produces lowered body resistance ⟶ development of illness

Note: ↑'d = increased.
  ↓'d = decreased.
Source: Cohen (1975).

conditions of the environment (for example, the balance between harm-producing stimuli and counterharm resources). Indirect support for this hypothesis is found in a study by Tuch (1975). Tuch's data show that para-menstrual women (that is, women about to have or who were having their menstrual period) more frequently sought medical treatment for their children, and yet their children were judged to be less sick and had been sick for a shorter period of time than the children of intermenstrual women (those who were between menstrual periods). Tuch suggests that the increased anxiety and irritability thought to be characteristic of paramenstrual women may have made them less able to tolerate their children's symptoms or to assess the severity of their children's illnesses.

The *personality dimension hypotheses* suggest that what may be involved in the links between personality and "disease" is a personality dimension that affects both the reporting of symptoms or negative life experiences and the seeking of medical treatment. Two types of dimensions are possible (Mechanic and Newton, 1965)—one involves a response tendency to report life difficulties and physical symptomatology (see also Sarason, de Monchaux, and Hunt, 1975), whereas the other involves a hypersensitivity to physical symptoms and other aspects of life. It is difficult to evaluate the response tendency hypothesis until studies are done that compare illness and illness behavior outcome variables in relation to self-reports of life events or personality. We just do not know if the relationships found between self-report independent and dependent variables are mediated physiologically or psychologically, and whether different relationships would be found if more objective measures were used.

The hypersensitivity view has been emphasized by Canter, Imboden, and Cluff (1966), who found that seeking of medical treatment could be predicted from high scores on personality scales that indicated somatic hypersensitivity, vulnerability to depression, low ego strength, and subjective report of many health-related complaints—that is, Hypochondriasis (Hs), a morale-loss scale, and a shortened ego-strength scale, all from the Minnesota Multiphasic Personality Inventory (MMPI), and the total score on the Cornell Medical Index. They termed these individuals "psychologically vulnerable" and suggested that perhaps their hypersensitivity resulted in increased treatment-seeking behavior: "It may be that the psychologically vulnerable person does not fundamentally get physical diseases any more often . . . but, rather, is more hypersensitive to the normal fluctuations in physical states. This hypersensitivity in the particular employment context of the study could be expected to impel such an individual to seek medical consultation more readily" (p. 349). One might expect such individuals also to be more sensitive to negative aspects of their environment and thus to report more negative life events.

Further support can be seen in the work of Hinkle and his colleagues (Hinkle and others, 1958), where personality differences were found between two small groups of Chinese immigrants showing either high or low incidence of self-reported illness. Low-illness subjects showed little conflict or anxiety and had reduced awareness of emotional problems as compared with those with a high incidence of illness. This suggests that those who report many illnesses may be more aware of and sensitive to emotions and the difficulties of life which could result in increased awareness of physical symptomatology. In addition, it has been found that focusing a person's attention on his or her symptoms (by asking the person to maintain an illness log) results in increased reports of symptomatology (Mechanic and Newton, 1965).

The work just reviewed suggests that a sharp distinction must be made between measures of illness and measures reflecting treatment-seeking behavior or illness reporting. Self-reports of illness or the use of medical facilities cannot be considered measures of "illness" unless medical examinations are carried out both on those seeking treatment and on a control group not seeking treatment for medical complaints. As mentioned earlier, this can be accomplished, although at considerable cost, by longitudinal studies that involve regular medical examinations. Until such studies are done, extreme caution should be used in interpreting findings and making recommendations about factors that produce illness based on studies that have only utilized measures of illness behavior.

Retrospective Reports of Life Events

The second methodological problem in research linking psychological factors and disease involves the inadequacy of looking for personality factors that may have an etiological link to disease by utilizing retrospective reports of life events or by assessing the patient's emotional state after a diagnosis is made. The knowledge that one is ill or the disease process itself may affect the independent variables hypothesized to be causal factors (see also Brown, 1974; Hudgens, 1974). Once disease has been diagnosed, increased expressions of hopelessness and helplessness are to be expected, and patients quite likely will respond differently to questions about their past experiences. For example, researchers once thought that Down's syndrome might be a result of emotional stress that occurred during early pregnancy because mothers of Down's syndrome children recollected such stressful events when asked about their pregnancy after the child was born. It was only after the discovery that a chromosomal defect produced this disease that such stress-related etiological hypotheses were finally discarded (Brown, 1974). Because the knowledge that one is ill affects one's emotional state, retrospective accounts of loss or stress or indicators of negative affect in patients who are ill certainly cannot be considered as causal variables. Many of the studies focusing on diagnosed cases have not utilized control groups or tried to minimize observer bias, raising further questions about the adequacy of designs that select patients for study only after diagnosis of illness has been made.

Studies that investigate a person's emotional state after he or she shows some clinical signs of illness, but before the diagnosis is made, cannot be considered free of a retrospective bias, especially in the case of cancer patients. As Davies and others (1973) suggest, the disease process in cancer may cause some psychological changes before the disease is fully manifest. Thus, investigators may be picking up the patients' increased sensitivity to their own disease, their suspicion that the symptoms have a bad prognosis, or psychological changes that have occurred as a result of the cancerous process. Indeed, studies by Fras, Litin, and Pearson (1967) and Kerr, Schapira, and Roth (1969) suggest that depressive symptoms may precede manifest physical symptoms of certain types of cancer. Friedman and his colleagues (1974) discuss other psychological states that may be prodromal symptoms of coronary heart disease rather than psychosocial risk factors for the emergence of the illness. Truly predictive studies, following large groups of healthy adults with no disease or cellular abnormalities present, are necessary to overcome these difficulties. Such studies may entail considerable expense but they are the only way to eliminate the biases of retrospective reporting of emotional state.

Generality Versus Specificity Approaches

Two broad points of view characterize the literature linking psychological factors and disease (Moss, 1973; Syme, 1967): a focus (Thurlow, 1967) on general susceptibility to illness (*generality* or nonspecific approach), and a focus on the development of specific illnesses (*specificity* approach). The general approaches posit hormonal-biochemical factors affecting a "general susceptibility to illness," which increases the probability of developing illnesses of many types. The specificity approaches focus on specific illnesses and implicate particular constitutional, psychological, or social variables in the etiology of these diseases.

The distinction between specificity and nonspecificity employed here is different from a distinction commonly found in the psychological literature on stress. For example, Lazarus (1966, 1974) and Mason (1971, 1974, 1975b) have challenged Selye's (1956; see also Selye, 1975) view that physiological stress reactions are a nonspecific response to any noxious stimulus. Lazarus and Mason argue that some stress reactions may be mediated largely by psychological processes and may be somewhat specific to particular types of cognitive appraisals (appraisals of threat or anticipation of activity or coping). Thus, their argument concerns the specificity or nonspecificity of the stimuli that can produce stress reactions—that is, whether all noxious stimuli result in increased physiological reactivity or largely those mediated by psychological processes. However, most of the medical literature relating stress or psychological factors to illness can be most clearly organized by looking at the outcome of the transaction—an increase in illnesses of all kinds or the development of one particular illness, such as heart disease. Thus, the basis of the distinction used to organize the research section of this chapter lies in whether generalized or specific somatic effects are predicted to result from the particular psychological factors under study. Generality theories hypothesize more general biological mechanisms which have negative effects on the system as a whole or on vulnerable organ systems, whereas most specificity theories focus on more specific biological mechanisms which, through their particular effects, are directly implicated in the development of a particular disease.*

General maladaptation theories take a third point of view in relating psychological factors to the development of disease—considering disease as merely one type of maladaptive behavior (along with juvenile delinquency, mental illness, and so on), which occurs as a result of disparities between the social structure and the individual's personality. Because of the broad scope of these theories and their limited ability to specify those conditions likely to lead to somatic disease as opposed to other types of maladaptive behavior, these theories will be mentioned only briefly.

Because research and theories from generality and specificity perspectives focus on different variables, they will be discussed separately. Under the generality approaches, we will look at loss events and the giving-up-given-up complex, accumulation of life changes, and stress-appraised life events. It is far beyond the scope of this chapter to review the vast literature relating psychological factors to the development of various specific illnesses. Our discussion of specificity approaches will focus on only two diseases in which psychological factors are hypothesized to play a role: coronary heart disease and cancer. See Weiner (1977) for a comprehensive review of the literature investigating the role of psychological factors in the etiology of various psychosomatic illnesses.

Generality Theories: Factors Thought to Increase Susceptibility to Diseases of Many Types

Loss Events and the Giving-Up-Given-up Complex

The notion of "giving-up" has often been implicated in studies showing sudden death after severe losses (Engel, 1968, 1971) or the breaking of a taboo (Cannon, 1942). Although anecdotal examples abound (see also Seligman, 1975), the biological mechanisms underlying this phenomenon are often disputed. Some suggest that the sudden death is due to myocardial infarction, or to bradycardia (slowness of heart action) occurring as a result of the oxygen-conserving or diving reflex (Wolf, 1967), or that it involves a vagal mechanism in reaction to loss of hope (Richter, 1957). Still others (for example, Barber, 1961) believe that "voodoo" deaths occur not because of biological mechanisms set off by feelings of giving-up but rather because of poison or organic disease or because the frightened person stops eating and drinking.

---

*The implicit argument, then, is a specificity argument in the sense that Lazarus (1966) and Averill and Opton (1968) use the term. That is, this approach seems to imply that particular stressors may be linked to the development of particular diseases, such as cancer. Whether such stressors might also be linked to the development of other diseases, such as heart disease or upper respiratory infection, is not evaluated in these studies and is one of the weaknesses of this approach.

In addition to anecdotal evidence and animal studies, another approach trying to link giving-up to the development of illness has been the work of Engel and Schmale (Engel, 1968; Engel and Schmale, 1967; Schmale, 1972; Schmale and Engel, 1967). They suggest that a giving-up-given-up complex in response to situations of loss may precede the development of illnesses of all types, in those with somatic predispositions. According to their view, if feelings of helplessness or hopelessness develop in patients who have experienced an actual, threatened, or symbolic loss, this can facilitate the development of existing somatic predispositions or external pathogens, resulting in disease. Thus, a psychological state of mind mediates the development of illness, although this state is not a necessary or sufficient condition—the person must be predisposed to the disease.

Although Engel and Schmale emphasize the occurrence of loss, more clearly it seems that what is involved is inability to cope in the face of negative environmental events. For example, Engel (1968, pp. 359-360) characterizes the giving-up-given-up complex as involving a "sense of psychological impotence, a feeling that for briefer or longer periods of time one is unable to cope with the changes in the environment, the psychological or social devices utilized in the past seem no longer effective or available." Although such states may occur occasionally in all of us, Engel believes that in prolonged states of helplessness or hopelessness, disease is likely to occur because the total biological economy of the organism is changed, making it less capable of dealing effectively with pathogenic processes.

Empirical evidence. The research investigating this theory has focused either on feelings of helplessness-hopelessness or on the occurrence of specific losses. The evidence that Schmale (1972) reviews in support of this view consists mostly of retrospective studies. One, for example, shows that from the interview responses of patients who are physically ill, evidence of a recent actual, threatened, or symbolic loss with feelings of either hopelessness or helplessness can be inferred in 80 percent of the cases (p. 23). Serious questions can be raised about the retrospective studies, as we have earlier discussed (and which Schmale acknowledges). Once disease has been diagnosed, increased expressions of hopelessness and helplessness are to be expected. Further, since most of these studies have not utilized control groups or tried to minimize observer bias, these studies provide weak support for their theory.

The only "predictive" studies reported are a series (Schmale and Iker, 1966, 1971) involving patients (all asymptomatic for cervical disease) who were hospitalized for a diagnostic cone biopsy because of repeated evidence of atypical cervical cytology (that is, suspicious cells). Predictions of cancer were made for those who suffered real or apparent losses with high hopelessness potential or expressed feelings of hopelessness (as determined through interviews). These predictions were subsequently borne out, suggesting that hopelessness potential is linked to increased probability of cancer of the cervix. However, this study is not predictive in the full sense of the word, since all patients were initially diagnosed as having some cellular abnormalities. As discussed earlier, the disease process in cancer may cause psychological changes before the disease becomes manifest (Davies and others, 1973). Thus, the hopelessness feelings may be a result of the cancerous process rather than a causal factor.

Other studies have focused on morbidity or mortality after the occurrence of a loss event, such as the death of a spouse. Some researchers have reported increased mortality among widows or widowers in the first six months after the death of their spouse (Ekblom, 1963; Young, Benjamin, and Wallis, 1963; see reviews by Jacobs and Ostfeld, 1977; Rowland, 1977), suggesting that they died of a "broken heart" (Parkes, Benjamin, and Fitzgerald, 1969). Rees and Lutkins (1967) compared the mortality rate of 903 close relatives of someone who died with a control group of 878. They found the death rate among bereaved relatives was seven times higher than in the control group during the first year after bereavement. The death rate was also significantly higher for males and was most significant for those who were widowers. However, Clayton (1974) did not find greater mortality for those who were widowed, as compared to a control group. Whether the increased death rate found in several of these studies was due to the effects of jointly sharing a deleterious environment or to the losses involved in widowhood has not been clearly established (Rowland, 1977).

The results are mixed regarding whether morbidity increases after the loss of one's spouse. Using retrospective reports of illness, Maddison and Viola (1968) found that during the year following bereavement, widows reported more physical symptoms such as headaches, indigestion, and chest pain, but that there was little change reported in the frequency or severity of major diseases. In a one-year follow-up, Clayton (1974) found that widows and widowers reported significantly more physical symptoms than controls on only three out of fifteen physical symptom variables (namely, blurred vision, shortness of breath, and palpitations) but did not report increased physician visits or more frequent hospitalization. The bereaved did report significantly more psychological symptoms commonly associated with depression (such as crying and loss of appetite). Parkes and Brown (1972) report similar results in a small sample; these investigators also found that hospitalization rates were higher for the bereaved group.

Focusing more narrowly on the issue of loss, Parens, McConville, and Kaplan (1966) report a predictive study with student nurses, relating their frequency of illness during the first year of nursing school with their response to separation from home, as measured by an adjustment scale and a depression inventory given six weeks after the start of the school year. Eight months later, it was found that those students who initially showed the worst adjustment to separation were ill most often (as measured by visits to the infirmary). Students with very high depression scores also showed more frequent illnesses, although the overall correlation was not significant. Other studies have not confirmed the relationship between loss and illness. Using a simple questionnaire to report "separation experiences," Imboden, Canter, and Cluff (1963, p. 433) reported that 25 percent of normal subjects in a sample of 455 employees at Fort Detrick, Maryland, reported a recent "separation experience," but that frequency of dispensary visits showed no significant differences between those who reported separation experiences and those who did not. Although some have suggested that the losses involved in institutional relocation hasten death among the elderly, the results of research studies are not clear cut or free from confounding variables. It does appear that relocation is related to increased mortality only for those initially in poor health (Rowland, 1977).

The work of Imboden, Canter, and Cluff (1963) underlines the necessity of including control groups and also points out the frequency of separation experiences in the lives of normal subjects. Actual, threatened, or symbolic losses and the necessity of giving-up *are* quite common in the life cycle, especially in changes from one stage to another, as most of these researchers mention. This suggests that such losses could quite easily be found in the history of most groups of people, especially if the interviewer is sensitized to looking for them; thus, control groups are essential. This also suggests that how one *copes* with "loss" may be more important than the *occurrence* of loss itself. This is implicit in Schmale and Engel's discussion, although some researchers emphasize the occurrence of loss as of primary importance (see later discussion of psychological factors in cancer). Future studies should address how coping abilities of the individual and social supports can mediate the effects of loss.

Biological mechanisms hypothesized. What are the biological mechanisms that could be involved in the giving-up-given-up complex? Schmale (1972) reviews studies that relate the helplessness-hopelessness affects to cardiac slowing or arrhythmias, drops in blood pressure, decreases in urinary water and sodium output, and so on. However, he and Engel favor the view that this reaction is linked to biological mechanisms of the conservation-withdrawal reaction that are associated with trophotropic (involving attraction and repulsion of nutritive substances by organic cells) activities of the central nervous system. Schmale (1972, p. 29) describes this reaction as follows: "The conservation-withdrawal reaction includes at the central nervous system level a preponderance of trophotropic influences with a predominance of parasympathetic activation and a relative sympathetic inactivity plus an overall mixture of hormonal influences which favor anabolic activity over catabolic activity. Such a combination of influences promotes internal survival at a reduced rate of functioning as well as protection against an unfavorable external environment." Thus, Schmale sees the conservation-withdrawal reaction as an adaptive mechanism, a way of withdrawing from an unfavorable external environment. However, he suggests that these reactions protect the organism from some consequences of stress but lead to increased vulnerability to others. This model is outlined in Figure 1.

The conservation-withdrawal reaction is one of two opposite biological patterns that Engel (1962) hypothesizes are found in response to a mounting need. The first-line biological defense—flight-fight—is characterized by energy expenditure and involvement with the environment. The second-line biological defense of conservation-withdrawal—which is characterized by energy conservation and withdrawal from the environment—arises only if the energy expenditure of the first reaction threatens the organism with exhaustion.

Although such a stage has been described behaviorally by various investigators as characterizing an infant's response to separation from its mother (Kaufman and Rosenblum, 1967; Spitz, 1945, 1946), the exact physiological mechanisms accompanying this stage have not been studied empirically and remain obscure. Kaufman and Rosenblum suggest that this second stage may be "kicked off" biochemically by the diencephalon in response to the persistence of high-energy distress. Studies are currently under way to investigate the physiological reactions accompanying such a depressed stage. Preliminary results (Reite and others, 1974) suggest that profound hypothermia (lowered body temperature) and bradycardia are found when separated infant monkeys appear to be "depressed." However, it is not clear how these bodily reactions might increase somatic vulnerability to all illnesses, as has been hypothesized.

Whether what Engel hypothesizes as a conservation-withdrawal reaction does accompany or produce a depressed state, or is related to helplessness-hopelessness feelings, still remains an untested empirical question, as does how such a biological reaction can increase somatic vulnerability. Much further research is needed to clarify whether separations and giving-up produce similar physiological responses and what the exact physiological mechanisms are (Denenberg, 1972; Hinde, 1972).

Accumulation of Life Changes

Holmes and Rahe and their associates (Holmes and Masuda, 1974; Holmes and Rahe, 1967b; Holmes and Rahe, undated; Rahe, 1972, 1974; Rahe, McKean, and Arthur, 1967; Rahe and others, 1964) have investigated the relationship between stressful life events and the onset of illnesses of all types. That is, they look at life stress in terms of life events or life changes that either are indicative of or require a significant change in the ongoing life patterns of the individual. A distinguishing characteristic of their approach is that they include life changes that are both positive (such as promotion, marriage) and negative in nature (divorce, arrest). Their Schedule of Recent Experiences (SRE) lists these various life changes, and the subject indicates how many times in the preceding two-year period each of these has occurred (Holmes and Rahe, 1967a). Each event is then given a Life Change Unit (LCU) score, and the sum of life change units during that period is determined. The LCU weightings for each life event were obtained by having diverse groups of subjects rate on the Social Readjustment Rating scale the amount of readjustment required in response to the various life changes listed (Holmes and Rahe, 1967b). These researchers have shown that life events cluster significantly in a two-year period preceding the onset of illness, and that the onset of illness can be predicted from the total number of life events (Rahe and others, 1964). Although most of the early studies involved retrospective reports of life change and of illness (see the review by Holmes and Masuda, 1974), subsequent studies (for reviews, see Rahe, 1972, 1974, and Rahe and Arthur, 1978), mostly with Navy men, have been predictive in nature, with retrospective reporting of life changes and predictive follow-up of illness (as determined by Navy records). The results of these more predictive studies support the earlier work, although only those life changes reported as having occurred during the previous six months were predictive of illness (Rahe, 1974) rather than those in the previous two years, as was true in the earlier studies. Significant relationships have also been found between reports of life changes and reports of psychophysiological symptoms and symptoms of depression (Markush and Favero, 1974; Vinokur and Selzer, 1975) and scores on several trait measures of anxiety (Reavley, 1974).

Although there has been considerable research using the SRE (Dohrenwend and Dohrenwend, 1974b; Gunderson and Rahe, 1974), the life change approach has come under considerable attack for methodological and theoretical reasons. Rahe (Rahe, 1974; Rahe and Arthur, 1978) has recently taken these criticisms into account in developing a complex model that provides less simplistic explanations of the relationships between life change and illness than the viewpoint originally proposed. Since this recent model emphasizes the appraisal of stress and other important intervening variables, these issues will be discussed in the next section of this chapter, which focuses on stress-appraised life events. Thus, some of the problems to be discussed here have been addressed in the new approach outlined by Rahe and Arthur.

Methodological problems. The methodology of studies using the life change approach has been sharply criticized (for example, Brown, 1974; Cleary, 1974; Dohrenwend and Dohrenwend, 1974a; Mechanic, 1974a, 1975; Rabkin and Struening, 1976; Sarason, de Monchaux, and Hunt, 1975; Wershow and Reinhart, 1974). First, many of the early studies were methodologically quite weak, involving retrospective accounts of life changes and retrospective reports of illness. In several cases where subjects were asked to report simultaneously on life changes and on past illness, the hypotheses being tested were undoubtedly clear to the subjects. Further, in these early studies, no guidelines were suggested as to what types of illnesses should be reported, and apparently subjects made their own judgments in this regard. Second, although significant results are often found, the magnitude of relationships is small. A correlation of .12 (as reported by Rahe, 1974, p. 80, in various Navy samples) is significant in samples of 800 but explains less than 2 percent of the variance. In some studies, the correlations are even lower, and characteristics of the occupational environment and demographic variables are found to be significantly better predictors of illness reporting than reports of recent life change events (Rahe and others, 1972). Third, the reliability of the Schedule of Recent Experiences (SRE) is lower than desirable (Cleary, 1974; Horowitz and others, 1977; Sarason, de Monchaux, and Hunt,

1975), especially in the Navy studies where it is about .6 (Rahe, 1974, p. 83). Fourth, it has been pointed out that many of the life events on the SRE could be considered presymptomatic manifestations of incipient illness (for example, changes in eating or sleeping habits) or consequences of illness, rather than antecedent life events, thus artificially inflating the association between such "life changes" and illness (Hudgens, 1974).

Fifth, it has become increasingly clear that groups of people vary significantly in their ratings (on the Social Readjustment Rating Scale) of the amount of readjustment that each life event requires and in the frequency with which they report the occurrence of particular life events on the SRE. Recent reports have cautioned researchers that sex, age, marital status, ethnicity, recency of experience, and other demographic and experiential variables may have significant influences on these measures and thus must be taken into account in efforts to increase the predictive validity of life change measures (Horowitz and others, 1977; Lundberg, Theorell, and Lind, 1975; Masuda and Holmes, 1978). Sixth, the indicators of illness in these studies are all subjective in nature. Thus, it is possible that what is being measured here is the relationship between reported life stress and various aspects of illness behavior, not illness, as Jacobs, Spilken, and Norman (1969) suggest, and as has been discussed at length earlier. Studies using adequate indicators of illness are necessary to clarify this important issue.

Theoretical problems. Cleary (1974) has questioned some of the basic assumptions of the SRE, such as whether LCU values accurately represent the pathogenic significance of a life event, whether these effects are additive, and whether these effects are best measured on a single scale. Cleary suggests that different life events may produce diverse physiological responses (as will be discussed later) and that it may be more important to explore the nature of these specific relationships than to look at life events and diseases in their broader contexts.

Although Holmes and Rahe and their colleagues theorize that all life changes, whether positive or negative, increase the probability that disease will develop, there is evidence that the undesirable events are the ones most strongly correlated with reports of illness symptoms (Liem and Liem, 1976; Vinokur and Selzer, 1975). More research is necessary to determine the relative impact of positive life events in increasing illness frequency. Another theoretical question concerns whether *no change* might have negative effects when, in the life cycle, change might have been expected (Gersten and others, 1974; Graham, 1974). One might imagine that not getting a promotion, not going to college, or not taking a vacation may have a negative impact on the individual, an issue not taken into account in this formulation. Other researchers (for example, Levi, 1974, and Frankenhaeuser, 1976) hypothesize that understimulation as well as overstimulation should lead to increased physiological activation.

Further, the life change approach emphasizes the negative effects of life changes and downplays the fact that a substantial number of people undergo many severely stressful events without developing illness (Hinkle,

1974). As Lazarus (1966) and others have pointed out, reaction to life changes or demands depends also on the capacity of the person to deal with the life changes, and on the nature of the surrounding environment, including the amount of social support available (Kaplan, Cassel, and Gore, 1977; Kaufman, 1973; Mechanic, 1974b; Nuckolls, Cassel, and Kaplan, 1972) and the institutionalized means for dealing with such changes (Goldschmidt, 1974). A theoretical formulation that ignores such important data is limited in its predictive value. It may be especially important to study those psychological factors (or modes of coping) that enable individuals to meet threatening situations without developing illness, rather than increasing the volumes of studies that focus narrowly on life events per se. Wershow and Reinhart (1974, pp. 400-401) suggest a similar viewpoint: "One might suggest a moratorium on papers employing the SRE and similar instruments. The point has been amply made that some relationship exists between change in life-ways, let alone stress, and illness. However, the relationship is a weak one. Some people become ill or are hospitalized and, as we have demonstrated, no discernible changes in their life have occurred. Others meet life changes in other ways, some withdraw into sleep, or leave the field in other ways; some may even find constructive ways of dealing with change. We would suggest that, among other steps, deviant cases be sought out, those who handle life changes well and those who break down on what seems to be little provocation, to learn more about coping mechanisms. . . . Trying to force the data into a stronger position than our favorite hypotheses warrant will only lead us further down the current cul-de-sac."

It is both theoretically and practically important to determine whether it is the actual *occurrence* of life changes, both positive and negative, or the person's *reporting* of or negative evaluation of such life changes, that is linked to either increased treatment-seeking behavior or incidence of illness. The importance of determining what variables are actually being tapped in such studies becomes clear when one hears (as the author has) that a health maintenance organization intends to counsel patients with large numbers of previous life changes to limit additional changes in an attempt to prevent illness. Similar advice has been offered in popular magazines and newspapers (for example, "Life's Good Times Can Be Dangerous," 1978). Such a suggestion to maintain the status quo seems quite inappropriate considering the weakness of the evidence and further ignores the possibility that *no* change might have even more deleterious effects. It becomes imperative to clarify these important theoretical issues before such interventions are made.

Biological mechanisms. Holmes and Rahe and their co-workers have not specified a specific physiological model to explain the relationship between life change and illness. Their view is that life changes (whether positive or negative in nature) require readjustment by the person that could result in increased physiological activation of various bodily systems. Over time, or if the changes are many in number, this could have a "wearing effect" on the body and result in illness. For example, Holmes and Masuda (1974, p. 68) state: "It is postulated that life change events, by evoking adaptive efforts by the human organism that are faulty in kind and duration, lower 'bodily resistance' and enhance the probability of disease occurrence." The model these researchers seem to be implicitly using is that of Hans Selye. We will, therefore, turn our attention to a discussion of Selye's General Adaptation Syndrome and diseases of adaptation.

One of the earliest theories linking stress to illness is that of Selye (1956), although Selye's focus was on animal research with stimuli that were physically noxious. However, his theory is often used as a model to illustrate the physiological mechanisms whereby stress can produce pathology. Selye suggested that *any* noxious stimulus (for example, heat, cold, immobilization) results in a particular biological response—the General Adaptation Syndrome (GAS)—characterized by increased pituitary-adrenal cortical hormone secretions (both inflammatory and anti-inflammatory hormones) which act as a system of "defenses" against the noxious stimulus. The GAS consists of three stages: alarm reaction, stage of resistance, and stage of exhaustion. During the alarm reaction stage, there is a trio of biological changes: enlargement of the adrenal cortex, atrophy of the thymus, and bleeding gastric ulcers. During the stage of resistance, there is increased resistance to the noxious agent but decreased resistance to other stimuli. If these defensive processes are prolonged, the animal may die or suffer irreversible bodily damage; that is, the GAS may result in what Selye terms "diseases of adaptation," such as arthritis and kidney disease. The disease process occurs usually as a result of the adrenal cortical and pituitary hormones, the inflammation processes (as in arthritis), or the lowering of bodily resistance. Thus, it is possible that many different diseases could result from the prolongation of the adaptive processes brought into play to deal with noxious stimuli. Depending on various constitutional or acquired weaknesses of the organism, different organs might be especially affected, and different diseases produced. It should, however, be emphasized that the GAS will not lead to disease unless the adaptive responses are prolonged or are somehow defective. The mechanisms involved in Selye's model are outlined in Figure 1.

It is not known exactly how these various noxious stimuli produce a similar physiological response. Selye's hypothesis has been described as follows: "In terms of physiological mechanisms, Selye's hypothesis was that the diverse stimuli or agents enumerated above, for example, cold, heat, exercise, and so on, all have a common quality of being 'noxious' to the organism and all activate some unknown common afferent system of one or more 'first mediators.' Such 'first mediators' then carry the message of exposure to 'noxious' agents through neural or humoral pathways to the integrative centers, which in turn, bring about the nonspecific response triad, including stimulation of the pituitary-adrenal cortical system" (Mason, 1975a, pp. 8-9).

Selye has emphasized the activation of the adrenal cortical hormones in response to stress, and the role of these hormones in lowering bodily resistance and producing other biological changes. It is important to remember that other hormonal systems also respond to stress, and their effects may be significant. Mason (1968a), for example, suggests that the metabolic effects of hormones are dependent not on the absolute level of any one hormone but on the relative overall balance among several hormones; he considers the pituitary-adrenal cortical system to be only one part of a coordinated overall pattern of endocrine responses. In his own work, Mason (1974) has found that different "patterns" or "profiles" characterize the neuroendocrine responses of rhesus monkeys to different noxious situations. Not only are levels of 17-hydroxycorticosteroids (17-OHCS) affected, but epinephrine, norepinephrine, testosterone, thyroxine, insulin, growth hormone, and other hormones also respond differentially to different noxious agents. Thus, although the GAS provides a model of how stressful events can reduce bodily resistance and damage various organs, it is not clear that this is the most important mechanism that leads to disease or that the adrenal cortical hormones play a preeminent role. Levi (1974), for example, has emphasized the role of the adrenal medullary hormones (epinephrine and norepinephrine) in responding to life changes and increasing the likelihood of disease.

There is considerable evidence that life events of either a pleasant or unpleasant nature result in increased physiological activation. For example, Levi (1965) has shown that both amusing and aggression-provoking films result in increased levels of adrenal medullary hormones (especially epinephrine). Rahe, Rubin, and Arthur (1974) review evidence that serum uric acid, cholesterol, and cortisol vary during different life events, with increased levels in situations involving, respectively, pleasant challenges, failure, and threatening demands. Theorell (1974) reports a modest but significant correlation between weekly reports of life changes and increased epinephrine and norepinephrine levels. Singer (1974) reviews substantial evidence that cardiovascular and psychoendocrine systems (see also Mason, 1968b, and Frankenhaeuser, 1971, 1975, 1976) show increased physiological reactivity in situations (whether of a pleasurable or threatening nature) where people are "engaged" or "involved." Thus, the evidence supports the notion that both positive and negative life events can result in increased physiological reactivity if the situation is one where the person is actively involved. However, it is still not known how responses of these physiological systems can affect one's "general susceptibility" to illness.

Stress-Appraised Life Events

Whereas the life change approach suggests that any life change, positive or negative, will increase the likelihood that illness will develop, other researchers have suggested that illnesses will be most frequent in people who undergo negative life experiences and who have difficulty successfully adapting to them. As discussed earlier, there is evidence that reports of negative life events are more strongly correlated with illness symptoms than are life changes of a positive nature (Liem and Liem, 1976; Vinokur and Selzer,

1975). Hinkle and his colleagues emphasized the role of negative life experiences in their studies investigating differences in illness frequency. These researchers (Hinkle and others, 1956; Hinkle and others, 1957; Hinkle and others, 1958; Hinkle and Wolff, 1957; see Hinkle, 1974, for a review) provide evidence that episodes of illness are not randomly distributed among the population. In several groups (career telephone operators, blue-collar workmen, Chinese immigrants) in which they studied the illness distribution episodes, it was found that about 25 percent of the members experienced approximately 50 percent of the episodes over a twenty-year period of the "prime of life," with another 25 percent experiencing fewer than 10 percent of the episodes (Hinkle and others, 1958, p. 278). Further, the more episodes of illness, the more variety of illness was found, the more organ systems were involved, and the more etiological categories (for example, metabolic, allergy) were included (see also Eastwood and Trevelyan, 1972). (One should, of course, keep in mind that there are nonpsychological reasons for clustering of diseases; the occurrence of an episode of one disease, such as diabetes mellitus, does increase the likelihood that episodes of another disease, such as urinary tract infection, will also occur [Hinkle, 1974].) These researchers further found that illnesses were not distributed at random over the life of a person but often appeared in "clusters." These clusters of illness, which "ran" for several years, most often appeared when a person was having difficulty adapting to his or her environment, as perceived by the person. That is, those with the highest susceptibility to illness were those who failed to adapt successfully to negative life situations (see Aakster, 1974, for a similar view). It thus appeared that many different negative psychological and social events produced a similar physiological result, namely an increase in general susceptibility to illness.

Mediating variables. The stress-appraisal viewpoint suggests that there is no simple or straightforward relationship between life change and illness, and that other mediating variables must be considered in predicting illness outcomes. These include biological predispositions to illness or a history of preexisting illness (Hinkle, 1974; Weiner, 1977), the person's appraisal of the situation, resources for dealing with the life event, the social supports received from others, the coping strategies used in dealing with the stress, and whether the life change results in significant modification of the person's activities, diet, and so on. For example, Hinkle (1974) has suggested that if there is no history of preexisting illness or susceptibility, or the person has certain psychological characteristics that "insulate" him or her from stressful life experiences, or the person's life activities do not change substantially, then illness will not result despite the magnitude of the social change.

Lazarus (1966) has emphasized the central role of *appraisal* (see the summary of his stress and coping perspective in Chapter Nine in this volume). Not everyone perceives life events in the same way; what may be stressful for one person may not be stressful for another. If a person has the resources to meet the challenge posed, has beliefs that result in a positive definition of the event, or does not perceive that danger exists, then no stress reaction will be evident. The meaning of the life change and people's feelings of satisfaction about their living situation are critically important, as Hinkle (1974) has emphasized. For example, in a study of refugees from the Hungarian revolution of 1956, Hinkle and his colleagues (1959) found that despite the social upheaval, physical dislocation, separation from family, and other changes, most refugees reported less illness following the revolution and their flight to the United States than prior to these changes.

Hinkle (1974) analyzed the personality factors that distinguished people who were rarely ill from those with frequent illnesses. He suggested that those who remain healthy show a lack of concern for other people and life goals, and lack of involvement in life affairs: "The healthiest members of our samples often showed little psychological reaction to events and situations which caused profound reactions in other members of the group. The loss of a husband or wife . . . or the failure to attain apparently important goals produced no profound or lasting reaction. They seemed to have a shallow attachment to people, goals, or groups . . . [and] behaved as if their own well-being were one of their primary concerns. An employed man or woman might refuse a promotion because he [or she] did not want the increased responsibility, refuse a transfer because it was 'too much trouble.' . . . As family members, such people might refuse to take the responsibility for an aged or ill parent or sibling, giving as an explanation a statement implying that it would be 'too much for me' " (1974, pp. 40-41). According to the portrait drawn by Hinkle, these individuals show little sensitivity to emotional states or involvement in life experiences, quite the opposite picture from that presented by the hypersensitive seeker of treatment discussed earlier in the illness behavior section.

These ideas are quite provocative, especially in pointing out the ways some individuals "insulate" themselves from potentially upsetting experiences. This most likely involves certain aspects of the self-regulation of emotions, as discussed by Lazarus (1975). However, because the analyses about the psychological insulation of healthy people are somewhat anecdotal in nature, based on impressions gleaned after the fact, the possibility of observer bias cannot be ruled out. Predictive studies are essential to test the hypothesis that those uninvolved in life are those most likely to stay healthy.

Other important factors may reduce people's vulnerability to disease or provide a buffer during times of stress. It has been suggested that those with many *personal resources*, assets, and competencies are better equipped to meet life challenges and to deal effectively with significant losses (Antonovsky, 1974; Beiser, Feldman, and Engelhoff, 1972; Murphy, 1974; White, 1974). There is some evidence that those who have sufficient *social supports* or social assets may live longer (Berkman, 1977), have a lower incidence of somatic illnesses (see reviews by Cassel, 1976; Gore, 1973; Kaplan, Cassel, and Gore, 1977; Pinneau, 1975, 1976), and less severe symptomatology (Luborsky, Todd, and Katcher, 1973), as well as higher morale and more positive mental health (Cobb, 1976). The implication drawn is that social supports "protect" the individual from developing illness, although some researchers suggest supports serve such a function only in situations of crisis or stress (Cobb, 1976; Kaplan, Cassel, and Gore, 1977). Supports are thought to modify the potentially negative effects of stress either by reducing the stress itself or by facilitating the individual's coping efforts. For example, Nuckolls, Cassel, and Kaplan (1972) found that neither high life changes nor low psychosocial assets were predictive of higher rates of complications in women delivering their first child, but that the interaction of both was important. Those women with high life changes and low psychosocial assets were most likely to have complications. Gore (1973) reports evidence that among men who lost their jobs, those with high levels of emotional support from their wives had fewer illness symptoms and lower serum cholesterol and serum uric acid levels, although all physiological and illness-related outcome variables were not significantly affected.

Although the general trend of the research investigating social supports is intriguing and mutually consistent, the research base is weak. There are numerous studies in which the expected relationships do not hold, and some of the most positive findings are open to alternative interpretations since other variables (such as the person's state of mental well-being or his or her "social marginality") may be confounded with the measures of support. Thus, it is important to disentangle the mental state of the individual from the actual or potential social support available, and to investigate further the mechanisms whereby social support is effective in reducing physiological symptomatology.

Numerous studies have shown that the way an individual *copes* may reduce physiological arousal in response to stress events. For example, successful defenses have been found to be effective in decreasing levels of 17-OHCS in persons in combat situations, in parents whose child is dying of leukemia, and in patients awaiting surgery (Bourne, Rose, and Mason, 1967; Friedman, Mason, and Hamburg, 1963; Katz and others, 1970; Price, Thaler, and Mason, 1957; Wolff and others, 1964). Others have suggested that being engaged in activity (that is, overt motoric activity), rather than remaining passive, can be highly effective in reducing threat and influencing the bodily precursors of disease. However, whereas most people prefer an active role in a situation of threat, it appears that such coping strategies result in increased physiological arousal, especially of the adrenal cortical hormones (Gal and Lazarus, 1975). For example, a study by Miller and others (1970) found a greater adrenal cortical stress response for pilots engaged in aircraft carrier landing practice as compared with the radar intercept officers, who have a passive role in the operation (that is, they monitor the radar from within the plane but have no direct control over the landing). However, the radar intercept officers reported more somatic complaints and a higher level of anxiety. Thus, the active person showed greater physiological activity and lowered psychological reports of distress. This is consistent with the work reviewed by Singer (1974), as discussed earlier, that active involvement in a situation of threat will result in increased autonomic and endocrine activity.

Hinkle (1974, p. 42) has stressed the notion that certain life patterns or *activities* must also *undergo change* if illness is to result: "If a culture change, social change, or change in interpersonal relations is not associated with a significant change in the activities, habits, indigestants, exposure to disease-causing agents, or in the physical characteristics of the environment of a person, then its effect upon his health cannot be defined solely by its nature, its magnitude, its acuteness or chronicity, or its apparent importance in the eyes of others." Weiner (1977) discusses how changes in diet or activity can be important mediating variables in certain psychosomatic illnesses.

Biological mechanisms hypothesized. Figure 1 outlines a simplified model of how stress-appraised events could lead to illness outcomes. There are two initial pathways possible: Stress appraisal could lead to coping behaviors that resolve the threat but have negative physiological consequences, or the coping strategies used in response to threat could be ineffective, thereby prolonging the stress and the physiological reactions to it. The activation of hormonal systems can have direct illness-producing effects, for example, by increasing blood coagulation (these effects will be discussed in the section on coronary heart disease) or can lower immunological response, thereby increasing susceptibility to illness (these effects will be discussed in the section on cancer). The appraisal of stress is key in this formulation; if no appraisal of stress is made, then coping and physiological reactions to a threat do not occur. Once stress is appraised, the coping strategies used and the successfulness of these strategies influence the physiological processes and outcomes. Lazarus and his colleagues (in press) elaborate on some of these issues in more detail. Weiner (1977) presents more complex models which illustrate the ways in which psychological and physiological processes may be linked (see also Lipowski, 1977).

Specificity Theories: Factors Thought to Predict Development of Specific Diseases

This section will provide an overview of specificity theories, focusing on two areas that have generated much research—coronary heart disease and cancer. Because of the vast literature in these areas, only a brief summary of studies will be provided. The discussion will emphasize the basic underlying mechanisms through which these relationships are hypothesized to occur.

Coronary Heart Disease

Psychological and social factors have often been implicated, along with biological factors, as precursors of coronary heart disease. Summaries of the literature (Jenkins, 1971, 1976; Keith, 1966; Marks, 1967; Russek, 1967; Smith, 1967) suggest a compelling number of studies supporting psychosocial influences, although many studies suffer from inadequate methodology (especially lack of predictive studies) and failure to rule out alternative explanations (Blackburn, 1974; Cassel, 1967; Jenkins, 1971, 1976; Keith, 1966; Marks, 1967). Despite the evidence, even today controversy is still strong between biologically and psychologically oriented cardiologists over the relative importance of biological risk factors and psychological or behavioral patterns (Perlman, 1975; Syme, 1967).

Somewhat different psychological factors seem to be implicated in the development of different types of coronary heart disease—myocardial infarction, "silent infarction," and angina pectoris. In myocardial infarction, an area of the heart muscle becomes necrotic or dies because of failure to receive sufficient oxygen or nutrition; this may be the result of a partial or complete occlusion of a coronary artery, usually due to a clot or thrombus. A "silent infarction" is an asymptomatic blockage with adequate development of collateral or bypass circulation. Angina pectoris, which is characterized by severe pains about the heart, results from an oxygen deficiency due to decreased or inadequate blood supply. Jenkins (1971) recommends that research studies treat angina pectoris, myocardial infarction, "silent infarction," and sudden death as four separate categories in order to disentangle those personality factors involved in one but not the other.

Jenkins (1971, 1976) provides thorough reviews of the literature on coronary heart disease. In this chapter, I will present only a brief summary of representative studies to illustrate the types of relationships that have been found. According to Jenkins' (1976) analysis, the most consistent psychosocial predictors of coronary heart disease are the occurrence of disturbing emotions, such as anxiety and depression, and a syndrome of traits and behavior—involving a competitive, striving, time-pressured life-style—labeled the "coronary-prone behavior pattern" or "Type A behavior" (Friedman and Rosenman, 1974).

Jenkins reviews numerous studies that find significant relationships between *Type A behavior* and coronary heart disease. Friedman and Rosenman (1974, p. 4) describe this behavior pattern as follows: "It is a particular complex of personality traits, including excessive competitive drive, aggressiveness, impatience, and a harrying sense of time urgency. Individuals displaying this pattern seem to be engaged in a chronic, ceaseless, and often fruitless struggle—with themselves, with others, with circumstances, with time, sometimes with life itself. They also frequently exhibit a free-floating but well-rationalized form of hostility, and almost always a deep-seated insecurity." Type B individuals, in contrast, are those with a more calm, relaxed style of living. As Jenkins (1976, p. 1034) emphasizes, Type A behavior is not a measure of stress but rather a coping style: "It represents neither a stressful situation nor a distressed response, but rather a style of behavior with which some persons habitually respond to circumstances that arouse them. . . . [It] is a deeply ingrained, enduring trait." This behavior pattern is assessed by means of a structured interview (Rosenman and others, 1964) or through a questionnaire—the Jenkins Activity Survey (Jenkins, Rosenman, and Friedman, 1967). The interview measure has been found to be a better predictor of coronary heart disease than the questionnaire.

Type A behavior has been consistently linked with increased incidence and prevalence of heart disease. For example, in a report on an eight-and-one-half-year follow-up of 3,154 men in the Western Collaborative Group Study, Rosenman and others (1975) confirm earlier findings (Jenkins, Rosenman, and Zyzanski, 1974b; Rosenman and others, 1970; Rosenman and others, 1964) that Type A behavior is strongly related to coronary heart disease incidence. They found that the incidence of coronary heart disease and the death rate from this disease were twice as high in Type A patients as in Type B. This higher incidence prevailed when subjects were stratified by other predictive risk factors (for example, parental history of coronary heart disease, smoking, high blood pressure, high cholesterol level). Thus, those exhibiting this harried competitive life-style are more likely to develop coronary heart disease even when the biological risk factors are controlled. Type A behavior has also been found to be predictive of degree of atherosclerosis as determined by angiography (Blumenthal and others, 1975).

Jenkins and his colleagues (Jenkins, Rosenman, and Zyzanski, 1974a; Jenkins, Zyzanski, and Rosenman, 1978) have recently reported evidence that different aspects of the coronary-prone behavior pattern may be found in individuals who subsequently develop myocardial infarction, angina pectoris, or "silent infarction." For example, they suggest that angina patients may be more reactive to their environment and more irritable, whereas acute myocardial infarction patients may be more time conscious and competitive on the job, though not so in personal interactions (Jenkins, Rosenman, and Zyzanski, 1974a).

Despite some contradictions in the data, there is considerable evidence that expressions of *anxiety, depression,* and reports of *psychophysiological symptoms* are related to the development of coronary heart disease, especially angina pectoris. For example, in a prospective study, Ostfeld and others (1964) found that those men who subsequently developed angina pectoris, as compared to myocardial infarction patients and those without heart disease, scored significantly higher on the *Hs* (Hypochondriasis) and *Hy* (Hysteria) scales of the MMPI and lower on Factor C of the 16PF (low indicating "dissatisfied emotionality"). That is, prior to developing angina, these people showed a greater tendency to complain of somatic symptoms of all types, a tendency toward repression and denial that could result in the development of somatic complaints as a way of resolving emotional conflicts, and a sense of dissatisfaction. Medalie and his colleagues (1973) found that subjects high in anxiety were twice as likely to develop angina pectoris as those low on their anxiety measure. Eastwood and Trevelyan (1971) report that those found, in a screening survey, to have psychiatric problems, mainly chronic anxiety and depression, were more likely to be diagnosed with possible or probable coronary heart disease than a control group of subjects without these psychiatric symptoms. Cardiological examinations were utilized to make the medical diagnoses. In a prospective study, Friedman and others (1974) found that those who later developed myocardial infarction, as compared with those free of coronary heart disease, had earlier reported symptoms of emotional drain and many minor physical complaints. However, when reanalyses were done eliminating those subjects who, at the time of the questionnaire completion, had physical symptoms suggestive of myocardial ischemia, the significant differences disappeared. These authors suggest that the psychological symptoms may have been prodromal symptoms of coronary heart disease, rather than predictors of the emergence of the illness.

Jenkins (1976) concludes that *work overload* and *chronic conflict situations* may be precursors to coronary heart disease, although the results are less consistent and the relationships may be weaker than for the variables discussed earlier. To illustrate, Theorell and Rahe (1972) found that patients with myocardial infarction had, prior to the infarction, been doing more overtime work and got less satisfaction from their jobs than a control group of healthy employees. Medalie and his colleagues (1973), in a prospective study, found that those with problems and conflicts relating to family, work, and finance were more likely to develop angina pectoris than those without such conflicts. In retrospective studies, positive associations have been found between the occurrence of *life changes* (as measured by the SRE or similar measures) and the development of myocardial infarction, but there are many inconsistent findings and the prospective studies tend to find negative results (for example, Theorell, Lind, and Flodérus, 1975).

In general, *demographic indicators* (such as education and occupation) are not consistent predictors of coronary risk. Certain combinations of social and demographic variables (such as status incongruity and cultural mobility) that were once thought to be predictive of the development of heart disease (Jenkins, 1971) are now thought to be valid predictors only under limited circumstances—for certain people, for certain types of heart disease, or in certain regions or eras (Jenkins, 1976).

Biological mechanisms hypothesized. What are some of the biological mechanisms that could link psychological factors to the development of coronary heart disease? In most of these studies, as with the generality studies, stress is implicated as an intervening variable, either via life situations thought to produce chronic stress or through personality characteristics or coping strategies that result in constant pressured involvements with the environment (Type A behavior). Social and psychological stress factors could increase heart disease through mechanisms of their own (for example, hormonal, fibrinolytic) or through affecting the so-called biological risk factors (for example, by increasing blood pressure, levels of serum cholesterol and other lipids, or smoking). Jenkins (1967, p. 143) poses some of these possibilities (see also Davis, 1974; Kagan and Levi, 1974): "Does anxiety raise lipid levels, while excitation and striving influence neurohumoral levels? Does repression of hostility slow down the elimination of lipids from the serum, rather than actually raise the input of lipids? Does smoking and psychological stimulation of the nervous system make the intima more susceptible to injury and infiltration or interfere with fibrinolysis, rather than directly affecting lipids and blood pressure?"

Exactly how these factors operate is still unknown. But the evidence seems strong that life situations usually accepted as being disturbing (such as experienced by medical students taking exams or men losing their jobs) or especially time pressured (such as experienced by accountants during deadline-pressing tax periods) are associated with increases in cholesterol and other lipids (Friedman, Rosenman, and Carroll, 1958; Thomas and Murphy, 1958; Wertlake and others, 1958; see also Rahe and others, 1971; Rahe, Rubin, and Arthur, 1974) and may be associated with increased blood pressure (Kasl and Cobb, 1970). Further, experiments in which laboratory animals were exposed to certain types of stress produced changes in cardiac tissue and increases in serum cholesterol (Caffrey, 1967; Jenkins, 1971).

It is still not known whether these life situations have direct effects on these biological risk factors or if there is mediation by other physiological mechanisms. Friedman and Rosenman (1974), for example, pinpoint the catecholamines (epinephrine and norepinephrine) as the central biological mechanisms influenced by Type A behavior, and which, through their effects, increase the risk of heart disease. According to Friedman and Rosenman, the Type A pattern—a continuous agitated involvement with the environment—results in increased secretion of epinephrine and norepinephrine and other hormones. If the struggle is a chronic one (as is typical for Type A), there will be a chronic excess discharge of these hormones, which is known to result in the following: increased blood level of cholesterol and other lipids; marked lag in ridding the blood of the cholesterol added to it through diet; and increased tendency for the clotting elements of the blood (platelets and fibrinogen) to precipitate out (see, for example, Simpson and others, 1974), thus building up the plaques (scarlike masses or thickenings) on the artery wall and further narrowing the passageway. The more that blood vessels are narrowed and clots formed, the greater the likelihood that these clots will occlude a coronary artery, resulting in angina pectoris or myocardial infarction.

Tasks that are especially demanding increase epinephrine secretion and heart rate (Frankenhaeuser and Johansson, 1976). Further, the evidence that Singer (1974) reviews, as mentioned earlier, shows that involvement is linked to elevated blood pressure and increased endocrine responses. If the individual's life-style involves intense day-to-day involvements, increased blood pressure and high endocrine levels would be expected. Rosenman (1973) has also suggested that Type A men have chronic hypersecretion of adrenocorticotropic hormone (ACTH), diminished adrenocortical reserve, and diminished growth hormone. This, he believes, could reflect functional alteration of the hypothalamic pituitary-adrenal axis. Thus, evidence supports the links between various psychological factors and biological changes, which, it has been shown, could increase the likelihood of coronary heart disease.

Cancer

In comparison to the heart disease literature, the evidence is considerably less clear that psychological factors are related to the etiology of cancer. Many inconsistent results are reported and the methodological problems (especially the lack of predictive studies) raise serious doubts about the findings. Studies focusing on cancer have either examined factors influencing the development of cancer or those that retard its spread once established. Concerning the *development* of cancer, it has, for example, been suggested that those who develop cancer are unable to express hostile feelings and emotions (Renneker and Cutler, 1952; Solomon, 1969b), are anally fixated (Mezei and Németh, 1969), make extensive use of repressive and denying defenses (Bahnson and Bahnson, 1966, 1969), are emotional and extroverted (Hagnell, 1966), are introverted (McCoy, 1976), report less closeness to parents (Thomas and Greenstreet, 1973), or have suffered a significant loss or separation from a significant person (Greene, 1954, 1966; Greene, Young, and Swisher, 1956; LeShan, 1959; LeShan and Worthington, 1956; Schmale and Iker, 1966, 1971). Others (for example, Bennette, 1969) suggest that cancer may be an alternative to the development of regressive psychoses, with an underlying pathology of alienation common to both; however, there seems to be no evidence whatever to support this position. Reviews of the literature have been done (Crisp, 1970; Fox, 1978; LeShan, 1959; Perrin and Pierce, 1959; Solomon, 1969b; see also Abse and others, 1974; and Bahnson, 1969), but, taken together, no strong consistent findings emerge that substantiate the relationship between specific psychological factors and the etiology of cancer.

Some researchers, rather than looking at "cancer patients" as a whole, have investigated the different personality patterns involved with patients who have cancer at different sites. For example, Kissen (1963, 1966; Kissen, Brown, and Kissen, 1969) suggests that lung cancer patients tend to bottle up emotional difficulties and have a diminished outlet for emotional discharge, although others have failed to find similar patterns (Abse and others, 1974). Others report that breast cancer patients show "abnormal release" (that is, either "extreme suppression" or, more rarely, "extreme expression") of anger and other feelings (Greer and Morris, 1975), are more inhibited, more orally fixated, and have an inner turmoil that is "covered over by a facade of pleasantness" (Bacon, Renneker, and Cutler, 1952), as compared with patients with cancer of the cervix (Stephenson and Grace, 1954), who are more impulsive and more overt in their sexual maladjustment (that is, dislike sexual intercourse and show high rates of divorce, extramarital affairs, and so on). However, these differences have not been confirmed by subsequent studies (see the reviews by Schmale and Iker, 1966, 1971).

Other studies have investigated psychological factors affecting the *course of the disease.* Longer survival rates from cancer have been associated with more frequent expression of hostility and other negative affects (Derogatis and Abeloff, 1978; Stavraky and others, 1968), mild intellectual impairment (which, according to Davies and others, 1973, helps reduce anxiety and despair over possible future difficulties), less inhibition and defensiveness (Blumberg, West, and Ellis, 1954; Klopfer, 1957; however, Krasnoff, 1959, failed to replicate these results), and reduced reality testing (Klopfer, 1957). For example, Blumberg, West, and Ellis (1954, p. 285) describe the patients with rapid growth of cancer as follows: "They were noted to be consistently serious, over-cooperative, over-nice, over-anxious, painfully sensitive, passive, apologetic personalities, and, as far as could be ascertained from family, friends, and previous records, they had suffered from this pitiful lack of self-expression and self-realization all of their lives." Although these results are not entirely consistent, they suggest that emotional expressiveness may be more often associated with a longer survival rate from cancer.

Methodological problems. Fox (1978) provides a most comprehensive discussion of difficulties with this research (see also Crisp, 1970; Perrin and Pierce, 1959, 1961). Space does not permit a detailing of the methodological problems involved or of the theories hypothesized, without any empirical support, to explain some of the relationships. For example, Bahnson (1969) tries to point out "isomorphisms" between psychological and physiological processes, while Bennette (1969) talks about "alienation" at the cellular and psychosocial levels. However, the most serious problems are the absence of predictive studies and the question of the methods used in measuring the psychological concepts involved. Some psychologists may not be satisfied with the psychological measures employed. For example, in the Bahnson and Bahnson (1969) study, the measure of repression used was whether positive adjectives were checked as descriptive of clicks of white noise. The use of positive adjectives was seen by the researchers as indicating that the subjects denied unpleasantness in the world around them and viewed it as a benign place where all is for the best. Kissen (1963) suggests that low scores on the neuroticism scale of the Maudsley Personality Inventory indicate diminished outlets for emotional discharge; however, Eysenck (1965) disagrees with this interpretation. Mezei and Németh (1969) use only the occurrence of the Rorschach responses "anus," "caudal bone," "rats," or "mice" as the indicators of anal fixation. Concerning the reliance on retrospective studies, as pointed out earlier, once cancer has begun its course, and especially once the diagnosis has been made, studies of psychological factors found at that time cannot appropriately be used to indicate etiology. Almost all studies reported are of this type. The few prospective studies that have been done do not examine similar variables, thereby preventing comparison of results. In addition, those retrospective studies investigating possible predisease "loss" have the same methodological problems as those discussed earlier in this chapter (such as observer bias), especially (for example, Greene, 1954; Greene, Young, and Swisher, 1956) where the person's entire life history is probed for evidence of loss. Other studies have used nonrepresentative samples. For example, Thomas and Greenstreet (1973) studied only medical students at the Johns Hopkins School of Medicine. Bahnson and Bahnson (1969) eliminated from their sample those patients who were consciously aware of their diagnosis, thus apparently excluding those who most likely would be nonrepressors.

The studies investigating psychological factors predisposing to cancer are methodologically quite weak, often cannot be replicated, and are occasionally quite narrow in their perspective. As Crisp (1970, p. 319) so aptly puts it: "Clinical literature in this field of premorbid personality factors leans heavily on theory and speculation which has outstripped data." Despite much literature reported and two conferences focusing on these issues ("Psychophysiological Aspects of Cancer," 1966; "Second Conference on Psychophysiological Aspects of Cancer," 1969), probably the best conclusion to be drawn from the review of this literature is that no clear link between specific psychological factors and the development of cancer has been shown at the present time (Salk, 1969b; Weiss, 1969). Predictive studies to be carried out before any possible cancerous process has begun are necessary in order to show clear etiological relationships with cancer development. The complexity of the factors affecting the growth of cancer, including the importance of environmental factors and the multiplicity of different types of cancer (Fox, 1978), appears to be so great that it seems unlikely any simple or clear-cut personality factors will be found (Salk, 1969a).

   Biological mechanisms hypothesized. Immunological mechanisms linked to psychological states are most often suggested as those underlying the development of cancer, with resistance to cancer depending on host-resistant factors in a way analogous to infectious diseases (Solomon, 1969b). That is, one theory suggests that when immunological surveillance is adequate, cancer cells are destroyed before tumor formation begins (Schwartz, 1975). Since it is known that immunological mechanisms are markedly depressed by adrenal cortical hormones, emotional stresses that increase the levels of corticosteroids could result in a decreased immunological response, thus allowing cells to flourish that might otherwise be destroyed (Southam, 1969). However, Solomon (1969a) points out that the link between adrenocortical activity and immunological response is physiologically complex. For example, in some circumstances, both high and low levels of corticosteroids suppress the immunological response, while intermediate levels enhance it. Further, the immune response is multifaceted, that is, many different antibodies with varying effects are involved, and small changes in environmental conditions can shift the patterns of resistance to various antigens (Weiss, 1969). Amkraut and Solomon (1974) describe the enormous complexity of the immune system and how various stress-responsive hormones increase or decrease aspects of immune response. These authors suggest that emotional factors may produce only small alterations in "immune balance," but this change in the balance between pathogenic events and bodily defense mechanisms can be sufficient to allow disease to occur. Schwartz (1975) and Stein, Schiavi, and Camerino (1976) also discuss the complexity of immune processes. Schwartz (1975, p. 183) concludes: "It is impossible to recount here the many other complexities of the problem of surveillance, such as the genes that determine protection against oncogenic viruses by nonimmunologic means ... the issue of immunity to oncogenic viruses versus surveillance to neoplastic cells ... or the lack of a high incidence of neoplasms in certain diseases characterized by anergy, such as sarcoidosis ... and leprosy.... Some neoplasms ... may indeed be eliminated by an immune response, whereas others may actually require an immune response for their pathogenesis."

Southam (1969) discusses how endocrine responses (both epinephrine and the adrenal corticosteroids) are influenced by the person's psychological state and may be factors in the metastasis (or spread) of cancer. In brief, he points out that circulating cancer cells in the body are not a problem to the organism; it is only when they implant in tissue and start to grow that the difficulties arise. Thus, factors that facilitate the embedding of cancer cells in tissues can increase the spreading of the disease. Psychic stresses can initiate smooth muscle contractions that could start the dissemination of cancer cells (as manipulation of the mass can do). These stresses could also increase the production of adrenal corticosteroids and the sex steroids, which affect the clotting mechanisms, thereby increasing the possibility that cells would actually go through the capillary lining, get caught in the surrounding tissues, and adhere. Each step of this process has been documented individually (for example, adrenal corticosteroids affect blood coagulation); the question remains whether all the steps of this sequence do occur and whether they are important in the spread of cancer.

Complexity of the Issues

The complexity of the relationships involved in the previously discussed literature must be underlined. First, the relationship between stress and the development of illness is by no means simple or straightforward. It may be that the effects of stress on particular individuals are influenced by the particular disease agents to which they are exposed. Laboratory work with animals suggests that certain forms of stress can lead to decreased resistance to some microorganisms and increased resistance to others. As Ader and Grota (1973, p. 401) illustrate: "Handling, for example, increases resistance to experimentally induced gastric erosions and retards the growth rate of a transplanted tumor, but handling decreases subsequent resistance to a transplanted leukemia and to electroconvulsive shock while having no effect on susceptibility to alloxan diabetes, encephalomyocarditis virus, or the spontaneous development of leukemia in AKR rats."

Reviews of this laboratory work show that the effects of stressful early experiences on later illness susceptibility further depend on the type of early stimulation given, the acuteness or chronicity of the stress, the developmental period when stimulation is experienced, the relationship between the stress and the time of inoculation, the measure (for example, weight loss, mortality, virus multiplication) used to reflect resistance, and the species of animal used (Ader, 1974; Friedman and Glasgow, 1966; La Barba, 1970). Friedman, Glasgow, and Ader (1969, p. 391) conclude from the animal data: "It also appears that no available single theory of stress can predict the effects that a particular form of stimulation will have upon host resistance and that even the direction of change in susceptibility is dependent upon the disease that the organism is experiencing. We believe that such findings also have implications for those investigating similar problems at the clinical level, in that life situations judged stressful, such as the loss of a loved one, might be expected to predispose tó some disease states and have a protective effect in others." Selye (1971) has also suggested that the same stressor can cause different lesions because of differences in conditioning factors. That is, stress may result in cardiac necroses if the organism was pretreated with certain hormonal or chemical compounds, and may prevent cardiac problems if conditioned with others.

Second, it should be reiterated that the actions of many of these physiological responses are quite complex (Amkraut and Solomon, 1974; Salk, 1969a; Solomon, 1969a; Weiner, 1977; Weiss, 1969); for example, the immunological response is multifaceted, and varying levels of adrenocortical and other stress-responsive hormones alternately increase or decrease aspects of it. (See Amkraut and Solomon, 1974, for an excellent detailed discussion of the various components and enormous complexities of the immune system and of the effects of various stress-responsive hormones in increasing or decreasing aspects of this multifaceted system.) Because of the complexities of these reactions, it is quite possible that no simple links between events and particular physiological patterns or diseases will be found.

Third, to get a clear understanding of the relationship between psychological factors and illness, it may be important to distinguish between those psychological factors that are linked to *precursors of disease* (Kagan and Levi, 1974), such as mild hypertension, those that lead to the *development of disease* itself, and those that affect the *onset and timing of particular symptoms of disease* (Luborsky, Docherty, and Penick, 1973). That is, different psychological factors may be involved in each of these categories; what relationships there are between these various factors needs to be investigated. For example, do the same psychological factors that produce mild hypertension also produce coronary heart disease and further bring on the symptoms of angina or cause a myocardial infarction? Or are slightly different psychological factors relevant to each of these manifestations? What other factors mediate this pathogenic development? These issues need to be explored.

Fourth, an important question concerns whether the best research strategy for studying the relationship between psychological factors and disease is to look for specific psychological factors relevant to the development of a particular disease (specificity theories) or to study diseases as a whole (generality approach). For example, the literature discussed earlier suggests that repression and denial characterize both cancer and coronary heart disease patients (although the evidence supporting these claims is quite weak). If this is so, then important data are lost and misleading theories developed if only cancer patients are studied in investigation of this link to disease. Luborsky, Docherty, and Penick (1973) claim that there is little specificity in the psychological state variables that precede the onset of particular *symptoms* of various psychosomatic diseases; how much specificity there is in those psychological factors that lead to the development of disease still needs to be explored. The recommendation can be made, therefore, that broad longitudinal studies should be carried out in which the incidence of many types of diseases, both minor and major, is investigated. Physiological measures should also be taken. Then aspects of these data can be studied to determine if specific psychological factors are related to different physiological levels of reactivity and/or to the development of specific diseases.

Fifth, this chapter has focused specifically on the relationships between psychological factors and somatic disease. However, some writers suggest much broader theories—general maladaptation models—that involve stress as an intervening variable in maladaptive responses of all types (Marks, 1967; Moss, 1973; Mutter and Schleifer, 1966; Reeder, Schrama, and Dirken, 1973). For example, Marks (1967) suggests that a lack of fit between the social structure and the individual's personality can produce chronic emotional stress, which can lead to maladjustment or adaptive responses of various kinds (such as somatic illness, mental illness, juvenile delinquency, and social protest). The factors that control these differential responses have not as yet been clearly delineated, although they undoubtedly include personality characteristics of individuals, their appraisal of situations, their coping abilities and response repertoire, and the social supports and resources available. How these factors interact and result in different responses must be specified before this general maladaptation model will become useful. However, this type of model does raise intriguing questions concerning the interplay between these levels, such as the question of how changes in physiological reactivity can affect mental states, social relationships, work performance, and so on, and what further interactions might occur. For example, does one form of maladaptive response preclude others, as in the hypothesis occasionally suggested that development of schizophrenia precludes the development of cancer?

The general maladaptation models underline some rather important notions, namely, that stress and coping can produce effects in several domains of functioning and that several different measures may be necessary in order to determine the impact of stress on an individual (Lazarus, 1966; Lazarus, Averill, and Opton, 1974; Lazarus and Cohen, 1977). That is, evaluation can be made in a physiological, psychological, or social domain, and these responses may reflect different aspects of adaptation. Thus, if disease, disrupted social relationships, mental distress, and criminal acts are all possible responses to stress, studies that examine the presence of only one of these responses may err in their conclusions about stress. This suggests the necessity of broad etiological population studies, examining several indicators of "adjustment." However, these theories also underline the importance of examining as many levels of response as possible in any study of the impact of stress.

Most of the literature relating psychological factors to disease emphasizes the negative effects of increased physiological activation. However, there may be positive consequences as well, and the interplay of these positive and negative factors needs further investigation. For example, Frankenhaeuser (1975, 1976) reviews studies that show that those who habitually secrete high levels of epinephrine have higher IQ and better school performance, are rated as happier and livelier, score higher on tests of ego strength, and perform better on certain laboratory tasks, as compared with those with low epinephrine levels. Frankenhaeuser (1976) and Gal and Lazarus (1975) also suggest that the magnitude of the physiological response may be an inappropriate measure of adaptation compared to the time necessary for the return to base-line hormonal levels. Thus, good adjustment may involve both efficient mobilization and demobilization of physiological systems.

Sixth, this author's analysis of different models relating stress to the development of illness or to increased treatment seeking was presented in Figure 1. Although the models are in very simplified form, they are useful for illustrating schematically how stress and disease might be linked. Weiner (1977) provides a detailed discussion and more complex models of physiological mechanisms that might link psychological factors and disease. Much further research is necessary to investigate the links hypothesized. Of great theoretical importance are some of the links suggested by the cognitively mediated endocrine/immunological mechanisms model, that is, the impact of various means of coping with stress on physiological reactions of all types. For example, what is the differential physiological impact (both short term and long term) of denying and suppressing strategies, of active confronting strategies, of strategies (for example, smoking) that reduce anxiety but have deleterious bodily effects? One could also investigate the effects of these strategies on other areas of life functioning, for example, how they might increase or decrease the number of subsequent stressful encounters. Research on such questions will help us better understand the interplay between psychological, physiological, and social domains of functioning, and how they are related to the etiology of disease.

5

Psychosocial Meanings of Unfavorable Medical Forecasts

Norma G. Haan

A concatenation of pressures and sensibilities is slowly but certainly moving the health care system to focus on the prevention of illness, or, if you like, on the maintenance of health. Not the least among these are economic pressures that call for rational use of health care dollars. As Marc Lalonde, Minister of National Health and Welfare for Canada, has pointed out, recent escalation in medical costs is in excess of economic growth, and "if unchecked, health care costs will soon be beyond the capacity of society to finance them" (1974, p. 28). The recent invention and use of unconscionably expensive, highly sophisticated, but effective, medical technologies have not substantially lengthened life expectancies. Instead, recent improvements in health indicators are primarily due to drops in infant mortality, whereas indexes remain high for "premature" deaths, many preventable because they are due to smoking, automobile accidents, suicides, poor nutrition, environmental pollution, and genetic disorders (Lalonde, 1974).

Note: The author thanks Carol Huffine for her critical reading of an earlier version of this chapter and for her suggestions.

113

Reducing mortality and morbidity are not our only goals; enhancing citizens' well-being is also in society's interest. For example, we now know that a malnourished mother is at risk of bearing a less "intelligent" baby who, in turn, has reduced prospects of being a full participant in and contributor to society (see, for example, Cravioto and Delicardie, 1970). Furthermore, as our society faces diminished natural abundance along with a higher portion of the population being aged, pressures will inevitably grow for citizens to be socially and economically productive. These reasons for increased emphasis on preventive medicine are oriented to society's view, but they harmonize with citizens' legitimate expectations that health professionals and the health care system will provide care as well as cures. Thus, some policy makers urge that the health system be reformed by switching priorities so that investments in preventive medicine are increased even if investments in curative medicine are decreased.

A major strategy increasingly being adopted by preventive medicine is the identification of persons at risk, followed by attempts to educate them in how to lessen or eliminate their vulnerability. The analysis of the social-psychological aspects of this educative interchange between health professional and citizen is the focus of this chapter.

The procedure of locating and informing those who are at risk involves, at the critical moment of interchange, attempts to persuade and motivate people to act in their own best interests. (See the chapter by Henderson, Hall, and Lipton in this volume for a discussion of the effectiveness of interventions designed to alter smoking, overeating, and alcoholism.) The content of this interchange is factual-biological in nature, but the structure and the ultimate success of the procedure depend on its social-psychological climate and the emotional states of the participants. Thus, health professionals clearly need to know more about clients than their physiological status. Indeed, the procedures of preventive medicine require a distinctively different set of assumptions, procedures, and understandings than restorative medicine generally uses or, at any rate, has deemed necessary or desirable to use for the past century. This does not imply that curative medicine has little to learn from the social psychology of preventive medicine. In fact, close examination of the interchange between client-patient and health professional leads me to propose in this chapter a different model of medical care and cure—one that depends on the psychology of people who are threatened with illness and their efforts to cope with this fact.

This chapter is concerned with the interchange between client-patient and physician during the critical period when clients learn that their forecasts or diagnoses are unfavorable. Clients, unlike patients, are not ill; they are only told that they may become ill. Little is known about the dynamic interplay between physician and client, so, assuming analogous meanings, I draw on the literature concerning the communication of diagnoses to patients and go on to analyze the meanings of these interchanges from both the patient's and physician's points of view. Because the assumptions of the biomedical model still permeate the thinking of health professionals and the procedures used by both curative and preventive medicine, I shall lay the groundwork for this analysis of the health professional-client interaction by examining the biomedical model and then evaluating the arguments of one of its detractors, Engel.

The Biomedical Model and Engel's Biopsychosocial Model

Despite common knowledge to the contrary, curative medicine usually operates on the basic premise that disease is exclusively biological in both origin and expression. Patients have complaints and/or symptoms that they describe to physicians, or their signs of illness are discovered in routine examinations. The patient is in pain, or feels he or she is malfunctioning, or is told that the latter is the case. The physician operates as the central figure in a hierarchy of personnel who attempt to diagnose the disease—fit the patient's pattern of signs to a known disease entity. On achieving a fit, the physician prescribes the procedures for combatting the illness and restoring the patient to health. The patient's role is to cooperate with the diagnostic procedures and palliative instructions. Usually (but not always or fully, as will be discussed later; see also Kirscht and Rosenstock in this volume), the patient is inclined to cooperate with the regime and be "patient" while the medical personnel do the work of bringing about a cure. Patients' motivation for accepting patienthood seems obvious—this is the proferred role; they are understandably troubled and overcome with their illness and almost always wish to be cured. However, as they accept patienthood, people mute their "natural" propensities to cope on their own behalf.* In other words, patients must react differently than they do when they have an ordinary problem in living. The pressures of tradition, the situation, patients' anxieties, and physicians' superior technical knowledge all merge to persuade patients to turn responsibility for themselves over to their physicians. Furthermore, physicians take this moral responsibility seriously. However, it is an unequal partnership that typically entails social-emotional hazards for both physician and patient. The consequences of this particular disproportionate assumption of responsibility are discussed throughout this chapter, and recommendations are eventually made for a different kind of moral balance between patient and physician that may better serve both.

Within the realm of psychological understanding, situations that en-

---

*The designation of coping used in this chapter is fully developed in Haan (1977) and differs from other definitions used in this volume. I identify coping as a process that represents reasonably accurate assessment of situation and self and reasonably accurate acts based on this information. Coping is presumed to be the normative and preferred way that people use to deal with their problems. A hierarchy of utility, which has some empirical support (Haan, 1977), is assumed: People will first attempt to cope but, failing to cope, they will move to use defensive strategies; if these fail, they will retreat to self-chosen fragmentation. In this sense, coping is qualitatively different from defensive actions in much the same way that Herzlich's (1973) findings, which are discussed later in this chapter, indicate that the experience of biological health is independent of and qualitatively different from illness.

force passivity and dependency are known to be debilitating. (See Lefcourt, 1973, for an excellent review of this literature.) Moreover, patients and their families do not always thoroughly accept this passivity and instead frequently engage in "secret" forms of coping. Nevertheless, this model of interchange is widely understood, accepted, and enacted in Western society by health professionals and lay persons alike. Parsons (1972) early analyzed, but did not criticize, how people are socialized to accept this sick role. Engel (1977) has recently argued that this form of physician-patient interchange is the "dominant folk model" of health care in the Western world and that it has acquired the status of a dogma.

Engel's (1977) criticisms of the biomedical model question this form of interchange. He gives six reasons why physicians' diagnostic and treatment procedures must take the "biopsychosocial" aspects of patients into account: (1) Psychosocial aspects must be considered in diagnosis, along with biological aspects, because patients with identical physiological patterns and laboratory findings vary in the severity of their illness. (2) Patients' reports of their symptomatic patterns must be understood and evaluated to secure reliable data to make accurate diagnoses. (3) Psychosocial factors often determine when patients and their families decide the patient is ill. (4) Psychosocial factors usually interact with the disease and affect its severity and course. (5) Clinical variations in rate of recovery occur among patients given identical treatments who have identical physiological signs of disease severity and identical physiological resources; psychosocial factors may account for variations in recovery rates. (6) The social-emotional relationship between physician and patient may influence the patient's rate of recovery.

Engel's recommendations are intended to improve the physician's traditional role performance: Diagnoses would be more accurate and treatment more effective if the physician were to take into account the total patient—his or her psychosocial views, beliefs, needs, and worries, as well as biological status. Nevertheless, Engel's analysis still assumes patients are wholly receptive, and especially so if they are well treated, and that in general they will be willing to supply physicians with the pertinent psychosocial information about themselves. In the present view, Engel's ill person is still "patient" instead of being obstinately active in his or her own behalf.

Preventive medicine does not often secure cooperative, captive audiences. Clients have no pain or impairment that motivates them to accept the self-resignation of patienthood. They are not always seen in hospitals nor are they often hospitalized. Therefore, they are not subject to the overt and covert determinations, and organized expectancies, that large, complex institutions generally use to ensure that clientele comply with standard procedures. Not being ill, clients have leisure to cope for themselves by actively seeking other diagnostic opinions in other locales, or by changing their way of life if they decide to lower their risks, or, less cooperatively, by defending themselves against the implications of negative forecasts by simply distorting or forgetting the bad news. Clients can do what patients find hard to do. They can maintain their options and autonomy because they can easily escape institutional control and their own anxieties. The moral responsibility for clients' care is their own, not the physician's. A doctor may point out the probability of a client developing lung cancer if he or she continues to smoke, but no one—not even the client—will hold the physician responsible if the client continues to smoke and subsequently develops the disease. The physician has discharged his or her responsibilities, as these are now defined by the medical world, by the simple act of telling the client. Furthermore, no differentiated guidelines exist for the way that the telling should be done, a critical consideration for the success of preventive medicine and clearly required by the recognition that all people—including clients—are incessantly active in making their own meanings of situations. The character of the telling is also a moral responsibility as it can be done in ways that damage people's lives.

The patient's position is different from the client's at the very core of his or her relationship with the health professional. This pivotal fact means that the procedures of the biomedical model are not only ineffective but also irrational when applied within the context of preventive medicine. In one way, the biological aspects of the client's status are peripheral to preventing his or her disability, although the medical facts provide the justification for the interchange between physician and client. In their present states of health, clients are not easily persuaded that their risk *is* a kind of illness or disability, that it belongs to them, that it is real, and that it can become an actuality. People are easily tempted to think that they may be one of the lucky ones who will not become a statistic. To understand why people do not readily take the "simple and logical" steps to prevent their risk being actualized, consider the phenomenological meanings of illness and health.

Psychological-Experiential Meanings of Illness and Health

Most useful here is Herzlich's (1973) empirical study, which focused on social-psychological meanings and implications of health and illness as states of being. Most previous analyses of this problem were done by medical sociologists who defined illness and health in terms of social roles. The most influential analysis has been that of Parsons (1972), who pointed out that the sick role is necessarily socially deviant. Sickness, he contended, can only be permitted by society after the doctor legitimizes the patient's need both to regress and accept the sick condition, because society's efficient functioning depends on contributions made by people who are healthy. (I am arguing throughout this chapter that patients' needs are more complex—at the same time they are tempted to regress, and may need to regress, they also will want to cope actively.) Psychoanalysis, in its focal concern with pathology, promoted the now widely held idea that illnesses are often "motivated." However, it seems unlikely that many people actively seek illness, although some may impart neurotic meanings to it, for example if they view illness as a punishment or as a relief (Lipowski, 1970). However, none of these analyses concerns people's ordinary constructions of the meanings of health and illness, nor do they help us penetrate our focal problem: What can a forecast of illness mean to a person who, for all intents and purposes, feels healthy?

Herzlich (1973) intensively interviewed both healthy and sick people about their definitions of health and illness and their notions of etiology. Her interviewees agreed that health comes from the person—it is an expected, normative, "natural" property of human existence. It exists when the person's ordinary way of life is in harmony with "nature." In contrast, illness was regarded as an intrusion, an external imposition that renders the person passive and powerless, instead of active and healthy. "Man becomes ill when his way of life overwhelms and constricts him" (Herzlich, 1973, p. 69). Thus, health is concordant with one's being, whereas illness is alien and discordant. Moreover, according to Herzlich's respondents, health has no genesis; it is the person. However, the genesis of illness is multiple in form; it is an intrusion, brought on by others or by toxicities. Herzlich's study demonstrates that people do not regard health and illness as symmetrical in meaning, as the medical model does. Illness is not seen as the lack of health, nor is health the absence of illness.

Herzlich's respondents further described health as a state of equilibrium that included the following themes: physical and psychological well-being, absence of fatigue, freedom of movement, good relations with others, and, on the organic level, "not knowing one's body is there." Still, health was not regarded as a state of perfection, but as the equilibrium that people maintain or want to restore when it is disrupted. Thus, when people face illness and concomitant physical and psychological inactivity, their self-views are disrupted. If they are to recapture self-sensibility, they need to make some sense—medically accurate or not—out of the fact of their illness within the context of their lives.* Herzlich (1973, p. 90) quotes Brissaud, writing in 1892: "The need to understand is so compelling that it may actually outdo the desire to be cured." However, the meaningful understandings that ill persons seek are not limited to the medical explanations of their conditions. Patients extend their formulations to embrace social-psychological implications for themselves and their lives. Some patients wholly distort or disregard medical explanations as do, for instance, laetrile users or members of some religions or cult groups.

The characteristic search of patients for the personal and social meanings of their diagnoses for their everyday lives is determined by the need to maintain their equilibrium and agency. These features of patients are especially striking, but we can also be certain they typify the clientele of preventive medicine. This line of reasoning has wholly different assumptions

---

*This line of reasoning is more fully developed for more ordinary contexts in Haan (1977), where ego activities are viewed as striving toward meaning by assimilatory and accommodative processes even when they are defensive or fragmenting. In these instances, equilibration may not be established and accommodation may overbalance assimilation or vice versa. The distressed person sacrifices allegiance to intersubjective reality in various degrees and ways to restore intrasubjective equilibrium. He or she chooses compartmentalization over disintegration.

from that of Engel. Engel's patient is tacitly regarded as entirely cooperative and receptive to the physician's ministrations and only noncooperative when the physician fails to be supportive. Thus, Engel's good physician is still benevolently in control. My "good physician" must be a partner who enters into an explicit moral bargain with the patient to facilitate recovery in ways the patient understands and endorses.* Patients' or clients' needs to formulate the meanings of their conditions in their own terms invariably make for more complexities in communication than are generally recognized. The next section considers the processes of these interchanges in greater detail.

General Considerations of Communication with Patients and Clients

Herzlich's findings were reviewed to make the point that persons are "blooming, buzzing centers of activity" (to merge statements of William James and Jean Piaget) who understandably regard the news or forecast of illness as an untoward, alien intrusion in their ongoing, everyday existences. Given society's disapproval of illness, people's personal propensity to avoid its intrusion, and physicians' benevolent paternalism, it is a tribute to human rationality that people assimilate as much information about their medical conditions as they do (particularly if they are not actually suffering) and that they frequently comply with physicians' instructions. However, patients are often secretly less compliant than they admit. Ley and Spelman (1967) and Sackett (1976) have summarized studies that suggest patients do not always assiduously follow their doctors' advice to take medications, to follow diet restrictions, or to keep clinic appointments for follow-up. For example, Sackett (1976) suggests that only about half of all patients take prescribed medications properly, whereas considerably less than half obtain recommended immunizations or attend scheduled appointments for treatment. Suggestions to lose weight or alter diet are rarely followed even if patients are enrolled in organized programs (see Kirscht and Rosenstock's discussion in this volume).

The Moment of Communicating the Diagnosis

The moment of communicating the diagnosis is clearly the worst for both physician and patient, a fact that is reported in a number of recent social-psychological studies (see, for example, Futterman and Hoffman, 1973). If significant life plans and social relations, such as marriage and

---

*Engel's analyses and mine have different views because of our reliance on different theoretical formulations. Engel's biopsychosocial model is based on systems theory applied to medical practice. He enjoins the physician to take the role of a system theorist and to act appropriately in terms of this knowledge. My analyses are based on a constructivist-interactionist view of the psychological person as persistently and obdurately constructing his or her own meanings (by attempting to cope or, with less social skill, defending or even choosing to fragment) and of the physician as inevitably caught up in this interactive process.

childbearing, must be altered (Sorenson, 1972), forecasts may also be traumatic. Recent work by Beeson (1977), for instance, indicates that pregnant women undergoing an amniocentesis were frequently the most upset when their obstetricians recommended prenatal diagnosis—the first intimation that the anticipated baby and their future motherhood might be in jeopardy. The delivery of genetic services in the province of Quebec (Clow and others, 1973) is so organized that no attempt is made to ensure that clients fully understand the meaning and risk of their genetic diagnosis until three or four weeks after it is first made. Clearly, the expectancy underlying this arrangement is that clients will assimilate the bad news during the waiting period, so later counseling can be directed to the factual aspects of their condition. However, this arrangement overlooks the fact that clients may badly need social-emotional support during earlier stages of the crisis, as they assimilate the diagnosis and forecast. Moreover, crisis theory suggests that clients may not be accessible at later dates because their defenses against dealing with the situation may already be consolidated.

A detailed and troubling account of a parent's reaction to a genetic diagnosis is included in the report of the First International Conference on the Mental Health Aspects of Sickle Cell Anemia: "He [the physician] could not know the impact his words had on me. I stood there trying to keep my composure amid the myriad feelings of guilt, inferiority, and the hopelessness that engulfed me. I desperately needed to see a glimmer of concern in his eyes. I needed to feel that this man, who glowed with pride at having made the correct diagnosis, cared even a little about me as a fellow human being. The almost smirk on his face made me know otherwise. This doctor, within the space of a few minutes, had taken it upon himself to play God, genetic counselor, and the deflator of my ego and my pride. It was a long time before the pall that came over my husband and me lifted. Our emotions ran from guilt, to shame, to self-hatred, and then to fear. How could we have done this terrible thing to our child? We were totally irrational. Perhaps if we had had more information on the disease we could have behaved more rationally, but I doubt that. The attitude of that doctor was what we were reacting to" (McKay, 1974, p. 66).

A classic definition of psychological crisis that well fits McKay's self-description is offered by Klein and Lindemann (1961, p. 127): "a sudden alteration in the field of social forces within which the individual exists, such that the individual's expectations of himself and his relationship with others undergo change." Within these contexts, it is understandable why physicians and patients are likely to become defensive and self-protective and thus less able to hear well and to respond, cogently and sensitively, to each other's statements and meanings.

From the Physician's Point of View

In examining physicians' roles in the interaction, we can see that a most salient fact of their professional lives is that they are the bearers of bad news. Clearly this role has hazards. In ancient Greece, bearers of bad news were sometimes killed on the spot. Medical education generally attempts to protect novitiates from stress by socializing students to assume and maintain stances of emotional detachment. However, this strategy is often not an effective way of dealing with stress in one's self or others because detachment impoverishes social understandings. Whatever our hopes might be that physicians are persons of iron, they have unusually high rates of suicide, drug addiction, and alcoholism (see, for example, Bressler, 1976; Bissell, 1976). Evidently, few attempts have been made to analyze systematically the causes for their distress, other than to suggest that they are overworked (however, see Cartwright in this volume).

Physicians' stress. The present line of reasoning highlights a psychological explanation for physicians' stress. Traditional medicine requires physicians to assume unilateral responsibility for patients. As a consequence, the moral balance between physician and patient is markedly one-sided and thus unstable. The doctor must do all and be all, and the patient takes little responsibility and need do little or nothing. Moral imbalances like these are usually seedbeds of misunderstandings (Haan, 1978). People who give much naturally expect much, but ill people and their worried families do not often think to be giving, particularly when they are specifically encouraged simply to be receptive.

The training of medical doctors does not prepare them to understand the role of "professional masochist"—giving much, receiving little, but knowing why—that psychotherapists use to protect their own mental health. Moreover, psychotherapists usually refuse to take unilateral responsibility, an obligation that puts physicians in the impossible position of needing always to succeed, irrespective of or even despite the patient. Given the realities of life and death, and being only human, physicians sometimes fail.

These kinds of stress that result from the biomedical definition of the physician's role do not occur in preventive medicine because the physician cannot take responsibility for the client's life. In fact, it may well be that many sensitive physicians escape the stress of close patient contact by moving into the public health field. However, effective prevention of later illness still requires that the physician tell the diagnosis, no matter how ominous, emotionally disturbing, or medically complex the condition may be. There are few careful studies concerning the processes of communicating forecasts within the context of preventive medicine, but many charge that physicians do not tell their patients about their conditions with sufficient clarity, detail, skill, and sensitivity. The difficulty is that most physicians are not trained to explain diagnoses to patients or clients in ways that would mobilize coping. Moreover, the health care system is not organized so that physicians are expected to take the time to work with patients in these ways. Other practical obstacles exist: the insufficient number of physicians, the character and costs of their training, and later of their time, and perhaps the selection procedures that recruit persons to medical training who are not always "natural" counselors.

This state of affairs is gradually being challenged by growing views that people have the right to understand their conditions and participate in

their treatment. The debate about patient information has moral tones—
patients have the "right" to understand their conditions and the physician is
"immoral" for not fully disclosing the information. For instance, one book,
which includes chapters by physicians, surgeons, theologians, and patients, is
titled, with a foregone conclusion, *Should the Patient Know the Truth?*
(Standard and Nathan, 1955). In interpreting his research, Freidson (1970a)
has argued that doctors' status needs are threatened by patients' questions
and therefore they discourage dialogue. This interpretation seems superficial.
If Freidson were correct, physicians' reluctance to communicate with patients would be morally suspect, given the considerable status they already
enjoy. However, there are other less certainly immoral but more emotionally
distressed reasons for doctors' reluctance to communicate bad news to patients.

The reason physicians do not always inform patients of bad news, or
do not generally do it well, is the distress physicians experience, a reaction
they unwittingly and understandably wish to avoid. Moreover, medical education actually provides students with specific defenses that avoid stress by
making intellectualized, detached positions quintessential, rather than teaching them how to cope with their unavoidable distress. As Bard (1970, pp.
107-108) comments: "Plagued by the guilt of bringing bad news, feeling ill-
equipped to handle the threatened emotional consequences of the information, burdened by his own confusions about life and death, and often feeling
pessimistic even when pessimism is unwarranted, most physicians work out
highly personal solutions to this question [of telling patients ominous diag-
noses]. The solutions are seldom based on rationality and logic." Further,
King (1962, p. 170) notes that "Continuous contact with suffering and
death is likely to conflict with strong psychogenic needs for inviolacy and
harm avoidance and to arouse anxiety."

Furthermore, people's distraught and defensive reactions tend to pull
like behavior from others, so physicians find themselves in emotionally con-
taminating situations with many patients. That chain reactions of mutually
transactive defensive responses occur among persons in small groups has been
demonstrated by Haan (1977) in a study of families. Teenagers imitate their
parents' preferred defenses significantly more often than they do their
parents' preferred coping processes. This is an expected result because defensiveness begets defensiveness, whereas forms of coping are more individually
and freely chosen. Bard (1970, pp. 102-103) has documented the fact that
patients in crisis face physicians with distortion, illogic, and illusion that bear
little relationship to their objective diagnoses. He reports that 48 out of 100
seriously ill patients in his study spontaneously blamed themselves or someone else for their illness, and 37 percent of these patients felt that interpersonal relationships were stressful enough to have caused the illness. These
assigned causes are not unusually distorted or pathological for distressed people; they only appear so when compared with the objective facts physicians
think patients should be considering. The fact is that "regressive reactions,
depression, and dependency are both appropriate and temporary for most

patients, and they can be regarded as a prelude to the process of emotional repair" (Bard, 1970, p. 105).

It seems possible to conclude that physicians and health professionals may avoid informing patients about their diagnoses in unwitting protection of their own social-emotional equilibrium, and not for the reason frequently given that the patient is better off not knowing too much about the illness. However, this procedure probably turns out, with some frequency, to protect neither patient nor doctor.

Communicating diagnoses and forecasts. With the aid of McIntosh's (1974) excellent review of the literature, we can now consider the empirical evidence that suggests that physicians' communications are often unwittingly determined by needs to diminish rather than deal with stress. Although physicians frequently say that their decisions about communication depend on the emotional status of each patient, McIntosh concludes that most of them follow a consistent policy of either telling or not telling. This conclusion suggests that physicians generally do not differentiate among the emotional states of patients because their professionalized detachment is actually a defensive maneuver that standardizes their reactions. Another defensive strategy is suggested by other studies McIntosh reviews. *Both* doctors and patients believe they are more able to bear the stress of an unfavorable diagnosis than others are. For physicians (and relatives of the patient), this supposition provides a rationalization for avoiding the stress of communicating to the patient. However, as the physician avoids stress, the patient's passivity is affirmed.

Other studies find that doctors frequently say they are reluctant to give an unfavorable diagnosis until it is certain for fear of making a mistake or worrying the patient unnecessarily. However, we can conclude that if the interval is of any length, patients will be hunting for their own meanings. Their greatest fear may not be "knowing" but instead "not knowing." When information is withheld, psychological vacuums are created that are filled by projections and unconscious fantasies that are liable to be more distressing than the reality. Given patients' obvious need to know about their condition, physicians' noncommunicativeness probably relates more to their own anxieties than to their understanding of patients' needs.

When they decide to communicate bad news, McIntosh summarizes, physicians often use indirect methods of "telling" that are thought to cushion the blow for the patient. This may not work in view of patients' active search for the meanings and implications of their conditions. Doctors may use euphemisms (a tumor instead of cancer) or medical jargon so they can reassure themselves that they have fulfilled their responsibility of telling the patient, although patients do not understand; they may hint at the nature of the difficulty; they may tell the patient the diagnosis but say it is uncertain when it is not; they may tell the patient's relatives on the supposition that they will tell the patient; or they may tell themselves that the patient will ask when he or she is ready to know. Directly avoidant strategies of self-protection were also observed in the studies McIntosh reviews: saying nothing, evading patients' questions, avoiding interaction, acting busy so patients feel their questions are taking the physician away from an important emergency, acting as if the patient's questions are complaints or too simple-minded, or creating social distance to maneuver patients into diffidence and consequent silence.

From the Patient-Client's Point of View

Several aspects of the general meanings of diagnoses and forecasts to patient-clients have already been considered: the feeling that illness is an assault and a foreign intrusion into a person's everyday existence; the social-structural arrangements of the biomedical model that conjoin and diminish the possibilities for patient-clients' being able to cope with their medical conditions as they do with the ordinary problems of living; and the acute distress at the worst moment of learning about a diagnosis. Now let us subject patient-clients' reactions to a finer-grained analysis.

The nature of the objective diagnosis. The objective nature of varying diagnoses plainly makes for differences in patient-clients' constructions of personal meanings and importantly determines their longer-term actions in working toward a cure or taking steps to prevent the actualization of incipient disabilities. Patient-clients will ask themselves (but not always their physicians), How life threatening is the illness or forecasted illness? Is it reversible? How imminent is its full onslaught? What was the fate of other people —people they know—who had the same diagnosis or forecast? Did their friends' impairment and course of onset or cure conform to the description the physician is now giving? Does this physician seem competent? What are the probabilities of *their* actualizing the outcome the physician is now mentioning? How much pleasure, how much of their usual life-style must be changed or given up to comply with the physician's planned course of treatment or implications for prevention? Will their social network of spouse, children, relatives, friends, and work associates support their following *or* ignoring the physician's recommendations? Is it possible that the diagnosis is simply wrong? What alternative courses do they have of verifying or disproving the diagnosis? What have other doctors previously told them about this condition, and do these statements jibe with what this physician is now saying? What is really going on in *their* body? What other measures has the physician overlooked or regarded as unimportant that they can take for themselves (like vitamin pills)? Will the physician be annoyed if he or she discovers that they have secretly acted on their own behalf? If they mention their own plan of treatment, will the physician be patronizing or accept it? We can rest assured that people consider all these and many other matters as they attempt to assimilate and accommodate to the intrusion of illness.

Studies reviewed by McIntosh (1974) indicate that the image the patient creates may influence how much information the doctor decides to give. Lower-class patients are told less than middle-class patients. Consequently, lower-class patients frequently use nurses as sources of information.

Some physicians argue that lower-class patients are not intelligent enough to understand. However, a careful study reported by Ley and Spelman (1967) suggests that the amount of medical information people retain is not related to the level of their IQ but is associated with their general interest in medicine. Relatives of patients were found to retain more information than several different kinds of groups, including patients.

Patient-clients' distressed reactions to diagnoses. Stress, like beauty, is partly in the eye of the beholder; consequently, the severity of stress cannot easily be quantified. The same stress has different effects owing to variations in people's condition at onset, their life history, and the varying ways in which they construct the meanings of the same event. Although we generally tend to think that stress results in response decrement—or, to use Lazarus' (1966) term, primitivization of response—this is clearly not always the result. Several studies of my own (Haan, 1977) that investigate the life stress of longitudinal samples suggest that people who have experienced a lot of stress (clearly not of the most nefarious type) were not conspicuous for their use of denial or avoidance; in fact, such strategies seemed patently unworkable for them. Instead, they had come to use mixed patterns of coping and defense, appearing less able to regulate their affect in coping ways but more able to cope in self-reflexive or intraceptive ways, such as being more empathic and more tolerant of ambiguity.

A review of the stress literature, which does not yet include adequate studies of long-term adaptations to stress, suggests that people generally have the most difficulty accurately assimilating the objective meanings of a stressor when: they do not anticipate it or they overanticipate it; they expect something different or better; the stress itself is ambiguous; they regard the situation as being similar to ones they did not handle well in the past; they are already in a distressed condition at the onset of the stress; and they are not able to secure vital information about the situation. People have a difficult time accommodating to stress when: they can do little or nothing to change or control it; the stress is prolonged; and they have had little previous experience in dealing with stress or the particular kind of stress involved (see Haan, 1977, pp. 156-193).

Little effort is required to extrapolate from these findings to patient-clients' conditions at the time of diagnosis or forecast. They may not have anticipated the diagnosis or they expected the worst and it came about; they hoped for a lesser difficulty than the one determined; they may regard their previous reactions to illnesses as less than adequate and are uncertain about their ability to accommodate to the present one; they are already upset by their condition or with personal matters extraneous to their condition; and, finally, the physician may not give them sufficient information or may not be able to translate the medical description into understandable, everyday words. Patient-clients may have difficulty accommodating to diagnoses and forecasts when they take no action in regard to their illness. Finally, some illnesses and risks involve prolonged stress, and many people, especially the young, have very little previous experience in coping with illness.

We have very little empirically based knowledge about people's temporal assimilations and accommodations to stress. Initial reactions of distress may not prefigure later defense negations of the objective knowledge of the diagnosis or forecast. Patient-clients' initial distress may signal that they are acknowledging the diagnosis, a logical preparation for coping with it. Although, in the medical world, stoical reactions are usually thought to be best, some physicians have practical knowledge of temporal accommodations to stress. One medical geneticist explained that a genetic counselor is helpful to families following diagnosis so they can "cry their eyes out." This geneticist regarded such a session as a necessary prelude to helping the family understand the medical condition and its forecast. Mothers who had borne malformed infants were interviewed by Hosack (1968), first in the hospital and then several times subsequently. Mothers who later coped with their infants' condition were initially more variable in their ego processes—both coping and defending—than mothers who both initially and later defended themselves against the knowledge of their baby's malformation. Folkins (1970) obtained related findings in a situation of simulated stress; defenders' physiological signs of being distressed were unrelated to the intervals of time they waited for the onset of stress, but copers were differentially reactive to the meanings of various intervals of waiting. Unfortunately, most physicians and health professionals (and psychologists!) operate with a model of tension reduction rather than with one of equilibrium. Consequently patient-clients' stoical, defensive reactions are regarded as proof positive that the patient or client is "taking the diagnosis well."

This view of patient-clients' assimilatory and accommodative activity at the time of diagnosis poses difficult problems for preventive medicine. The fact that clients' disabilities are not yet actualized makes it easier for them to rationalize and deny their forecasts, particularly if they value risk-taking behavior. If clients do not permit themselves to hear, and thus do not assimilate and accommodate to the information given, or if doctors' own anxieties cause them to garble or impoverish communications, clients may later become statistics of morbidity or mortality. As an example, an intelligent mother related in a recent meeting in a San Francisco Bay area hospital that she had had three Down's syndrome children before her physicians' communications were sufficiently clear and explicit that she understood what was happening to her babies. However, informed clients who choose to act in ways that maximize risk are not always being defensive and irrational. For instance, a couple may so want a baby of their own that they will, after careful consideration, choose to go ahead with a pregnancy despite their genetic risk. In these situations, the goals of society conflict with those of the individual. The ethical issues posed will be considered in detail later.

The central psychological questions for preventive medicine concern clients' processing of their forecasts—whether they will cope with their diagnosis by directly confronting it (adopt babies, use prenatal diagnosis, or change life-styles to lower their blood pressure), or defend themselves against the implications that their bodies are different than they had thought, or fragment and become psychiatrically ill. As Bard (1970, p. 109) comments, "Many of the lives saved by advances in medical science are doomed to psychological invalidism—which could be minimized by sound psychological preparation."

Some mass educational methods used by preventive medicine may have more deleterious effects on the population at large than the diseases they seek to prevent. For instance, a group of cardiovascular specialists ("Can Hypertension Be Induced by Stress?" 1977) recently wondered whether the public's new and easy accessibility to mobile blood pressure units might not be actually producing mass hypochondriasis and hypertension, given the high reactivity of blood pressure levels to worry or concern. As another example, hundreds of people stood in line for hours several years ago during a severe rainstorm to be screened for Tay-Sachs disease immediately after a Marcus Welby program that was concerned with this genetic disorder. Although the television program obviously worked as persuasion, it is an example of psychological overkill.

Crisis Intervention Theory and Practice Applied to Diagnostic Situations

Having recognized that patient-clients are frequently distressed at the time of diagnosis, let us now consider the implications for medicine of the comparatively new work concerning crisis intervention and therapy for persons within medical settings. In the most general sense, we can say that a crisis exists when a person faces obstacles to important life goals and these difficulties are not readily overcome by customary methods of solving problems. Clearly, a serious diagnosis or forecast is such an obstacle.

Several frequently observed aspects of crisis states are similar to the patient-clients' situations at the time of diagnosis: (1) the sudden onset following revelation of ominous information; (2) the short period of the client's accessibility to help from others; (3) the possibility that the client may engage in defensive maneuvers that result in partial assimilations and distorted accommodations or, alternatively, that the client may use coping strategies that permit reasonably accurate assimilations and realistic, pragmatic accommodations; (4) the probability that once the client chooses a course of resolution, it will be continued, so strategies of coping are set in motion or maladaptive defenses and symptoms are "fixed"; and (5) the likelihood that the newly diagnosed illness or risk will have an impact on the family and that members will be variously supportive or nonsupportive of the client.

A crisis state is one of cognitive confusion. People have difficulty clearly defining or formulating the reasons for their distress and framing questions that would give them the information they need. Rusk (1971) notes that injured systems become closed (repressing and denying); however, this is only one general strategy of self-protection. Persons may remain open but chaotic—rationalizing the difficulty, compartmentalizing or isolating it, displacing it, projecting it, and the like. Whatever the method, many distressed persons clearly need help, and many are remarkably open to help from others who can tolerate expression of feelings, who are explicitly empathic, who are optimistic about the possibilities of new adaptations, and who reduce cognitive confusion by corroborating the facts, meanings, and implications of diagnoses.

Mental health workers have come to the conclusion that states of intense crisis are self-limited, usually lasting only from one to six weeks. As Moos and Tsu (1977, p. 7) wrote, "A person cannot remain in an extreme state of disequilibrium . . . some resolution, even though temporary, must be found and some equilibrium reestablished." However, these resolutions can be poor ones that are purchased at the cost of negating reality and producing psychological symptoms.

When a diagnosis is presented, the physician's (counselor's or therapist's) ultimate aim is to help clients achieve an objective formulation of their condition. This requires that the clients' coping be facilitated. Rusk's (1971) recommendations for methods of crisis intervention can be redrawn to apply to this situation: (1) Helping clients express their feelings about their diagnoses is a step toward helping them assess and organize their reactions and feelings, so they can take these into account and treat them as valid data as they work toward resolution. (2) Being explicitly empathic provides consensual validation that others can understand, if only partially, how it feels to have this diagnosis. (3) Emphasizing the positive aspects of the situation and the clients' strengths helps them recognize and assess their capabilities of coping with their condition. (4) Fostering clients' criticisms of the counselor's interpretations and suggestions supports their agency and their own appraisal of their condition. (5) Exuding hope and calm confidence communicates to clients that other people believe these problems are solvable. One other aspect of crisis intervention, as it relates to illness or the threat of illness, is mentioned by Futterman and Hoffman (1973): The mutual interchange between client and counselor should remind clients of their essential and "natural" commitment to life, despite their present necessity to redefine the meanings of their lives.

Basic to working with clients with unfavorable forecasts is understanding the meaning of illness as an intrusion that threatens to make them passive. Thus, Rusk's (1971, p. 251) admonition: "The golden rule for the therapist in crisis intervention is to do for others that which they cannot do for themselves and no more!" To do more for persons, in a crisis of illness or threatened illness, is to rob them further of their sense of self-determination, whereas to do less is to abandon them to their illness, defenses, and potential disorganization.

That ill people take steps to restore their own agency and activity is clear. But equally clear are the observations that health professionals frequently regard patients' and clients' efforts to restore their agency as inappropriate and troublesome. Futterman and Hoffman (1973) aptly describe parents' efforts to cope after their child has been diagnosed as having leukemia. They have a thirst for information and search for people with similar experiences who will help them understand the facts and their own reactions and help them formulate the meanings of their situation. They question medical personnel intensively, read exhaustively, attempt to locate potential supportive resources, and reassess the events prior to the onset of illness in an attempt to find causes and thereby make the illness rational and sensible. They talk with other experts and shop for other doctors and other treatments. These parents have strong needs to participate actively in the care of their child—again a form of reestablishing their own agency. However, it is only recently that the organizations of hospital wards in Western medical care have begun to make arrangements for families to participate in pediatric patients' care. These arrangements are narrowly seen as support for the child, rather than as ways of supporting their families' coping.

Parents' and patients' needs to cope often take two other forms frequently regarded as irrational. Hospital personnel observe that some patients and parents would rather feel responsible for their child's difficulty (or patients for their own)—they actively brought it about—than conclude that the cause was adventitious and beyond control. Thus, some parents want to take hold of fate and redo it, so they begin to plan to have another "well" baby. On later accommodation to the child's illness, Futterman and Hoffman (1973) observe, many parents deliberately set out to take steps to restore equilibrium in the family, for the sake of all concerned, by attempting to adhere to familiar routines and continuing the usual forms of family interaction. Other activities include conscious regulation of the ways they express emotions—monitoring, regulating, and modifying feelings in the service of the family's equilibrium.

Social-Psychological Aspects of Genetic Diagnosis, Forecasting, and Counseling

The Politics and Ethics of Genetic Services

The increasing number of genetic services is evidence of society's growing interest in preventing later disabilities by locating, diagnosing, and informing persons or families about their genetic risks. No other area of preventive medicine is growing as rapidly or seems to hold such promise of preventing suffering and saving health care dollars. The growth of genetic services in recent decades has been facilitated by significant advances in genetic research and the development of practical and comparatively inexpensive diagnostic technologies. The social efficacy of applied genetics lies in the hope that the number of impaired children can be reduced. Such children place substantial financial burdens on society. For instance, the lifetime cost of caring for a person with Down's syndrome may be in excess of $400 thousand. Thus, in the parlance of politicians and health planners, genetic services are "cost effective."

We can reasonably assume that the best interests of society will coincide with the interests of most persons' preferences to bear healthy instead of impaired children, when they have the choice and if all other matters are equal. However, the assumption that society's and the individual's interests harmonize is not only superficial but dangerous—critical exceptions occur. Some people have important rational reasons—religious, personal, and social —for deciding to take chances. Critical ethical questions are raised by preventive medicine's new intent to locate and confront healthy people with the potentiality of illness. There is danger that society in protection of its interests will deprive individuals of theirs. Thus, a central question of public policy is how society should organize and deliver genetic services—to whom, when, with what sociopsychological expertise, and with what safeguards for individuals' well-being. These matters will probably be worked out as official public health policy within the next ten to twenty years.

Common Situations for Genetic Diagnosis and Counseling

People will seek or find themselves receiving genetic diagnosis in a wide variety of circumstances. They may want a diagnosis because they think they are carriers of a genetic defect, either because of their family history or because they belong to an ethnic group that has a higher incidence of a disorder than the general population. They may already have had a stillborn or surviving baby with a disorder or a baby identified as having a disorder in the increasingly prevalent newborn screening programs. The mother may undergo a prenatal diagnosis because of family history or because she is past thirty-five years of age, the point when the risk of bearing a child with Down's syndrome markedly increases. People may be referred for diagnoses by physicians, public health nurses, or paraprofessionals who work in communities, or they may be self-referred. Whatever the case, persons of different social class and educational background are unequally informed about the possibilities of genetic diagnosis and thus have unequal opportunities to receive genetic information. At present, more middle-class than lower-class persons go to medical centers for genetic diagnoses and are more often self-referred. More lower-class people are likely to be seen in mobile screening units for a specific disease, such as sickle cell anemia.

The Usual Organization of Delivery Services

In all these instances, interchanges between health professionals and clients take place around the main goals and activity of genetic services: the genetic diagnosis of individual clients and/or their families. Diagnosis is almost always done by physicians who have specialized training in genetics and who, more often than not, are associated with university research hospitals. Although the quality of the medical work is undoubtedly high, the biomedical model of physician-patient interchange and the effects of the large hospital setting undoubtedly flavor the form and content of communications. Clients are seen as patients in the sense that they have a biological difficulty (or luckily do not). The physician uses procedures—clinical and laboratory—to determine whether the client's picture matches a known entity and whether impairment is potential, present, absent, or probably present, and forecasts are presented in terms of probabilities; patients are variously informed about their diagnoses. However, in sharp contrast to bio-medical contexts, the client is solely responsible for taking the initiative for his or her own "treatment."

Most discussions of genetic counseling recommend that communications concerning the diagnosis be factual and neutral with respect to the client's decisions concerning childbearing. However, the very organizational structure of services is based on the implicit expectancy—and the hope, if these services are to be effective—that clients will choose to act "rationally" in terms of their now-known genetic risk. They should not have babies if their risk is high and perhaps not if it is moderate. In other words, the organizational basis of the services, if not the expressed sentiments of the personnel, is the supposition that the clients are like patients—receptive.

Most critical to the main argument of this chapter and true to the bio-medical model is the implicit mandate that the physician is responsible for *only* that part of the client's life that comes under medical purview. If clients, for whatever reason, are unable to accept the logical implications of their diagnoses, physicians need not feel responsible. They have discharged their responsibility by making the correct diagnosis and informing the client. To fulfill their responsibility of information giving, geneticists often use graphic illustrations or write letters to the client several weeks after counseling. Responsibility does not necessarily extend to how clients are told, whether they understand or how they feel about their diagnosis or what impact it may have on their everyday life. In fact, most clients are seen only once and follow-up counseling is usually regarded as a tender-hearted and expensive frill. Moreover, this approach gives the personnel assurance that the taxpayers' money is not being misused. Costs to society for a moderate-sized genetic service are easily justified within any one year if only a few clients are deterred from having disabled babies, and enough clients appear to respond stoically in compliance with the role of good patient, so the social-emotional costs are not clearly evident. That the biomedical model determines the widely held view of genetic counseling is illustrated in this statement made by an influential medical geneticist: "Genetic counseling involves determining the risks of recurrence of a particular disorder in various relatives and explaining possibilities open to a couple in view of these risks, the prognosis, and availability of treatment. . . . The amount and nature of the information imparted should clearly be related to the educational background of the parents" (Emery, 1974, pp. 642, 644). Within this context, we can readily see why genetic counseling is usually and simply viewed as the delivery of the diagnosis and does not often include the kinds of activity and interchanges between client and professional that are usually implied by the word *counseling*.

Social-Emotional Meanings of a Genetic "Defect"

To consider the impacts of counseling in greater depth, we need to analyze the special social-emotional meanings of a genetic defect. For centuries, the fantasies of humankind have included the specter of the "bad seed"—the marked person—whose birth and existence unmask ancestral sins. Although parents cannot reasonably hold themselves responsible for their genes, people prefer believing that their acts determine their fate to believing that illness and disability are random. (Increasing availability of genetic information, contraception, and prenatal diagnosis could eventually build "rational" social pressures that parents are responsible for the birth of impaired babies; in this event, parents could literally be held responsible for the action of their genes.) Moreover, genetic diagnoses are so technical and genes so intangible and mysterious that lay persons have few common sense ways to check their diagnoses and must take them on faith. A genetic defect is believed a stigma, though normal people generally carry two to six defective recessive genes—a statement often used by geneticists to reassure clients. The question for the individual is still "Why me?" People's distressed reactions to genetic disorders must also be understood within the sociohistorical context of recurrent and repugnant social ideologies that stress the purity of the race, inferiority or superiority of stock, eugenics, and euthanasia. A social psychology of personal defectiveness and blemishes permeates our thinking as a general fear of castration (Shore, 1975), so healthy people often reject ill or disabled people in subtle ways. A number of social psychological studies have found that people with visible handicaps suffer more discrimination than ethnic minority groups. All these fears and fantasies affect how people who are carriers or who have a disorder feel and think about themselves and how they negotiate their social roles (Sorenson, 1972). If they have a bad seed, should they marry? Will a potential spouse find them acceptable? If they marry, should they have children? If they have a child with a genetic disorder, are they responsible? Will their spouse then reject them?

The central but often implicit issue among geneticists and ancillary personnel concerning the delivery of genetic services is simply whether or not clients experience stress at the time of diagnosis. Although this question is easily investigated, it has not been. The practical corollary question is, If clients are frequently distressed, how much preparatory and follow-up counseling should be offered and at what level of expertise? The usual answer is that few clients become distressed, and the ones who do are properly referred to psychiatrists. However, mental health workers know that people in crisis are not readily referred to someone else at some place else because they regard referral for a reality problem as rejection in itself. Furthermore, many people regard psychiatric referral as stigmatizing. Recall Bard's (1970) comment noted earlier: "Many of the lives saved by advances in medical science are doomed to psychological invalidism."

Review of Studies Evaluating Genetic Diagnosis and Counseling

Investigations of genetic counseling should be done to describe and explain the processes of clients' experiences in order to ascertain, at a minimum, the levels of stress they receive, the distress they experience, and the forms and patterns of counseling that facilitate their coping with their diagnoses and forecasts. Most evaluations published so far are concerned only with specific outcomes of genetic counseling: Do clients remember that diagnosis and, if they are of high risk, does this information appear to prevent their having children in the future? Although my focus is on the social-psychological effects of genetic counseling, we can regard the retention of the objective facts of diagnosis and forecast as more than a matter of economic efficiency; it may also be viewed as an index of clients' distress at the time the facts were conveyed. However, forgetting is only one kind of maladaptive reaction to stress. Clients can "act out" their understanding of their diagnoses in various distorted ways—by not having children when their risk is low, dissolving their marriages, developing various psychosomatic symptoms, and the like.

We turn now to review several examples of psychosocial studies of genetic diagnosis and counseling. In evaluating the adequacy of these studies, it is important to consider the nature of the clientele, the criteria for assessing outcomes, the measures of clients' coping or defending, and whether or not actual counseling was done. The outcomes usually examined are clients' understanding of the diagnosis, whether they were deterred from having children, and their negative emotional reactions, like depression or anxiety. In addition, some studies analyze various demographic characteristics of the participants.

Carter and others (1971) investigated, on follow-up, whether 455 British families, out of an initial 558 who had genetic counseling, understood their diagnoses and were deterred from having children. Apparently, all participants had had a child with a genetic disorder and almost all had initiated the inquiry themselves, so this sample was probably especially receptive and ready to deal with their diagnoses. The actual sample studied contained a higher proportion of upper and middle classes than was representative of the population at large. The investigators assert that "the couples had understood and still remembered the risks they were given"; however, no criterion for establishing the couples' level of understanding or methods of calculating incidence of understanding are described. Incidences of later childbearing are analyzed, but only 421 out of the total 455 couples are included, without breakdown for social class or level of understanding (1971, pp. 283-285). The incidence of deterrence after counseling was 40 percent (N = 169). However, 60 of these couples had a low risk of bearing a child with a defect. (The authors note that low risks were of the order of 1 in 20.) Among the couples who were undeterred, 61 had a high risk and 192 a moderate or low risk. Thus, 121 couples (29 percent of the total 421) did not make what these authors label "sensible and responsible" decisions—60 low-risk parents avoided having children and 61 of high risk did have children. No systematic attempt was made to assess the social-emotional effects of the experience; however, the divorce rate among the contacted families was apparently 2.6 percent (text not clear), compared to the British average of 1 to 2 percent for women of comparable age. The authors observe that the incidence of divorce among the 103 families they were unable to locate may have been higher. These investigators' sanguinity about the "effectiveness" of genetic counseling that they think their study reveals typifies interpretations based on statistical, instead of humane, definitions of criterion. An incidence of 121 couples who did not make "sensible and responsible" decisions is not regarded as "large." However, some portion of these couples might have coped with their diagnosis if they had had adequate counseling. The question arises as to why inadequacy in utilizing social-psychological practices should be any more acceptable than medical malpractice.

Sibinga and Friedman (1971) took great care in assessing the degree to which parents understood the nature of phenylketonuria (PKU), which their children had. With the help of a research assistant, 79 parents, who had regularly visited the clinic for more than six months, filled out an essay-type questionnaire concerning the genetic causation, pattern of symptoms, prognosis, and treatment of PKU. Only 19 percent of the parents gave adequately correct answers for all sections, but 48 percent were correct in regard to the genetic bases of PKU. The parents' educational level did not relate to the adequacy of their understanding nor to their tendencies to distort their answers. Thus, we can conclude that these parents' educational sophistication had little to do with their ability to assimilate emotionally loaded information about their disabled children. The investigators additionally found that if both parents had adequate understanding of PKU, their child gave evidence of better social and mental functioning. To assess levels of parents' understanding of PKU, Fisch and others (1977, p. 12) surveyed 20 families who had children with this disease. Although most or all parents were undoubtedly told of the genetic basis of PKU, 70 percent did not retain this information.

Reiss and Menashe (1972) investigated the retention of risk figures in 35 couples who had children with congenital heart disease. They found that only 5 couples (14 percent) could remember one to four months later their risks of recurrence if they had another baby.

Emery, Watt, and Clark (1972) investigated deterrence of pregnancy in a follow-up study of 53 women with Duchenne muscular dystrophy (carried by women but manifested in sons). Of these women, 41 were considered high risks and 39 of them had avoided pregnancy. The authors comment that these results suggest that "most parents act responsibly when told the risks . . . but a small proportion seemed undeterred and we feel that responsibility for this must lie, at least in part, with the genetic counselors" (p. 150). However, the authors do not propose that genetic counseling would be improved by socio-psychological support, but only by clearer delivery of the facts.

In studies of 100 families, 50 each from Scotland and Ireland, McCrae and others (1973) investigated whether parents who had offspring with cystic fibrosis understood the genetic basis of the disease. The authors assumed some genetic report had been given to all parents at the time of diagnosis; nevertheless, 47 to 84 percent of the mothers or the fathers in the two countries complained that "the instruction" they had received was insufficient. Moreover, approximately 80 percent of the parents in both countries did not actually have complete or "excellent" understanding of the disease's genetic basis. A considerable number (24 to 40 percent in different samples) reported they felt guilty for having transmitted the disease, and 79 percent of the mothers described themselves as depressed (1973, pp. 141-142).

Reynolds, Puck, and Robertson (1974, p. 182) studied adequacy of understanding and deterrence of pregnancy in 98 (out of an original sample of 300) clients who had been diagnosed as having different kinds of genetic diseases and who were willing to cooperate in a follow-up study. They found that 84 percent had "adequate" understanding of their diagnosis and 16 percent did not. These findings are tenuous for three reasons: (1) The high rate of attrition means the sample is probably biased; those persons who were willing to be interviewed were probably among the most satisfied with their counseling experience. (2) The interview schedule was sent to the participants before they were seen, and it included the question, "What were you told in the genetic counseling session?" An unknown number of persons probably took the opportunity to prepare their answers before the interviewer from the diagnostic center arrived. At any rate, functional knowledge was clearly not measured. (3) No mention is made as to whether interviewers presented themselves as independent evaluators (a design flaw that was apparently not considered in any of these studies); consequently, the respondents probably did not feel free to reveal their dissatisfactions. Forty-four percent of the mothers were not deterred from becoming pregnant after counseling (36 of low risk but 7 of high or moderate risk); 7 women, all in the low-risk category, underwent amniocentesis (1974, pp. 183-184). Five couples divorced following counseling, and two of these couples indicated that their fear of having a defective child was the cause. Again, a statistical rather than psychological evaluation of the adverse effects of genetic diagnosis is the ground for the investigators' conclusion that no damage occurred.

To determine clients' understanding of their diagnoses, Hsia (1974) surveyed "about 200" families who had received genetic counseling. He found that approximately 90 percent stated they felt counseling was conducted at a level they could understand, and most (number not stated) indicated their questions had been satisfactorily answered. Recall of their risks was "good" for 75 percent and fair for 20 percent (criterion not stated). Approximately 50 percent of the families had already made their decisions about future childbearing before they were counseled, suggesting that this sample was unusually well informed before counseling (1974, pp. 105-106).

Hsia comments that most young parents made their decisions on "non-genetic" bases.

Gath (1977) investigated the impact of the birth of a Down's syndrome baby on 30 couples who were matched for socioeconomic status and family structure with 30 couples who had had a normal baby. Grief was mentioned by all the Down's syndrome parents in the first interview and by 90 percent of them two years later. Marital breakdowns and severe disharmony occurred with 30 percent of the Down's parents but with none of the control parents. Sexual dissatisfactions were reported by 27 percent of the Down's couples but only 8 percent of the controls (1977, pp. 405-408).

To investigate several effects of genetic counseling, Morris and Laurence (1976) followed 160 couples, almost all of whom had babies with neural tube malformations. The sample was of higher socioeconomic status than the source population. A two-hour interview was held with each couple; over one third reported the counseling session had been upsetting. Couples of very high risk (greater than 1 in 10) and of very low risk (1 in 70) retained the most accurate information. The remaining 79 percent had less "predictable" recall, particularly, the investigators conclude, if they were seen "too soon" after diagnosis. Nevertheless, 83 percent reported that the genetic counseling session had been helpful; many of the displeased couples appeared to adopt the patient role because they felt the physician should have told them whether to have another baby (1976, pp. 158-159). Consistent with the view that genetic counseling should be solely directed toward the goal of insuring that clients retain their risk figures, Morris and Laurence recommend that counseling be done six months after the diagnosis.

To investigate the emotional impact of cystic fibrosis on families, Allan, Townley, and Phelan (1974) interviewed 50 mothers out of a clinic list of 174 for about three hours each. "Almost every mother" stated she had heard nothing after the doctor had indicated the nature of the illness. Thus, they had "considerable confusion" about the genetics of the disease, which they reported led to discord with their husbands and/or with the child's grandparents. Only 4 had sought information for 16 siblings of marriageable age.

In the most psychologically detailed study yet reported, adequacy of understanding, deterrence, and other outcomes were studied by Leonard, Chase, and Childs (1972) in a follow-up of 61 families who had received genetic counseling because their offspring had cystic fibrosis, PKU, or Down's syndrome. Although the range of social class was considerable, the sample appears to match the national average. In direct interviews, 44 percent of these families demonstrated "imperfect" memory of the genetic information given them—claiming they were never counseled, agreeing they had been counseled but saying they were unable to remember because of the emotional shock, stating they had never been able to understand genetics or probabilities, denying they were the natural parents, claiming their offspring was normal, and the like. Thirty-four percent reported that the diagnostic experience had adversely affected their sex lives (1972, pp. 435-437). Their understanding of the genetic bases of their child's disease was significantly related to their educational level. However, whether they actually had more children or not related only to their religion and the mother's age.

Blumberg and Golbus (1975) examined the emotional reactions and personality status of 13 women who had undergone amniocentesis and selective abortion. Their husbands were also seen. Eleven of the 13 women and 4 of the 11 men (not all fathers were available) spontaneously mentioned their depressive reactions to the abortions. Moreover, of the 6 people who did not mention depressive reactions, 3 had profiles on the Minnesota Multiphasic Personality Inventory that indicated that they tended to deny emotional problems. Consequently, the authors conclude that depressive reactions may have been as high as 92 percent for the women and 82 percent for the men (1975, p. 192). They note that these incidences of depression are considerably higher than those reported in studies of abortions performed for other reasons. The investigators give two reasons why aborting a defective fetus may be especially difficult: By necessity, prenatal diagnosis and abortion are done during the second trimester after quickening establishes the fetus in the parents' mind as a "potential future child"; and the parents' sense of guilt and shame in the case of a genetic disease is greater and makes the moral decisions involved more difficult.

Apparently only one study (Antley and Hartlage, 1976) has so far directly assessed the emotional effects of genetic counseling in a systematic design. Levels of anxiety, hostility, and depression were investigated in 43 parents who had borne Down's syndrome babies 6 weeks to 18 months prior to counseling. Assessments were made before and after the parents received counseling—usually only one appointment—and their precounseling scores were compared with a control group of nursery school parents, students, and job applicants. Prior to counseling, the parents of the Down's children were significantly more anxious, hostile, and depressed than the control group. After counseling, they were significantly less anxious and depressed than before, but not less hostile. Despite these improvements for the group as a whole, 26 percent became more upset after counseling (1976, p. 263). The authors analyzed these cases individually and pointed out that each client had particular extenuating circumstances. They suggest more sessions of counseling may have been needed.

Methodological Criticisms of These Studies

These studies include most of the published formal investigations concerning the social-psychological effects of genetic diagnosis and counseling. As empirical inquiries, they leave much to be desired. Common methodological requirements for social-psychological investigation and reporting were often not followed:

1. The representativeness or the effects of unavoidable biases in samples were not analyzed. These concerns are particularly important when

results are reported for clinic populations of mixed diagnoses, socioeconomic statuses, religions, and ages of fertility, who are self-referred or
physician referred, who undergo different kinds of counseling experiences, and who do or do not have a child with a genetic disorder at the
time of counseling. All of these factors will have very different effects on
the clients' assimilation, accommodation, and eventual coping. When the
effects of sample identity are not analyzed, general conclusions about the
financial or emotional cost effectiveness of genetic counseling can not be
drawn.

2. In many instances, the methods of data collection were not reported or
    were mentioned only in an offhand fashion, so evaluation of whether
    clients' understandings and reactions were assessed in reliable or sensitive
    and cogent ways is difficult.

3. Research subjects' willingness to report whatever interviewers want to
    hear—a problem well known and analyzed as an artifact in psychological
    research (Rosenthal and Rosnow, 1969)—was not recognized, so the
    highly satisfactory evaluations given by clients in some studies may be
    due to the fact that their interviewers were representatives of the consult-
    ing clinic and were pulling, consciously and unconsciously, for clients to
    endorse the services.

4. Research studies were not designed to evaluate differences among various
    genetic counseling problems. In most studies, factors such as having a
    child with a disorder, receiving a diagnosis of a disease or a diagnosis that
    one is a carrier, and receiving or not receiving consultation or coun-
    seling after a diagnosis were all treated as if these were equivalent experi-
    ences.

5. All kinds of genetic counseling were treated as if they were identical and
    provided the same experiences to all clients. Some experiences called
    counseling are properly regarded as consultations. No descriptions of
    counselors' training or experience were given nor was the number of
    counseling sessions usually reported, although they were surely almost all
    one session.

6. Only one study (Antley and Hartlage, 1976) can be said to have eval-
    uated, directly, the effects of genetic counseling separate from the effects
    of diagnosis. These investigators assessed clients after diagnosis (but in
    some cases, many months later), made evaluations before and after coun-
    seling, and used a control group. However, their control group was in-
    appropriate. Choosing a control group for a sample that receives genetic
    counseling is a difficult matter because of ethical considerations. If re-
    sources are available to study a group of noncounseled, but genetically
    diagnosed clients, then resources would surely be available to counsel
    them. The next best choice may be a group of matched families who have
    received consultations, but not counseling, in regard to a child with a
    nongenetically based disease of comparable social and emotional signifi-
    cance.

Substantive Import of the Findings

Putting these methodological criticisms and recommendations aside, let us consider what these studies suggest about the reactions of clients to genetic diagnosis and counseling. The following social disruptions or malfunctions were observed: unhappy marriages, marital sexual dissatisfactions, increased divorce rates, discord with grandparents, high-risk mothers becoming pregnant, low-risk parents avoiding pregnancy, young parents making their decisions on "nongenetic" bases, and parents' physical health being affected.

Descriptions of personal malfunctioning are more extensively documented, despite the necessity of our frequently relying on the retention of the facts of a diagnosis as the only index of emotional stress. In the studies reviewed, the following indicators of personal malfunctioning were observed: parents of PKU children did not retain and often distorted important medical and genetic information despite having been clinic visitors for some time; couples with children having congenital heart disease did not retain the risk figures; other parents had imperfect memory of several diagnoses; parents did not understand the genetic basis of cystic fibrosis; parents felt guilty and depressed about a child with a disorder or about their decision to undergo selective abortion; parents reported that their mental health was affected; higher levels of anxiety, hostility, and depression were found in parents of Down's children than in a control group.

Taken altogether, and despite their methodological weaknesses, these studies provide some answers to the question of whether clients and families are stressed by learning of their genetic diagnosis. Obviously, they often are. However, these studies do not provide an answer to the next question: What form should delivery services take to ensure that clients cope with their diagnoses and forecasts? Investigations will have to be considerably more sophisticated to answer the latter question, and the work should be done by social scientists as independent evaluators. Understanding the effects of delivery services is not only a humanitarian but also a practical consideration, because a side benefit of improved counseling may be that a number of clients will be better able to hear and retain the information presented to them. If they do not, there is no way that they can consider or act in their own best interests, whatever these might be.

Conclusions

This chapter has delineated the sociopsychological concomitants of preventive medicine's growing interest in identifying and informing seemingly healthy persons who are at risk in order to help them take steps to reduce their vulnerability. Surely, no one quarrels with the general idea that people need and even have a right to accurate, scientifically based information and predictions about themselves. However, the position that preventive

medicine must take in relation to its clientele, the forms of interchange between client and health professional that it entails, and the likelihood that the
biomedical definition of patient's and doctor's roles will continue to be generalized to the client bring the need for sociopsychological understandings of
clients into bold relief.

My central argument is not merely an extension of Engel's that the
patient should be wholly understood as a biopsychosocial being (Engel,
1977). More critically, I point to the extensive documentation in psychological research that people deeply need to avoid the intrusion of illness and its
concomitant sense of powerlessness and that, contrariwise, they need to
maintain a sense of their own options and of their own capacity to control
their fate. Because people decide for themselves what to do, they easily
defeat—if they so choose—the goals of prevention, overtly or covertly. This
view of people and their need to cope is not consistent with either the biomedical model's or Engel's definition of the patient's and the physician's
roles. These prescriptions for medical intervention place physicians in the
counterproductive, emotionally and morally untenable position of taking
unilateral responsibility for the passive-receptive patient. Because this one-
sided moral bargain runs counter to people's psychological nature, both
physicians and patients are confused and stressed, and they interact defen-
sively. Thus, it is widely believed and documented in the studies of genetic
counseling that communications between doctors and patients and patient
compliance are generally poor.

If this line of reasoning is correct, it has important and radical implications for the ways in which health care services are presently delivered—the
implications for preventive medicine differ only in being more salient. These
recommendations are not new; they began with Szasz and Hollender (1956)
and are very much part of the present thinking. I extend this line of thought
by arguing that participatory medicine has a social-psychological basis in
facilitating patients' coping. Health care services based on the recognition of
people's activity in their own behalf would no longer provide services to persons defined as patients but would instead work with clients who are taken
into full, responsible partnership in achieving their care and their cures and
in preventing their risks from being actualized. This recommendation does
not mean abandoning often regressive, ill persons to suffer their crises of
diagnosis by themselves. In fact, support to help them cope at these times is
seen as not only a pragmatic but also a humanitarian measure. It does not
mean physicians will be less responsible but rather responsible in a different
way. It does demand that physicians understand the lengths to which people
will go to maintain their initiative and ward off helplessness.

6 ⤧

Changing Self-Destructive Behaviors

Judith B. Henderson

Sharon M. Hall

Helene L. Lipton

⤧ Health care professionals from a wide variety of fields are beginning to confront the issue of changing people's day-to-day habits and behavior patterns. Those without a social science background sometimes make the naive assumption that once a person understands how to enhance his health status—whether it be by using seat belts, engaging in prophylactic dental care, changing diet, smoking, alcohol, or exercise patterns, taking a prescribed medication, or following a treatment plan—a change in behavior will follow. Ironically, even the design of the large, national Multiple Risk Factor Intervention Trial to study coronary risk reduction was based on the premise that all subjects would change smoking, dietary, and other habits if told to do so by a physician (Henderson and Enelow, 1976). Practitioners who have attempted to inform and/or persuade people to take appropriate action are shocked and disillusioned to realize that most people regularly engage in

Note: Preparation of this chapter was supported in part by 1 H81 DA 01978 from the National Institute on Drug Abuse.

behavior that will cause them later pain and expense. It is the conclusion of many who are not social scientists that people simply cannot change habits and that self-destructiveness is inevitable (Burnum, 1974).

The purposes of this chapter are: to confirm that, indeed, most behaviors are not easy to change, and to bring some conceptual, theoretical, and empirical understanding to the conditions under which one could expect to succeed in changing behavior. Existing theoretical models are examined for their applicability to the self-destructive behaviors of obesity, cigarette smoking, and alcoholism. The empirical literature is reviewed and some of the more promising intervention strategies are presented. These particular self-destructive behaviors were selected for discussion because each is clearly a serious health hazard and each has a literature of at least some experimental intervention studies.

The current interest and involvement in trying to define, analyze, and change self-destructive behaviors stem from a basic shift in the patterns of morbidity and mortality in this country and in other modern, industrialized cultures. The major health problems facing the medical profession in 1900 were influenza, tuberculosis, and gastroenteritis. After the causal organisms were identified and immunizations developed, these infectious diseases were, to a large extent, prevented and cured, so that by 1970 the leading causes of death were the chronic diseases and accidents. Noncommunicable or chronic diseases such as malignant neoplasms, vascular lesions of the central nervous system, coronary heart disease, and the cardiovascular complications of hypertension are now the problems that require innovative approaches in prevention, control, and cure.

There is growing evidence that detrimental life-style patterns and day-to-day health habits are linked to the probability of developing these and other chronic diseases. Furthermore, self-destructive habits may influence not only the development of disease but also general levels of physical and mental well-being. Some examples of relationships that have been confirmed to varying degrees in existing empirical literature follow:

1. Several prospective studies indicate that hypertension, cigarette smoking, and a diet high in saturated fat, cholesterol, and sugar contribute to an individual's risk of coronary heart disease. Obesity, lack of physical activity, and various life stresses, including behavioral coping mechanisms such as Type A Behavior Pattern (Rosenman and others, 1976), also appear to contribute to coronary risk status (Carlson and Bollinger, 1972; Inter-Society Commission for Heart Disease Resources, 1970). Many of these behaviors and resulting physical conditions may, in turn, interfere with quality of life and overall well-being.

2. The relationship between diet and weight and increased incidence of diabetes mellitus is well established (Carlson and Bollinger, 1972; Inter-Society Commission for Heart Disease Resources, 1970). Adverse psychological consequences are also associated with obesity and malnutrition by virtue of their possible interference with one's work, social activity, and sexual life (Stuart and Davis, 1972).

3. There is a great deal of evidence linking cigarette smoking to health hazards such as lung cancer, emphysema, chronic bronchitis, and diseases of the heart and blood vessels (World Conference on Smoking and Health, 1967).
4. Alcohol abuse manifests a number of physical complications, such as liver cirrhosis and kidney diseases, as well as related loss of social and emotional functioning in areas of employment, marital and other family relationships, and integration into the community (National Institute of Alcohol Abuse and Alcoholism, 1974).

The predominance of high-risk and self-destructive behaviors has far-reaching and complex implications. It has been estimated that forty to eighty million people in the United States are overweight and lacking in proper nutrition (Stuart and Davis, 1972, p. 1). About fifty million are smokers (Statistical Abstracts of the United States, 1976, p. 117), and approximately nine million are either alcohol abusers or alcoholics (National Institute of Alcohol Abuse and Alcoholism, 1974, p. 7). It has been estimated that $11.5 billion are spent annually in the United States for health care costs associated with cigarette smoking (Sommers, 1976, p. 1), and that alcohol abuse and alcoholism have an associated annual cost of $25 billion (National Institute of Alcohol Abuse and Alcoholism, 1974).

The control of self-destructive behaviors is especially difficult because they are largely outside the scope of traditional medicine. Physicians usually see, treat, and cure sick people, and people usually seek a physician's consultation if they are sick and expecting to receive treatment that will lead to a cure. Unfortunately, much self-destructive behavior is not accompanied by unpleasant symptoms in the early stages and goes unnoticed by individuals. In addition, self-destructive behaviors have to be considered in their entirety —that is, they may be risky or dangerous but may also bring benefits to the person. Some benefits may be obvious and compelling, such as those derived from an occupation that has environmental or safety hazards (coal mining, law enforcement, or chemical manufacturing), but also supports an individual, or recreational activities that are dangerous (mountain climbing, skateboarding, or hang gliding) but provide needed relaxation and physical activity. Other benefits may be compelling to the individual but less clear to others, as in the case of smoking, consuming alcohol, overeating, or taking psychotropic drugs to cope with stress and tension. Still other benefits an individual could accrue are the social rewards of conformity to self-destructive group behavior such as poor eating, smoking, and alcohol habits, which may be supported by subcultural norms.

Even if a physician is made aware of an individual's self-destructive behavior, the most he or she usually can do is to advise behavior change. The individual is then left with the responsibility for making difficult changes in often rewarding life-styles with minimal change in symptomatology, little social support, and, frequently, social disapproval (Baric, 1969).

Some obvious implications of the problem of modifying high-risk behaviors are the need for changes in the role of consumers and health providers. Consumers need to be reeducated to assume responsibility for taking preventive actions with or without a physician's advice. Physicians need to learn how to help people make difficult changes in habits by drawing upon professionals in the behavioral sciences and related fields. The entire health community needs to cooperate in creating national health-promoting policies and in providing services to help people learn how to make changes in their lives. These tasks involve enormous challenges to health professionals, public health services, and the population in general.

Major Issues in Research on Self-Destructive Behaviors

The literature on self-destructive behaviors that is most relevant to this discussion focuses on attempts to change habits through intervention. The actual substance of the interventions is derived from the various theoretical models of behavior to be discussed later. But the research methodology itself in the areas of obesity, smoking, and alcoholism raises a number of similar issues. They are: individual variability among subjects, premature termination from treatment or dropout rates, long-term maintenance of change, generalizability of results across different populations, and cost effectiveness. These issues will be discussed first because they are crucial to the evaluation of interventions derived from the theoretical models.

Individual Variability

The question of individual variability is one of the greatest challenges to researchers studying obesity, smoking, and alcoholism. Most investigations of behavioral weight control strategies, for example, have been characterized by marked individual variability in degree of weight loss (Penick and others, 1971). The exploration of this variability and attempts to specify effective predictor variables generally have not yielded clinically useful findings. However, some variables have been shown to have unusually strong relationships in initial studies or some degree of replicability. With respect to obesity, variables worthy of further study include mood disturbance (Hall, Bass, and Monroe, 1978), family involvement (Mahoney and Mahoney, 1976; Brownell and others, 1977), age of onset (Stunkard and Rush, 1974), and self-reported alteration of eating habits (Mahoney, 1974b). Generally, studies of smoking behavior have been unable to locate stable predictors, although some research indicates that the involvement of "significant others" may predict success (Bornstein and others, 1975; Lawson and May, 1970).

In alcoholism studies, the best predictors of outcome success are social stability, including marital and employment status (Baekeland, Lundwall, and Shanahan, 1973; Bowen and Adroes, 1968; Dubourg, 1969; Gerard and Saenger, 1966; Gillis and Keet, 1969; Goldfried, 1969; Kish and Hermann, 1971; Kissin, Platz, and Su, 1971; Mayer and Myerson, 1971; Pokorny, Miller, and Cleveland, 1968; and Rosenblatt and others, 1971), and socioeconomic status (Gillis and Keet, 1969; Mindlin, 1959; Trice, Roman, and Belasco, 1969). Psychological variables with favorable prognostic significance in alcohol treatment include dependency (Blane and Meyers, 1963), superior intellectual and emotional functioning (Mindlin, 1959; Rossi, Stach, and Bradley, 1963), moderate levels of self-punitive "conscience structures" (Walton and others, 1966), high affiliative needs and group dependence (Trice and Roman, 1970), and client motivation (Linksy, 1970).

Future research needs to address itself to the specification of traits or combinations of traits that can be used as predictor variables, as well as to the subsequent modification of these variables and the determination of which individuals benefit by which treatments. Unfortunately, although there are some associations that are of statistical significance, only a small part of the actual variation in behavior is accounted for, thus making the relationships too weak to be of clinical significance. Worthy of attention, but little studied, are biological variables such as differences in fat cell structure in obese individuals (Bray, 1970) or physiological responses to nicotine administration in the case of smokers. These variables are only recently being considered and there are no data available on whether nicotine is the addictive substance in cigarettes or whether fat cell differences can predict later changes in body weight.

Premature Termination

Another variable of interest in evaluating treatment programs for self-destructive behaviors is premature termination or dropout rates. A high premature termination rate may greatly decrease the overall effectiveness of a treatment if the outcome for all those inducted into it is considered methodologically. The unavailability of individuals for follow-up measurement creates a "subject mortality" bias in results. Study results are further complicated by a lack of uniformity in the way researchers deal with dropouts (Jeffrey, 1975). Some exclude dropouts from all analyses; others include them until they drop out and exclude them from further analyses; and still others include dropouts in all analyses.

In obesity research, differences in attrition rates within treatment modalities seem to be due neither to subject variables nor to specific treatment procedures or reported experimental variables (Hall and Hall, 1974). Given the great variability in premature termination rates and the paucity of knowledge regarding determinants, it would seem necessary to conduct systematic research in this area to identify possible variables to explain differences. It has been suggested that examining the impact of expectational and attitudinal variables may prove fruitful in this regard. For example, Nash (1976) found that the most likely client to drop out of a commercial weight loss program was the person who had dropped out previously. This finding was then linked with clients' expectations of failure and self-attribution of personal weakness.

Long-Term Maintenance

One problem in studying addictive behaviors is that behavioral changes are not stable over time. There is a general tendency for relapse to occur, but there are no longitudinal data available on the rate or the course of recidivism. In addition, most controlled studies of addictive behaviors do not include follow-up periods exceeding one year. Thus, the long-term impact of treatment methods is difficult to assess. In obesity research, for example, the few controlled studies that have follow-ups of one year or more generally have found that the originally observed differences between groups were no longer significant (Foreyt and Kennedy, 1971; Hall and others, 1977; Harris and Bruner, 1971; Kingsley and Wilson, 1977; Stunkard, 1977a). Similarly, the findings for alcoholism and smoking indicate high levels of recidivism after the initial treatment period has ended (Bandura, 1969; Hunt, Barnett, and Branch, 1971). Little empirical and systematic investigation of those who recidivate has been conducted. Research is needed to determine the optimal follow-up treatments and whether and in what ways those who maintain change differ from those who do not.

Factors contributing to loss of treatment effects have been hypothesized. One explanation is that in many studies active treatment periods are limited to two or three months. This relatively short period of time may not be sufficient for many individuals to acquire and maintain new behaviors. Also, individuals may vary in the length of time they need to learn and firmly establish new behaviors, suggesting the need for individually tailored programs (Musante, 1976). Treatment length, generally, has been found to be positively related to outcome in outpatient treatment studies (Fox and Smith, 1959; Gerard and Saenger, 1966; Kissin, Platz, and Su, 1971; Ritson, 1969).

Another factor contributing to loss of treatment effect could be a person's dependency on a therapist or group for encouragement and support in applying various self-management techniques and in sustaining commitment and motivation. In obesity research, two approaches have been suggested to ameliorate this problem. One approach provides for periodic contact with clients during follow-up in the form of booster sessions (Hall and others, 1975; Hall and others, 1977; Kingsley and Wilson, 1977). The other approach reduces direct contact with a therapist during active treatment by substituting written materials in the place of oral instruction. The efficacy of this latter approach has been examined (Hanson and others, 1976) and the results showed that the reduced-contact treatment did not differ significantly from more intensive treatments at ten weeks, and that low-contact subjects continued their weight losses at one year. A recent review (Hall and Hall, in press) indicates at least four factors in successful maintenance: continuing support; simple, specific treatment techniques; prevention of dependency on the therapist; and increased self-attribution of change.

Studies have generally failed to address themselves to the issue of *what* is being maintained. In obesity research, for example, most subjects lose moderate amounts of weight, but rarely reach goal weight. If particular strategies produce maintenance of this loss, it is important to analyze whether these strategies are maintaining eating habits that keep weight down or a set of behaviors that produce rapid and potentially dangerous weight losses immediately before scheduled weigh-ins.

Generalizability of Results

The generalizability of the results of most studies in the areas under discussion is unknown. Carefully controlled experimentation with adequate sample sizes is rare (Bandura, 1969). Many studies, especially those of alcoholism, are often carried out in treatment centers in which all those requesting help are treated without experimental controls. Most weight reduction studies have employed small groups of mildly overweight female subjects drawn from a campus population (Hagen, 1974; Harris and Bruner, 1971; Harris, 1969; Wollersheim, 1970). It is uncertain whether treatment results for this kind of college-educated population can be generalized to clinical settings with other moderately or severely overweight middle-aged males and females. Indeed, there is already some indication that behavioral studies using noncollege student populations have produced less striking results than studies using college students (Horan and Johnson, 1971; Meyer and Henderson, 1974; Tyler and Straughan, 1970), although evidence of this point is conflicting (Hall and others, 1974). Further, there is some evidence that when weight control techniques are introduced into large population groups through commercial institution auspices, the outcomes are less effective than those achieved with smaller groups in university settings (Levitz and Stunkard, 1974).

Researchers need to pay closer attention to the impact of social variables, most notably socioeconomic status, when designing, recruiting for, and conducting programs designed to modify self-destructive behaviors. For example, in obesity research, more attention should be focused on clients of lower socioeconomic status. This shift in emphasis can be justified for several reasons. First, there is a clear inverse relationship between social class and the prevalence of both malnutrition and obesity (Stuart and Davis, 1972). Second, several recent studies have shown that a greater proportion of persons of higher socioeconomic status already are concerned with or are presently following some dietary regimen, suggesting that socioeconomic status influences the likelihood that action will be taken without intervention (Stuart and Davis, 1972). The reasons for this relationship are by no means clear. One possible hypothesis might be that hardships of poverty reduce motivation to engage in improved eating behavior. If this is found to be the case, then greater attempts have to be made to increase motivation. However, another possible explanation may lie in the relative nonavailability or accessibility of nutrition or weight-reducing programs in poor communities. The fact that the overwhelming majority of studies have been conducted with homogeneous middle-to-upper-class populations would tend to corroborate the latter view. There is clearly a need to diversify the research populations on variables like social class, age, and sex, thus enhancing the external validity of such studies.

It has been suggested that one of the reasons for the high premature termination rates and relatively limited success of many weight reduction, smoking cessation, and alcohol treatment programs may be the fact that only the most intractable cases come to the professional's attention. This assumption has never been questioned or systematically investigated. It could be argued that those who volunteer for treatment are among the most highly motivated to change their behaviors, and those who do not participate might represent a large number who have "given up the struggle" and have adopted a defeatist attitude. There is a need for systematic research to determine whether and in what specific ways those who join programs differ from those who do not. Knowledge of these factors would enable professionals in the field to make more accurate assessments of the generalizability of their research results.

Cost Effectiveness

The issue of cost effectiveness has rarely been addressed in obesity, smoking, or alcohol research. In his recent review, Mahoney (1975) noted that in a Stanford-based study in which subjects received self-help books through the mail, the cost was less than $2 per subject. However, this is one of the very few cases in which the issue of cost has been raised. Therapeutic approaches should be evaluated not only on effectiveness but also on efficiency. A treatment program that is moderately effective but costs inordinate amounts of time and money, when compared to standard routine care, may not be worth the additional expenditure of human and monetary resources. At a minimum, it would seem that researchers should report the cost of the clinical aspects of the intervention per patient, so that studies can be compared on efficiency as well as effectiveness (Jeffrey, 1975; Jeffrey and Christensen, 1972).

Models of Self-Destructive Behavior

The question of why people engage in behaviors that are injurious to their health can be analyzed by examining some of the literature on human development and behavior. The psychological models with the greatest relevance to self-destructive behaviors are the rational model and its variants, the psychodynamic model, and the social learning model. These particular models are chosen for review in this discussion because they have generated relatively complete conceptualizations with respect to self-destructive behaviors. They also have served as the theoretical basis from which the most significant intervention strategies for changing behavior have been developed and have generated the most published research and case reports. Other models that would seem to provide a potential for developing such interventions are discussed briefly.

To provide a unifying thread, one behavior, overeating, will be examined from the perspective of each of the models, looking in turn at explanations of the etiology of the behavior, interventions implied, and the outcome of these interventions both generally and in terms of the major research issues. The review of smoking and alcohol literature follows the discussion of models.

Rational Model

The rational model derives from the literature of eighteenth-century rationalism. It assumes that human behavior is guided by an objectively logical thought process. Thus, this theory would hold that given appropriate information about the health risks of various behaviors and the health-protective qualities of other behaviors, individuals will modify their actions to preserve their health. Self-destructive behavior would be explained primarily in terms of lack of appropriate knowledge of risks and hazards involved in engaging in such behavior.

At least two variants of the rational model have been adopted by health care providers and educators. Both emphasize the importance of rational decisions in the continuation or termination of self-destructive behaviors. The first variant, the more general decision-making model, assumes that people assess the personal, social, and psychological costs and benefits of their actions and the resulting cost-benefit ratio determines behaviors. Although the factors entering into this decision may not be in full awareness, or fully verbalized, the model assumes that the decision is central in determining further behavior (Janis, 1975b). If a decision to change is made, but an individual fails to carry out his or her plan, the theory suggests that there is interference from cognitive defenses. These rationalizations minimize the self-destructive aspects of the behavior or exaggerate withdrawal symptoms (Janis and Mann, 1977), and cognitive interventions to counteract the rationalizations are needed (Reed and Janis, 1974).

Another variant of the rational model is found in the Health Belief Model, which, in brief, suggests that individuals' perceptions of their health influence changes in health-related behaviors. Modification of self-destructive behavior would involve modifying perceptions of the severity of the behavior and one's own susceptibility to its complications and sequelae as well as the extent to which one believes in the efficacy of the proposed plan to change behavior and the perceived barriers that would make change difficult or unpleasant (Becker, 1976).

The intervention approach for weight reduction in obesity suggested by the rational model is the provision of information about nutrition, exercise, and input-output energy ratios. Actual interventions have consisted of specific diet plans and nutrition education. These programs can be quite inexpensive and can reach large numbers of people, but their poor weight loss results can produce an unfavorable cost-benefit ratio. Dropout or premature attrition rates vary but have run as high as 80 percent of the initial sample in some studies. The individual variation in study populations is also high, so that many, if not most, obese individuals in nutrition education programs fail to lose clinically significant amounts of weight (Stunkard and McClaren-Hume, 1959). A primary problem with such information provision approaches is that many individuals lack the skills to adhere to the standards the information suggests would be desirable. Combinations of such informational approaches with training in behavioral skills seem to produce optimal outcome (McReynolds and others, 1976).

The rational/informational approach is widely used by health professionals and is trusted because of its inherent logic. Unfortunately, as the example of obesity intervention shows, the practical results of applications of the rational model to addictive behaviors are disappointing. Both large-scale information campaigns and small-scale controlled studies show that an information-only treatment is generally not a very effective method of changing behavior (Meyer and Henderson, 1972). Part of the problem with the rational model is that it offers an oversimplified notion of the change process; it deals only with cognition while ignoring the evaluative, affective or behavioral aspects of an individual's psychological makeup.

The Health Belief Model improves upon the rational model in that it identifies different types of information that can have greater or lesser persuasive appeal. It also acknowledges that information can be provided in indirect ways, for example, via past treatment experiences. However, this model has generated little intervention research in self-destructive behavior designed to test it directly. In fact, most efforts to validate the model in general have been retrospective: Current health beliefs have been compared to previous health behaviors (usually, compliance) and the results have generally been in the expected direction (Becker and Maiman, 1975). Interestingly, however, the results from more recent prospective studies have produced inconsistent findings, suggesting that health beliefs may result from, rather than cause, changes in health behavior (Taylor, in press).

Rational approaches need to be used creatively within the context of a more comprehensive change strategy. Information and knowledge may be necessary although not sufficient conditions for change. For example, in any change strategy, individuals have to have information about what it is they are trying to do. Additionally, however, the person needs to have the motivation to change, the skills necessary to change, and the ability to maintain change over time.

Psychodynamic Model

The psychodynamic model holds that within an individual there are conflicting tendencies between instinctual, rational, and moralistic forces which develop early in life. Most of these conflicts are assumed to be out of conscious awareness and thus not readily dealt with or verbalized. The essential conflict between the psychodynamic model and other models is that the former views the unconscious conflict as the root of the self-destructive behavior problem. The behavior is a symptom and if it is eliminated without in-depth evaluation, it is expected that another symptom will emerge. Psychodynamic interventions require an examination of an individual's emotional past to find underlying causes for maladaptive behavior. Self-destructive behaviors would be seen as symbolically fulfilling a deep emotional need within the individual, and behavior change would come about through the insights into an individual's thoughts and feelings gained from psychoanalysis or other variants of insight-oriented psychotherapy.

With respect to our example of obesity, the psychodynamic model has produced not one, but several conceptualizations of etiology. Early writers assumed that one underlying conflict was the primary factor. Conflicts proposed included excessive oral dependency needs, rejection of pregnancy, and "psychological cannibalism" as causes of obesity. Applications of classical psychoanalysis to obesity have generally not been considered a viable treatment by contemporary writers, including psychoanalytically oriented ones. A leading contemporary theorist in obesity has produced a model that emphasizes the diversity of factors in this area of study (Bruch, 1973). However, like more traditional analytic writers, Bruch emphasizes that obesity is determined by unconscious psychological factors arising from experiences early in life. She assumes pathological obesity is due to unconscious struggles about control over one's life and a learned inability to recognize hunger. The latter factor results from inappropriate parenting and the use of food by the parents to satisfy needs other than hunger. Bruch's intervention of choice remains individual, long-term psychotherapy.

The analytic or insight approach does not lend itself easily to evaluation or research since it is difficult to document unconscious processes. Most writers assume it is not applicable to all obese individuals, only to those who seek psychiatric help. Therefore, its generality is limited to what would seem to be a particularly disturbed subgroup of obese individuals. Controlled studies of its effectiveness are not available, and the case studies presented often provide little outcome data. Issues such as individual variability, maintenance, and premature attrition cannot be addressed until preliminary attempts at assessing outcome have been made. In any event, the intervention is an expensive one, usually involving long-term individual psychotherapy. Group intervention is possible at a lower individual cost, but it is not the treatment of choice and is often seen as a prelude to more intensive individual approaches (Buchanan, 1973). Less traditional adaptations of the psychodynamic approach to insight-oriented groups have been minimally effective (Holt and Winick, 1961; Slawson, 1965).

Social Learning Model

The learning theories formulated by Pavlov and Skinner form the basis for social learning theory. The mechanisms for learning are expanded to include modeling or imitation of the behavior of others (Bandura, 1969, 1976;

Bandura and Walters, 1963) and reinforcement based on subjective expectations regarding the future 'consequences of one's actions (Rotter, 1954; Rotter, Chance, and Phares, 1972). The role of social reinforcement by other people is emphasized, and even the vicarious reinforcement experienced as a result of observing another person receive approval or disapproval has been found to have a profound influence on the behavior of the observer (Bandura, 1969).

The social learning theorist would argue that individuals engage in self-destructive behavior because they have learned that this behavior is an acceptable coping mechanism and/or is socially rewarding. Children are especially susceptible to learning detrimental dietary, smoking, or alcohol habits by modeling the behavior of adult or peer models in their lives or in the media. Once a behavior has been learned and is a part of an individual's behavioral repertoire, it is then maintained by social reinforcement or intrinsic rewards.

The social learning approach to intervention focuses directly on the self-destructive behavior to be changed. It is specific, directive, predictive, time-limited, and focused on solving one problem at a time. An underlying assumption is that the individuals can learn and maintain new behaviors if they make a commitment to take responsibility for changing their behavior. To change behavior, the task is to reduce the reward value of an old response pattern and to establish a new behavior with a high reward value by means of selective reinforcement and modeling. Models can be especially effective in demonstrating and inducing individuals to try new behaviors. Guided participation by the model further enhances the change process by providing chances to practice new behaviors with social support and encouragement (Bandura, 1969, 1971; Bandura and Walters, 1963).

The change process can be specified in terms of: (1) outcome goals set by the individual and health professional and sequenced objectives that break down the goals into specific target behaviors; (2) a behavioral analysis of the conditions under which a given response or set of responses occurs; (3) rewards and punishments that will be selectively received; (4) feedback and evaluation of the success of the program; and (5) revision of goal activities, or rewards based on evaluation data.

Social learning theorists generally have assumed that obesity is due to the learning of faulty eating patterns (Ferster, Nurnberger, and Levitt, 1962; Stuart, 1967). Intervention strategies dictated by this approach are the learning of new eating habits. New learning must include not only accurate knowledge about nutrition and energy consumption but also new skills with which obese individuals can manipulate their own environments. Interventions include food and weight monitoring, methods for reducing the stimuli that evoke eating, self-reward strategies, ways of modifying the act of eating itself, and the development of substitute behaviors.

Starting with early studies by Ferster, Nurnberger, and Levitt (1962) and by Stuart (1967), the social learning approach has produced a vast research literature. It has been thoroughly reviewed at various points in its history (Bellack, 1975; Hall and Hall, 1974; Stunkard, 1972, 1977a; Stunkard and Rush, 1974). These reviewers have repeatedly concluded that the social learning approach remains the most promising one in the treatment of obesity, not only in weight change but also in low rates of premature attrition. The issue of its effectiveness is not as simple as these conclusions might indicate, however. First, behavioral approaches appear to produce larger variability in results than those produced by other methods (Hall and others, 1977; Penick and others, 1971). As noted above, efforts to isolate variables that predict this variability have not been markedly successful. In addition, long-term maintenance is a serious and well-recognized problem within the field (Brightwell, 1976; Brightwell and Sloan, 1977; Hall and others, 1974, 1975, 1977; Stuart, 1977; Stunkard, 1977a). Efforts have been made to devise strategies to enhance maintenance. These include booster sessions (Hall, Bass, and Monroe, 1978; Kingsley and Wilson, 1977), development of simple environmental controls, such as using special plates or storage areas (McReynolds and others, 1976; Weiss, 1977), and methods that reduce therapist dependency (Hanson and others, 1976). Although each of these approaches would seem to have some merit, no conclusion about their efficacy or generalizability can be drawn at this point (Hall and others, 1974; Levitz and Stunkard, 1974).

In spite of the assumption that behavioral methods are quite cost effective, cost-benefit analyses of behavioral approaches are not frequently reported. The approach does lend itself well to both group and individual treatment, with and without professional leaders. The one comparison of group and individual treatment reported by Kingsley and Wilson (1977) indicated that individual treatment actually resulted in poorer long-term weight loss than group methods. Comparisons of individuals attempting change without professional help have not always been conclusive, but evidence tends to show that they may produce favorable outcomes. If so, low contact methods may be more cost effective than more intense methods (Hanson and others, 1976).

Other Models

There are other proposed models that can be applied to the explanation of, and intervention in, self-destructive behaviors. Attitude theory provides a model of the multidimensional processes involved in thought and action by identifying cognitive, affective, and behavioral components (Rokeach, 1966-1967). The preferred strategy for changing attitudes is to create cognitive dissonance by increasing awareness of conflicts among knowledge, feelings, and behavior (Abelson and Rosenberg, 1958; Festinger, 1957; Osgood and Tannenbaum, 1958). It is the conclusion of many social scientists that attitude theory is limited in applicability because most changes in attitude follow behavioral changes, and, therefore, the focus should be on the behavior itself instead of on opinions and attitudes (Janis, 1975b).

The recent conceptualization of the "at risk" role (Baric, 1969) has updated traditional formulations of roles related to health and illness (Kasl, 1975b) and has generated considerable interest among researchers in chronic diseases because of its emphasis on individual responsibility and permanent life-style change. It is hoped that intervention strategies that take this model into consideration will be presented in the future.

Discussions of behaviors such as overeating and alcoholism are not complete without some mention of self-help groups such as Weight Watchers or Alcoholics Anonymous (AA). These groups developed as "common sense" lay organizations and their development has not reflected influence by the social sciences. They implicitly assume that interpersonal support and a coherent philosophy about one's disorder are of greatest importance in treatment interventions. Although some of their strategies do have theoretical underpinnings and they report successful outcomes, they have generally not undergone systematic evaluation.

Summary of Research on Obesity

In summarizing the research generated by the various models of obesity and/or overeating, it seems justified to conclude that the psychodynamic model fares the least well. Reports lack methodological rigor and do not supply even basic information about outcome. Since these reports are no more than case studies, little can be said about the usefulness of the technique except that, owing to its expense, it is unlikely that it will ever gain wide acceptance for these not psychologically impaired obese.

With respect to the nutrition education proposed by the rational model, regardless of the outcome of the provision of such education alone, it would seem that an accurate knowledge of nutrition is an important component of any treatment devised for obesity. Behavioral approaches can teach eating skills, but sensible goals toward which such skills can be directed can only be formulated when knowledge of optimal eating is available. In fact, one might argue that social learning approaches have been able to show success only because the general public has some knowledge of nutrition. To take the case to the extreme, no matter what eating control skills one taught an individual who believed that lard and sugar made up a satisfactory low-calorie diet, it is not likely that such a person would lose much weight.

The social learning approach has generated the most and the best controlled research on obesity and overeating. Although it currently is evaluated by most authorities as the most effective treatment both in terms of outcome and attrition, the fulfillment of this early promise on the clinical level is yet to be determined. Crucial issues of generalizability, individual variation, and maintenance remain unresolved.

Summary of Research on Smoking and Alcoholism

The major theoretical models that have influenced the treatment of obesity, smoking, and alcoholism have been reviewed, using the research on obesity to show their applicability. The research on smoking and alcoholism will now be summarized within the context of the three models.

Smoking

The rational approach explains smoking as a failure to understand the effects of smoking on health. This approach suggests that effective provision of information about the deleterious effects of cigarette smoking is the crucial intervention. Two lines of evidence are available from which this intervention can be evaluated: the effects of education campaigns on smoking, and changes in smoking as a result of the Surgeon General's report.

Most educational campaigns have been conducted in high schools and colleges, using arguments against smoking that are health related. Generally, these campaigns have been markedly unsuccessful (Andrus, Hyde, and Fischer, 1964; Monk, Tayback, and Gordon, 1965; Wayne, Montgomery, and Pettit, 1964). It has been suggested that adolescents do not feel vulnerable to long-term health problems and that the type of information provided in these campaigns was inappropriate. Recently developed research on smoking prevention and cessation that emphasizes physical attractiveness and interpersonal variables may be more successful (Evans, 1975).

Although overall levels of smoking have not changed drastically in the fourteen years since the Surgeon General's report was released, smoking is beginning to decrease among men thirty-five to sixty-five years of age, where risk of lung cancer and coronary heart disease is highest. Unfortunately, this decrease is offset by increased smoking rates among adolescents and women (Jarvik and others, 1977). Although the data seem to indicate that information provision alone is ineffective, better matches between target populations and message content may result in relatively more effective change procedures. The methods used to study the effects of information provision do not lend themselves to an analysis of generalizability, maintenance, or individual variation. Outcomes have not been sufficiently favorable to permit a useful cost-benefit analysis.

Smoking has not been of great interest to contemporary psychodynamic theorists. Earlier writers viewed excessive smoking as the result of underlying conflicts stemming from childhood. Masochism (Green, 1923) has been suggested as an underlying cause, as has hostility toward parental figures which manifests itself in smoking and is assumed to be symbolic masturbatory activity (Bergler, 1946). The standard intervention is long-term analytic psychotherapy to resolve hidden conflicts. Overall, the evaluation of analytic treatment for smoking is similar to that for overeating. Although several case studies have been reported (Green, 1923; Bergler, 1946, 1953; Szasz, 1958), controlled studies are not available. Basic outcome issues, including premature termination, have not been addressed. Again, as with obesity, the model originated from work with a disturbed subset of individuals and is probably too expensive and limited in generalizability to be of much use when dealing with the majority of smokers.

As in the case of obesity, most well-controlled research in smoking cessation has been conducted from a social learning perspective. A social learning analysis conceptualizes smoking as a habit maintained by a variety of factors, including the physiologic effects of nicotine, social reinforcement, and anxiety reduction. Such a formulation leads to several intervention strategies; some seem more promising than others. Strategies used include: electrical aversion procedures, where smoking urges or actual smoking behaviors are paired with electrical shock; rapid smoking, where clients smoke every six seconds until they reach a point just short of nausea; and a variety of self-control procedures, such as confining smoking to a specific area, gradually decreasing situations where smoking takes place, contracts between smokers to decrease smoking, and self-administered shock or punishment in the client's home environment. Lichtenstein and Danaher (1976), in their comprehensive review of the literature on behavioral approaches to smoking cessation, tentatively concluded that rapid smoking shows the greatest promise for smoking cessation but that maintenance of abstinence is a major issue.

When applied in a clinical setting, rapid smoking generally produces abstinence rates of 90 percent or greater at termination; at six months, abstinence is usually around 60 percent. Although no clinically useful predictors of individual variability in abstinence are available, these rates are consistently higher than those obtained with educational procedures or those reported by other smoking cessation treatments in general, including other behavioral ones, in which abstinence rates at six months are often nearer to the rate of 20 percent cited by Hunt, Barnett, and Branch (1971, pp. 455-456) as typical of the field. The one long-term follow-up available, however, yielded disappointing data. Abstinence rates ranged from 35 percent to 24 percent at follow-ups from two to six years (Lichtenstein and Rodrigues, 1977, p. 111). Strategies to enhance maintenance have been evaluated, but results are inconclusive at best (Colleti and Kopel, 1977; Kopel, 1974). Similarly inconclusive results have been produced when self-control strategies, designed to improve maintenance, are added to rapid-smoking treatment (Danaher, 1977).

Generalizability of rapid smoking poses some interesting problems. It has been suggested that the technique causes such rapid intake of carbon monoxide and nicotine that it may be dangerous, especially for individuals with cardiac and pulmonary disorders (Hall, Sachs, and Hall, in press; Horan and others, 1977; Sachs, Hall, and Hall, 1978), and that all individuals who apply for the treatment should receive physical examinations to rule out these disorders. The obvious implication is that those whose health is most endangered from smoking would be the least likely to be accepted into a smoking cessation program of this type.

Because of the small number of sessions required, almost total cessation rates, and low attrition rates—usually less than 10 percent of the total sample—rapid smoking is quite cost effective. It can be offered in groups, as well as individually. It would seem possible, if safety issues are favorably resolved, that the treatment could be modified to be primarily self-administered. In summary, information dissemination alone, suggested by the rational model, is not an adequate treatment technique in smoking. As in obesity, however, it seems to be a necessary but not sufficient condition for change: How many of those who have quit smoking via rapid smoking would have done so had they not believed that smoking is related to lung cancer? The usefulness of the psychodynamic approach appears limited in much the same way in smoking cessation as in obesity, in terms of both cost and generalizability.

Rapid smoking appears to be the most efficacious treatment available. However, problems of maintenance and, more importantly, problems of safety are unresolved. The latter may ultimately limit the use of the technique to that segment of the population for which smoking is least dangerous—young, healthy smokers—and may exclude those at highest risk for health problems. Although other behavioral approaches appear promising, such as punishment of smoking urges (Berecz, 1974), there are not enough data on which to evaluate them. Some writers (Adesso, 1977) have suggested that controlled smoking is a goal to be considered as an alternative outcome for clients who cannot or will not abstain. A similar point of view is being debated in the field of alcoholism and is discussed in the following section. The true utility of this approach awaits determination of what level of cigarette intake, if any, is not injurious to health.

Alcoholism

The rational approach emphasizes the alcoholic's lack of information about the effects of his or her drinking. The appropriate intervention would include information about the causes and consequences of drinking and perhaps information about how to stop drinking. Informational approaches are usually included as components of multifaceted treatment programs. However, given the devastating, immediate feedback of excess alcohol consumption for the alcoholic, it is generally assumed that additional information via formal programs will in itself not result in marked changes; therefore, no attempts have been reported where information alone is the intervention modality.

Psychodynamic writers conceptualize the alcoholic as a self-centered person who is fixated at the oral stage of development and who has problems with dependency as well as a history of poor relationships with parents. Again, intensive psychotherapy is the suggested cure, if the alcoholic is sufficiently motivated to become involved in it—which is often not the case. In general, research indicates that there is little empirical evidence for the efficacy of psychotherapy (Hayman, 1956; Hill and Blane, 1967; Levinson and Sereny, 1969; Moore and Ramseur, 1960; Voegtlin and Lemere, 1942) or group therapy (Baekeland, Lundwall, and Kissin, 1975; Ends and Page, 1957, 1959; Mindlin and Belden, 1965; Wolff, 1968).

As is the case with smoking, a social learning analysis of the etiology of alcoholism emphasizes the use of the drug to avoid problems, to relax, and to experience a modified physiological state. While the addictive aspects of drinking are not denied, major importance is given to the effects of imitation or modeling of others' behavior and social reinforcement as factors in the development and maintenance of excessive drinking. Most evaluations of social learning approaches focus on aversion therapy and indicate wide variation in success rates (Anant, 1967; Edlin and others, 1945; Kant, 1945; Miller, 1959), although nausea-producing substances seem to be the most effective aversion stimuli (Blake, 1965, 1967; Farrar, Powell, and Martin, 1968; Hsu, 1965; Laverty, 1966; Sanderson, Campbell, and Laverty, 1963). Approaches that go beyond extinction of drinking and attempt to establish alternative coping behaviors (Bandura, 1969) through the use of operant reinforcement procedures report encouraging results in terms of achieving abstinence or controlling drinking (Hunt and Azrin, 1973; Lovibond and Caddy, 1970; Sobell and Sobell, 1972, 1973).

Alcoholism treatment evaluations indicate little, if any, significant difference among treatments (Emrick, 1975; Wallgren and Barry, 1970). A recent report to Congress on the "state of the art" of alcoholism treatment and research concludes that all approaches have discouraging results and that the mechanisms of alcohol intoxication and addiction remain "outstanding fundamental questions" (National Institute of Alcohol Abuse and Alcoholism, 1974).

Alcoholism research is in a much more primitive state than is the case in the other self-destructive disorders. Part of the problem may be the lack of separation between research and treatment programs, which often results in a reluctance to withhold treatments from control subjects or to randomly assign subjects to different treatments. Evaluation is complicated further because, unlike treatments developed for smoking and obesity, alcoholism treatments almost always have combined modalities. Most treatments include counseling, in both individual and group contexts, and the use of drugs as an adjunctive therapy. Family therapy is being added to many programs to facilitate changes in aspects of the social system that may be supporting alcoholic behavior. Alcoholics Anonymous is often used in conjunction with formal treatment programs. All promising approaches seem to be included in a single treatment strategy which precludes controlled study.

An issue that is the focus of much controversy in the field of alcoholism, as in smoking research, is that of abstinence versus controlled use as a treatment goal. Recent research appears to indicate that at least some alcoholics can control their drinking in a variety of situations and that, following treatment, some alcoholics do drink moderately and may improve social functioning while doing so (Lloyd and Salzberg, 1975; Miller, 1977). This is in direct contradiction to the traditional view that alcoholism involves a diseaselike progression of symptoms and that, because alcoholics cannot regain control over drinking, total abstinence is the only acceptable goal of treatment. Clearly, further research is needed on this controversial issue.

Conclusions

At present, the behavioral model appears to be the most promising in terms of the development of useful treatment interventions in cases of smoking, obesity, and, possibly, alcoholism. The contribution of the rational model to the decision to enter a treatment program and to set goals must also be noted. Empirically, the psychodynamic model has fared least well, but it seems premature to discard the potential of the model for developing intervention strategies in the future. Specifically, two points bear further thought: First, the psychodynamic model is intuitively feasible—after all, there is something quite irrational about misusing substances to the point of death or refusing to adhere to a simple treatment regimen that would aid one in terminating the use of such substances. It makes sense to explore further the importance of such emotionally based "resistances" that hinder the implementation of behavioral change strategies. Second, as we have noted, behavior modification frequently produces tremendous interindividual variability. It is possible that at least some of the variability is due to emotional factors that prevent adherence to the self-management regimen. In addition, it should be remembered that the failure of traditional analytic methods in effecting behavior change in self-destructive behaviors is a reflection of the adequacy of the interventions derived from the model to this point. It is possible that more appropriate interventions will be derived that will provide needed enrichment to other techniques.

Methodologically, more attention needs to be focused on the unresolved research issues raised in the foregoing sections. There is a great need for carefully designed and well-controlled studies that build on each other and that deal in detail with problems of subject variability, dropouts, generalizability of study results, cost effectiveness, and long-term maintenance.

It is our conclusion that a more comprehensive, conceptual perspective is needed that takes into account all of the social, cultural, political, and economic influences affecting individual health behavior. Specifically, the individual needs to be viewed in light of the beliefs and values of the society in which he or she lives. For example, it is clear that the very same self-destructive substances that health providers are attempting to control are often supported politically and economically by powerful lobbies, supportive legislation, and well-financed advertising campaigns. The population is bombarded with products considered to be health hazards, such as cigarettes, alcohol, and foods high in saturated fat, cholesterol, sugar, salt, and calories. In addition, traditional concepts of health and illness often do not include individual responsibility for preventing serious illness. Rather, there is a belief in the ability of the medical profession to cure illness after the onset of symptoms. Children in the society learn through modeling of adult behaviors that self-destructive patterns can be generally accepted and socially appropriate. It may be a more sensible approach to attempt to prevent individuals from starting a self-destructive behavior in the first place since, clearly, changing adult behavior is a difficult and often unsuccessful endeavor. Programs designed to educate and influence the behavior of children and parents may well be a most cost-effective approach. In any case, intervention programs need to deal with the powerful influences of the media and other channels of communication from the manufacturers of high-risk products.

7

Why People
Seek Health Care

Irwin M. Rosenstock

John P. Kirscht

This chapter will focus on theory and data concerning the ways in which people reach their decisions to use or not to use health services. In this effort, we will summarize but not emphasize descriptive data on how people and which people use various health services. We will, thus, not be concerned with estimating the total number of visits to providers or facilities according to sociodemographic classifications but will, instead, focus on explanations of utilization rather than on the extent of utilization.

Several definitional problems need to be resolved before an orderly presentation is feasible. These include definitions of the various kinds of behavior to be explained and what is meant by use or utilization.

With respect to the kinds of behavior to be included, we use a distinction first reported by Kasl and Cobb (1966). Drawing on categories defined earlier (Mechanic and Volkart, 1961; Parsons, 1951b), they distinguish three classifications of health-related behavior. The first, *health behavior*, is defined as activity undertaken by individuals who believe themselves to be healthy for the purpose of preventing disease or detecting disease in an asymptomatic state. This is in contrast with *illness behavior*, defined as activity undertaken by individuals who feel ill for the purpose of defining the

161

state of their health and of discovering suitable remedy, and with *sick role behavior*, which includes activity undertaken by those who consider themselves ill for the purpose of getting well. While the present chapter will consider all three of these types of behavior, sick role behavior is discussed in greater detail in Chapter Eight.

It is very likely that the three-part specification of health-related behavior first posited by Kasl and Cobb should be expanded to include the concept of the "at risk" role described by Baric (1969). The individual at risk is somewhere between the state of health and the state of experiencing symptoms. People at risk include those engaged in certain activities that increase their risk of illness to a much higher degree than that of the rest of the population. Baric's examples include "middle-aged men who are obese, smoke cigarettes, and have a raised blood pressure, drivers of cars who also enjoy alcoholic drinks, people who are working with lead or certain kinds of oils" (1969, p. 27). It is clear, though Baric does not say so explicitly, that the risk must be perceived as such for it to have any impact on the decision making of the person at risk. That is, the middle-aged, male cigarette smoker who has no awareness of his increased risk of heart disease will not consider himself to be at risk and will therefore take no action on that account.

With respect to the meaning of use or utilization of health services, it seems useful to consider not only the occurrence or nonoccurrence of a single contact with a health provider or agency but also to consider delays in seeking care and the problem of dropouts in the seeking of care. Although those who drop out are clearly of major importance in sick role behavior because they may not be receiving care for their conditions, they are also important in accounting for utilization of preventive and diagnostic services. Moreover, some attention should be given to the outcome of referrals and to so-called inappropriate use of services.

The distinction between health and illness is blurred both from the patient-client's point of view and the provider's point of view. From the client's point of view, it is rare, if indeed it ever occurs, that one is continuously free of bodily stimuli that are capable of being interpreted as symptoms. In fact, symptoms occur much of the time in virtually all people (Mechanic, 1972b; Zola, 1973). We will deal later with the role of symptoms in explaining health-related behavior and with group differences in symptom definitions. At this point, it needs only to be noted that most people are frequently in a position to describe themselves as having symptoms. How many of us never experience a twinge of pain, stiffness of muscles, a cough, sneeze, more fatigue than usual, and so on? Yet, Kosa and Robertson (1975, p. 43) point out that one widely accepted view is to define illness in the patient's terms: "Whoever feels ill should be regarded as sick." These authors emphasize the importance of attending to the subjective base leading any prospective patient to the doctor. Most decisions to seek care are self-initiated and have a voluntary component. However, they point out, such a criterion raises a problem of its own, that of distinguishing between a "bio-negative feeling" (p. 43) and a so-called objective state of disease. At the opposite pole from the purely subjective definition of illness is the simplistic medical view that illness is any state that has been so diagnosed by a competent professional. Such a definition also poses problems. Many, in fact most, illnesses are never brought before professionals (Kosa and Robertson, 1975). In other cases, professionals are not unanimous in their diagnosis. Clearly, neither definition of illness is entirely satisfactory.

Another approach that has some intuitive appeal has been to consider interference with normal functioning as the hallmark of illness. The person who can function reasonably effectively in his or her societal roles can be regarded as healthy. But this approach, too, has difficulties. For one thing, it does not take account of the at-risk role; the obese hypertensive who also smokes and drinks but is currently fulfilling all role demands and expectations would be regarded as healthy according to the disability criterion. It is also apparent that decisions about illness definition are heavily influenced by nonphysiological states. This influence can be illustrated by an example. Apply the disability criterion to two men who have had recent severe myocardial infarctions, one of whom is a laborer and the other a white-collar worker. The white-collar worker would have to be regarded as healthy (or at most, at risk) if, as is probable, he could return to his job, while the laborer would have to be regarded as sick if a change in occupation were required.

Complicating the definitional problem of health and illness is the changing nature of the prevalent illnesses. Up to fifty years ago, the leading causes of morbidity and mortality in the United States were the acute infectious diseases. In the last half century, however, the chronic diseases have assumed increasing importance. Many diabetics, hypertensives, survivors of heart attack, arthritics, and others do not usually feel ill and can function effectively in their social roles. Are they to be regarded as sick or healthy?

A developing view of disease causation holds that a great many social, psychological, physical, and environmental variables are involved (Kosa and Robertson, 1975). The field of social epidemiology is dedicated to the view that disease occurs only as a consequence of such interactions, and it would appear that in the future such concepts will assume increasing importance. That is, it seems likely that disease will come to be seen as incorporating physiological elements—including genetic factors—and social and psychological predispositions, as well as influences from the social or physical environment, all of which come together in producing conditions defined as disease.

Another perspective for viewing health and illness is the normative-statistical one. Both ends of any dimension of normality, of course, focus on deviations from some standard (Mechanic, 1968). However, they have different implications with regard to the proportion of a population that can be regarded as deviant or sick. The normative approach is so called because it applies norms to the situation being considered. In the case of normative definitions, the standard is usually an arbitrary one, frequently set by providers but sometimes by lay persons. The physician who decides that a client is obese by reference to an internal standard of normality is using a normative definition. The individual who regards a given amount of alcohol consumption as abnormal is also using a normative definition. However, deviance may be regarded in a statistical sense as variations from the arithmetic mean or some other measure of central tendency. Thus, if a person who is 20 percent heavier than the average weight for height in the population is declared to be overweight or obese, a statistical definition has been used. In the statistical approach, the average is normal by definition, and the number of persons who are called abnormal is limited. In the normative approach, everybody or the majority may be deviants from the norm and therefore abnormal or sick.

In the subsequent discussion of research on use of health services, it will be necessary to accept the authors' stated or implied definitions of health and disease, which may vary widely from study to study. However, in efforts to *explain* health-related behavior, we shall generally adopt a phenomenological, that is, client-centered point of view.

Approaches to Explaining Health-Related Behavior

McKinlay (1972) has identified six major theoretical orientations that characterize most of the research directed toward explaining health-related behavior: economic, sociodemographic, geographic, sociopsychological, sociocultural, and organizational. These are presented briefly to show the reader the range of explanatory schemes that characterize research on health-related behavior.

The Economic Approach

The emphasis here is on the impact of financial barriers on seeking health care. McKinlay concludes that this approach is good as far as it goes—certainly financial barriers to care are important—but it has been shown that even when such barriers are reduced or eliminated, fairly wide variations still exist among income and ethnic groups; the poor tend to underutilize compared with the nonpoor.

The Sociodemographic Approach

In this approach, utilization rates are analyzed for various easy to identify subgroups. We learn from such studies that utilization tends to be higher for females, is correlated with age, income, and education, and is lower for nonwhites than whites. The problem with this approach is that no explanation is offered of *why* differences exist, and any obtained relationship is inevitably explained in other terms. Also, this approach typically provides no analysis or explanation of the wide variations that exist within groups; for example, while females use health services more than males, a great many females use them rarely and many males use health services frequently.

The Geographic Approach

This approach examines the association between geographic proximity of services to clients and utilization rates. McKinlay concludes that there is no clear evidence that geographic convenience within metropolitan areas is of great importance. Of course, it is well known that utilization rates are higher in urban than in rural areas (Aday and Andersen, 1974).

The Sociopsychological Approach

In this approach, the emphasis is on motivation, perception, and learning. The Health Belief Model, described in Chapter Three, exemplifies the social psychological approach. This model will be applied to preventive health behavior, illness behavior, and sick role behavior later in this chapter.

The Sociocultural Approach

The sociocultural approach, not vastly different from the sociopsychological approach, emphasizes values, norms, beliefs, and life-styles. This approach focuses on the differences among various socioeconomic groups.

The Organizational or Delivery System Approach

This approach emphasizes the elements of a system that foster or impede utilization. For example, researchers have suggested that large organizations, in order to survive, may neglect clients in greatest need of their services, that is, those with more difficult problems to treat or those whose ways of life are different from those of the providers. It has also been observed by researchers in this area that the delivery system may be so arranged as to maximize the convenience of the providers at the expense of the clients, who may be shuffled around from agency to agency and forced to submit to what has been called the "revolving door" approach to health services delivery (Levine and others, 1969).

Relationships between the individual and medical care services also affect the extent to which services will be obtained. It is known that the quality of the encounter between the patient and the provider will modify patient behavior. A study by Francis, Korsch, and Morris (1969) found that the extent to which patient concerns were met in the interaction with physicians related both to patient satisfaction and to subsequent adherence to medical recommendations. The degree of patient satisfaction itself is affected by the relationship to the source of care. Becker, Drachman, and Kirscht (1974) report that continuity of care was an important predictor of satisfaction with a source of care. While medical need and absence of barriers directly affect choice of services for an illness disturbance (Anderson and Bartkus, 1973), it is also true that conditioned reactions will affect perceptions of the value of services offered. In a study of illness behavior, Hallauer (1972) found that reinforcement given for this behavior directly related to how it was expressed.

Utilization of Preventive Services

Any effort to explain preventive health behavior requires an initial consideration of several underlying issues. One issue, which has never been satisfactorily addressed, is the question of whether the concept of health per se constitutes a cognitive structure (such as hunger) or whether it is without phenomenological meaning for most people, constituting rather a construct invented by analysts. The question is whether behavior can be better explained by invoking the concept of health and attributing some organizing and motivating characteristics to it or whether behavior is better explained by considering particular kinds of health-related matters that may be poorly related or unrelated to each other.

This, of course, is an empirical matter but one that has not been well studied. We do not know with any great degree of assurance whether people can be arrayed along a dimension of health consciousness or possession of a health concept in a manner that will be useful in explaining or predicting their subsequent behavior. There is evidence (Becker, Drachman, and Kirscht, 1972b) that a tendency to be aroused by health-related stimuli and a general concern for health has value in explaining mothers' decisions to adhere to a prescribed regimen for their children. But in another setting (Becker and others, 1975), general concern with health did not explain peoples' decisions to participate in a program to detect the Tay-Sachs trait. It should be noted that the first of these studies concerned behavior under conditions of diagnosed illness, whereas the second concerned behavior while in the healthy state. Perhaps health consciousness helps to explain illness or sickness behavior but is less valuable in explaining preventive behavior. It has been shown (Haefner and Kirscht, 1970) that although there were positive correlations among four preventive health actions that were studied, these correlations were quite modest. This finding supports the notion that general health orientation has no strong explanatory or predictive value for preventive health behavior. It should, however, be noted that the four preventive actions studied (chest x rays, medical and dental visits in the absence of symptoms, and toothbrushing after meals) were not selected to represent the universe of actions that could have been studied. Other behavior might have shown stronger or weaker intercorrelations.

While there is uncertainty as to whether knowledge of a person's behavior in one health-related situation improves the accuracy of prediction of an unrelated health behavior, there is little question that such knowledge is of virtually no value in predicting behaviors that are not commonly thought of as health behavior, but which could affect health (Williams and Wechsler, 1972). For example, the person who regularly seeks medical checkups in the absence of symptoms is no more likely to use seat belts regularly than the person who does not obtain such checkups—nor is the person who uses seat belts, or buys insurance, or keeps a fire extinguisher in the home, any more or less likely to be careful of diet, exercise regularly, or visit the dentist regularly.

A second question concerns behaviors that may have impact on health but which are undertaken or avoided for reasons clearly unrelated to health. Toothbrushing seems to exemplify such a behavior. Adults who habitually brush their teeth shortly after arising each day and have done so since childhood probably learned the behavior during early socialization and continued it for reasons unrelated to dental health. In the adult, the behavior is triggered by the various stimuli that become associated with the toothbrushing response—waking up, experiencing an undesirable taste, and the like. Probably a great many of our behaviors that have implications for health are of this habitual sort. Our patterns of eating have large habitual components reflecting nearly automatic, rather than reasoned responses to particular stimuli. Habits, rather than conscious planning, influence greatly the types of foods we prefer, the amounts we eat, and the speed of eating. Our immediate responses to symptoms are almost certainly habitual—whether we attend to them or disregard them, whether we mention them to a friend or immediately reach for the phone to call the doctor.

The foregoing considerations have important implications both for understanding, predicting, and modifying behavior. Appeals to children to adopt specific, healthful behavior patterns should not be restricted to those connected with health motives—if indeed, health motives exist—but should rather appeal to the entire panoply of motives and incentives relevant to the issue. The ethical issue, of course, always has to be considered. Unlike dentifrice manufacturers, health professionals cannot promise that use of a particular toothpaste will improve one's sex life, but within our cultural and subcultural values, we can ethically state that the likelihood of more attractive teeth will be enhanced by the regular use of dental hygiene procedures, including toothbrushing. What we are saying is if there is no overall health dimension influencing a wide variety of behaviors and if many behaviors that affect health are automatic and not based on "health motives," those who wish to modify behavior should be prepared to appeal to the motives that do exist to guide current behavior. While the issue of whether the global concept—health—has valuable psychological organizing characteristics is unsettled, it is almost certainly true that specific health threats do have such characteristics. These will be discussed later.

A third issue concerning preventive health behavior relates to the ways in which people seek satisfaction of a dominant or regnant motive. An important dimension in choice of action is that of self-care versus professional care. Parents who are motivated to prevent a particular disease, say polio, in their children, may do so by obtaining professional help (immunization), or they may seek to prevent the disease through their own actions, for example, through prayer, by keeping their children away from swimming pools during the polio season, and the like. The current movement in the direction of self-care (Levin, 1977) generally relates to the views held by policy makers that strains on the health care system could be reduced if people were encouraged to handle "minor" problems on their own and if they did not use emergency rooms for nonemergency conditions. However, the rationale underlying self-care also includes an implicit notion that the way people handle these minor nonemergency conditions will be in accord with what the professionals would do if they were given responsibility. The advocates of self-care, while acknowledging the fact that humans have always used self-care more than professional care, apparently disregard the fact that the choice of action made by the individual, based as it is on cultural and subcultural values and norms, may or may not be in accord with modern medical wisdom. This issue is introduced here to illustrate the point that the nature and the direction of behavior aroused by a motive cannot be predicted from a mere knowledge of the nature of the stimuli arousing the motive and from identification of the motive itself. Dietary fads, perhaps, provide the best current examples of the range of things people will do to prevent illness. The widespread use of vitamin C and of garlic are but two examples of behaviors not generally endorsed by the medical establishment which people have adopted in their desire to prevent disease. (All of us would probably agree that the heavy use of garlic prevents a number of things, but there might be less agreement as to what exactly it prevents.)

Demographic Variations in Preventive Health Behavior

Analyzing the major findings of studies on the patterns of use of preventive and detection services permits certain summary generalizations about the association of personal characteristics with the use of services. In general, such services are used most by younger or middle-aged people, by females, and by those who are relatively better educated and have higher income (though perhaps not the very highest levels of education and income). Striking differences may nearly always be found in acceptance rates between whites and nonwhites, with whites generally showing higher acceptance rates, although occasional exceptions occur (Borsky and Sagen, 1959; Kasl and Cobb, 1966; Kegeles, Lotzkar, and Andrews, 1959; Somers and Somers, 1961; U.S. Department of Health, Education, and Welfare, 1960a, 1960b, 1977).

It has been suggested that the frequency of health supervision visits is increasing—that is, of visits to practitioners in the absence of symptoms (Alpert and others, 1970). A question may be raised as to whether such increases, if indeed they are occurring, show the typical social class gradient, with those of higher income accounting for most of the increase. There are no definitive data on the subject, but inferences can be drawn from a combination of findings from several sources. Herman (1972) notes, as have many others, that although higher rates of disease and mortality still persist among those with very low incomes, their frequency of visiting the physician is considerably lower than for the more affluent, healthier group. It is commonly known that even when immunizations are free, higher-income families show a much better rate of protection than do poorer families. Moreover, whereas ambulatory services generally show a lower utilization rate by lower-income households, poor people are overrepresented among hospital patients; their hospitalization rates are as high as, or higher than, those of upper-income levels and their length of stay longer on the average. This probably reflects the failure to receive treatment at earlier stages of disease and disability.

Although some of these data are not as recent as one would like, there seems to be no reason for concluding that the poor, as yet, are showing any marked increase in their likelihood of seeking preventive health services, compared to their prior behavior or to the behavior of the more affluent. This is not to say that the removal of economic and social barriers will not increase the use of health services; indeed, it may well do so. In an experiment oriented to use of both preventive and curative services (Alpert and others, 1970), it was shown that after exposure to comprehensive, personalized health care, low-income families (median income of $4,100) became more satisfied with the services received, reported an increased likelihood of using a family doctor or pediatrician for selected medical problems of children, and reported a greater likelihood of using the telephone as a first contact. Nevertheless, it is still questionable whether such attitudinal changes will result in patterns of use of preventive health services that are like those of the more affluent.

The work of Monteiro (1973) suggests that the poor do not always have lower utilization of services. Using data from the 1968 National Health Survey, she demonstrates that persons with incomes between $3,000 and $10,000 made fewer visits to physicians than those with either lower or higher incomes. These data do not distinguish preventive from curative visits. Monteiro also reports a study in Rhode Island, conducted in 1967, 1968, and 1969, with a follow-up in 1971, that confirms the national data. The author herself notes that there may be wide differences as to what is defined as illness, a topic she did not study. Thus, the poor may tolerate more severe morbidity before restricting their activity and, in fact, go to the doctor with much more serious illness than the nonpoor. Since it has been shown that the poor have substantially higher levels of morbidity than the nonpoor, if income were unrelated to utilization one might expect that the poor would visit the physician much more often than the nonpoor. Other crucial criticisms can be leveled at Monteiro's interpretations, for she merely used gross counts of doctor visits, a measure that has always been regarded as fairly crude. If she had studied the purposes of the visits or the use of other professional providers—for example, dentists—she would likely have found what has so often been reported in the National Health Survey and by other investigators, namely, that the poor show substantially lower utilization than the nonpoor of each of the following kinds of primarily preventive services: routine physical examinations (under age seventeen); visits to pediatricians (under age seventeen); visits by women to obstetricians; visits to dentists within the past year and, within that category, rate of dental restorations versus extractions; obtaining tests for cervical cancer; seeking regular chest x rays; obtaining polio immunizations; and brushing teeth regularly.

What Monteiro's study seems to show is that publicly financed care will increase utilization among poor people experiencing substantial medical need. However, other research shows that the level of utilization for less disabling conditions, and the use of preventive services, remains highly correlated with income—the poor receive far less of such services than the nonpoor. It may also be emphasized that within comparable income categories, utilization of services tends to be substantially higher for whites than nonwhites (U.S. Department of Health, Education, and Welfare, 1977). Even where preventive services are designed expressly for low-income groups, there is evidence that the relatively more advantaged within those groups (that is, those with a higher level of education) will respond more frequently, and the services will be utilized by persons who are not members of the target group but who are already predisposed to use the available preventive care (Elinson, Henshaw, and Cohen, 1976).

Why People Use Preventive Health Services

If we can take it as demonstrated that the poor and nonwhite use preventive health services less, how are we to understand this difference? While a variety of theoretical models have been formulated to account for illness and sick role behavior, far less attention has been given to the study of preventive health behavior and, consequently, fewer explanatory models have been proposed. It is not surprising that the Health Belief Model has received the most attention in this area because that model was originally developed solely to account for preventive health actions. However, there have also been efforts to interpret variations in preventive health behavior in terms of differing characteristics of the social groups to which individuals belong. A variety of such formulations have been developed. According to Langlie (1977), perhaps the earliest and most widely known is one developed by Suchman (1964) which Langlie names the Social Network Model. In fact, the Suchman model to which Langlie refers was specifically directed toward explaining illness behavior. Suchman himself proposed a separate model for preventive health behavior (1967), which will be described later. But let us consider Langlie's reference first, since it does have implications for preventive behavior.

In Suchman's view, the core of the model refers to the location of the individual in a group structure varying from parochial to cosmopolitan. Such groups display health orientations that differ along a dimension of popular (folk) to scientific. Parochial groups exhibit traditional family orientations, ethnic exclusivity, and friendship solidarity. They are presumed to have popular or folk health orientations and therefore to be less likely to adhere to the norms of the medical profession than are cosmopolitan groups. In the same vein, Green (1970) hypothesizes that the relationship between socioeconomic status and preventive health behavior is due both to a higher likelihood of interaction with nonkin, which increases the likelihood of encountering people who display preventive behavior, and to more "scientific" preventive health behavior norms within the higher social strata. More recently, components of social network models have been shown to help explain preventive health behavior. For example, Bullough (1972) found lower levels of utilization of preventive care to be partly attributable to the direct consequence of poverty (that is, inability to pay and a low educational level) but reinforced by the subculture of poverty, including feelings of powerlessness, hopelessness, and social isolation. She found that poverty and minority ethnic identification are related to such feelings of alienation. It is important to note that in her study dental care was primarily dependent upon income, but all the other failures to obtain care by mothers for themselves and their children were most likely due to alienation arising from membership in the subculture of poverty and minority status.

As indicated, most research designed to explain preventive health behavior has been, in one way or another, influenced by or has employed variables in the Health Belief Model. There have been studies of participation in cancer-screening programs (Kegeles and others, 1965), polio vaccination programs (Rosenstock, Derryberry, and Carriger, 1959), dental care (Kegeles, Lotzkar, and Andrews, 1959), tuberculosis-screening programs (Hochbaum, 1958), penicillin prophylaxis (Heinzelmann, 1962), influenza vaccination (Leventhal, Hochbaum, and Rosenstock, 1960), genetic screening programs (Becker and others, 1975), and many others.

The details of the Health Belief Model will not be given here since they are described in Chapter Three. The reader will recall that the major components of the current formulation of the model (which has been somewhat modified from its original formulation) include health-related motivations, subjective estimates of susceptibility to and severity of illness, and subjective estimates of the benefits or efficacy of any proposed regimens minus the perceived barriers to taking such action. It is also believed that sociodemographic and structural variables influence the perceived susceptibility and severity of various states of ill health, as well as the perceived benefits of and barriers to specified preventive action. Three significant studies will be described briefly. The first, by Hochbaum (1958), is selected because it is the first to have employed major components of the Health Belief Model; the second, by Becker and others (1975), because it is one of the most recent on preventive health behavior; and the third, by Haefner and Kirscht (1970), because it represents an effort to modify selected health beliefs and, consequently, behavior.

Hochbaum (1958) studied more than 1,200 adults in three cities in an attempt to identify factors underlying the decision to obtain a chest x ray for the detection of tuberculosis. He tapped beliefs concerning susceptibility to tuberculosis and beliefs in the benefits of early detection. Perceived susceptibility to tuberculosis contained two subelements—the respondent's beliefs about whether tuberculosis was a real possibility in his or her case, and the extent to which he or she accepted the fact that one may have tuberculosis in the absence of all symptoms. Perceived benefits of early detection tapped respondents' views about how much difference it made in the prognosis whether tuberculosis was detected early or late. According to Hochbaum's findings, of the group of persons that exhibited both beliefs—that is, belief in their own susceptibility to tuberculosis and the belief that overall benefits would accrue from early detection—82 percent had had at least one voluntary chest x ray during a specified period preceding the interview. Of the group exhibiting neither of these beliefs, only 21 percent had obtained a voluntary x ray during the criterion.

Belief in one's susceptibility to tuberculosis appeared to be the more powerful variable studied. For the individuals who exhibited this belief without accepting the benefits of early detection, 64 percent had obtained prior voluntary x rays. Of the individuals accepting the benefits of early detection without accepting their susceptibility to the disease, only 29 percent had had prior voluntary x rays (1958, p. 10).

Hochbaum failed to show clearly that perceived severity plays a role in the decision-making process. This may be due to the fact that his study was not designed to identify perceived severity with any high degree of accuracy and his measures of severity proved not to be sensitive. However, his data are in accord with the widespread view that the relationship of perceived severity with health behavior is curvilinear. He identified sixteen individuals who seemed intensely afraid of tuberculosis; none of them had had a single voluntary x ray during the preceding eight-year period. In addition, those respondents who appeared indifferent to the disease were among those who tended not to feel susceptible and, consequently, not to take x rays. Finally, those who exhibited some "mid-range" level of fear participated to a slightly greater extent than those at the very high or low end of the scale.

Becker and others (1975) applied the Health Belief Model to the area of genetic screening. Beginning in 1971, an identified Jewish population in the Baltimore-Washington area was invited to participate in screening for the Tay-Sachs trait, which has a frequency of about 1 in 30 Jews of Ashkenazi ancestry (compared with 1 in 300 among non-Jews). Tay-Sachs disease, an incurable condition that is always fatal in early childhood, can be diagnosed prenatally through amniocentesis at a stage when abortion is feasible. Thus, the situation presents all the conditions for observing the role of the components of the Health Belief Model in predicting preventive health behavior. Furthermore, since this relatively rare disease and the diagnostic test for it were largely unknown to the lay public, it is a reasonable inference that the majority had had little contact with the disease, with screening, or with amniocentesis and that they had few relevant beliefs about it in advance of the program.

Multiple educational approaches were used to saturate the communities with accurate and clear information about the screening. Since lists of the target population were available, it was believed that all members of the target group—couples of childbearing age—were exposed to at least some of these educational activities. As applied to the Tay-Sachs situation, the explanatory variables were defined as follows: "Health motive" was, for the first time, explicitly introduced as a variable in the model to explain health behavior. In the present case, this motive was considered to include two components: a positive response indicating a desire to have (additional) children, and a set of generalized items about typical health behavior, such as the frequency with which the respondents thought about their own health and whether they generally went to a physician right away if they felt ill. Another variable, "perceived susceptibility," included respondents' beliefs that they could carry the Tay-Sachs gene and transmit it to their progeny. Perceived severity of the disease was not directly measured in this study. However, the perceived impact of learning that one was a carrier was measured in terms of how it would affect future plans to have (additional) children. The definition of perceived benefits was in terms of a personal evaluation of how much good it would do potential carriers to be screened for the trait: Did they really need to know or want to know their carrier status? Costs or barriers to action were not directly measured in this study.

All adults who appeared for screening, some 7,000 in the first year, were asked to complete a brief questionnaire just before going through the screening process; 500 of these were selected at random as the participant sample. In addition, 500 questionnaires were mailed to a random sample of nonparticipants who had been invited in for screening; here the response rate was 82 percent. It should be noted that nonrespondents as well as respondents had received intensive informational material on Tay-Sachs disease and screening.

The analysis showed that the participants, compared to nonparticipants, were significantly younger, had had fewer children, were less likely to have completed their families, and were slightly better educated. The participants and nonparticipants differed sharply on the measure of health motivation—82 percent of those who expressed the desire to have future children participated in the screening program, while less than 19 percent who did not desire future children participated (1975, p. 6). There was no significant difference in participation according to general health behavior. Mean score on perceived susceptibility to being a carrier was highly correlated with participation in the screening program, whereas perceived impact of learning one was a carrier was negatively associated with participation.

Among those individuals who indicated that they planned to have more children, the nonparticipants more than the participants indicated that the discovery that either husband or wife was a carrier, or that both were carriers, would change their future child-planning behavior; frequently they reported they would have no additional children. One possible interpretation of this finding related to beliefs exhibited by participants and nonparticipants about the transmission and detection of Tay-Sachs disease and about reproductive alternatives. More of the participants had learned that carrier status in only one member of the couple poses no dangers. However, in response to the question on the impact if both parents were found to be carriers, although participants were again less likely to change their reproductive plans than nonparticipants, they did indicate they would reduce the number of children planned or they would use amniocentesis (fetal diagnostic test) in order to continue to have children. Very few of the nonparticipants displayed knowledge of the availability of amniocentesis; rather, they tended to indicate that in the event either member or both members of a couple were found to be carriers, they would not have further children.

Since more participants than nonparticipants learned about the "fetal diagnostic test," it may be inferred that screening resulted in considerable benefits for participants: (1) They could rule out the possibility that both partners carried the recessive gene. (2) If both proved to be carriers, amniocentesis could rule out the possibility that the fetus had the disease. (3) If the child were diseased, they could elect to abort it. Whereas nearly all the study respondents held attitudes favoring abortion in the event that a fetus had Tay-Sachs disease, the nonparticipants did not see as much benefit in screening, presumably because most of them had not learned about amniocentesis even though the information was provided to them.

Haefner and Kirscht (1970) attempted experimentally to increase people's readiness to follow preventive health practices by presenting them with messages about selected health problems. These messages were intended both to increase their perception of susceptibility and/or severity regarding the health problems and to strengthen their beliefs in the efficacy of professionally recommended behavior. As measured by a questionnaire administered soon after the messages, the experimental treatment was successful (compared to several control groups). Significantly more persons exposed to such messages visited a physician for a checkup in the eight months following the experimental manipulation, in comparison with a control group not exposed to the messages. This significant difference held only for visits made in the absence of symptoms, that is, preventive health behavior. For individuals reporting actual symptoms during the interval, the rate of physician visits was the same in the experimental and control groups. While income as such was not measured, the sample was drawn from a universe of nonacademic university employees, a group above the poverty level but, in general, far from affluent. This study provided direct evidence that it is possible to modify the perceived threat of disease—that is, the combination of perceived susceptibility to and severity of diseases—as well as the perceived efficacy of professional intervention, and that such modification leads to predictable changes in health behavior.

By way of closing this section, it seems appropriate to consider Suchman's (1967) early paper on preventive health behavior. Specifically, he studied factors influencing acceptance of an accident-preventive measure—a protective glove—among sugar cane cutters in Puerto Rico. Acceptance of the glove was found to be associated with a number of beliefs, including (among others) concern about having an accident, belief in one's vulnerability, belief in the efficacy of the glove, and beliefs about the convenience and comfort of the glove. These measure the essential elements of the Health Belief Model.

Illness Behavior

Demographic Variations

Having considered health-related behavior in the absence of symptoms, we turn now to a consideration of behavior undertaken in response to symptoms. In looking at utilization of services, illness behavior cannot be distinguished from sick role behavior because the available data do not distinguish between those with undiagnosed and those with diagnosed symptomatic conditions. A review of the data on utilization of diagnostic and treatment services suggests a pattern quite similar to that obtained in connection with preventive and detection services. In general, more females than males visit the physician and the dentist and incur hospitalization, even when hospitalization for pregnancy is excluded. Higher socioeconomic groupings (defined in terms of educational and income level) are also more likely to obtain medical, dental, and ambulatory hospital services, although the associations between income and utilization are becoming less marked in recent years (Aday and Andersen, 1974; Lerner and Anderson, 1963; Somers and Somers, 1961; U.S. Department of Health, Education, and Welfare, 1977). With reference to race, whites show much higher utilization rates than nonwhites in all three utilization categories—physician visits, dental visits, and hospitalization, though length of stay is greater for nonwhites who are hospitalized. As indicated earlier, poorer persons are overrepresented among hospital patients. Since the majority of poor persons are white, there is no discrepancy between the findings concerning hospitalization and poverty and hospitalization and race.

With respect to access, Aday and Andersen (1974) conclude that children are more likely to have a usual source of care that is convenient to them than are adults. Older adults, fifty-five and above, more often than others travel over an hour to reach care. Nonwhites less often have a usual source of care than do whites, and their care (travel time, appointment waiting time, and time spent in the office) is less convenient. Inner-city residents and rural farm dwellers are less likely to have a regular source of convenient care. People below the poverty level are more likely to have no regular source of care, to have to travel more than thirty minutes to obtain services, and to wait more than thirty minutes in the doctor's office than are the nonpoor.

Why People Use Medical Services

The basic problem of illness behavior concerns what individuals do in the presence of symptoms and why they do it (Kasl and Cobb, 1966). Short of initiation of professional treatment, there are many definitional and re-medial behaviors taken in the effort to cope with episodes of health dis-turbance. Many of the episodes are transitory and minor, but some eventuate in the adoption of the sick role and entail professional care. Some episodes will result in a decision to do nothing or to self-medicate, even though, from a professional medical point of view, the condition required professional attention. The timing of decisions to seek care is a further aspect of illness behavior (Zola, 1973), and there is some evidence that certain people will typically wait longer before acting on a disturbance (Becker, Drachman, and Kirscht, 1972b). The behavior that takes place in trying to define the state of one's illness is critical in the process leading to treatment, particularly be-cause so many of the decisions are self-initiated or at least lay initiated—hence, the importance of understanding illness behavior in relation to the utilization of health services, what conditions are seen professionally, delay in seeking care, and the use of nonprescribed medications and nostrums.

The function of illness behavior is that of defining one's health state in the presence of a health disturbance. The ways in which people go about defining their health state are extremely varied. First, reactions may range all the way from deciding to ignore the disturbance to seeking immediate pro-fessional care for the condition. There clearly are some conditions involving health—such as intractable pain, fractures resulting from accidents, or severe bleeding—in which the demand is so strong and urgent that virtually every-one in the population would immediately decide to seek care (Mechanic, 1968). Short of such urgency, however, there are many symptoms and con-ditions that are sufficiently vague to permit considerable latitude in interpre-tation and decision making (Fabrega, 1974). Second, the type of care sought for a health disturbance may be quite variable. Does one seek help from a physician, a chiropractor, a homeopath? Third, with respect to the forms of illness behavior, in many cases the health disturbance is seen as requiring the legitimation or approval of other persons in the environment prior to the sufferer's seeking care or acting on symptoms (Zola, 1966). The decisional processes and the alternatives available, taken together, permit considerable latitude in what is actually done in the face of many health threats. Let us consider now how actual behavior emerges from experience with symptoms and from social factors constraining response.

There are a number of known differences in response to health dis-turbances. First, there are differences in the ways in which symptoms are experienced. It has been pointed out that, contrary to what many people believe, symptoms occur much of the time in virtually all people (Mechanic, 1972b; Zola, 1973). It has also been pointed out that symptoms vary greatly in their clarity as cues, that they are subject to substantial situational influ-ences and meaning (Ross, Rodin, and Zimbardo, 1969), and that their recog-nition is highly influenced by learning patterns of behavior reflecting, to some extent, cultural patterns (Koos, 1954; Zborowski, 1952).

Virtually all of the research in the area of symptom occurrence is retrospective. In a large-scale prospective study of well adults, recruited by the American Cancer Society, Hammond (1964) found a high incidence of complaints for a twenty-four-hour recall period. About half of the sample in his study reported having headaches, over a quarter had indigestion, and nearly a third had a cough. Similarly, the extensive study of symptom occurrence by Roghmann and Haggerty (1972), utilizing a diary method, found that a significant portion of adults noted symptoms in a twenty-four-hour recall. About a third of all the days on which the reports were made had some stress reported, and the occurrence of stressful events was related to the frequency of report. It should be noted that these health disturbances represent only the ones that people found worthy of mention.

In addition to variation in the interpretation of symptoms, there is considerable variation in the response that is made to a given symptom experience. Some studies find marked differences according to socioeconomic status in what people say ought to be done about symptoms (Banks and Keller, 1971; Hetherington and Hopkins, 1969). Other studies, however, have found little difference in the socioeconomic dimension (Feldman, 1966; Guttmacher and Elinson, 1971). In the Banks and Keller study, there was high agreement among respondents on the relative ordering of a symptom list in terms of what should be done, but class differences in readiness to act. Feldman (1966) reports that most people in a national survey responded that one should see a doctor for most of the conditions he listed. In general, where questioning refers to what people *should do*, as in the Feldman study, there is agreement to advise "see a doctor." However, where the question asks what *would you do*, there is less tendency for the respondent to say "see a doctor," and the responses vary by socioeconomic status. A rather large number of people apparently say that they would take care of a serious health problem themselves, provided it is their problem.

Major differences in symptom reports are associated with sex; women uniformly report more health disturbances than do men (Andersen and others, 1968; Haggerty and Roghmann, 1972; Nathanson, 1977; Verbrugge, 1976). Also, the occurrence of stress is associated with a greater incidence of symptom reports (Kasl and Cobb, 1966; Mechanic, 1972b; Rahe, 1974). Tessler, Mechanic, and Dimond (1976) have shown that psychological distress is causally related to subsequent physician utilization in a prepaid group practice.

Use of medical services is not the most usual response to symptoms. Most episodes are self-treated or treated within the family (Haggerty and Roghmann, 1972). Self-treatment is an alternative to seeking medical care and an alternative that has at times been viewed with alarm (National Analysts, 1972). Seeking advice in response to an illness episode is also not limited to advice sought from health professionals (Freidson, 1961; Suchman, 1966). "Lay referral" refers to a process of discussion of health disturbances with other people, and the seeking of legitimation for a decision to take on at least some components of the sick role (Zola, 1973).

What are some of the factors related to whether an individual will decide to seek professional help in the presence of symptoms? One obvious impetus to action is represented by the severity or *perceived urgency of the condition*. Richardson (1970), in a study of Office of Economic Opportunity neighborhoods, found that the perceived severity of the condition was the most influential factor affecting whether medical services were sought. In that particular study, respondent ratings of severity correlated rather well with independently obtained physician ratings of severity; this kind of correlation is not often seen in studies that compare respondent perceptions of disease and independent physician views of conditions (Becker and Maiman, 1975).

A second obvious factor involved in the decision to take an action is *availability of paths of action* open to individuals who are experiencing an episode. Alternatives are available unevenly throughout the population for various reasons (Andersen, 1968). In taking account of the *costs* of different courses of action, people are apparently constrained both by the roles that they typically occupy in their lives and by the expectations of others to whom they are significantly related (Twaddle, 1969). Robinson (1971) considers the effects of cost in relation to social position, based on an intensive study of actions taken by families when symptoms occur. The question is, When is it permissible for the individual to engage in illness behavior? Robinson concludes that the threat of an illness is weighed against the threat of role loss, in terms of both short- and long-term gains and losses. A person in a new job or during a critical work period may well ignore symptoms that would be treated professionally in other circumstances. Although Richardson (1970) noted that with severe disturbances, the (direct) cost of seeking care did not affect the decision, he also found that, for less severe conditions, costs clearly entered as a factor in seeking professional help. Among the so-called enabling factors discussed by Aday and Andersen (1974) are having a usual source of care and having resources necessary to seek care (such things as money, transportation, and so on). These enabling factors would reflect, to some extent, the alternatives available to the individual in making a decision to act during a health disturbance.

"Readiness to use services" is a concept that has been given varying definitions, ranging from Hochbaum's (1958) "psychological readiness" (a combination of health belief elements) to reported inclination to seek care right away versus waiting in the presence of symptoms (Mechanic and Volkart, 1961). Similarly, "orientation to care" appears in several forms in the literature on use of services. The concept appears to refer to the general value put on medical care. In its most abstract form, the concept is nearly the inverse of alienation and powerlessness. Ludwig and Gibson (1969) compared a group of older persons who had not received medical care for six months with a group that had. Neither type nor number of symptoms differed between the groups. Both income and "recent welfare contact" related positively to receiving care. So did their measure of orientation to care. The authors suggest that situational factors create negative orientations, which, in turn, may serve as rationalizations for failure to seek care. In another study on older persons, Hyman (1970) concluded that a negative orientation to medicine was responsible for the fact that persons with low incomes are less ready to seek care. Such an orientation would also lead to discontinuity in care, further increasing the chance of untreated episodes of ill health.

Delay in Seeking Diagnosis

Delay in seeking care has been studied principally in relation to cancer (Kalmer, 1974). Clements and Wakefield (1972) have noted that nondelay in initiating care for cancer is related to seeking care for any type of symptom, thus indicating that patterns of delay may be typical of particular individuals, unlike patterns of health behavior discussed earlier. An extensive review by Antonovsky and Hartman (1974) of this literature concerning delay has noted that the findings are not entirely consistent or clear. In general, lower socioeconomic status and low educational levels are frequently, but not always, associated with delay. However, it is difficult to know whether socioeconomic status or education is the more powerful factor since the two are highly interrelated. No other sociodemographic factor provides a basis for firm generalizations about delay.

With respect to knowledge about cancer and the consequences of symptoms, Antonovsky and Hartman (1974) conclude that knowledge interacts with affective orientations. Thus, they found that knowledge about cancer symptoms, when combined with a high level of anxiety or fear, leads to greater delay, whereas knowledge with a low level of anxiety leads to less delay. If anxiety is related to beliefs that cancer cannot be prevented or cured, this finding would appear to be closely related to the Health Belief Model variable regarding the perceived benefits of action. The authors report a variety of studies on the role of various emotional reactions (for example, fear, guilt, fatalism, shame) on delay. The reported results are somewhat equivocal, however. It would seem that reinterpretation of these findings in terms of Health Belief Model components might yield more comprehensive explanations. For example, fear might be related to perceived severity and fatalism or to perceived susceptibility or benefits. According to Antonovsky and Hartman, personality variables have generally not been useful across studies in accounting for delay. Certainly, IQ does not appear to be associated nor do measures of neuroticism. However, hypochondria has been implicated in a tendency not to delay. Contrary to these authors' expectations, greater delay was found among persons who scored relatively high on a scale to measure independence and forcefulness in approaching tasks and resistance to diversion by stress. Studies of coping styles have not proved useful in distinguishing delayers from nondelayers. Antonovsky and Hartman report that delayers more often believe in divine healing, whereas nondelayers have acquired habits of paying attention to symptoms and have faith in the medical profession. The authors were unable to find research on the effects of social influence on delay, though they correctly point out that such influences have been found to be important in other areas of preventive health behavior. Finally, they conclude that a comfortable relationship between patient and doctor at the very least removes a barrier and facilitates nondelay or participation in preventive examinations.

Explanatory Theories

As indicated earlier, there are a variety of explanations for health-related behavior in the literature. Since these have been recently reviewed by McKinlay (1972) and Kirscht (1974), the review will not be repeated here. However, the main types of explanation that seem appropriate to illness and sick role behavior will be outlined briefly.

One class of explanation for illness behavior relates to the *cultural background* of the individual. The basic hypothesis is that differences among cultural groups result in variations in the interpretation of symptoms, in the vocabulary in which symptoms are expressed, and in differential readiness to act on symptoms. Such cultural differences among various ethnic groups have been discussed extensively by Zola (1973) and Mechanic (1968). For example, Zola found cultural differences in interpretation and response to symptoms between Americans of Irish and Italian descent. One way of looking at cultural differences is that there exist different norms for behavior in the face of the health disturbance among different cultures. These norms are learned and internalized in the process of socialization (Litman, 1974), producing characteristic ways of experiencing and acting on health problems. To some extent, one could use a cultural interpretation in explaining sex differences (Mechanic, 1972b). Differences between male and female responses to symptoms are known to become socialized at a relatively early age. Similarly, familial differences in decision making with respect to health and illness can be regarded as an expression of cultural differences (Litman, 1974). Zola's (1973) explanation for cultural differences in illness behavior revolves around the way in which illness episodes are treated by people. Decisions to act on symptoms are affected principally by the extent to which the symptoms interfere with the ordinary roles of the individual and by the process of legitimation for seeking care on the part of other people in the individuals' environment.

Since culture can only operate on individual behavior by influencing motivations and perceptions, it is entirely possible that the effects of culture can be specified by the sociopsychological approach. The major concepts utilized in the sociopsychological approach involve beliefs, motives, and perceptions; these concepts center on views of people concerning the appropriate paths of action to take in the presence of disturbances to health, on their perceptions of barriers in the environment to action, and on their subjective interpretations of the symptoms themselves. The sociopsychological approach attributes psychological rationality to people. This approach is perhaps best illustrated by the Health Belief Model (Kirscht, 1974; Rosenstock, 1974); applications of the Health Belief Model to the area of illness behavior have been reviewed by Kirscht (1974). Evidence for the relationship of the perceived value of actions to social characteristics seems fairly clear. In a national study, beliefs about the efficacy of taking actions to prevent or ameliorate several diseases were directly related to income, education, and occupational level (Kirscht and others, 1966). More general pessimism, alienation, skepticism, and fatalism also appear to be associated with less income and education (Hyman, 1970; Suchman, 1965). It is not clear whether the barriers associated with low income and education (that is, costs) reduce the perceived value of a possible benefit or condition a general negative reaction toward the possibility of intervening. Application of the Health Belief Model to behavior of mothers on behalf of illness in children yielded findings that lend support to the approach (Kirscht, Becker, and Eveland, 1976), although much more extensive application is needed.

Selection of a particular means of care in response to an illness episode can also be explained in terms of health benefits. Some writers distinguish between the primary symptom response (that is, the need for care) and the secondary response of what service to use (Franklin and McLemore, 1970). Two studies, both investigating student use of university health services in relation to all medical care obtained, included scales of attitudes toward the health service (Anderson and Bartkus, 1973; Franklin and McLemore, 1970). There was at least partial support for the notion that attitudes regarding the specific health care system determine the choice of services in an illness episode.

General beliefs and expectancies concerning the value of taking action with respect to health threats reflect the personalitylike construct of internal-external control. Control refers to the person's level of expectancy that outcomes depend on one's actions. As applied to health-related behavior, the notion is that people differ systematically in their beliefs about the efficacy of acting (Dabbs and Kirscht, 1971; Leventhal, 1970; Mechanic, 1972b; Wallston and others, 1976). In general, more coping responses are expected from those with higher levels of belief in personal control over health. Coping strategies with respect to illness and threats to health thus represent an area of considerable interest (Lipowski, 1969; see also the chapter by Cohen and Lazarus in this volume).

One other approach to explanation for illness behavior might be termed a *situational or eclectic approach.* The writings of Aday and Andersen (1974) illustrate this approach in their discussion of factors affecting access to health care. Their model includes predisposing, enabling, and need factors as determinants of response to a health disturbance. Differential access to care is principally a function of the enabling factors, which include the resources available to the person for health care (such things as money, a regular source of care, transportation, and health insurance). To the extent that enabling factors are not present, health care will not be obtained. By extension, it can be said that in the face of a health threat, people will use those services that their resources permit them to obtain. Another factor affecting illness behavior is stress. The presence of situational stresses of various kinds is thought to affect the perception of symptoms, making them more salient and/or more serious in their impact on the individual (Kasl and

Cobb, 1966; Mechanic, 1972b). Further, there is evidence that psychological distress is associated with increased use of medical services (Tessler, Mechanic, and Dimond, 1976). The mechanism by which stress operates to affect symptom perception is not well understood. However, a related aspect of each person's unique situation, which counters the effects of stress just described, involves the interference of difficult life circumstances with decisions to obtain treatment for symptoms. It has been found, for example, that difficult and taxing personal circumstances act as a barrier to seeking medical care (Kirscht, Becker, and Eveland, 1976), and that the extent of personal problems in an individual's life affects the degree of compliance with the medical regimen (Becker, Drachman, and Kirscht, 1972b). The experience of stressors, whether from external circumstances, psychological problems, or illness itself, will vary across individuals. Some of the confusion in the literature may result from these offsetting effects of stress.

Sick Role Behavior

The efforts to describe and explain sick role behavior, that is, activity of those who consider themselves ill for the purpose of getting well, are largely covered in the section on illness behavior. However, a number of issues have not been covered and will be dealt with here. Becker (1974b) has noted that most research aimed at understanding sick role behavior has yielded an unsystematic multiplicity of findings. He ascribes part of the problem to reliance on a medical model of patient behavior that focuses on certain enduring (usually demographic) characteristics of the patient, the nature of the illness as defined medically, and characteristics of the regimen.

More generally, sick role behavior has been viewed in the context originally set forth by Parsons (1951b, 1972). Parsons posited the "sick role" as a construct to account for the rights and duties of the sick person in the context of American values. Since then, the concept has generated a great deal of discussion and research; however, while it has proved to be an intriguing concept, many questions remain about its usefulness in explaining and predicting behavior and its utilization in efforts to modify behavior.

Parsons' discussion begins with the notion that the sick person suffers a disturbance of capacity. Once the incapacity is recognized, the sick person moves into the sick role. According to Parsons, occupants of the sick role are exempt from responsibility for the incapacity since it is beyond their control and they are therefore exempt from normal social role obligations. However, the legitimation of the sick person's exemption from usual obligations requires that the occupant of the sick role recognize that to be ill is inherently undesirable and that he or she feel obligated to try to get well. Finally, the person in the sick role has an obligation to seek technically competent help and to cooperate in the process of getting well.

In a review, Segall (1976) shows that while Parsons' concept has been widely, often uncritically accepted among medical sociologists, empirical work with the concept has uncovered many difficulties. For one, the model does not appear to account for psychiatric dysfunctions. Secondly, the chronically ill patient does not appear to be encompassed by the sick role; indeed, by definition, the chronic illnesses are not curable and the requirement on the patient would therefore be more one of adjusting to the condition than trying to get well. In addition, the exemption from usual responsibility in chronic illness would ordinarily be partial rather than complete. Thus, the theoretical usefulness of the "sick role," as defined by Parsons, is restricted primarily to acute physical illness. In its original form, the sick role would appear to have limited value in accounting for behavior among the physically disabled, the aged, and the mentally and physically handicapped. It has also been pointed out that Parsons' views should not be applied to the alcoholic, since to do so might legitimize alcoholism by removing the individual's responsibility for behavior (Roman and Trice, 1968). While alcoholism is clearly a disease, society may not be ready to regard it as legitimate.

It has also become clear that it is possible for sick persons to adopt some part, but not all, of the elements of the sick role. The very existence of the problem of compliance described in the next chapter demonstrates that many persons who are sick are not fully cooperating in the process of getting well, though they may be quite willing to give up some or all of their usual role obligations.

The sick role concept has not been useful in accounting for sociocultural differences in sick role expectations. Indeed, one effect of the concept has been to draw attention away from such variations in illness behavior (Gordon, 1966). Twaddle (1969) concluded that Parsons' concepts apply only to a minority of people, and Berkanovic (1972) considered them not at all useful for social psychological analysis.

In summary, the sick role concept has intrigued medical psychologists and sociologists for a quarter of a century. Its simplicity and apparent comprehensiveness have tempted many investigators and guided much research, and some of Parsons' concepts may, with appropriate modifications, still prove useful in explaining behavior and providing a basis for behavior modification. Nevertheless, the original formulation of the concept has had quite limited value in increasing knowledge.

Dropping Out of Treatment

The extent and determinants of dropping out of treatment have not been well studied except in the psychiatric area. Nevertheless, there are indications that premature dropping out is probably a significant problem in disease control. For example, it is reported that 37 percent to 50 percent of tuberculosis patients drop out of treatment against medical advice (Drolet and Porter, 1949; Wilmer, 1956). In hypertension, from 20 to 50 percent drop out in the first year, most of them during the first two months (Armstrong and others, 1962; Caldwell and others, 1970).

Why do people drop out? In a thorough review of the psychiatric literature, Baekeland and Lundwall (1975) conclude that not all dropouts are lost to treatment since many of them seek treatment elsewhere. Moreover, they believe some persons drop out because their health has improved, perhaps spontaneously. The generalizability of the latter finding to organic problems, however, is unknown. They also conclude that likelihood of dropping out is related to social isolation or lack of affiliation, negative therapist attitudes and behavior, low personal motivation, long waiting time for treatment, low socioeconomic status, young age, female sex, and social instability.

While derived from studies of psychiatric settings, these findings (with the exception of sex and perhaps age) seem to be quite similar to those identified as influencing compliance behavior. It should be emphasized that features of the treatment setting and system of care are involved in the problem of dropout. Relatively simple changes in the system, such as reminders and continuity, have demonstrated notable effects toward keeping patients in treatment for alcoholism (Baekeland and Lundwall, 1975). Similarly, modification of clinic procedures toward more personalized, convenient care has proved valuable in reducing the dropout of hypertensive patients (Finnerty, Mattie, and Finnerty, 1973; Stekel and Swain, 1977).

The Fate of Referrals

It has long been known that many clients referred by one agency for care at another never receive care at that agency. Levine and others (1969), for example, have shown that most children referred to child guidance clinics for service fail to obtain service at those clinics. Cauffman and others (1974) have probed this problem and emerged with some surprising findings. The overall aim of their project was to develop and implement an on-line computer system for making referrals for health care throughout the Los Angeles area, using a comprehensive health service data bank to which health workers in various agencies would be linked by terminal devices. Thirteen diversified agencies in the East Los Angeles Health District participated in a feasibility study of the system. Over the study period, data were collected on a total of 471 consumers, each with a single referral. It was found that over 40 percent of consumers referred for care did not receive care. Some of these appeared for care but did not receive it, perhaps for good medical reasons, but 34 percent of the total group did not show for care.

Only two factors studied showed significant relationships to showing or not showing for care: (1) whether the consumer was given a specific appointment with a provider; and (2) whether the consumer was given the name of a person to see at the provider's office. Those consumers given specific appointments and/or a named person to contact were more likely to show than other consumers. These findings are reasonable and the action implications seem obvious.

A number of variables did *not* distinguish shows from no-shows. These included: sex, age, type of health problem, possession of a Medicare or Medi-Cal card, convenience problems (including transportation, language, child care, parking, financial), time lag between referral and appointment, distance, and type of provider. Some of the nonfindings are surprising, especially those concerning convenience problems in obtaining care. It seems worthwhile to replicate a study of referral outcome to see whether those findings will be confirmed. At this time, however, it is clear that referral failures are widespread and it is likely that the rate of no-shows could be reduced by giving clients specific appointments with named providers.

Overutilization

In attempting to interpret the increasing demand for health services over the past few years, growing attention has focused on the problem of overutilization or inappropriate utilization of health services (Dunnel and Cartwright, 1972; Lave, 1974). These concerns are largely based on physicians' judgments as to what is appropriate utilization. Thus, it has been noted that the emergency room is increasingly used for nonemergency services. However, a look at the data on use of emergency services suggests that the picture is ambiguous.

It is clear that the way in which a service is used depends on alternatives available. Persons who lack a regular source of care are more likely to go to an emergency service for a wide range of medical (and nonmedical) problems (Alpert and others, 1969; Kelman and Lane, 1976). Where there is a regular source of care, emergency services are less likely to be used. As we have seen earlier, having a source of care is strongly associated with income; therefore, the use of emergency services for primary care by the poor is not hard to understand. In the Kelman and Lane (1976) study, which compared two suburban groups with the same income levels (one with and one without a regular physician), two thirds of those who had a personal physician came to the emergency service for treatment of an accidental injury; of those without their own doctor, over half sought treatment for an illness which, in a majority of cases, had lasted over twenty-four hours. The study by Kahn, Anderson, and Perkoff (1973) on children brought to an emergency service suggests that a major factor in precipitating visits is the perception that the condition has worsened.

Thus, while the use of the emergency room may be inappropriate from the point of view of the health profession, it may be quite appropriate from the point of view of the client. On a more general level, it seems that questions of appropriateness of use frequently are based on a medical model of physical disease. What often fails to be recognized is that patients do not visit physicians because they are sick but because they are concerned, and that concern needs to be dealt with. In this context, it is not easy to judge what ought to be regarded as appropriate utilization of professional health services.

Summary

We have considered briefly the extent and kinds of actions people take to prevent illness or its progression (preventive health behavior), their behavior in response to symptoms (illness behavior), and their behavior in response to diagnosed disease (sick role behavior). Also considered were the individuals "at risk" who are aware that their life-style increases their probability of contracting chronic diseases, but who are not (yet) symptomatic. The distinctions between health and illness are not clear cut, either from the point of view of the client or of the provider. A variety of approaches to explaining health-related behavior were described, of which sociopsychological and cultural approaches appear to have been the source of the most productive explanatory research, although aspects of the organization of health services are of considerable importance in influencing client behavior.

In considering preventive health behavior, there is as yet no firm evidence that the concept of health per se has any unitary organizing meaning for most people, although it has become increasingly clear that a variety of more specific health conditions or threats do have such meaning. Accordingly, the attempt to assess the role of general health motivations has yielded mixed results. Similarly, the search for a preventive orientation within people has yielded somewhat ambiguous results; there seems to be no strong evidence that persons who take preventive actions in one area are more likely to take preventive actions in other areas than would a group failing to take a particular preventive action. We also indicated that a variety of behaviors that may affect health are probably undertaken for reasons unrelated to health. Finally, we noted that the choice of methods to deal with the health threat will depend on the individual's beliefs about the efficacy of various alternatives. These may or may not be in accord with professional views about appropriate actions.

Utilization patterns in the area of prevention show considerable consistency across studies. In general, preventive health services tend to be used more by younger or middle-aged people, by females, by those relatively high on educational attainment and income, and by whites. Public financing of preventive health services would probably not materially change the patterns of use of such services among the poor, though it is likely to increase utilization among poor people experiencing substantial medical need.

Models to explain preventive health behavior have not been as abundant as those to explain illness or sick role behavior; indeed, preventive health behavior has not been the subject of as much study as have other kinds of health-related behavior. Nevertheless, two kinds of explanatory schemes have some currency in the preventive area. What has been termed the Social Network Model considers preventive health actions to be a function of the group structure in which individuals find themselves as well as of the psychological consequences of membership in subcultures, such as the subculture of poverty and identification with minority groups. A second kind of sociopsychological approach to the explanation of preventive health behavior has been offered by the Health Belief Model, the most widely employed in this area. As translated in the health area, the major components of the model include health-related motivations and subjective estimates of the benefits or efficacy of any proposed regimens minus the perceived barriers to taking such action. Sociodemographic and structural variables have an influence on these various subjective estimates.

Concerning illness and sick role behavior, consideration was given both to access to care and to actual utilization. With respect to access, children are more likely than adults, especially older adults, to have a usual source of convenient care. Adults over the age of fifty-five, nonwhites, and poor persons are more likely than their opposite numbers to have no usual source of care and to experience relatively longer waiting times in the providers' offices once they do seek care. Concerning actual use, middle-aged and older adults have the lowest levels of utilization. Whites consistently have more physician contacts, and females make greater use of health services than do males. While the poor and the nonpoor have similar utilization rates overall, when proxy measures of medical need are introduced, the poor use fewer services than the nonpoor.

In trying to explain utilization in the presence of symptoms or illness, we noted that most people, regardless of socioeconomic status, subscribe to the notion that a great many symptoms and conditions should be seen by a doctor; however, when asked what they would actually do if these symptoms occurred, a socioeconomic gradient appeared, with those lower on the scale less likely to indicate that they would, in fact, see a doctor. Low socioeconomic status is also associated with delay in seeking diagnosis of symptoms.

A variety of explanatory frameworks or variables have been introduced to explain utilization of services in illness and sick role behavior. One class of explanations includes cultural or subcultural background of the clients. In addition, the Health Belief Model has been applied with some success in accounting for variations in illness and sick role behavior. Various personality constructs have promise for explaining such behavior, especially such constructs as locus of control and self-esteem. An approach that has considerable currency may be termed an eclectic model. It includes sociodemographic, sociopsychological, economic, geographic, and organizational factors. These are specifically subdivided into predisposing, enabling, and need (that is, illness level) factors. The Social Network Model has also been applied to explaining illness and sick role behavior.

The classical sick role model was described and its limitations noted. Specifically, the model appears more adapted to acute physical illness than to chronic illness or to psychiatric dysfunction. Clearly, sick persons may adopt some part but not all of the sick role elements. Moreover, focus on the sick role tends to draw attention away from sociocultural variations in behavior under illness conditions. In general, it tends to be a static concept, not taking account of subcultural differences and individual differences or of the dynamic processes people go through in decisions about how to behave.

Specific reference was made in this chapter to the problem of dropouts from treatment and to the fate of referrals. Large proportions of people drop out of treatment during early phases of their treatment, and a great many who are referred from one place to another never show for care. Of those who do, a much smaller proportion, but nevertheless a substantial proportion, apparently fail to receive care. Appropriateness of utilization was also considered. A modified Health Belief Model shows some promise in explaining behavior of such persons in connection with their illnesses.

Since this chapter has been written by two psychologists, it is not surprising that we conclude that sociopsychological models have shown and continue to show the greatest promise in accounting for all health-related decisions, including preventive health behavior, illness behavior, and sick role behavior. To be sure, the current model, while useful, does not account for as much variance in behavior as could be desired. However, an important start has been made. Future research should be directed toward increasing the conceptual and operational precision of the concepts already identified, and toward incorporating such additional variables into these models as will permit more accurate predictions of health-related behavior.

8

Patients' Problems in Following Recommendations of Health Experts

John P. Kirscht

Irwin M. Rosenstock

Although many of the harmful effects of disease agents and potentially disabling conditions are preventable or treatable, not all of these are currently being prevented or treated. Deaths from communicable diseases for which there are simple, effective immunizations still occur; venereal disease is a growing problem. Diseases of nutritional deficiency still take a toll in the health and strength of large numbers of people who live in the world's most affluent country, and life-style patterns known to be deleterious are followed by millions. A major factor in this gap between what health technology makes possible in the way of prevention and control and actual health outcomes is that health recommendations are not followed.

Because the topic "health recommendations" covers so much ground—ranging from a single prescription written by a physician as treatment for a specific diagnosis to public warnings or exhortations by health experts regarding common threats to health—it is necessary to restrict this discussion to a few types of problems. In the recent past, there has been a rapid growth

189

of interest in the issue of patient compliance or adherence to medical regimens. "The gap," noted one investigator (Sackett, 1976, p. 9), "between the therapy prescribed by the physician and the therapy actually taken by the patient is distressingly wide for self-administered regimens." This aspect of the fate of health recommendations deals with patients and clinical recommendations. It has focused primarily on the extent to which patients comply with advice within a framework of expert authority where the advice is taken to be sound and efficacious for the individual.

Beyond this problem of patient adherence, there are myriad suggestions from health professionals directed at classes of people thought to be at risk. For example, the Surgeon General of the U.S. Public Health Service issued a formal warning in 1964, based on an accumulation of evidence, that cigarette smoking was harmful to health. The American Heart Association recommends reducing cholesterol in the diet; the Cancer Society advocates screening programs for the early detection of cancer. Fluoridation of water supplies is urged by the American Dental Association. Public officials, professional organizations, medical writers, and health promoters of varying qualifications, including those selling products that are linked with health, all contribute to the stream of recommendations. With all this, none of the advice is followed in full, and some of it, not at all. Much of the discussion that follows will focus on the behavioral effects of advice given to a patient by a provider of a health service, although broader forms of recommendations will also be touched on.

Patient Adherence

Magnitude and Scope of the Problem

While estimates of adherence to recommendations vary widely, there is firm evidence that substantial nonadherence occurs in every circumstance where some form of self-administration is involved. Averaging results over many studies of medications, Sackett (1976, p. 16) suggests that 50 percent of the patients do not take prescribed medications in accordance with instructions. Some 20 to 40 percent of recommended immunizations are not obtained. Crude averages from many studies show that scheduled appointments for treatment are missed 20 to 50 percent of the time. Where changes in habitual behaviors are recommended, as in dietary restrictions, cessation of smoking, and increase in physical activity, there is still greater noncompliance: Programs designed to deal with smoking are considered unusually effective if more than one third of entrants have reduced their smoking at the end of six months; large percentages drop out of weight control programs; and dietary restrictions are often observed primarily in the breach.

There is, of course, wide variability in the results of studies done regarding patient adherence, depending on the population studied, the type of recommendations, the treatment setting, and so on. Examples of adherence research will help provide some idea of the scope of the problem:

1. High levels of blood pressure are present in an estimated 15 percent of the adult population. Effective treatment is available through use of medications and dietary restrictions. A few years ago, it was estimated that only one of eight persons with essential hypertension (high blood pressure of unknown cause) had achieved blood pressure control; yet this condition is regarded as the number one risk factor for coronary heart disease and stroke. Wilber and Barrow (1972, p. 658) reported that, in screening some 6,000 people in Atlanta, 23 percent were found to have elevated blood pressure levels or already diagnosed hypertension. Of those, 57 percent reported that they were currently under treatment for the condition; yet 37 percent of the current patients in treatment had uncontrolled blood pressure. A large portion of this problem is due to difficulties in adherence, including failure to initiate or stay in treatment (Foote and Erfurt, 1977). Because hypertension is typically a symptomless, noncurable condition, and control requires a lifelong regimen, often with unpleasant side effects, it is a likely condition for nonadherence.

McKenney and others (1973, p. 1107) studied fifty patients under treatment for hypertension at a neighborhood health center. Prior to an intervention through the pharmacy service, the patients' intake of prescribed medications was followed for seven months by means of pill counts. About 65 percent of the recommended pills were taken. Only ten of the patients took at least 90 percent of the dosages prescribed.

2. Adherence to penicillin regimens for acute infections in children is an important aspect of pediatric care. Becker, Drachman, and Kirscht (1972b) followed 125 pediatric patients, all of whom were under treatment for acute middle-ear infections and all of whom received a ten-day course of penicillin. The medication was free. It was possible to check, through analysis of urine samples, for the presence of the drug about midway into the ten-day period. By that time, over one half the mothers were no longer giving the medication to their children.

Utilizing private practices, Charney and others (1967, p. 190) tested 459 children, ages two to twelve, who were given ten-day courses of penicillin therapy for pharyngitis or otitis media. Urine samples were collected and analyzed after either the fifth or ninth day of treatment. Of the patients tested, 81 percent were receiving the drug after five days, and 56 percent over the full ten-day period. Compliance was better for treatment of pharyngitis than for ear infections.

3. Failure of patients to remain in treatment or to keep appointments is a major problem in outpatient services. Tagliacozzo, Ima, and Lashof (1973, p. 23) followed a group of 195 adult patients receiving outpatient care for chronic conditions, principally for hypertension and diabetes. All of the patients received a medical work-up and a diagnosis; all were told to return for regular follow-up appointments; most were prescribed drugs and needed to return for renewal of prescriptions. After this entry into treatment, 49 percent had terminated by the fourth scheduled visit. Although the number dropping out lessened subsequently, there was a continual shrinkage

of the group receiving medical care over the entire twenty-seven months of the study.

Even in a prepaid medical care plan, appointment keeping poses problems. Over a variety of different services in the Portland Kaiser Health Plan, Hurtado, Greenlick, and Columbo (1973, p. 190) noted that of the total scheduled appointments for a year, 16.3 percent were failures—8.5 percent attributed to the patient's not showing up at all, and 7.8 percent owing to cancellation by the patient on the day scheduled.

4. Hospitalization does not guarantee that a regimen is followed. Wilson (1976) described a number of instances in which hospitalized children failed to receive the proper dosages of medications; instances of both underdosage and overdosage are described. These were failures of the system of care because of faulty drug records and lack of systematic control by the therapists. However, many hospitalized patients can exercise choices about their regimens. Roth and his co-workers have conducted a series of studies regarding adherence in a Veterans Administration hospital. In one research study (Roth and Berger, 1960), 75 patients in the gastrointestinal ward who were prescribed a liquid antacid were followed. It was possible to measure consumption of the liquid unobtrusively. Although patients were supervised in a general way, actual intake of the medication was left to the individual. Less than half of the amount prescribed was taken. Further study of ulcer in-patients (Caron and Roth, 1971, p. 63), who were prescribed special diets but took their meals in the hospital dining room, showed that the average patient took the proper diet on three fourths of the days observed. One quarter of the patients, however, followed the diet 60 percent of the time or less.

As these examples show, adherence varies, but it averages less than 100 percent in every report of regimens that involve elements of choice or opportunity for variation to occur. The existence of such variation often shocks health workers, who may assume that good compliance is the norm. If a therapy is worthwhile, which in itself may be an untested assumption (Stimson, 1974), then its benefits cannot be gained in the absence of adherence. The efficacy of some drugs depends on maintenance of proper blood levels, which cannot be achieved if dosing is erratic or incomplete. One possible ramification of nonadherence is that if a course of therapy is apparently ineffective, the therapist may try more heroic measures or shift treatment without a true evaluation of the effects of a given course of treatment. It is apparent that the professionals are often unaware of the extent and magnitude of nonadherence. Studies of physicians' ability to predict compliance in patients reveal only chance levels of accuracy (Haynes, 1976).

A further ramification of adherence levels relates to procedures for establishing efficacy of therapeutic maneuvers. Drug trials are required before a medication can be legally utilized. Proper comparison of treated with untreated groups, or among varying dosage levels, assumes that the treatment actually takes place. As Goldsmith (1976, p. 150) notes: "It can be seen that incomplete compliance can have a devastating effect, both upon the sample-size requirements for showing real differences between treatment and control groups and upon the ability to conclude that treatments have clinically significant effects."

Adherence—Diversity of Behaviors and Situations

Even a strictly medical definition of adherence as "the extent to which patient's behavior coincides with the clinical prescription" (Sackett, 1976) includes a wide array of different behaviors. If the concept is broadened to encompass any type of health recommendations made by health professionals, there is indeed a problem in specifying its referents. Such recommendations range from relatively simple, one-time actions (an immunization) to repeated short-term behavior (taking medication for an infection) to complex patterns (exercise) to long-term modification of habitual actions (substitution of a diet low in saturated fats) to avoidance of certain substances and behaviors (cessation of cigarette smoking). There is, then, a dimension of behavioral complexity among different regimens.

Health recommendations come from different sources. Some advice is given by an individual physician or nurse to an individual client. Some comes from a professional source but is offered to a class of people (Dr. Zilch recommends an inoculation against influenza); some, from impersonal sources (the Heart Association or Health Department). Often, public advice has an element of controversy, as in the swine flu campaign of 1976, general recommendations for checkups (see Spark, 1976, for a negative view), breast cancer screening, or dietary advice. There is little question that the source of a health recommendation is an important component of the influence process. Most people have considerable faith in physicians, especially their own physicians, as dispensers of advice (Aday and Andersen, 1975; Freidson, 1970), and express high degrees of satisfaction with the care they receive. Beck and others (1974) noted in their study of genetic screening that people preferred to have a physician recommend the procedure, but very few physicians knew about or advocated the testing. Since much medical advice is presented in face-to-face situations, it has the added advantage of personalized communication—typically a more effective mode of influence (Leventhal, 1973).

As with other types of influence, recommendations regarding health are directed at people who vary in their receptivity and circumstances. Some behaviors are advised for individuals not currently experiencing symptoms or disease states but rather are oriented toward preventing future occurrences. As might be expected, there is wide variability in preventive or detective behavior. For example, a national study found that 46 percent of the adult population had a voluntary checkup in the absence of symptoms within a five-year period (Haefner and others, 1967, p. 453); among women invited to participate in breast cancer screening in the Health Insurance Plan of New York, 65 percent were screened (Fink, Shapiro, and Roeser, 1972, p. 329); in the genetic screening program reported by Beck and others (1974), less than 10 percent of the target group participated. Since most preventive or detective procedures are discretionary and involve out-of-pocket costs, it is not surprising that they are typically associated with socioeconomic status (Rosenstock, 1974). Even where direct monetary barriers are removed, however, educational level remains an important correlate of preventive behavior (Fink, Shapiro, and Roeser, 1972; Green, 1970). Typically, women are more likely to engage in prevention (Rosenstock, 1974), possibly reflecting their greater concern for health and awareness of health information. The fact that requirements for preventives reduce social differences in acting—for example, where the law specifies that children entering school must be immunized—emphasizes that there are social differences in readiness to act on a recommendation.

When people are ill, the presence of symptoms forms a focal event for reacting to advice (Kasl and Cobb, 1966). Where the course of acting includes attempts to relieve symptoms, recommendations are usually followed more faithfully (Haynes, 1976). The other side of the coin is that premature termination of a regimen is often associated with the disappearance of symptoms. In a study of children given penicillin for an acute infection, mothers most frequently cited remission of symptoms as the reason for stopping the medication (Becker, Drachman, and Kirscht, 1972b). Treatment of asymptomatic chronic conditions is thought to pose special problems. In every program of screening for hypertension, a substantial portion of those with elevated blood pressures are found to be aware that they have the condition (Wilber and Barrow, 1972). Some never followed up previous referrals; many dropped treatment. While symptom occurrence is not a sufficient condition for adherence, it is a factor in personal readiness to act on medical advice. With older groups of people more subject to chronic illnesses, it is common for the individual to be under treatment for several conditions (Kirscht and Rosenstock, 1977), adding to the dimension of complexity in the sick role.

It should be noted that the individual's *interpretation* of symptoms is more likely the key to understanding the role of symptoms in behavior. Symptom occurrence is ubiquitous and most are dealt with outside the medical care system (Haggerty and Roghmann, 1972). That people may not act on apparently severe symptoms is noteworthy, as illustrated by the research on delay in seeking care (Antonovsky and Hartman, 1974); those who delay longer are typically of lower socioeconomic status or have high levels of health-related fears.

In summary, the behaviors entailed under the rubric of health recommendations are diverse and variable in their demands on the individual. Advice comes from different sources, through different modes of contact, and falls on persons with different characteristics, inclinations, and widely varying personal circumstances. In trying to sort out the factors related to adherence to health recommendations, we shall need to keep in mind the different dimensions represented in the problem.

Measuring Adherence

A conceptual definition of adherence contains at least two parts—the recommendation and the behavioral performance, judged in the light of the recommendation. An important issue in the study of the fate of professional recommendations is measuring the behaviors involved. As in most areas of human behavior, there are difficulties associated with making the concepts of interest operational.

Relatively simple are those behaviors in which a formal record is made of an individual's public actions. Thus, assessment of appointment keeping or of an immunization may be straightforward; however, even here not all visits and services are recorded. Use of services over periods of time or for specific purposes is somewhat more difficult to measure, and losses occur because people change sources of care or because record systems are always less complete and accurate than might be imagined. Studies of populations utilizing several sources of care make the use of records more difficult; so do nonstandardized and haphazard record systems.

Those behaviors, usually private, that are not subject to regular entry in medical records—most of the interesting ones relative to health recommendations—pose measurement problems of still greater magnitude. By now there is a considerable literature on assessment of medication behavior (Gordis, 1976). Measures vary in their apparent validity and directness. Ideally, we would like to observe the extent to which patients consume prescribed drugs. With that generally not possible, investigators utilize pill counts or assessments of physiological traces of drugs through blood or urine tests (markers or by-products may also be used). Pill counts are not easy to do and pose a series of problems. For example, medications are not always kept in their original containers, supplies are divided up, containers are not returned on request; moreover, frankly acknowledged pill counting is probably reactive: subjects may deliberately dissemble. Physiological assessments have advantages but may be costly and alter behavior if patients know they are being tested. In addition, the presence of a drug in the body is dependent on its pattern of uptake and physical characteristics of the individual, so that variation occurs in blood level of a drug even under conditions of perfect compliance.

Many investigators rely on self-report by the patient—an obvious source of information but one that is subject to several sources of invalidity (Gordis, 1976). Self-report may yield overestimates of adherence to recommendations (Gordis, Markowitz, and Lilienfeld, 1969a), although some studies of medication adherence in which self-report was compared with other methods of assessment have yielded accurate results (Feinstein and others, 1959; Francis, Korsch, and Morris, 1969). Other types of behavior related to health recommendations are quite difficult to measure except through asking questions: for example, eating behavior, physical activity, noting symptoms, alcohol consumption, and smoking. In each of these, the task for a patient is not simple, as in trying to reconstruct what was eaten over a period of several days. Moreover, the danger of overreporting "good" behavior is always present.

What ought to be measured in studies of adherence needs to be clear. Medical interest focuses on health outcomes, such as blood pressure, reversal of a disease process, body weight, or control of diabetes. Measures of outcomes are typically not direct measures of patient behavior (taking medication, eating certain foods, or taking temperature), although the outcome measures may be taken as indicators of patient adherence. Becker and others (1977b) report a study of dietary compliance among a group of obese children. Weight change was used as a principal index of eating practices, but with the recognition that it was a proxy measure. In addition, measuring adherence involves decisions about when and how often to take measures. Single assessments may contain a lot of noise, especially if the behaviors are complex. Roth, Caron, and Hsi (1971) followed ulcer patients over a period of two years in order to measure intake of a prescribed antacid. Interest in the modification of life-style habits, such as diet and smoking, has shifted toward taking longer-term measures (Kasl, 1975b). It should be noted that the issue of behavioral consistency in adherence over time is an empirical question; often, however, we assume consistency by taking measures only once or a very few times.

The other referent of the concept of adherence—the recommendation—should not be forgotten. Medical advice dispensed to patients is subject to several interpretations: (1) the objective recommendation (usually not known to anyone for certain); (2) the recorded advice, if any (say, an entry in a medical record or on a prescription form); (3) what is reported by the patient; and (4) what is reported by the health professional. Ideally, there should be a close match among these; in fact, they do not always correspond well (Hulka, Cassel, and Kupper, 1976). Ley and Spelman (1965) have shown that the patient typically remembers only a fraction of the advice given. Hulka's work has concentrated on the congruence between the reports of patient and physician as it affects compliance. With other types of professional recommendations, there is always a question regarding their initial perception and retention by an individual. There is, in one sense, no behavioral adherence problem regarding a recommended immunization if the person is unaware of the suggestion. However, the general problem of influence by health professionals on behavior includes the full range of transactions, whether communication was successful or not.

Adherence and Psychosocial Factors

In this section, we will investigate relationships of adherence behaviors to personal, social, and situational variables. After discussing some generalizations that have support in research, we will examine an array of specific psychosocial characteristics and present studies that help fill in the more abstract summarization of outcomes. Historically, the search for correlates of adherence has been descriptive rather than explanatory. In many studies, a common aim was to identify groups of nonadherers, often with a hope that identification would solve the problem. For that reason, much of the research was essentially atheoretical, and many variegated factors were investigated whose reason for inclusion was, at best, only implied. Well-elaborated hypotheses have been the exception rather than the rule.

Haynes' (1976) review of "determinants" of compliance with medical regimens, covering some 185 original research reports, summarizes a variety of factors: demographic characteristics of patients; features of the disease, the regimen, and the therapeutic source; aspects of patient-physician interaction; and sociobehavioral characteristics of patients. He concludes that only a small number of variables have demonstrated consistent relationships with patient adherence. Among these factors (all associated with lower rates of compliance) are: a "psychiatric" diagnosis; the complexity, duration, and amount of change involved in the regimen itself; inconveniences associated with operation of clinics; inadequate supervision by professionals; patient dissatisfaction; "inappropriate health beliefs"; noncompliance with other regimens; and family instability. This summary is noteworthy for what it does not include—the many variables studied that have not yielded consistent relationships with adherence across different situations and regimens, such as demographic factors, personality characteristics, knowledge, health status, social norms, and patient-provider interactions.

Other reviewers have noted that few associations are found between adherence and ordinary social characteristics of patients, such as age, sex, and education (Becker and Maiman, 1975; Kasl, 1975b). It is often stated that a "defaulting" personality does not exist, because personalitylike measures have had little success in predicting compliance and because measures of different aspects of adhering have, in general, shown relatively low levels of association. Kasl (1975b) notes that characteristics of the regimen and the nature of the patient-provider relationship have yielded relationships with compliance, although sociodemographic characteristics of patients are not reliable predictors. The review by Becker and Maiman (1975) reaches much the same conclusion, with the additional note that the Health Belief Model is demonstrably predictive of the extent to which regimens are followed.

To discuss the various factors that have been investigated in more detail, we will present information about personal and social characteristics of patients, patient knowledge, characteristics of the regimen, features of the patient's social situation, and interactional factors between patient and provider.

Patient Personality

In discussing personality correlates of adherence to medical recommendations, it is necessary to make a distinction. The term "defaulter" recurs in the literature, its earlier connotation being that of a peculiar constellation of enduring personal traits that made the individual noncompliant. There is by now widespread agreement that the existence of the defaulting patient is a myth (Blackwell, 1973). We must, however, distinguish this conception from the idea that some personality characteristics may be associated with differential likelihood of adherence.

Although a number of personalitylike measures have been utilized in studies of adherence, they have not been strikingly successful in predicting compliance. An exception is psychiatric diagnosis of schizophrenia or personality disorder (Haynes, 1976); other psychiatric categories have not been successful predictors of adherence. A number of studies have used measures that revolve around personal control and alienation. Davis (1966) reported that a measure of anomie was unrelated to compliance among a group of cardiac patients; Gordis, Markowitz, and Lilienfeld (1969b) found such a measure unrelated to following a penicillin regimen for rheumatic fever patients. However, there is some evidence that those with greater belief in internal control are more likely to try to gain information about a health condition (Seeman and Evans, 1962; Wallston, Maides, and Wallston, 1976) and to follow advice where self-management is especially important, as with diet (Kirscht and Rosenstock, 1977). Internality as such may not lead one to follow advice: Dabbs and Kirscht (1971) found internality associated with failure to obtain a flu vaccination.

In reviewing studies on dropping out of treatment, Baekeland and Lundwall (1975) identified a series of factors that relate to patients' terminating therapy. Although much of the review concerns studies of psychotherapy, it also includes studies of medical treatment, alcoholism programs, and drug trials. Aggressive or passive aggressive behavior patterns, dependence, and denial are generally associated with dropping out. As a group, however, these personalitylike factors are less predictive than other aspects of the situation, such as social isolation and discrepancies between patient and provider expectations.

Social Characteristics of Patients

Standard demographic categories are not consistently related to compliance. It seems well established that men and women do not differ systematically in following medical advice for illness; in the case of preventive health measures, however, women are more likely to "adhere" (Rosenstock, 1974). Age is also typically uncorrelated with compliance in the sick role, although older adults are less likely to engage in preventive actions. Younger adult patients have been reported as more likely to break appointments in general medicine clinics (Hurtado, Greenlick, and Columbo, 1973; Jonas, 1971). Continued attendance after diagnosis of a chronic disease was unrelated to age in a group of 159 patients (Tagliacozzo and Ima, 1970). Medication compliance is not consistently related to age (Davis, 1968; Hulka, Cassel, and Kupper, 1976), although adolescent diabetics are apparently among the poorest adherers (Gordis, Markowitz, and Lilienfeld, 1969b). In the case of children, compliance is unrelated to the age of the mother (Becker, Drachman, and Kirscht, 1972b).

Measures of social structural variables, such as educational level, income, and occupation, show mixed results; when related at all to adherence, higher levels are associated with greater adherence. In terms of keeping appointments, Tagliacozzo and Ima (1970) reported that continued attendance for treatment of chronic conditions is positively related to education; Caldwell and others (1970) found that patients dropping out of treatment for hypertension have less education, income, and lower occupational level. Dropping out of treatment for alcoholism and dropping out of psychotherapy are associated with lower socioeconomic status (Baekeland and Lundwall, 1975). Adherence to a therapeutic regimen, however, is not consistently related to socioeconomic level. For example, Hulka, Cassel, and Kupper (1976) reported that medication errors of various types made by a group of patients under treatment for chronic illness were not related to educational level. Becker, Drachman, and Kirscht (1972b) noted that the education of the mother was unrelated to adherence to a penicillin regimen for the child and to keeping appointments, although positively associated with learning the regimen and knowing the date for a follow-up visit.

Information

It might appear that level of knowledge should be associated with greater adherence. For general medical knowledge, however, few studies have found consistent associations (Haynes, 1976). A study by Gordis, Markowitz, and Lilienfeld (1969b) of rheumatic fever patients yielded no relationships between a test of knowledge about the condition and following the prescribed drug regimen. Kirscht and Rosenstock (1977) obtained scores from hypertensive patients on a set of items concerning high blood pressure and found them unrelated to taking medications or following dietary advice. Sackett and others (1975) also found that knowledge scores relative to hypertension did not predict adherence. In a study of contraception (Siegel and others, 1971), knowledge of contraceptive methods was not related to continuation after one year. However, in a study by Tagliacozzo and Ima (1970), which included a test of information about the causes, symptoms, and complications of four chronic conditions, higher levels of knowledge were associated with continuing in treatment. The relationship, however, was conditional upon other factors; for example, it predicted best for those with little illness experience, low anxiety, and reported high interference with activities.

A different kind of "knowledge" does appear related to adherence—namely, the extent to which the patient knows what behavior the regimen requires, and how and when to perform it. Such knowledge is a necessary, but not sufficient condition for following the regimen. A number of studies have found that this kind of information relates positively to adherence (Becker, Drachman, and Kirscht, 1972b; Hulka, Cassel, and Kupper, 1976). Hypertensive patients who were not sure of the condition for which they were under treatment were less likely to be adhering with prescribed drugs or dietary advice (Kirscht and Rosenstock, 1977).

Features of the Regimen

Since recommendations for treatment vary in their demands, in terms of complexity of execution, duration, and extent of behavior change, a number of investigations have assessed the nature of the regimen in relation to

adherence. Generally, the more the patient is told to do, the greater the likelihood of failure (Blackwell, 1973). For example, there is more failure when
many doses of a medication are prescribed. In a study of drug errors by 180
outpatients being treated for a wide range of different conditions, Latiolais
and Berry (1969) found that the more drugs a patient received, the more
errors were made—both overdosing and underdosing. In a study by Hulka,
Cassel, and Kupper (1976) of diabetic and congestive heart disease patients,
error rates increased both with the number of drugs and with the complexity
of the medication schedule. Duration of treatment also tends to be negatively associated with levels of adherence (Haynes, 1976).

In a panel study of cardiac patients, Davis and Eichhorn (1963) noted
that the patients tended to make those changes that required the least adjustment. Modifications of personal habits were least well followed. Modification of habitual behaviors, such as diet, smoking, and alcohol consumption,
is difficult at best (McAlister and others, 1976) and high rates of dropout are
typical in programs seeking to change those behaviors. Baekeland and Lundwall (1975) stress the losses from long-term treatment programs, although
they note that a number of dropouts turn up again—a phenomenon that
needs much more attention.

While adherence to related aspects of a regimen may be associated,
behavior across unlike demands is usually not highly related (Kasl, 1975b).
In particular, keeping appointments may show little association with adherence to medication. A study by Roth, Caron, and Hsi (1971) of ulcer out-
patients taking medications and keeping appointments found that adherence
rates to the two drugs prescribed were strongly related but showed no association with keeping appointments. Caron and Roth (1971), in a study of
ulcer patients in the hospital, reported no association between following a
diet and taking prescribed antacid. Becker, Drachman, and Kirscht (1972b)
found slight associations between appearing for a follow-up visit and giving
prescribed penicillin to an ill child, and between following a diet for obesity
and keeping appointments with a dietitian (Becker and others, 1977b). In
the latter study, weight change was unrelated to keeping clinic appointments
over a year's period. Perhaps the best that can be said is that response generalization occurs to some degree, probably along dimensions of similarity.

Social Situational Aspects of Adherence

As Davis (1968) has pointed out, recommendations for health-related
behaviors are not made in a social vacuum but are filtered through the social
roles people play. Expectancies for behavior are shaped by others, and behavior is directed and modified through their reactions. Among the significant influences on compliance of cardiac patients, Davis noted the effects of
family and friends. As an example of role factors, Davis found, in his study
of farmers with heart disease, that those whose work orientation was high
were much less likely to adhere to physicians' recommendations about curtailment of work activities. In their study of appointment keeping by chroni-

cally ill patients, Tagliacozzo and Ima (1970) reported that where there was a high degree of interference with daily activities, the patients were less likely to stay in treatment. In this case, following the advice apparently would have interfered with important activities of the patients. Another expression of this difficulty is found in the study by Becker, Drachman, and Kirscht (1972b); mothers in taxing personal circumstances were less likely to give their children the complete course of penicillin for an acute infection. Family instability is mentioned by Haynes (1976) as a clear-cut contributor to not following advice; many of the studies cited deal with failures to keep follow-up appointments in pediatric services. Kirscht, Becker, and Eveland (1976) present data showing that in use of medical services for children the symptom level is critical, but, with illness level taken into account, barriers such as difficult social circumstances become significant.

Recent interest in the social situation as related to health behavior is evidenced by the growing emphasis on the concept of social support (Caplan and others, 1976). The degree to which significant others provide support for behavior is regarded as critical. In a study of hypertensive patients, Caplan found that adherence to the regimen was related to the help and approval of others. Family influence has been noted by several investigators as a factor in adherence (for example, Donabedian and Rosenfeld, 1964). This has been true also for preventive behaviors (Haggerty and Roghmann, 1972). According to Green (1970), preventive medical actions are significantly related among family members. It is Green's view that normative expectancies within groups account for the clustering of preventive behaviors. Elinson, Henshaw, and Cohen (1976) report findings from a study of screening programs in a low-income population that support this view.

In earlier studies of patients under treatment for tuberculosis, it was observed that a prominent correlate of nonadherence was social isolation (Kasl, 1975b). Those who live alone or have few contacts with others are less likely to follow medical recommendations. For example, Porter (1969) observed fifty-eight patients on long-term treatment in a general practice and found that the only social characteristic related to nonadherence to drug therapy was social isolation. Concern with medication errors made by isolated, chronically ill patients is evidenced in the literature (Neely and Patrick, 1968). In reviewing a wide range of studies on dropping out of treatment, Baekeland and Lundwall (1975) also concluded that social isolation is a very important problem.

Relationships of Patients to Providers

Features and effects of the system through which patients interact with professionals have a marked effect on outcomes. It has been demonstrated that the language and concepts of the medical field are not widely understood (Pratt, Seligmann, and Reader, 1957). Not only are many of the technical words not shared by patients but also many commonly used bits of advice do not convey meanings as intended—"reduce salt intake" or "take the medicine on an empty stomach" may not be interpreted correctly. McKinlay (1975) demonstrated that terms commonly used by physicians vary considerably in whether they are understood; but even more, he found that the physicians use terminology that they themselves believe is not understood by patients. A bizarre facet of the terminology game is that physicians have been found typically to *underestimate* the level of knowledge actually possessed by the patient. Even in the interpretation of instructions on prescriptions, there is considerable ambiguity (Mazzullo, 1976, p. 24): In a sample of medical-service patients who were asked to interpret instructions on drug labels, only 36 percent correctly stated what "every six hours" is supposed to mean. Interpretations of what is meant by "evening" and by "with meals" varied considerably.

The role of patient satisfaction with medical care has received considerable attention (Aday and Andersen, 1975). Although general satisfaction with the medical system is not very predictive of particular behaviors, evaluations by patients of specific visits for care do relate to adherence. In the studies by Becker, Drachman, and Kirscht (1972b) and by Francis, Korsch, and Morris (1969), both involving mothers of children with acute illnesses, satisfaction with a particular visit related positively to medication adherence and to keeping appointments. It should be noted, however, that patient satisfaction is a vague concept and has been measured in a wide variety of ways. Most assessments of satisfaction find patients highly satisfied with most aspects of care; further, criticism of the system is positively related to educational level (Kirscht, Becker, and Eveland, 1976), suggesting that many measures of satisfaction are not tapping motivational factors.

There are relatively few studies of the interaction between patients and providers. Davis (1968) studied the content of such interactions using broad categories for coding behaviors. He reported that for the adult patients studied, deviations from normatively expected patterns of relationships were associated with nonadherence. For example, the combination of active, aggressive patients with the same type of physician was considered deviant. However, Francis, Korsch, and Morris (1969), using tape recordings of encounters between mothers and physicians in a pediatric service, found that adherence was higher when the physician was seen as friendly and when the visit met the mothers' expectations.

Hulka's approach (Hulka, Cassel, and Kupper, 1976) emphasizes the interactional nature of compliance. In a study of 350 patients (with diabetes or congestive heart failure) of 46 private physicians, these investigators found that patients tend to be compliant "to the best of their knowledge," but have various types of misinformation. Knowledge of the regimen and its function was related to fewer errors. One source of error was the apparent failure of communication, measured by the match between what the physician said was prescribed and what the patient reported as the regimen.

Svarstad's study (1976, pp. 226-227) of patients and physicians at a neighborhood health center emphasizes the interactional nature of medical recommendations. She noted many instructional failures: Some medications were never discussed, few indications were given on how long to take medications, and written instructions were incomplete at best. Among patients with accurate information, 60 percent adhered while only 17 percent with misinformation did so. Key elements found in the interactions were efforts of the physician to instruct and motivate the patient and patient ability to comprehend and provide feedback. A conclusion is that no one method works magic—for example, the exercise of authority by the practitioner was not, by itself, effective—but that both parties contribute to successful or unsuccessful outcomes.

Conceptualizations of the Adherence Process

While much of the research related to following health recommendations has not derived from theoretical propositions, some is conceptually oriented and has attempted to develop explanatory bases for the area. In general, the concepts applied have derived either from more psychological or more sociological orientations. We will discuss first the health belief approach, then social and behavioral explanations.

The Health Belief Model

This model seeks to explain specific decisions made regarding health behavior in terms of the value of that behavior for coping with a threat. The model was developed in the 1950s to deal with preventive behaviors (the history is described in Rosenstock, 1974): Under what circumstances will individuals voluntarily act to ward off a future health problem? The cognitive elements comprised: (1) beliefs about the nature of the threat in terms of its perceived subjective severity if it should happen and the personal susceptibility to that danger; (2) beliefs that specific actions had benefits in protecting against the threat; and (3) beliefs about the barriers or costs associated with taking an action. An action was thought to be more likely where, in the presence of a threat, the action was seen as efficacious and possible at a tolerable cost. Obviously, the preventive must be available to the individual, and the threat must be perceived. Barriers to acting included all perceived impediments—cost, inconvenience, pain, and so on. With respect to preventive behavior, such as obtaining immunizations, checkups, and screening, the elements of the health belief model have received considerable support as predictors of decisions to act or not act (see, for example, Becker and others, 1975). A recent study (Cummings and others, in press) of immunization for swine flu is illustrative. Nearly 300 residents of a county in Michigan, including urban, suburban, and rural areas, were interviewed by telephone prior to the availability of the vaccine, using a random digit dialing technique. Health beliefs, information about the vaccine program, demographic characteristics, and intent to act were all obtained. Three to four months later, at the conclusion of the health department's effort to vaccinate adults, the same people were reinterviewed to assess whether they had been inoculated, their reasons for acting or not acting, and their reactions to the campaign. Each of the health beliefs, taken separately, yielded significant associations with intention and behavior: the perceived severity of swine flu, vulnerability to it, the amount of protection believed to be afforded by the shot, and the perceived ease of obtaining the vaccine as well as its safety. Taken together, the set of elements yielded a multiple correlation of .5 with the dichotomous measure of behavior. As has usually been found, receiving the vaccine was highly associated with measures of socioeconomic status, but a significant relationship between health beliefs and the behavior of receiving the vaccine remained after the effect of socioeconomic status was removed.

Application of the health belief model to illness and sick role behavior has also yielded some positive results. Where an illness has been diagnosed and a course of therapy recommended, the individual's perception of the threat represented by symptoms or by the future course of the condition becomes central. It is in relation to this threat that possible actions and their costs can be evaluated when decisions are made. A recommendation by a health professional becomes one possibility, to be judged by its perceived value for dealing with the threat and in the light of barriers to acting.

Becker and Maiman (1975) have reviewed much of the literature on patient adherence from the point of view of the health belief model, and Becker and his colleagues have applied it to studies of adherence to regimens for acute illness (Becker, Drachman, and Kirscht, 1972b) and to obesity (Becker and others, 1977b). The model has also been applied to studies of adherence to hypertensive regimens (Kirscht and Rosenstock, 1977).

Other psychosocial variables can be incorporated into the framework provided by this model. Background characteristics condition the beliefs people hold about particular threats and about the value of taking an action (Kirscht and others, 1966), and a variety of forces in the individual's situation can act as facilitators or inhibitors of paths of acting. At present, the model seems least applicable to behaviors that are strongly habitual. Kasl (1974) noted that factors predicting initiation of some action, such as a decision to quit smoking, may not relate to success in carrying out that decision over the course of time. Further, the role of professional encounters and social influences are not explicitly handled in the model. There are, however, two aspects of behavior in relation to illness that are illuminated by considering such a perceptual-cognitive model. First, people can only act on what they believe to be the case, even though this may not correspond with what professionals think they have made perfectly clear. Johannsen, Hellmuth, and Sorauf (1966), in discussing cardiac patients' adherence to recommendations, concluded that the major difficulty lay in the patient's psychological readiness; they found many instances of what are described as "distortions" of the situation. Second, medical recommendations by no means encompass all health actions taken. People deal with most health matters without medical advice. Haggerty and Roghmann (1972) collected extensive health diary information from 512 families. They found large amounts of symptom occurrence and self-treatment, noting, for example, that one out of three children will already be on some form of medication when first seen by a physician and, more generally, that "the doctor's control over disease-relevant behavior is limited" (p. 114).

Social Role and Context Models

Social factors are clearly implicated in adhering to health recommendations. There are several formulations or frameworks within which these factors can be viewed. One is through the concept of the sick role and its obligations, especially regarding other role obligations. A second is in terms of social facilitation for adherent behavior, and the third is viewing behavior as the outcome of an interaction process, especially that between patient and provider.

Parsons' (1951a) classic statement of the ideal form of the sick role in our society has had a major effect on subsequent thinking concerning the social nature of illness. As a complement to exemption from normal obligations, the sick person is supposed to seek competent help and to cooperate in becoming well again. It is clear that behavioral enactment of the role will actually vary, even assuming relatively widespread acceptance of the nature of sickness. Some forms of "illness" are disputable (for example, mental illness) in terms of how they are regarded, so that the application of the obligations and rights is not clear. Variations in the way sickness is defined have been noted by a number of investigators (Segal, 1976) and, in particular, the applicability of the traditional sick role concept to chronic disease and behavior problems has been questioned. Parsons' description of the role, however, is in the context of a social system in which actors occupy a number of roles, and the very connotation of sickness as a form of deviance is that it creates trouble for the society. Hence, behavior in sickness must be shaped in part by other roles that are involved.

Norms about sickness or about its variants are not completely shared either between patients and professionals or among different groups. Hence, individuals vary in their expectations as to what they themselves or others should do. Following medical advice may not be the norm (Twaddle, 1969). Perhaps most important, sick role behavior represents the resolution of conflict, both among the sick person's various obligations and between that person and significant others. In general, we would expect that where elements of the regimen conflict with other norms, there would be lesser adherence to those elements. Vincent (1971) applies this conflict notion to compliance with a glaucoma regimen. In their study of cardiac patients, Davis and Eichhorn (1963) noted that those patients with a high work orientation were least likely to accept modifications of their behavior. A study of patients in a rehabilitation program (Ludwig and Adams, 1968) found evidence that those whose pre-illness status was more independent were less apt to complete the rehabilitation activities. These examples indicate that normative considerations play a role in adherence.

The general hypothesis in the social support framework is that the quality of relationships among those involved in a social network is a major determinant of behavior. Perhaps the best elaborated expression of this viewpoint in relation to health is the paradigm of Caplan and others (1976). Starting with the notion that behavior represents goal seeking, and the evaluation of an action is in terms of its utility for achieving goals, the model postulates that input provided by others acts on the individual's motives, learning, and relationships to the environment. Social support is defined as activities that help the individual move toward goals; it may be in tangible or symbolic form. Social-emotional ties can also help buffer strains from the environment.

In terms of adherence to medical recommendations, significant others, including professionals, can facilitate or impede movement toward goals by helping to define the role of adherent behavior, by aiding or hindering the behavioral process, and by providing feedback on the behavior itself. This formulation is related to the process outlined by Kosa and Robertson (1975), who note that illness episodes create needs both for solution of the problems or task and for reduction of anxiety about the episode. Significant others are especially important in meeting the emotional needs of the person.

Caplan and others (1976), in a pilot study of 200 hypertensive patients attending an outpatient clinic for treatment, found that patients who were highly motivated to comply with their regimen also had a high degree of support from their physician and from their spouses, although the measures of social support did not relate directly to adherence. The highest levels of adherence were observed in those patients with perceived self-competence, augmented by support from others. A small-scale experiment indicated that supportive group relationships led to better adherence.

It should be remembered that the social support model does not necessarily predict higher adherence to medical recommendations but only that the direction of forces provided by others is an important determinant of behavior. Significant others may provide influence in the direction of non-adherence. In a study of acceptance of treatment for tuberculosis among Mexican-Americans, Nall and Speilberg (1967) reported that greater social integration was associated with not following the treatment.

As an approach, social interaction does not represent a well-elaborated model but, rather, an emphasis on the importance of joint forces, in contrast to focusing solely on patient characteristics to produce behavioral outcomes. If there are important assumptions of this approach, they take the form of emphasis on patient behavior as influenced by an interactive system in which the professional has a specialized role in defining the health problem and shaping patient behaviors.

Francis, Korsch, and Morris (1969) focused on the communicative acts that took place between the mothers of ill children and physicians. To the extent that mothers' concerns were expressed and dealt with in a friendly fashion (reflected by satisfaction with the encounter), adherence was better. Both parties were active determiners of the process. Some findings of

Becker, Drachman, and Kirscht (1972b) were analogous—belief of the mother in the correctness of the diagnosis for an ill child and satisfaction with the encounter were associated with successful information transmittal and greater adherence. A study of adult patients by Hulka, Cassel, and Kupper (1976) concluded that accuracy of information, some understanding of purpose, and agreement regarding the medical advice were necessary for adherence to occur. Svarstad's (1976) work goes further in emphasizing accurate perceptions by the patient concerning what is expected, which depend on explicit interactions about the nature and purpose of a regimen. Efforts on the part of the professional to facilitate interaction and comprehension result in better adherence. Podell (1975) similarly stresses the need for the physician to seek an understanding of the patient's perspective. A common theme is that the patient has a more active role within a system of relationships. There is the flavor, however, that the participants are not equals, that professionals have specialized knowledge, that many patients fail to react or ask questions, but, nevertheless, that adherence is jointly determined. Many of the writings by pharmacists reflect the same point of view (McKenney and others, 1973).

An aspect of some behavioral formulations is closely related to patient-provider interaction. Contracting between individuals is an example of an interactive system in which specific behaviors are agreed to by each of the participants, based on the idea that social commitments influence behavior. One role of the professional (not universally accepted) is to provide help in formulating realistic ways to achieve goals and to monitor an agreement. Stekel and Swain (1977) showed the value of contracting with hypertensive patients to help them achieve compliance. A key part of their procedure was to encourage patients to write the contract and to assist them in analyzing the process into manageable steps (for example, in changing eating patterns to attain weight loss). All the patients complied with the contracts they had shared in preparing.

Interventions and Adherence

Much of the work on adherence described thus far represents associations between psychosocial factors and behavior in naturally occurring situations. Evidence from correlational research may be highly suggestive, but a more rigorous test of a formulation is through effective experimental manipulation. In the literature on adherence, there are a number of attempts to modify behavior patterns by systematic intervention, and we now turn to what has been found.

Patient Education

We noted previously that the relationship of knowledge and adherence is not clear because the concept of knowledge has been used to cover too broad a range of information. Attempts to provide information about the nature of illness and its treatment, at a fairly abstract level, have generally not affected adherence to medical recommendations. Sackett and others (1975) and Kirscht and Rosenstock (1977) reported attempts to inform hypertensive patients concerning the condition, both studies utilizing control groups that did not receive the information. While there was a difference in knowledge on the part of those who were informed, no difference appeared subsequently either in adherence behaviors or blood pressure levels. In both studies, adherence was assessed months after the intervention. Tagliacozzo and others (1974) introduced a special nurse instruction for patients with chronic diseases attending an outpatient clinic; a control group received the regular care procedures. It is not entirely clear what was taught in the intervention group, but it was formally structured to cover specific information about diseases and treatments. In terms of main effects on staying in treatment, adhering to advice, or even changing attitudes, there was little impact. However, some interactive effects occurred: "The experience appears to increase compliance among those with more knowledge of illness, multiple illnesses, high anxiety, favorable attitudes toward the clinic and those who felt their illness was serious" (1974, p. 603).

In a study of obese children attending a clinic (Becker and others, 1977b) mothers of the obese patients were randomly assigned to one of three groups: a threatening communication condition, a low-threat communication, and a no-communication control. The messages were delivered orally in a standardized format, following an initial visit to the clinic. Subsequently, each patient received dietary counseling and reappointments to the clinic. The groups receiving the communications lost significantly more weight than the controls through all four of the follow-up visits, and the group receiving the more threatening message did better than that receiving the low-threat version. For the entire sample of mothers, initial health beliefs regarding health threats, the child's susceptibility to illness, and the benefits of weight loss were predictive of subsequent success in reducing weight. In this instance, providing "persuasive" information resulted in better adherence to a diet.

Information intended to inform people about their regimen has demonstrated utility in relation to adherence. In connection with a neighborhood health center, McKenney and his associates (1973) selected fifty hypertensive patients. One half met monthly with the pharmacist, the other half continued with the usual level of care. The meetings included discussion of medications, educational efforts, evaluation of progress, and counseling regarding treatment. The members of the intervention group significantly increased not only their knowledge but also their adherence and control of blood pressure. After a five-month period, the intervention ended, and all patients were followed for a period of time; their compliance and blood pressure reverted to prestudy levels. Clearly, more than information was provided to the patients; for example, the pharmacist made a series of recommendations to the treating physicians, which may itself have altered the situation, providing a more supportive environment for adherence (Caplan and others, 1976). Other instances of successful educational-counseling efforts are summarized by Sharpe and Mikeal (1975) and by Schwartz (1976). Not all instructions given about regimens necessarily enhance compliance: Malahy (1966) reported no differences in medication errors made by a group of patients given brief instructions after seeing a physician as compared with randomly assigned controls who did not receive the special instruction.

Provision of information and reasons for regimens shade over into interventions designed to facilitate adherence, either by adding to the forces for acting or by removing factors that hinder or impede action. Those interventions that increase convenience—for example, better labeling, dose dispensers, simplification of regimens, and individual appointments versus block scheduling—generally yield better adherence. Psychologically, such maneuvers should help provide paths of action with fewer barriers or greater facilitation of the recommended behavior. An example is a study (Lima and others, 1976) in which patients given antibiotic prescriptions also received special reminders, such as a sticker to be put on the refrigerator; there was a control condition. As measured by bottle checks, the reminders nearly doubled adherence. The influence of barriers is illustrated by a study in which adult patients given child-resistant medicine containers experienced significantly greater difficulty in opening them and poorer adherence than a control group given conventional bottles (Lane and others, 1971).

Reminders have been quite successful in lowering appointment failures. Gates and Colburn (1976, p. 265) compared phone reminders, letters, and a no-contact control condition for patients with appointments scheduled at a neighborhood health center. Among the controls, there was a 38 percent failure rate, whereas only 9 percent and 10 percent respectively of the phone and letter groups were judged failures. The authors note that the reminders have differential effectiveness in that more patients were reached by letter. Similar results were noted by Shepard and Moseley (1976) for clinic patients at Children's Hospital in Boston; they found that more patients were reached through the mails, at about one half the cost of the telephone strategy.

Social Support

Interventions specifically designed to influence adherence through supportive actions by others have been relatively rare. We noted earlier the study conducted by Caplan and his co-workers to implement a "buddy" system. There have been some promising attempts to demonstrate the effectiveness of group support on adherence. Green and others (1977) conducted group sessions at a clinic with patients suffering from asthma, a condition known to be influenced by psychological and situational factors. Even with relatively brief group meetings, the participants had significantly fewer emergency room visits and their subsequent attacks were of less severity than those of controls who did not meet together. Rosenberg (1976) discusses other instances in which the use of group discussion by patients resulted in lower need for emergency and hospital services.

Modifications in Providing Care

Changes introduced into the system of care may enhance adherence through providing a greater degree of support and clearer expectations for a patient. Thus, awareness of the problem of dropouts in treatment for hypertension has led to attempts at changing the way in which medical care is provided. Finnerty and others (1973b) set up modified clinic procedures—including definite appointments, better monitoring, and more sensitivity to patients' needs—that led to dramatic reduction in losses. Wilber and Barrow (1972) utilized home visits by a nurse that seemed to result in greater compliance and better management of blood pressure. Fletcher, Appel, and Bourgois (1974) introduced a special follow-up of patients found to be hypertensive on a visit to the emergency service at Johns Hopkins Hospital. The usual referral of a randomly selected group of patients was augmented by special contact to remind and assist. Compared to controls, 21 percent more returned for follow-up, although better blood pressure control was not achieved in the experimental group.

Facilitating roles played by clinic workers have some support in studies. A family health management specialist was tried out in a large acute care pediatric clinic (Fink and others, 1969). All new patients over a four-month period were randomly assigned to a control group or to intervention by the specialist, who met with the family and provided education and coordination in addition to some nursing services. In terms of medication adherence, appointment keeping, following other recommended procedures, and understanding, the experimental families did significantly better.

At a more ambitious level, there have been two experimental tests of the generally accepted truism that "continuity of care" is always better. Both were studies of pediatric services and yielded conflicting conclusions. Gordis and Markowitz (1971) studied a continuous care system, set up for a randomly assigned group of children who received penicillin prophylaxis for rheumatic fever. Care was provided by two pediatricians, who handled all medical problems of the children. Control children were given the usual clinic care, being seen by different physicians at each visit. Adherence to the penicillin regimen was tested over fifteen months through collection of periodic urine samples taken on a random schedule. There were no differences between the groups. One peculiar finding was a decrease in compliance for both groups from the one-year baseline period to the experimental period. The second study (Becker, Drachman, and Kirscht, 1974) involved setting up two sides in a large pediatric care center: One was staffed by a panel of physicians and with assignment of families to a particular physician; the other was the usual clinic setup with rotating staff and subclinics. Families were randomly assigned to the continuous or discontinuous system. After a year, both patient and staff reactions were assessed. In this case, the continuous care system yielded significantly greater adherence (appointment keeping) and satisfaction on the part of patients, as well as staff satisfaction with both work situation and with patients.

A system change that deserves much wider testing involved the introduction of educational sessions for physicians treating hypertensive patients at the Johns Hopkins General Medical Clinic (Inui, Yourtee, and Williamson, 1976). Physicians were assigned to treatment or control groups as a function of the day of the week on which they served at the clinic; in all, sixty-two physicians participated. After information was obtained from a sample of patients, through interviews and record review, tutorial sessions were conducted with twenty-nine physicians, using information about compliance and beliefs derived from the patients themselves. Subsequently, a second sample of patients was assessed. Those patients under treatment by the "educated" physicians showed greater knowledge about their regimen, more appropriate beliefs concerning hypertension, greater compliance in taking medications, and significantly better blood pressure control than did control patients. The two groups did not differ on keeping appointments or on reported dietary adherence. Data were also collected indicating that the tutorial sessions modified physician behavior; for example, experimental physicians spent more time in educational activities during patient encounters. Changes in physician behavior, or in the way care is provided, obviously represent complex interventions. They modify the social situation in the process of giving care and probably affect the nature and amount of information transmitted.

Self-Help

We will not review applications of self-help techniques to health problems, such as behavior therapy, except to discuss briefly some trials related to adherence. Work with patient contracts for hypertensive treatment was described previously (Stekel and Swain, 1977). In this case, the intervention involved changes in the system of care, in interaction patterns between patients and providers, and in the degree of active participation by the patient in the regimen itself (demonstrated by Schulman, 1977, in her follow-up study of the patients involved). The idea of self-control or self-monitoring has been widely discussed; examples of applications are found in Katz and Zlutnick (1975). Sackett and his colleagues (1975) employed home blood pressure units as part of an intervention with noncompliant hypertensive patients, finding better compliance and control of blood pressure. However, a study by Carnahan and Nugent (1975) of a group of hypertensive patients given home blood pressure kits found very modest reductions in blood pressure, as compared with control patients; of course, theirs was not a study of compliance but of outcome.

Modes of Contact in Prevention and Screening

Many health recommendations made outside of clinical settings in which treatment is being delivered involve the problem of how people are reached. Mass campaigns of various types have been conducted, although rigorous evaluations are not very common. There is widespread agreement that personal contact is more likely to result in influence transmission as compared to impersonal media. The latter, however, are much cheaper and more pervasive (Swinehart, 1968).

In terms of large-scale efforts to influence preventive behavior, the Stanford three-community study is one of the most ambitious (Maccoby and Farquhar, 1975). Since 1972, three California towns have been involved in the research: One receives no special communication efforts; one receives an intensive broadcast and print mass-media campaign; and the third receives the media efforts plus intensive counseling of high-risk persons. Multiple assessments, including interviews and examinations, have been conducted. Throughout, the focus has been on reduction of risk for cardiovascular disease: smoking, dietary intake, weight, hypertension, and physical activity. The results for dietary behavior have been promising (Stern and others, 1976), with evidence for reduction of the intake of fatty foods most marked in the intensively instructed group but also significant for the mass-media campaign.

This study represents one of the most intensive efforts at community-wide trials of health education. Other controlled studies of mass media have not yielded very successful outcomes. A careful evaluation of a community exposed to a television campaign to induce use of seat belts showed no difference in observed belt use from a group not exposed to the messages (Robertson and others, 1974). Using a quasi-experimental design, Udry and others (1972) tested a mass-media effort concerning contraception. A six-month campaign yielded no differences between experimental and control communities on attendance at family-planning clinics, sale of contraceptives, or incidence of unwanted births. Thus, use of mass media needs to be approached with caution, especially in terms of what changes or effects can reasonably be expected.

Studies of specific efforts to influence participation of groups in health behavior have yielded some positive findings. In studies of notification by schools to parents that screening had detected a condition in the child needing follow-up, Gabrielson, Levin, and Ellison (1967) found that likelihood of parental action increased with more, and varied, contact efforts. Every additional effort at contact for participation in breast cancer screening yielded more response (Fink, Shapiro, and Roeser, 1972). In recruitment of community residents for blood pressure screening, four different contact procedures were compared, plus a control, in comparable inner-city areas (Stahl and others, 1977). Home visits yielded the greatest number of previously undiagnosed hypertensives as compared to letters and gift offers. However, in this instance, the more "passive" measures were more successful in turning up people who already knew they were hypertensive but were not currently in treatment. A number of the findings suggest that greater influence will be exercised if the communication strategy and themes are tailored to particular target groups. Kirscht, Haefner, and Eveland (1975) compared three different forms of mailed materials inviting participation in a multiphasic screening program: a "usual" but rather uninformative letter and brochure, a threat-oriented version, and a positive health version.

Overall, the latter two yielded higher proportions of response, but virtually all of the differences were due to women's responding to the positive health theme.

Some Ethical Issues in Adherence Interventions

The area of adherence to health recommendations raises questions about the ethics of both research and practice. Concern with ethical issues is evolving rapidly, with an emphasis on individual rights that was hardly thought possible about ten years ago. In the research area, there are persistent difficulties in measures of adherence, for reasons noted previously. Because of these, it has been tempting to develop covert assessments in which the individual is not an informed participant. Testing for tracer substances used to measure medication compliance has frequently been done without knowledge of the patient. Pill counts have been taken in various studies at unexpected home visits or patients requested to return medication containers, apparently on pretexts. Most published studies involving such procedures appear to have been done without explanation to the patients rather than with any active deception. However, Gordis' (1976) discussion of measuring compliance notes the possible reactivity of direct assessment of compliance where the patient becomes "suspicious," implying that passive deception, at least, is required. We believe that such practices are clear violations of patient rights.

More difficult, however, is the question of how much information should be given in seeking consent from prospective participants. The problem of consent exists no matter what form of data collection is utilized. Much information that bears on the study of adherence is available in medical, dental, and pharmacy records. Most patients are probably not aware of the nature and extent of existing data; requests to consult records certainly need elaboration for an informed decision. Even where an investigator is utilizing straightforward questions concerning an individual's behavior, there may be subtle pressures to respond, particularly if the questioning is done in a context where a connection is seen between obtaining care and responding. Beyond guarantees of anonymity and procedures set up to prevent any future harm from identification of individual responses, investigators must be responsible for monitoring sources of pressure on potential participants.

While it may go without saying that a recommendation should be reasonably efficacious, it should also be added that interventions should be reasonably free of potential harm. This issue comes up in connection with strategies that may be regarded as coercive or in the use of emotion-arousing themes regarding threats to health or consequences of noncompliance. Many professionals are concerned about the use of threats in connection with health communications. We believe there is nothing inherently wrong with graphic description of health consequences, but that attention needs to be directed toward accuracy and use of caution in arousing fears about consequences that cannot be averted. Virtually every message about health carries an implied threat and raises the need for reassurance.

A more subtle problem connected with adherence is that of conceptual perspective and the uses to which information is put. Research on adherence is generally applied research; investigators have some responsibility for the nature and possible effects of interventions developed from information gathered about adherence, and for the direct and indirect effects of interventions that are tested. Whether recognized or not, attempts at change involve assumptions about that which is to be changed. Since the subject of adherence research is people, approaches and perspectives are not ethically irrelevant. Stimson (1974) presents detailed objections to much of the research on patient compliance on the grounds that it implies by conceptual stances that the patient is the culprit and we have caught him out. While we have utilized the health belief approach to adherence and believe that it helps explain whatever behavior occurs, and not just medically approved behaviors, there is still the fact that the model has not been put into a sufficiently large context. The danger is that a focus on individual factors will shape a framework in which other contributors are ignored. Specifically, attention should be devoted to the medical care system, the behavior of professionals, economic problems and inequities, and problems of access. Selectivity is involved in any perspective, including both investigators and professional use of information.

Education about health may be regarded as having two components: information necessary to make informed decisions, and behavioral skills necessary to act on that information. It would seem that health professionals have not only the right but also the obligation to provide information to an uninformed client or public and to make a responsible effort to provide it in a manner that assures it will be received and understood. Then, for the motivated client or population who wish to act on the knowledge, the professional would seem to have the further obligation to give instruction in behavioral skills necessary to satisfy those motives. To illustrate, the coronary patient (or general public) may not be fully aware of the relationship between cigarette smoking and heart disease. It becomes an obligation of the health sciences to educate both patients and the public on that matter. Then, for cigarette smokers who wish to cut down smoking or to give it up entirely, it is a further responsibility of the professional to assist them in doing so using whatever ethical means the state of the art offers.

It appears to us that the only serious ethical question arises in the case of clients whose motives are such that they do not wish to modify a particular behavior. It is our view that in such cases it is inappropriate to attempt to change motives (even if it were possible). Any informed person who wishes to engage in any personal practices that are not conducive to good health, should, if those practices do not constitute a danger to others, be free to do so.

Overview

The following table is offered as an overview of relationships between adherence and selected psychosocial factors. In the table, many of the char-

Table 1. Adherence Behaviors

	Following Prescribed Regimen	Staying in Treatment	Prevention
Social characteristics			
Age	0	+	—
Sex	0	0	+ (female)
Education	0	0	+
Income	0	0	+
Psychological dispositions			
Beliefs about threat to health	+	+	+
Beliefs about efficacy of action	+	+	+
Knowledge of recommendation and purpose	+	+	+
General attitudes toward medical care	0	0	0
General knowledge about health and illness	0	0	+?
Intelligence	0	0	0
Anxiety	—?	—	?
Internal control	0?	0	+
Psychic disturbance	—	—	?
Social context			
Social support	+	+	+
Social isolation	—	—	—
Primary group stability	+	+	+
Situational demands			
Symptoms	+	+	NA
Complexity of action	—	—	—
Duration of action	—	—	—
Interference with other actions	—	—	—
Interactions with health care system			
Convenience factors	—	—	—
Continuity of care	+	+	+
Personal source of care	+	+	+?
General satisfaction	0	0	0
Supportive interaction	+	+	?

Note: Many of the 0 entries represent inconsistent findings; in the case of education, for example, there are positive relationships to medication compliance in several studies but no relationships in many others.

acteristics discussed previously are listed, in abbreviated form, on the left side. The three columns represent different behaviors: adherence to prescribed regimens, staying in treatment, and taking preventive actions. The entries indicate our judgment and synthesis as to the *general* relationship between the listed factor and the particular behavior form, as follows: positive association (+), negative association (—), no definite association (0), uncertainty (?), and not applicable (NA). Obviously, the entries are judgmental and oversimplified but are intended to convey a view of the current status of knowledge concerning adherence.

9

Coping with the Stresses of Illness

Frances Cohen

Richard S. Lazarus

"When a person is incapacitated by a serious acute illness and has to enter a hospital . . . for initial emergency support, he is not only severely debilitated by physiological imbalance, but his whole psychological adjustment is in severe turmoil. He is faced with the sudden termination of his customary life-style, which has abruptly passed out of his control. He suffers pain, strange symptoms, and a frightening disruption of physiological processes that were once either automatic or taken for granted. He is afraid of getting worse or even of death and dying. He must leave his immediate future up to the 'experts,' most of whom he has never met before. He is concerned about the disruption in his family, friend, and work circles and its consequences; and he worries about his capacity to reenter these circles. He faces an uncertain future in which resumption of normal activity is questionable for him. He is concerned about whether he can make major changes to accommodate any physical residues of his illness. Finally, he questions the reasons why he became ill and what he can do to prevent a recurrence" (Gruen, 1975, p. 223).

Developing symptoms of illness and undergoing medical treatment can be highly stressful events. Many people take for granted their health and abilities to carry out daily activities and to fulfill social roles. Since this view of oneself as being healthy, able, and having a normal physique is central to most people's image and evaluation, becoming ill can be a shock to a person's sense of security and to his or her self-image. Not only does it threaten the customary view of oneself, but it further underscores that one is indeed vulnerable (to illness, and perhaps then to other problems), that life is uncertain, that one may have little control over events, and that one's life may be changed in major respects. As a result, adjustment to an illness or injury which is life-threatening or potentially disabling may require considerable coping effort.

The aim of this chapter is to provide a theoretical overview of the stress and coping perspective so as to set the literature on coping with illness into a meaningful context, to highlight important issues that deepen our understanding of the coping process, and to present and discuss important empirical research studies that focus on coping in health care situations. Space limitations prevent the attempt to offer anything even approaching a thorough review of the literature on the stresses of illness and on coping with them. We shall address the following general questions: What are the stresses involved in illness and in medical treatment? What coping mechanisms are used to deal with these stresses? What is adaptive coping in the face of serious medical problems? How can interventions be made to facilitate patients' coping efforts?

Understanding these issues is important not only from a theoretical perspective but also because of their many practical ramifications. There is much clinical evidence that despite similarities in medical condition, patients differ greatly in their course of medical recovery. It is quite possible that this reflects the relative success or failure of different patterns of coping with the threats of being ill and being treated. Our view is that cognitive factors are central in determining the impact of stressful events (Lazarus, 1966; Lazarus, Averill, and Opton, 1970, 1974; Lazarus and Launier, 1978) and that the ways individuals interpret or appraise a situation affect coping and the emotional, physiological, and behavioral reactions to stressful experiences.

We shall begin with a description of our theoretical framework for analyzing coping, providing a selective overview of the issues inherent in the concept. For additional treatments of coping, the reader is referred to Coelho, Hamburg, and Adams (1974), Haan (1977), Lazarus (1966), Lazarus (1978), and Lazarus and Launier (1978). After presenting the framework, we will consider the types of stresses potentiated by illness and medical treatment, suggesting that these be viewed as posing a series of adaptive tasks requiring coping. The last section reviews research focusing on: (1) the processes of coping in illness; (2) the relationship between coping dispositions, coping processes, and medical outcomes; and (3) the effects on outcome of various psychological interventions designed to influence coping strategies.

Theoretical Framework

Cognitive factors play a central role in emotion and adaptation, affecting, for example, the impact of stressful events, the choice of coping patterns, and the subjective, physiological, and behavioral reactions. The process of cognitive appraisal mediates psychologically between the person and the environment in any stressful encounter. That is, the person evaluates whether a situation is damaging, or potentially damaging, on the basis of his or her understanding of the power of the situation to produce harm and the resources he or she has available to neutralize or tolerate the harm.

There are two types of appraisal: Primary appraisal is an evaluation of the significance of an event for one's well-being (stressful, benign-positive, or irrelevant), whereas secondary appraisal is an evaluation of coping resources and options. These processes may be conscious and deliberate, unconscious, or at the fringe of consciousness (see, for example, Weisman's, 1972, concept of "middle knowledge"). Appraisals of stress are of three types: harm/loss referring to damage that has already occurred; threat referring to anticipated or future harm; and challenge in which the focus is placed positively on potential gain, growth, or mastery rather than negatively on the possible risks. The way a person construes an encounter (appraisal) is, in short, the psychological key to understanding coping efforts in that situation and to understanding the emotional reaction, which waxes and wanes and changes in quality with the flow of events and the shifting pattern of appraisal.

Definition of Coping

Coping is defined as efforts, both action-oriented and intrapsychic, to manage (that is, master, tolerate, reduce, minimize) environmental and internal demands, and conflicts among them, which tax or exceed a person's resources (Lazarus and Launier, 1978). Coping can occur prior to a stressful confrontation, in which case it is called anticipatory coping, as well as in reaction to a present or past confrontation with harm. In our view, insufficient attention has been paid to anticipatory coping. In a series of recent papers, the importance of anticipatory coping activities has been heavily emphasized (Lazarus, 1975; Lazarus and Cohen, 1977; Lazarus and Launier, 1978; Folkman, Schaefer, and Lazarus, in press). The key point is that while we are sometimes accidentally confronted by a situation having major relevance for our welfare, we also engage in the active regulating of our emotional reactions, selecting the environment to which we must respond, shaping commerce with it, planning, choosing, avoiding, tolerating, postponing, escaping, demolishing, manipulating attention, and so on. Cognitive behavior therapists who encourage "rehearsal" as a way of preparing for a stressful encounter (see Meichenbaum, 1977) are dealing with anticipatory coping in their treatment procedures.

We do not make a sharp distinction between "defenses" and "coping," as Haan (1963, 1969, 1977) and Kroeber (1963) have done. These writers view defenses as distorting reality, rigid and pulled from the past, while coping is seen as flexible, adaptive, oriented to reality, and moving toward the future. To us, such a distinction reflects value judgments on the part of the observer and involves inferences that the observer may not have sufficient information to make (see, for example, Sjöbäck, 1973). Further, defensive and coping processes may interweave as people deal with situations of threat, and it may be difficult if not impossible to separate these strands (Murphy, 1974; White, 1974). For example, Murphy describes how children intertwine active coping and defense mechanisms in a pattern described as a "two-steps-forward, one-step-backward process" (p. 76) in trying to master common childhood fears. Vaillant (1976) provides illustrations of how immature and mature defenses (the latter might be labeled coping by Haan) are intermixed in efforts to deal with situations of conflict. And elsewhere, Lazarus (1978) has speculated that normally or even optimally functioning persons use an admixture of problem-solving and intrapsychic (palliative) modes of coping which can be highly serviceable in managing situations in which morale, social functioning, and somatic health depend on more than mere mastery of a short-lived harm or threat. As the terms are used throughout this chapter, "coping" or "coping processes" include any efforts at stress management, including processes that can be called defenses.

Functions of Coping

A distinction should be made between problem-solving efforts to cope with the threat itself (that is, to deal with the obstacles and opportunities present in the environment or in oneself) and efforts to regulate the emotional distress (see Hamburg, Coelho, and Adams, 1974; Lazarus, 1975; Lazarus, Averill, and Opton, 1974; Lazarus and Launier, 1978; Mechanic, 1962a; Murphy, 1974). Lazarus and Launier refer to the former as the instrumental or problem-solving function and the latter as the palliative function. Caring for a wound, quitting a stressful job, fortifying one's house against a storm, or seeking advice about medical treatment are all attempts to alter the troubled person-environment relationship in a stressful transaction. On the other hand, practicing meditation, undergoing biofeedback, taking drugs, or denying or avoiding unpleasant facts, all represent efforts to regulate the emotional responses themselves.

These two functions of coping can be mutually facilitative, as in the case in which reducing the emotional distress may enable the person to study more effectively for a crucial, upcoming exam (see Mechanic, 1962a). However, one function can get in the way of the other, as when denial that a breast lump could be anything serious leads to delay in seeking medical evaluation (instrumental actions) and increases the risk of advanced-stage cancer (Katz and others, 1970), or when such denial results in testing one's physical condition during a heart attack by climbing flights of stairs to reassure oneself that there is nothing seriously wrong (Hackett and Cassem, 1975). Purely palliative coping efforts, especially those involving reality distortion and seeming "irrational," are often perplexing to health professionals. The two functions of coping and their intricate relationships must be kept in mind if one is to understand the varied patterns of coping seen in people with serious illness.

Coping Modes

We identify four main modes or forms of coping: information seeking, direct action, inhibition of action, and intrapsychic (or cognitive) processes. *Information seeking* is one of the most basic forms of coping in situations that are novel and of which knowledge is limited, or under conditions of ambiguity. The person tries to find out whether problems exist and what, if anything, must be done. In the context of illness, as we shall see later, some patients are insatiable in their search for information about their problem, whereas others avoid it and prefer to place themselves in the hands of someone they can trust. What to do about such individual differences is an interesting and important practical problem. *Direct actions* include arguing, running away, putting oneself on dialysis—in short, doing something about the problem. However, often the wise coper refrains from actions that are impulsive, poorly grounded in information, or potentially dangerous or embarrassing. Therefore, the obverse of direct action, *inhibition of action*, can legitimately be thought of as a mode of coping. *Intrapsychic processes* include denial, avoidance, intellectualized detachment, putting a good face on a bad situation, and any of a wide variety of what are traditionally thought of as defenses. These modes are particularly important in the context of illness because, so often, little can be done directly by the patient (as when hospitalized for diagnosis or surgery) except to allow therapeutic procedures to be applied and to find some serviceable way to think about what is happening. The more helpless the person is, the more he or she must depend on cognitive or intrapsychic modes of coping. A fifth mode of coping could be added here, namely, *turning to others* for help and succor (Chapter Ten in this volume). There is growing evidence that ailing persons do better in many ways if they can maintain and utilize social relationships. Social supports appear to enhance the possibilities for effective coping (Cobb, 1976; Dimsdale and others, 1978; Kaplan, Cassel, and Gore, 1977).

Others have identified coping strategies in the health care setting in overlapping but different ways, and at present there is no widely agreed upon system for describing coping. Researchers who study coping in health care situations often focus their attention on those strategies that seem to emerge from the data obtained; thus, the mechanisms described in various studies differ. For example, coping strategies have been described for patients with serious illnesses (Lipowski, 1970), families of children with polio (Davis, 1963), patients with severe burns (Hamburg, Hamburg, and deGoza, 1953), patients who are dying (Weisman, 1972), women coping with menopause (Hamburg, Coelho, and Adams, 1974), women facing a breast biopsy (Katz and others, 1970), and so forth.

Some researchers list strategies thought to be common to many health-related situations, although there is often little overlap in the strategies given. For example, Lipowski (1970) suggests that minimization and vigilant focusing are the two central cognitive coping styles; these can be expressed behaviorally in one of three ways, that is, by tackling, capitulating, or avoiding. Moos and Tsu (1977) list the following strategies or skills as common to illness situations: (1) denying or minimizing the seriousness of a crisis, (2) seeking relevant information, (3) requesting reassurance and emotional support, (4) learning specific illness-related procedures, (5) setting concrete limited goals, (6) rehearsing alternative outcomes, and (7) finding a general purpose or pattern of meaning in events. Working with advanced cancer patients, Weisman and Worden (1976-1977) list the following as general coping strategies: rational-intellectual methods, shared concern, reversal of affect, suppression, displacement, confrontation, redefinition, fatalism, acting out, negotiating feasible alternatives, tension reduction, stimulus reduction, disowning responsibility, compliance, and self-pity.

Haan's (1977) system, alluded to earlier, provides a taxonomy of generic ego processes, which includes discrimination, detachment, means-end symbolization, delayed response, sensitivity, time reversal, selective awareness, diversion, transformation, and restraint. Each of these ego processes can be observed in a coping version, a defensive version, and as a form of ego fragmentation. For example, concentration is the coping version of the ego process of selective awareness, denial is the defense form, and distraction/ fixation the fragmentation form.

As one can see, some classificatory schemes, such as our own, are rather broad, with only four major categories, though with many more specific ones within each division. Others, such as Haan's, are restricted to ego or cognitive activity, that is, are intrapsychic exclusively. Still others (for example, Moos and Tsu, 1977; Weisman and Worden, 1976-1977) arise in the special context of the medical setting and are not necessarily designed to extend to other types of stressful encounter. Much needs to be done to sharpen and improve our present systems of classification of coping processes.

Assessment of Coping

Intervention research and practice related to prevention, treatment, and education require a knowledge of which coping patterns are successful, the ways in which they work, and the conditions under which they work. However, in order to gain this understanding, we need to be able to assess such patterns, and this is where technology is, as yet, quite inadequate to the task. For this reason, we should take some time to spell out some of the issues involved in the assessment of coping.

Dispositional Versus Process Approaches

An important distinction must be made between two ways of evaluating coping—that is, assessing coping as a disposition, trait, or style, or as a process (Averill and Opton, 1968). Both methods of assessment have been used in research on coping in medical situations.

Coping *dispositions* refer to tendencies of an individual to utilize a particular mode or pattern of coping in a variety of stressful encounters. Research on coping dispositions has focused mostly on narrow coping dimensions, such as a tendency to avoid or seek out threatening information (the repression-sensitization dimension of Byrne, 1961, 1964), although broader cognitive styles (such as cognitive controls and neurotic styles) have also been examined (see, for example, Gardner and others, 1959; Shapiro, 1965). To measure coping dispositions, the tendency of the person to use one or another coping process is usually assessed independently of the stressful event by a questionnaire or projective technique. This test behavior is treated as a trait measure and considered as a predictor of the coping behavior observed in some stress situation, such as coping with surgery. For example, in a study by Andrew (1967, 1970) a sentence-completion test was used to measure the tendency of a person to use "coping" (sensitizing) or "avoiding" strategies. Responses to these sentences were scored and used as a measure of whether subjects would be utilizing avoiding or coping strategies in response to a forthcoming surgical operation.

Alternately, one can study the coping *processes* individuals actually use in coping with a particular stressful situation. The individual's behavior is observed as it occurs in that stressful situation and the mode of coping inferred from it. For example, Cohen and Lazarus (1973) interviewed patients preoperatively and rated whether they sought or avoided information about their illness and the anticipated operation. Other researchers have interviewed patients awaiting breast biopsies or general surgery, or during their child's terminal illness, and evaluated the defenses those patients used or were using and the successfulness of those defenses (Katz and others, 1970; Price, Thaler, and Mason, 1957; Wolff and others, 1964).

One weakness of the dispositional approach is its assumptions regarding consistency in coping behavior. Little evidence exists that there is much consistency in mode of coping from one situation to another (Palmer, 1968; Wiener, Carpenter, and Carpenter, 1956). Situational factors, including demands of the situation, coping options available within it, social supports, and so on, also have important effects on the coping strategies an individual uses (see also Block, 1968). To the extent these conditions affect the coping processes, trait measures will have limited predictive power. As it turns out, only weak or nonsignificant relationships have been found between measures of coping dispositions and the actual coping behavior observed (Austin, 1974; Cohen and Lazarus, 1973; Hoffman, 1970). This raises serious questions as to what such coping tests are actually measuring (see Lazarus, Averill, and Opton, 1974; Woods, 1977).

Not only can questions be raised about the consistency of coping from one situation to another, but it is also likely that within a stressful encounter, such as major illness, several different stages of coping may be observed, each with its own pressures leading to the use of different modes of coping. For example, Hofer and others (1972a, 1972b) suggest there may be highly significant individual changes in coping, and in psychological stress reactions, during different periods of a stressful life situation. Parkes (1972) has described how individuals initially refuse to accept the loss of a loved one, but through subsequent oscillations between denial and reality-testing can gradually come to terms with it. Bereavement is a particularly useful model for illustrating coping as process and the notion of stages. Horowitz (1976) also describes how patterns of denial and intrusive thoughts may alternate in reactions to stressful life events. Mages and Mendelsohn (Chapter Ten in this volume) outline the different demands and strategies found in the various stages of cancer, arguing that such coping should be seen as a developmental process. This variability in coping processes from one time period to another lends support to the argument that dispositional tests of coping provide inadequate measures of actual coping. It also suggests the importance of studying coping processes in the same individual over time, a theme developed extensively also by Lazarus (1978) and Lazarus and others (in press).

Moos (1974b) has provided an overview of dispositional measures and procedures that have been used to assess coping. Researchers hoping to assess coping behavior in real-life situations are often distraught by the unknown validity and reliability of such measures, by other researchers' seeming indifference to issues of process and validity, and by the range of coping behaviors assessed in different studies. For example, one of the coping styles most commonly assessed is the polarity or dimension of repression-sensitization (Byrne, 1961, 1964; see also Epstein and Fenz, 1967), and the closely related concepts of repression-isolation (Gardner and others, 1959; Levine and Spivack, 1964), avoidance-coping (Andrew, 1967, 1970; DeLong, 1970; Goldstein, 1959; Goldstein and others, 1965), and denial-intellectualization (Lazarus and Alfert, 1964). However, many questions have been raised about the validity of these measures (see Lazarus, Averill, and Opton, 1974). Further, although the theoretical basis of these various polarities or dimensions appears to be similar, research reveals low or nonsignificant correlations among them (Cohen and Lazarus, 1973; Levine and Spivack, 1964).

Difficulties in Assessing Coping

To assess coping processes requires measurement strategies that are quite different from those employed in measuring coping styles or traits. Assessment of coping as a process requires developing means of describing what the person is doing and thinking in specific encounters. Trait measures may ask questions about what a person usually does but they do not focus on what a person actually is doing. They are also usually focused on a limited class of coping modes; rarely do they cover the full ground of the four modes cited earlier (information seeking, direct actions, inhibition of action, and intrapsychic processes).

There are a number of difficult problems that must be faced if one is to assess coping as it takes place (as a process) in naturalistic settings. We shall briefly discuss a few major ones—specifically, how to assess coping as a constellation of many strategies, how to obtain information about coping, difficulties in assessing specific coping processes, and evaluating coping effectiveness.

Coping as a constellation of many acts. Coping is not a single act but rather a constellation of many acts and thoughts, triggered by a complex set of demands that change with time. What is needed is a way of describing and categorizing the combinations of things a person did or thought during the period of encounter. Such a pattern description could then be used to compare one person or group with themselves and with others (ipsative-normative analyses). For example, in a quarrel with a spouse, a person may use humor, denial, threats, anger, attempted detachment, information seeking, avoidance of implications, self-depreciation, tears, expressions of love, criticism, and so forth. How is this "mode of coping" to be described? We need first to develop methods to assess and describe the various interpersonal, intrapsychic, and problem-solving maneuvers used in one situation, and second to find ways to categorize the constellation of coping processes found, both in that situation and over time. Only then will we be able to begin to assess the coping processes used by an individual in more complex situations, such as in coping with the threat of surgery or heart disease.

The clinical setting has a tradition of doing this type of evaluation, as in the case of Berne's (1964) transactional analysis, in which not only are the types of interchanges described but also interpretive names are given that reflect the type of interpersonal game (implying the motivation or function) being played. The problem is not that such description has not been attempted, but that what has been done is not systematic or measurement-oriented so that it can ultimately be used in research on coping with illness or other long-term stressful encounters. Lazarus and his associates are currently trying to develop methods for handling this assessment problem systematically.

How to obtain information about coping. It is probably not fruitful to ask most people to tell us how they coped, except perhaps in the case of a limited number of persons who are familiar with concepts of coping and are capable of introspection and verbalization in the classic tradition of Wundt. Defense mechanisms, according to the classic definition, are unconscious; most people may be unaware of the particular coping strategies they are using. At the present time, we do not know what relationships there are between self-report and observer-based assessments of coping processes. Yet self-report can be used by observers to make inferences about how people cope. We can ask people to tell us what they thought or did—for example, whether they wanted to do something even though they knew such action could not change the situation; whether they sought information or the company of others, tried to see things in a positive light, saw the situation as hopeless, tried to avoid thinking about the problem, and so forth. Guidelines can then be established for observers to use in making judgments about coping. Previous research using process ratings of coping (avoidant versus vigilant modes) found inferences could be made with good reliability between raters when clear criteria are established (Cohen, 1975; Cohen and Lazarus, 1973).

We need to know much more about the relationship between self-report and observational, inferential sources of knowledge. Future research efforts must try to correlate information from these two sources in order to understand better the usefulness of each of these measures of coping. The relationship between such patterns and outside criteria can then also be examined.

Difficulties in assessing specific coping processes. When we speak of denial, avoidance, and other intrapsychic coping processes, it is as though we know clearly what these processes are and how they are to be assessed. Such clarity, however, does not exist, and in practice their assessment is filled with ambiguity and confusion. There are two problem areas. One involves making incorrect classification because insufficient data are obtained in the research setting. The other involves treating coping as an achievement rather than as a process.

The mechanisms of denial and avoidance illustrate the first problem. Although they are quite different processes psychologically, they are often confused or considered to be similar. Denial is the effort, sometimes successful, sometimes not, to negate a problem or situation. The person states something that indicates that he or she is not angry, sees no negative implications of an illness, does not believe death is imminent, and so forth. Avoidance involves acceptance of the reality of the threat, but there is a deliberate effort not to think about it. That is, in avoidance the person does not deny the facts or implications of an illness but, whenever possible, refuses to talk or think about them. The assessment problem is that often in research on the subject, especially where the assessment is superficial, the avoidance of discussion of a topic may lead the researcher to classify the process as denial although no negation has occurred.

Second, and more important, our typical trait-centered, static research paradigm leads us to treat denial as a coping achievement, not a process—that is, we tend to speak of deniers rather than of denying. This is misleading because a process like denial is subject to uncertainty, challenge, or even dissolution, and its use may differ in discussions with different people. For example, a cancer patient may give direct evidence in an interview that he or she is denying imminent death. Yet upon leaving the office and encountering another professional, the same patient may burst into tears, overwhelmed by the thought of death. What happened to the denier?

On the one hand, the first clinician may tend by his or her manner and personal vulnerabilities to encourage denial, in a manner described insightfully by Hackett and Weisman (1964). This may implicitly threaten the patient with the loss of an important human relationship, so the patient "denies" to meet that person's expectations. On the other hand, in an interaction with a more accepting and less vulnerable person, the patient may reflect his or her true feelings. This may be an unconscious process, in which a patient seems to believe one thing on the surface but somehow "knows" at some dim and perhaps even unverbalized level that death is imminent; Weisman (1972) has elaborated on this concept of "middle knowledge." Alternately, ill people may seek to have different needs fulfilled by different people —hoping for reassurance from one and an opportunity to ventilate feelings with another. This mix of interpersonal relationships may help the patient maintain morale while facing painful realities. Another possibility is that in the first interaction the patient is trying to see the situation in favorable terms, but eventually this proves to be unsuccessful. Listening to one's own statement of this may subsequently make it impossible for the patient to believe what he or she has just said.

The conceptual confusion lies in treating a process of coping as a static state of mind rather than as a constant changing transaction. Depending on the moment, the circumstances, the evidence, the social pressures, and one's personality, such a construction remains always in flux. Only severely disturbed persons display well-consolidated defenses that constantly resist uprooting. One could look at the problem as a continuous effort at creating meaning (Frankl, 1955, 1963). This is similar to the way Erikson (1956) views the struggle between the two poles of the developmental polarities he has outlined. One does not usually arrive fixedly at one or the other pole of thought but is constantly in tension between the two.

Not only does this idea of constant tension between polarities, of fluctuations in construing what is happening in one's existence, represent a dramatically different view of coping than the more traditional emphasis on trait, style, or achieved structure, but it also calls for a very different research strategy. One must observe the coping pattern employed by an individual at diverse moments, and across different types of encounters, in order to make an accurate description. Our mistake has been prematurely to freeze people analytically into postures and styles; that may not represent accurately their characteristic coping patterns. For such a style to be a valid representation, one must study the individual in greater depth and breadth of encounter than possible in a single sampling and recognize the frequently transient nature of the coping process and pattern found.

Evaluating coping effectiveness. The final difficulty on which we wish to comment is perhaps the most complex and tenuous of all, and it is also the aspect of coping that has been given the least attention. This issue is how to determine whether coping behavior is effective or adaptive. The adaptiveness of any behavior is always a value question and must be answered from a particular point of view, concerning a particular point in time, and in reference to a particular situation. First, one must determine *in what domain* (psychological, physiological, social) adaptability is to be measured, and within that domain what is considered optimal. For example, those involved in efforts to change Type A behavior because it predisposes to greater risk of cardiovascular disease than for persons who are less pressured, aggressive, and achievement-oriented, often forget that for the Type A person the alternative may be to give up a social value to which he or she has made a lifelong commitment in favor of another which, for that person, is anathema. Is lowered risk of disease more important than personal satisfaction? There is no longer any doubt that values are inextricably tied to the evaluation of coping effectiveness. We have to ask, "Coping effectiveness for what?" "And at what cost?" The stakes include somatic health or illness, psychological morale, and social functioning. It is clear that sometimes one of these is achieved at the expense of the other. Fulfilling deeply entrenched social and personal values as a Type A may increase both morale and risk of illness. However, being insulated from others in human relationships might facilitate somatic health (see Chapter Four in this volume), but also decrease those emotional satisfactions and involvements that help make life worthwhile.

Second, *long-run versus short-run* determinations of effectiveness must be distinguished. For example, denial defenses may be adaptive for parents of children dying of leukemia prior to the child's death (Wolff and others, 1964) but may be devastating to the parent after the child dies (Chodoff, Friedman, and Hamburg, 1964). These defenses may also reduce feelings of anxiety and hydrocortisone levels before a breast biopsy but increase the likelihood that any cancer that is present has progressed to a more advanced stage, since denial is also related to delay in seeking treatment (Cameron and Hinton, 1968; Katz and others, 1970). Denial is associated with reduced mortality in the coronary care unit (Hackett, Cassem, and Wishnie, 1968) but also with a tendency to resist medical advice related to work, rest, and smoking one year after infarction (Croog, Shapiro, and Levine, 1971).

Third, the usefulness of any coping mechanism can only be ascertained *in reference to a particular situation*, and one must be wary of making generalizations about the effectiveness of particular strategies from the study of only one situation. For example, Hackett and Weisman (1964) found that persons suffering from a myocardial infarction seemed to benefit psychologically from denial, although incurable cancer patients could not. That is, denial was more effective in the situation with the greater possibility of a positive outcome. Cohen and Lazarus (1973) found that patients who avoided or denied information about a forthcoming elective surgical operation showed faster and less complicated recovery from surgery than patients who sought information about their operation. However, Layne and Yudofsky (1971) suggest that with more serious operations, such as open heart surgery, preoperative denial may result in increased postoperative psychotic reactions, because the denial mechanism is inadequate to deal with the aftermaths of the physical assault of such surgery and with the nature of the intensive care unit environment (however, see Morse and Litin, 1969).

The great dilemma is that, just as we know little about the patterns of coping most people use, we also are not clear about which patterns of coping work for certain types of persons, how they work, and the specific sets of circumstances under which they are effective. Research efforts must be directed at these important questions if we hope to be able to make suggestions about beneficial interventions for people coping with illness. In prevention efforts directed toward patients who are physically ill, the absence of clear understanding of these issues poses a serious handicap.

Stresses of Medical Illness and Treatment

Coping never occurs in a vacuum but implies the question, "Coping with what?" Let us turn now to the stresses potentially created by illness and treatment. We say "potentially" because their relevance and importance varies with the illness, the patient, and the treatment setting.

Being ill can involve threats not only to life and physical well-being but also to one's self-concept, belief systems, social and occupational functioning, values, commitments, and emotional equilibrium. Since efforts to cope may be directed toward these threats, as well as toward doing something about the physical illness itself, our discussion of coping with illness will benefit from a greater understanding of the different threats that can occur. Based on a synthesis of material presented by Hamburg, Hamburg, and deGoza (1953), Mages and Mendelsohn (Chapter Ten in this volume), Moos and Tsu (1977), Visotsky and others (1961), and other writers, such threats can be categorized as follows:

1. Threats to life and fears of dying itself
2. Threats to bodily integrity and comfort (from the illness, the diagnostic procedures, or the medical treatment itself)
   a. Bodily injury or disability
   b. Permanent physical changes
   c. Physical pain, discomfort, and other negative symptoms of illness or treatment
   d. Incapacitation
3. Threats to one's self-concept and future plans
   a. Necessity to alter one's self-image or belief systems
   b. Uncertainty about the course of the illness and about one's future
   c. Endangering of life goals and values
   d. Loss of autonomy and control
4. Threats to one's emotional equilibrium, that is, the necessity to deal with feelings of anxiety, anger, and other emotions that come about as a result of other stresses described
5. Threats to the fulfillment of customary social roles and activities
   a. Separation from family, friends, and other social supports
   b. Loss of important social roles
   c. Necessity to depend on others
6. Threats involving the need to adjust to a new physical or social environment
   a. Adjustment to the hospital setting
   b. Problems in understanding medical terminology and customs
   c. Necessity for decision making in stressful and unfamiliar situations

Most health professionals focus on efforts to reduce threats to life and bodily comfort. However, stresses that interfere with one's self-concept, future plans, emotional equilibrium, or social roles must also be dealt with

by the patient and may have a negative impact on the course of the illness
and on morale and social functioning. Even when progression of the illness
has been halted and cure is expected, extensive coping efforts may still be
necessary. For example, serious physical illnesses that are disfiguring may require significant changes in one's self-image, changes that may be difficult to
accomplish for people for whom bodily health and integrity are an important feature of their self-concept.

Mattsson (1972) has discussed many of the problems children face in
adjustment to serious illnesses. The following account from Hathaway
(1943, pp. 41, 46-47) of a girl bedridden during childhood because of a
tubercular infection of the spine illustrates difficulties related to the self-
concept:

> When I got up at last . . . one day I took a hand glass and
> went to a long mirror to look at myself. . . . But there was no
> noise, no outcry; I didn't scream with rage when I saw myself. I
> just felt numb. That person in the mirror *couldn't* be me. I felt
> inside like a healthy, ordinary lucky person—oh, not like the
> one in the mirror! . . .
>
> Over and over I forgot what I had seen in the mirror. It
> could not penetrate into the interior of my mind and become
> an integral part of me. I felt as if it had nothing to do with
> me. . . . In the place where I was standing, with that persistent
> romantic elation in me, as if I were a favored fortunate person
> to whom everything was possible, I saw a stranger, a little, piti-
> able, hideous figure. . . . Every one of those encounters . . . left
> me dazed and dumb and senseless every time, until slowly and
> stubbornly my robust persistent illusion of well-being and of
> personal beauty spread all through me again, and I forgot the
> irrelevant reality and was all unprepared and vulnerable again.

Threats connected with the medical environment are particularly salient for health psychology and deserve some special attention here. Special
hospital environments such as isolation units and open-heart surgery recovery rooms may have sensory deprivation or monotony effects; witnessing attempts at resuscitation of patients having a cardiac arrest may be terrifying
to other coronary care unit patients (see Kornfeld, 1972). More basically,
many patients are confused by the customs and language of the medical
world, by the loss of autonomy and control they experience in the hospital
environment, by the amount and complexity of information presented to
them (for example, Golden and Johnston, 1970), and by the need to make
decisions about medical treatment that involve balancing of many conflicting
factors. Hunt and MacLeod have elaborated on the difficulties in assimilation
of factual material (see Chapter Twelve in this volume), though we think
that emotionally laden information may present even greater problems for
the patient than they have described. Janis and Rodin (Chapter Nineteen in

this volume) also discuss some of the important factors that influence decision making in situations of crisis. We address some of these here.

Increased legal pressures to obtain "informed consent" from patients undergoing medical procedures can exacerbate their problems by forcing the patient to contend psychologically with some degree of risk. Certain diagnostic medical procedures illustrate this dilemma—that patients may have to make decisions about and take the responsibility for undergoing medical procedures that are themselves fraught with danger. For example, invasive radiological procedures such as arteriograms, although potentially lifesaving because of their diagnostic function, also involve numerous risks to life and to physical well-being. In an arteriogram, a catheter is inserted, most often, into a leg artery and threaded through the blood vessels to the area of interest. If a cerebral problem is suspected, the catheter would go through the vessels to the major arteries in the brain. When the problem area is reached, a contrast media is injected and x rays are taken. If blood vessels are found to be clogged and narrowed, or if the test reveals there is a tumor or aneurysm (ballooning out of the blood vessel or heart wall), surgery might be recommended as a result. However, the risk of having serious complications from an arteriogram has been estimated as 2 to 10 percent, depending on the area under study (O. H. Cohen, personal communication, 1978), and the risk of dying from the procedure averages 1.7 percent (Abrams, 1971, p. 24). This may not seem much epidemiologically speaking, but it may carry heavy weight in the patient's mind. The catheter could produce direct physical trauma (by penetrating a blood vessel); calcified plaques could be knocked off the side of blood vessels and float through the bloodstream, resulting in the blocking of important blood vessels in the leg (necessitating an amputation) or the brain (resulting in loss of certain cerebral functions, such as eyesight); one could have an anaphylactic shock reaction to the contrast media, or die from cardiac arrest.

A clear description of the risks involved in even simple medical procedures is thought widely to be capable of deterring many patients from accepting such lifesaving treatments (Ravitch, 1974); as a result, many physicians do not fully inform patients of the risks involved, or leave that discussion to a time immediately preceding the procedure (which makes it awkward for the patient to refuse). Others suggest that those who are informed of possible complications of drugs or medical treatment may actually have more of such complications as a result, though there is no evidence to date that such effects occur (Cohen, 1975; Myers and Calvert, 1976). There is evidence, however, that most patients forget substantial amounts of the information presented about serious risks (Horwitz, 1976).

Individual Differences

Although there are many potential threats in situations of illness, individuals vary in their appraisal of them. For example, certain threats, such as loss of personal autonomy, come about because of changes in the life pattern experienced in a hospital (Brown, 1965; Kutner, 1958; Meyer, 1958). However, whereas for some being removed from the active involvement of work and family may be threatening, for others who view their usual social world as hostile, because of its many responsibilities and frustrations, going to the hospital may be a welcome relief (Johns, Dudley, and Masterton, 1973). The loss of a breast will have a different meaning to different women depending on how much it is seen as a symbol of femininity and what meaning femininity has to each person (Bard, 1952). Clearly, various personality and other characteristics, such as a person's sense of confidence, his or her attitudes, beliefs, and personal resources, all affect the appraisals of threat that are made (see also Kahana and Bibring, 1964; Lipowski, 1969).

Lipowski (1970) has described the strikingly different ways individuals view illness, and how this meaning can influence emotional and coping reactions (see also Kahana and Bibring, 1964). He suggests that illness may be viewed as: challenge (a life situation with particular tasks to be mastered), enemy (an invasion by harmful forces), punishment (just or unjust), weakness (a sign of failing), relief (respite from life demands or conflicts), strategy (a coping technique for securing attention from others), irreparable loss or damage, or value (an opportunity for growth and development). Different threats may be involved in each. For example, the person who sees illness as punishment may be relieved if he or she also views it as providing the opportunity for atonement but may become upset if there is no such opportunity. Such meanings may add considerably to the sense of threat—for example, when illness is seen as weakness or damage—but may also reduce threat—for example, when illness is a relief from other burdens (see also Lipowski, 1975). Pritchard (1977) discusses how these different meanings can affect patients who are undergoing hemodialysis.

Adaptive Tasks of Illness

Although illness is commonly appraised as threatening, many patients view these events not as threats but rather as challenges or tasks to be mastered. Thus, it may be helpful to examine the adaptive tasks that must be dealt with for a satisfactory adjustment to illness (see Hamburg and Adams, 1967; Hamburg, Hamburg, and deGoza, 1953; Mages and Mendelsohn, Chapter Ten in this volume; Visotsky and others, 1961). This will also provide a framework for understanding the focuses of patients' coping efforts and the types of interventions that might be beneficial.

Synthesizing the contributions of the authors mentioned above and others, the adaptive tasks of illness are: (1) to reduce harmful environmental conditions and enhance prospects of recovery, (2) to tolerate or adjust to negative events and realities, (3) to maintain a positive self-image, (4) to maintain emotional equilibrium, and (5) to continue satisfying relationships with others.

1. Efforts must be made to neutralize harmful environmental conditions where possible and to act in such a way as to aid recovery. It may be easier to deal with these tasks if patients have a satisfactory understanding of the medical problem and of what must be done to recover from it. For example, patients may need to rest, follow dietary or exercise regimens, or alter destructive life-style patterns. Kirscht and Rosenstock deal with some of these issues in their discussion of adherence in Chapter Eight.

2. A second set of tasks involves making some adjustment to negative events and realities that result from the illness. It may take considerable time for patients to understand the negative implications of the illness and to mourn losses of parts of the body, functions, or potentials. Patients may avoid or deny negative realities, tolerate or even accept such losses (see, for example, Kübler-Ross, 1969), or replace or compensate for them where possible.

3. Maintenance of self-image is one of the most important tasks, since illness is a direct assault on the usual view of self. To maintain a sense of self-worth and preserve as much as possible the continuity of their life pattern, most patients try to gain a sense of control over their lives by actively making choices and preserving as much self-sufficiency as is possible. In some way, although the process may be slow, most people are able to integrate the experience into the rest of their lives, altering their self-concept to be in alignment with the new reality.

4. Maintaining emotional equilibrium is a fourth task. Depression, fear, anxiety, and anger are normal responses to situations of threat and loss, but, if they are severe, such emotions can be overwhelming, stifle efforts to cope, interfere with support from others, and may possibly impede medical recovery. Thus, patients usually try to avoid being overcome by negative emotional states. In addition, feelings of hope and positive morale are valuable for a sense of well-being and may aid recovery processes (see, for example, Cousins, 1976; Frank, 1975; Mason and others, 1969). To maintain a positive mental outlook without being incapacitated by depression, fear, and other negative emotions also facilitates the management of other concrete tasks, including following a treatment regimen and meeting family and work responsibilities.

5. Maintenance of satisfying social relationships is among the most important tasks of the ill person. Relationships with family, friends, and others must be continued despite disruptions in normal roles produced by the illness. Patients may have to learn to accept a degree of dependence without adversely affecting their self-concept. In addition, they usually try to build a working relationship with medical personnel who treat them.

Relevant Research

We are now ready to examine some of the relevant research that has dealt with issues and concepts outlined above. Such research represents mostly incomplete beginnings in the study of coping and illness, from which ultimately serviceable concepts of intervention could be derived. However, such research points to some valuable directions in which to look for principles of intervention.

We will first discuss some major studies that describe the coping strategies used in response to serious illness and their effects on psychological adjustment. In general, the descriptive studies have used process ratings of coping—that is, an individual's behavior is observed as it takes place in the stressful situation of illness and as it changes over time, and the mode of coping is inferred. We will then review studies investigating the relationship between coping and physical recovery from illness. Some of these studies have used process measures whereas others have employed trait measures of coping. As we shall see, in many cases different relationships to outcome variables are found when one rather than the other measure is used. This suggests that there are important differences in the behaviors assessed by trait and process measures.

Modes of Coping with Illness

There has long been interest in how people cope with serious or disabling illnesses, and there are innumerable first-person accounts that illuminate these processes: to mention just a few, coping with polio (Linduska, 1947), deafness (Warfield, 1948), amputation (Baker, 1946), blindness (Criddle, 1953), arthritis (Perkins, 1964), breast cancer (Kushner, 1975; Rollin, 1976), and collagen disease (Cousins, 1976). Case histories describing various reactions and strategies are also available, for example, Janis' (1958) discussion of coping with surgery and Rosenbaum's (1975) description of coping with the treatment process in cancer. Most of the early research is entirely descriptive, though some studies try to assess the effectiveness of particular coping strategies in the situation under study.

Descriptive accounts. Hamburg, Hamburg, and deGoza (1953) and Visotsky and others (1961) have provided some of the earliest and most insightful descriptive research accounts of patients' coping efforts in the face of life-threatening illnesses, such as severe burns and polio. For example, different coping mechanisms were observed in the period of physical emergency after severe burns were incurred than in the recovery phase thereafter. In the acute period, many patients seemed consciously or unconsciously to avoid thinking about unpleasant experiences or feelings or showed little expression of emotion regarding their illness. Hamburg, Hamburg, and deGoza (1953, p. 7) describe one manifestation of this emotional constriction: "It was impressive indeed to see a patient who was almost covered with bandages and very weak and badly discolored act as if he had accepted this unfortunate occurrence as a part of nature, without apparent regret, resentment, or recrimination."

Other frequent but less common coping strategies used in the initial period were denial (of the injury or of the consequences of it), rationalization, development of conversion symptoms, distortion of reality through

delusions or hallucinations, regression, rumination over the traumatic experience itself, withdrawal from interpersonal contact, and the use of religion to
help achieve resignation or acceptance. The authors suggest that the function
of most of these defenses was to minimize awareness of emotionally painful
factors which might otherwise have overwhelmed the patient. During the
convalescent period, hope, pride, restoration of interpersonal relationships
and self-esteem, testing of key figures in the environment, and attempts to
regain active participation were common. The researchers concluded that,
overall, many patients made a quite successful adjustment despite some evidence of transient psychotic episodes or periods of moderate depression and
anxiety.

Visotsky and his colleagues (1961) have described the coping behavior
found in patients with severe poliomyelitis. Avoidance and denial were common strategies during the acute phase: Over half of the patients studied did
not recognize that they had polio or were skeptical of the diagnosis. In the
chronic phase of the illness, avoidance and denial became much less frequent, although some patients took several months to become aware of the
implications of the illness, such as its crippling nature. Other coping strategies used during the chronic phase included religiosity, projection of concern, emotional constriction, "bargaining," setting intermediate goals,
lengthening time perspectives, testing of hospital staff and family members,
and efforts to be physically active. Patients not only employed diverse strategies but also often seemed to intermingle them or use them successively.
Sometimes they appeared to hold certain strategies in reserve in case a particular one was not effective.

Visotsky and his colleagues, more than other observers, have emphasized the sequencing of coping strategies and the stepwise nature of the
changes. Efforts are first made to minimize the impact of the event through
denial of the nature and implications of the illness. This minimization allows
the patient to make a gradual transition to the difficult tasks ahead and reduces feelings of depression. As patients eventually begin to seek information about their illness and face its long-term consequences, depression tends
to increase, suggesting the beginnings of a mourning process. Visotsky and
others (1961, p. 447) also emphasize the slowness of these transition periods, suggesting that most patients go "through a series of successive approximations . . . leading to ultimate recognition of a painful reality. . . . The loss
of cherished capabilities thus occurs in small increments, with some personality reorganization taking place in each intermediate phase. . . . It appears
that the stepwise nature of this transaction makes the whole process more
bearable." Thus, while many issues that are first denied are worked out in
the first few months of the illness, others may not be resolved until a year or
more later. Visotsky and his colleagues also point out that hope, emotional
support from others, and the sense of being needed are sustaining forces in
adjustment to severe illness.

Other descriptive studies support these earlier findings, especially regarding the frequent use of denial or avoidance processes in the initial adjust-

ment to illness. Wright (1960) provides a comprehensive discussion of the psychosocial situations that confront persons with physical disabilities and elaborates on the coping processes used in dealing with these disorders (see also Cobb, 1973; McDaniel, 1969). Others have described the coping processes used by cancer patients (Bard, 1952; Druss, O'Connor, and Stern, 1969; Hinton, 1973; Holland, 1973; Shands and others, 1951; Weisman and Worden, 1976-1977), stroke victims (Espmark, 1973), burn patients (Andreasen and Norris, 1972), myocardial infarction patients (Cowie, 1976; Hackett and Cassem, 1975), patients undergoing hemodialysis (Abram, 1970; Short and Wilson, 1969), patients awaiting a breast biopsy (Katz and others, 1970), and women coping with menopause (Hamburg, Coelho, and Adams, 1974), to mention a few areas of focus. The early studies of the processes of coping with illness highlighted the types of coping strategies used in these crisis situations and suggested how these strategies might aid psychological adjustment. Subsequent studies, which we will review shortly, investigated whether coping would also benefit physical recovery from illness.

Possible mechanisms linking coping and recovery. In looking for links between psychological factors and recovery, the assumption most often made is that individuals who are ill prepared or utilize maladaptive coping styles will become anxious, angry, or depressed in coping with illness. These negative feelings, especially anxiety, may be reflected in postoperative emotional episodes, may cause increased use of pain medications, or may decrease bodily resistance (thereby increasing the likelihood of infections) or increase the number of minor "conversion symptoms."

Regarding pain medications, for example, Drew, Moriarty and Shapiro (1968, p. 827) have shown that there is a close relationship between anxiety (" 'pain' augmented by emotional overlay") and pain ("somatic pain"), and that an examination of postoperative drug usage patterns cannot differentiate the two types of responses. In a comparison of patients having general surgery with those having relatively painless but very threatening eye surgery, they found more medications were taken in the latter group, suggesting that the number of pain medications sought is not related solely to severity of the pain (see also Beecher, 1959). Numerous others have also suggested that there is a large psychological element in postoperative pain (Boyar and Gramlich, 1970; Petrie, 1967; Sternbach, 1968; Wright and Holmes, 1963; Zborowski, 1952; see also Weisenberg, 1975, 1977). It has also been found that only two thirds of patients hospitalized for major surgery received analgesics postoperatively (Jaggard, Zager, and Wilkins, 1950) or had pain that could not be relieved by a placebo (Papper, Brodie, and Rovenstine, 1952).

One would also expect psychological factors to affect physiological reactivity, with subsequent effects on bodily resistance. For example, Bursten and Russ (1965) found a significant positive relationship between ratings of preoperative discomfort-involvement and plasma corticosteroid levels in patients awaiting hernia surgery; Price, Thaler, and Mason (1957) found similar results with thoracic surgery patients. Other studies have found that successful use of defenses can lower levels of these hormones (Bourne, Rose, and Mason, 1967; Friedman, Mason, and Hamburg, 1963; Wolff and others, 1964). Since corticosteroids are thought to reduce bodily resistance (see, however, Chapter Four in this volume), one might expect patients using such defenses to be less susceptible to infections postoperatively.

There are other ways in which coping can affect recovery, other than through direct hormonal action. For example, recovery may be slowed if coping involves habits which, themselves, interfere directly with health, such as smoking postoperatively or insisting on being physically active when such activity is damaging (as in recovery from myocardial infarction). The course of recovery is not only a matter of physical healing and the return of strength and energy but also involves a complex of behavioral events that could be influenced by coping. Coping strategies can interfere with adaptive behavior that would hasten recovery, as when denial of disability prevents the patient from making the special efforts needed in physical rehabilitation tasks. Additionally, certain interpersonal styles may affect transactions in the health care environment, thereby influencing the behavior of medical personnel for better or worse. Cancer patients who are complaining and demanding may have their symptoms monitored more closely, allowing further treatments to be initiated if recurrence is thought to occur; in contrast, those who are more passive and less sensitive to small bodily changes may delay seeking medical advice until more serious damage has been done. Patients who try to radiate a sense of health and well-being may convince physicians to discharge them earlier from the hospital; other patients at a similar stage of recovery remain longer in comparison.

Other writers have suggested that the will to live and the maintenance of morale may not only aid patients' determination to persevere with unpleasant medical treatments but also may have direct physiological effects. For example, in 1964 Norman Cousins, former editor of the *Saturday Review*, was diagnosed as having a serious collagen disease with virtually no chance of recovery. Cousins reasoned that if negative emotions had negative physiological effects, then positive emotions might have positive effects on bodily processes. The treatment regimen he proposed for himself—in addition to massive doses of Vitamin C, the discontinuance of all painkillers and anti-inflammatory drugs—included a program of laughter therapy, which consisted of watching old Candid Camera vignettes and being read selections from books of humor (Cousins, 1976). Whether the Vitamin C, laughter therapy, his active participation in his own treatment, or the cathartic effect of a "belly laugh" was critical in producing his unexpected cure is unclear. Nonetheless, it is possible that positive emotions could have beneficial effects on recovery in ways we do not yet understand (see Lazarus and others, in press).

In looking at the effects of coping on recovery, two different research approaches have been followed. One relates the use of specific coping strategies to physical outcome measures (*nonintervention* studies). The other introduces psychological interventions designed to alter coping strategies in the medical situation and determines their effect on medical outcomes (*intervention* studies).

Nonintervention Studies

There are three different ways coping-related variables are assessed in nonintervention studies. Some assess the use of particular *coping strategies* directly in the situation under study. Others focus on the outcome of inadequate coping, that is, on the occurrence of particular negative *emotional states* (or on events thought to produce these emotional reactions). A third approach measures *personality traits* or dispositional characteristics, the assumption being that such traits predispose to certain emotional states—for example, by affecting appraisals and subsequent emotional reactions to various situations (Lazarus, 1966)—and produce coping strategies that are counterproductive for many reasons.

*Recovery from nonsurgical illnesses.** The following independent variables have been examined in studies relating psychological factors to recovery from nonsurgical illnesses: depression; active participation coping strategies; inhibition versus expression of emotion; anxiety; occurrence of additional stresses; and existence of psychological impairments. For more detailed discussions of some of this literature, see Cohen (1975), Imboden (1972), and Kahana (1972).

Several studies have suggested that those who are *depressed* take longer to recover from illnesses or are more likely to die from serious illnesses. (Giving-up has also been related to the etiology of illness; see Chapter Four in this volume.) Such a lowering of psychological morale is thought to affect physiological processes in a deleterious way, to interfere with the mobilization of energy, or to result in unwillingness to cooperate with treatments that may be painful or require physical effort. The research shows fairly consistent negative effects of depression on recovery outcomes. Patients with higher scores on the Depression (*D*) scale of the Minnesota Multiphasic Personality Inventory (MMPI) have been found to be less likely to survive a myocardial infarction for at least five years (Bruhn, Chandler, and Wolf, 1969), to have a more complicated hospital course of recovery from myocardial infarction (Pancheri and others, 1978), and to take longer to recover from brucellosis (Imboden and others, 1959), tuberculosis (Calden and others, 1960), and influenza (Imboden, Canter, and Cluff, 1961).

Imboden, Canter, and Cluff (1961) argue against the idea that a physiological link is involved in cases of infectious disease. They suggest that clini-

---

*In our review, we do not include studies of the relationship between coping and recovery from the so-called psychosomatic illnesses (see Weiner, 1977, for a review of this literature). Since psychological variables are thought to play an important role in the etiology and exacerbation of these diseases, we would expect the course of the disease to be more easily influenced by psychological factors. The relationship between coping and recovery can be more clearly understood through a review of studies of illnesses whose etiology may be less strongly psychologically based.

cal signs of depression such as fatigue may merge with the usually transient symptoms such as tiredness and weakness commonly found with influenza and other infectious diseases. Because the person attributes his or her psychological symptoms to the continuation of the disease process, the "symptoms" persist longer, making it difficult for patient and physician to determine the endpoint of the disease. Although the studies using the *D* scale of the MMPI show fairly consistent negative effects, Rosen and Bibring (1966) found that patients rated as depressed did not have a more difficult hospital course of recovery after a myocardial infarction. This inconsistency of results may reflect differences in the way depression was assessed (trait versus state measures), in the outcome measures examined, or in the nature of the diseases studied.

The opposite of depression—taking an *active, involved role*—has been linked with faster recovery from severe burns. In their study, the authors (Andreasen, Noyes, and Hartford, 1972) indicate that they originally believed that an active, aggressive life-style would interfere with adaptation to the patient role of forced dependency and passivity: "We began with the suspicion that the life-style helpful in coping with the vicissitudes of modern civilization, involving qualities such as independence, aggressiveness, and high energy levels, poorly prepares the individual who has been seriously injured for coping with the forced dependency, passivity, and monotony of prolonged *patienthood.* Yet we repeatedly observed individuals who defied our predictions and, after a brief period of depression or anxiety, rapidly learned to cope with the new stresses of hospitalization by using their old familiar defenses and adaptive mechanisms" (p. 523). Thus, in this research, active involvement resulted in a smoother psychological and physiological course of recovery. Boyd, Yeager, and McMillan (1973) suggest somewhat similar findings for patients recovering from reconstructive vascular surgery.

Taking an active, involved role may aid adjustment in one stage of illness but not in another. Patients who prefer an authoritarian approach by hospital staff show better emotional response to hospitalization (DeWolfe, Barrell, and Cummings, 1966). Tuberculosis patients who are active fare better in the community after hospital discharge but do less well in adjustment to the hospital environment (Vernier and others, 1961). Women who are independent and autonomous (as defined by a body image measure from Holtzman inkblot responses) show greater delay in seeking treatment for symptoms of breast or cervical cancer (Fisher, 1967; Hammerschlag and others, 1964). It appears that active involvement aids in rehabilitation from illness but can result in delay in seeking treatment or greater emotional distress in the early stages of disease. Whereas such patients may be upset by the confinement of the hospital environment, they may also be willing to make the special efforts needed to hasten their rehabilitation from serious illnesses.

Inhibition versus expression of emotion has been studied as a factor in cancer, tuberculosis, and respiratory disease. The "bottling of emotions" is thought to have negative effects on bodily processes, although it is not clear that inhibition necessarily involves "bottling" or that there is a physiological mechanism to explain such effects. Those who readily express emotions may also be more likely to seek treatment when symptoms first appear, which, as we shall see, could have a positive or negative effect on outcome, depending on the variable assessed. Longer survival rates from cancer have been associated with more frequent expression of hostility and other negative effects (Stavraky and others, 1968; Derogatis and Abeloff, 1978) and less inhibition and defensiveness, as measured by the Rorschach (Blumberg, West, and Ellis, 1954; Klopfer, 1957; however, Krasnoff, 1959, failed to replicate these results). Calden and others (1960) found that patients rated as "good, cooperative" had a slower recovery from tuberculosis than those rated as "nonconforming, recalcitrant." However, using MMPI data, Cuadra (1953) found the opposite results. In a study of patients with irreversible diffuse obstructive pulmonary syndromes, Dudley and others (1969) suggest that successful use of denial, repression, and isolation, which protects patients from potentially upsetting environmental inputs, was related to better psychological and physiological adjustment. Strong emotional reactions in these patients were associated with increased respiratory symptoms and physiological decompensation to which patients could not adjust.

Kinsman, Dirks, and their associates found that asthma patients who were emotionally labile, extremely sensitive, and easily defeated required a longer hospital stay and a more intensive posthospitalization steroid drug regimen (Dirks, Jones, and Kinsman, 1977; Dirks and others, 1977; Kinsman and others, 1977). Tuberculosis patients high on this dimension also required longer hospitalization (Dirks and others, 1977). However, both those asthma patients who were high or low on this MMPI Panic-Fear dimension were rehospitalized more than those in the middle (Dirks and others, 1978). Dirks and his colleagues (1978) suggest that patients high on this dimension exaggerate symptoms and discomfort, which influences physicians' decisions regarding drug treatment and rehospitalization. Because those low on the scale minimize their discomfort, symptoms might be aggravated to the extent that rehospitalization would be necessary.

These various studies investigating the expression of emotion illustrate why one must consider carefully the outcome variable to be measured and the mechanisms thought to influence recovery. Those who express their emotions may draw attention to themselves and their symptoms, resulting in more diagnostic tests, greater frequency of hospitalization, and more intensive drug regimens, all of which could improve their chances of surviving a disease like cancer. However, in other illnesses, such as obstructive pulmonary syndrome, emotional expression can directly exacerbate symptoms and hasten the disease process. Thus, the adaptiveness of emotional expression would differ according to the nature of the illness and the outcome measure examined (mortality versus length of hospitalization).

Anxiety is often thought to increase levels of hormonal activity, with deleterious effects on bodily processes; however, the evidence is mixed that anxiety results in slower recovery from illness. Pancheri and others (1978) found that patients who were higher on state and trait measures of anxiety had a more complicated hospital course of recovery after myocardial infarction; other investigators did not find similar results using process measures of anxiety (Rosen and Bibring, 1966). In addition, anxiety in coronary care unit patients has not shown conclusive relationships to their mortality while the patient is in the hospital (Vetter and others, 1977).

If ill patients are burdened by *additional stresses* or have fewer resources upon which to draw, one might expect they would have more difficulty in adjustment to illness. Several studies support this proposition, although others find that stresses or assets alone do not have direct effects on recovery outcome variables. Patients who had to cope with stresses other than their physical illness had a slower recovery from illness than those without such additional problems (Querido, 1959). Pancheri and others (1978) found that those with many work-related problems had more complicated recovery after myocardial infarction. De Araujo and others (1973) note that to predict steroid regimens in asthmatics, it was necessary to take into account both the life experiences of patients, as measured by the Schedule of Recent Experiences (Holmes and Rahe, 1967a), and their personal attributes, as measured by the Berle Index (Berle and others, 1952), a scale that taps areas such as employment adjustment, age, marital status, previous health, and emotional support. Those with a low Berle Index and many life changes needed significantly higher doses of steroids.

Those with *psychological impairments*, or who were "more disturbed psychiatrically," as measured by the MMPI, Bender-Gestalt, or a deprivation scale, were found to have intractable symptoms of duodenal ulcer (Lothrop, 1958; Pascal and Thoroughman, 1964; Thoroughman and others, 1964; Weiner, 1956) or more complications after myocardial infarction (Pancheri and others, 1978), whereas those low on the ego strength scale of the MMPI were found to have a more prolonged recovery from mononucleosis (Greenfield, Roessler, and Crosley, 1959). Dudley and others (1969) found that the number of psychosocial assets alone did not predict mortality from irreversible diffuse obstructive pulmonary syndrome; significant results were obtained when physiological deficits were also taken into account.

What conclusions can we draw from these studies of nonsurgical illness? Results differ from study to study depending on the nature of the disease, the way the independent variable is measured (trait versus process measure), and the type of outcome variable examined. Certain consistencies do emerge. Those high on trait measures of depression have a slower and more complicated recovery from infectious diseases and myocardial infarction, although no physiological link is necessarily involved. Those who take on active roles have more difficulty adjusting to the hospital environment but show better long-term rehabilitation after serious illnesses. Expression of emotion can exacerbate respiratory symptoms and therefore hasten physical decompensation in certain diseases, or draw attention of physicians to medical problems, resulting in increased treatment efforts which may prolong survival from other diseases. Those who have additional stresses or fewer psychological assets have more prolonged and complicated recovery from a number of illnesses. No conclusions can be drawn about the relationship between anxiety and recovery from nonsurgical illness.

Recovery from surgery. Much has been written about the psychological stresses of surgery (Abram, 1967; Adriani and Lief, 1963; Cooley, 1961; Corman and others, 1958; Deutsch, 1942; Hiatt, 1963; Janis, 1958; Kutner, 1958; Meyer, 1958, 1967; Renneker and Cutler, 1952; Titchener and Levine, 1960), and there is abundant research in this area. One of the advantages of doing research on recovery from surgery is that there are more clear-cut physical indicators of outcome, which are easily obtained (from hospital charts).

Two different types of outcomes are evaluated (see also Wolfer, 1973). One approach looks at recovery in the psychological domain and focuses on the presence or absence of *negative emotional states* postoperatively (for example, Janis, 1958). This approach is especially common in studies of open-heart surgery cases, where psychotic reactions occur in a significant number of patients. The second looks at more *physical aspects of recovery*, described in the next paragraph.

The research to be reviewed is complex. One reason for this is the great variation in the types of outcome measures utilized. In the studies to be reviewed, these include at least one of the following: number of postoperative emotional reactions, length of hospital stay, number of analgesics taken, number of sedatives taken, self-reported pain, a weighted sum of the number of minor medical complications that occurred, respiratory functioning, vital capacity impairment and chest complication scores, vomiting and/or nausea, blood pressure and pulse readings, urinary retention, bowel difficulties, ambulatory functioning, number of elevated temperatures, chest x ray reports, and mortality. Because of the variety of indicators used, we will try to summarize results without going into detail about the specific outcome measure examined. Methodological inadequacies of particular studies will not be addressed here. A full discussion of this literature can be found in Cohen (1975).

The diversity of measures makes it difficult to replicate results (since researchers rarely use similar measures) and to know how to weigh negative and positive findings. If a scale indicating proneness to anxiety is positively correlated with postoperative vital capacity impairment and chest complication scores in one study, and a trait measure of anxiety is related to self-reported pain on the first but not the third postoperative day, and yet other trait measures of anxiety fail to show significant relationships to urinary or bowel difficulties, number of elevated temperatures, or number of analgesics taken postoperatively—what are we to conclude about the influence of trait anxiety on postsurgical outcomes? In addition, whereas most studies focus on general elective surgery, such as hernia and gall bladder, some studies use operations that may have special psychological meanings (such as hysterectomy) or are of high risk (open-heart surgery). Still other researchers use an extremely wide range of surgical procedures, for example, from dilation and curettage to gastrectomy. Thus, if severity of operation differs between different treatment or coping groups and recovery measures are not standardized, misleading results can be obtained (Cohen, 1975).

The following independent variables have been examined in nonintervention studies of recovery from surgery: level of anticipatory fear; depression; information seeking; life changes; trait measures of repression-sensitization, anxiety, dependence, and ego strength; internal-external locus of control; and personality scale scores. Few of these overlap with variables used in studying recovery from nonsurgical illnesses.

Janis (1958) has presented the first research study of psychological process variables and recovery, focusing on the relationship between preoperative and postoperative emotional states. A curvilinear relationship was found between level of *anticipatory fear* and postoperative emotional reactions. Patients with high anticipatory fear were more likely to have emotional outbursts and to be anxiety ridden or fearful after the operation, whereas those with low fear were most likely to show anger and resentment. Those with moderate fear had the fewest emotional episodes postoperatively. Janis argued from these findings that a moderate amount of anticipatory fear is necessary to prod a person to begin the "work of worrying." By mentally rehearsing potential unpleasant events and by gaining information about what to expect, the patient can develop effective forms of coping with the subsequent deprivation.

Janis' findings of a curvilinear relationship between preoperative anxiety level and postoperative emotional difficulties have never been replicated. One study (Opton, n.d.) found high preoperative fear and postoperative hostility, anger, and resistance to a "good patient" role to be so rare that these variables could not be investigated for their possible relationships with the course of recovery. Most studies using questionnaire or self-report measures of preoperative anxiety level have found a positive linear relationship between preoperative anxiety level and postoperative negative emotional states in general surgery patients (Cohen and Lazarus, 1973; Johnson, Leventhal, and Dabbs, 1971; Sime, 1976; Wolfer and Davis, 1970; see also Abram and Gill, 1961). That is, high-fear patients have the most emotional disturbance postoperatively, and low-fear patients the least. Contradictory results have been found in the case of open-heart surgery. Whereas Layne and Yudofsky (1971) found low-fear patients to have the greatest incidence of delirium after open-heart surgery, Morse and Litin (1969) found them to have the least. Contradictory results are also found when self-report measures of fear are related to physical outcomes of recovery (Cohen and Lazarus, 1973; Johnson, Leventhal, and Dabbs, 1971; Sime, 1976).

Other studies using process measures of anxiety have also found high-fear patients to have the worst postoperative adjustment. Kimball (1969) found that those patients who were anxious had a more complicated physiological and psychological postoperative course after open-heart surgery (however, no statistical analyses were presented). Yet Kornfeld and others (1974) found no relationship between a process measure of anxiety and incidence of postcardiotomy delirium. Eisendrath (1969) suggests that grief and fear play a role in the death of kidney transplant patients; most of those who died following renal transplantation had, prior to the surgery, expressed a sense of abandonment by their families or experienced panic and a sense of pessimism about the outcome. (However, since these data were obtained retrospectively, the possibility of observer bias cannot be ruled out.) Those who took longer to return to an active life-style after reconstructive vascular surgery for occlusive disease had higher levels of anxiety preoperatively (Boyd, Yeager, and McMillan, 1973).

Although there are some inconsistencies in results, most process measures of anxiety show a positive linear relationship with postoperative psychological adjustment. Those who are most anxious preoperatively have the most difficulty after surgery. This does not necessarily mean that anxiety interferes with the adjustment process in surgery. The same personality state or response style may be manifesting itself in two different periods of a crisis situation.

The effects of *depression* on recovery from surgery have also been studied, but the results are not as clear cut as in the case of nonsurgical illness (although similar mechanisms have been hypothesized). Kimball (1969; see also Tufo and Ostfeld, 1968) found that patients who were rated as depressed preoperatively (process measure) showed greater mortality following open-heart surgery (although no statistical analyses were done). Ratings of patient "acceptance" (that is, feelings of optimism, trust, and confidence) before a retinal operation were found to be positively related to speed of healing of the surgical wound (Mason and others, 1969); the seriousness of the retinal detachment did not influence healing speed. However, those high on the D scale of the MMPI did not have greater mortality from open-heart surgery (Gilberstadt and Sako, 1967; Henrichs, MacKenzie, and Almond, 1969; Kilpatrick and others, 1975). Kornfeld and others (1974) found only a statistically suggestive relationship between ratings of depression and incidence of postcardiotomy delirium. A questionnaire measure of depression did not predict complications of delivery of a child when variance due to health problems was controlled (Erickson, 1976). This inconsistency of results may reflect the difference between trait and process measures. Process measures of depression may be easily influenced by other factors, such as severity of the illness or preoperative organicity, which have direct effects on medical outcomes (Kornfeld and others, 1974). These variables must be controlled when process measures of depression are utilized. In general, depression does not show as strong a relationship to recovery from surgery as it does to outcome of nonsurgical illnesses.

Janis (1958) and others have suggested that by gaining information about what to expect and becoming aware of potential threats, patients can develop effective ways of coping with the threats involved in surgery. However, many patients and health professionals believe that "ignorance is bliss." Cohen and Lazarus (1973) investigated the relationship between recovery from surgery and *avoidance or vigilance toward seeking information* about the medical condition and surgery, as measured in a preoperative interview. The results showed that those who knew the most about their operations (the vigilant) had the slowest and most complicated recovery from surgery. The latter finding was subsequently replicated (Cohen, 1975). A hypothesis offered to explain these results was that vigilant copers were those who utilized a strategy of actively trying to master the world by seeking information. This style turns out to be maladaptive in the postoperative situation where there is nothing the individual can do to "master" the situation actively. Kornfeld and others (1974) express a similar view in explaining why patients who were dominant and self-assured had a greater incidence of delirium after open-heart surgery. Cohen and Lazarus (1973) further suggest that elective surgery may be one of those stressful occurrences that can be more effectively dealt with by avoidant-denial forms of coping than by vigilant ones, since although many threats occur in the surgical context, few actually materialize.

Sime (1976) used two different questionnaires to investigate information seeking and the amount of information received. She found no significant relationship between these measures and postoperative negative affect, number of analgesics, or length of hospital stay. She did find significant interactions with level of preoperative fear. High-fear patients who reported receiving little information and moderate-fear patients who reported receiving much information showed the poorest recovery. The differing findings may reflect differences in interview-based and questionnaire-based assessments of information and information seeking and in the types of outcome measures utilized.

Whether the burden of additional stresses or *life changes* influences outcome of surgery has been examined in a few studies, using the Holmes and Rahe (1967a) Schedule of Recent Experiences, or an abbreviated version of it (Rundall, 1976). Although stress was related to slower recovery from nonsurgical illnesses, no significant relationships between life changes and recovery from surgery have been found (Cohen and Lazarus, 1973; Rundall, 1976). Nuckolls, Cassel, and Kaplan (1972) found no direct relationship between life-change scores and the number of complications in delivery of a first child; there was, however, a significant interaction with psychosocial assets. Those with many life changes and few assets had more complications of delivery. Thus, it may be necessary to take into account both the stresses to which a person is exposed and the resources he or she has to cope with the additional stresses.

We will now review some studies relating trait measures of coping, anxiety, and personality to outcome of surgery. One might hypothesize that those who characteristically repress unpleasant facts, who are prone to anxiety, who feel little sense of personal control, and so on, would have a more difficult recovery from surgery. However, the results show very few consistent significant relationships between trait measures and recovery variables. Few positive associations have been found between *repression-sensitization* measures and psychological or physical recovery variables (Cohen and

Lazarus, 1973; Minckley, 1974; Walseth, 1968). Scores on Andrew's version of the Goldstein avoidance-coping SCT were found to be positively related to the number of postoperative pain medications but not to other physical or psychological indicators of recovery (Cohen and Lazarus, 1973).

Largely negative results have also been found for trait measures of *anxiety* (from the Institute for Personality and Ability Testing Anxiety Scale or the 16 Personality Factor questionnaire) and physical indicators of recovery (Bruegel, 1971; Rothberg, 1965). Although Bruegel found no significant relationship between number of analgesics taken and anxiety, Chapman and Cox (1977) did find a positive correlation between Spielberger's trait anxiety measure and patient's self-reported pain on the first but not the third postoperative day. The Neuroticism scale (indicating proneness to anxiety) on Eysenck's Personality PEN Inventory was found to have a significant relationship to measures of postoperative vital capacity impairment and chest complication scores (Parbrook, Dalrymple, and Steel, 1973).

A trait measure of *dependence* was found to have no significant relationship to measures of physical recovery (Rothberg, 1965). Giller (1962) found a significant negative correlation between *ego strength* and the number of pain medications taken postoperatively. Johnson, Leventhal, and Dabbs (1971) found that those scoring as *internals* on the Internal-External Locus of Control Scale (that is, those who felt a greater sense of personal control) took more postoperative analgesics; however, Smith (1974) found no relationship between scores on this scale and psychological or physical measures of recovery.

Inconsistent results have been found in studies relating MMPI scales to mortality from open-heart surgery. Gilberstadt and Sako (1967) found that those who died following open-heart surgery were less guarded, had more energy (or some organic disability), and were more socially introverted than those who survived (that is, had lower L and K scores, higher F, Pa, Ma, and Si). These patients were significantly older, however. Henrichs, MacKenzie, and Almond (1969) found male survivors of open-heart surgery had significantly lower Pt and anxiety scale scores than nonsurvivors, whereas female survivors had lower Hs and repression scale scores. However, Kilpatrick and others (1975) found no significant differences on any MMPI scales between survivors and nonsurvivors of open-heart surgery. They found that indexes of organicity and of cardiac impairment were most predictive of mortality. Cohen (1975) found that personality trait factors derived from the California Psychological Inventory (Gough, 1956) and the Adjective Check List (Gough, 1952) were related to physical recovery from surgery. Those who were inhibited, cautious, and methodical stayed longer in the hospital, whereas capable, conscientious, conforming individuals who like to work toward defined goals and who minimize worries and complaints had more minor medical complications postoperatively. It is difficult to draw conclusions about the usefulness of trait measures because of the inconsistency of results, but, in general, they appear to have very little ability to predict outcome of surgery.

Overall, the results of studies of surgery are not clear cut. The tremendous variability in physical indicators of recovery used makes it difficult to obtain definitive results; therefore, we shall emphasize the consistencies that emerge. Those who have high levels of anticipatory fear before an operation seem to have more emotional difficulties postoperatively. However, this may merely be evidence of one personality state or response style being expressed in two different time periods. Whereas questionnaire measures of depression consistently fail to relate to measures of recovery, those high on process measures of depression have more complicated recoveries from surgery. This relationship may reflect the influence of the state of physical health on both process measures and medical outcomes. Those who seek information or who are vigilant preoperatively may show more complicated recovery from surgery since there is nothing that can actually be done to master the situation actively. Most trait measures show nonsignificant or inconsistent results in relationship to outcomes of surgery.

Intervention Studies

Information has long been considered valuable as an aid to adjustment to stressful situations. As already noted, Janis (1958) believed that information was necessary to challenge people's reassurances and help them to begin to do the "work of worrying." Laboratory work has shown that a subject's physiological response to a stressful situation can be made more benign by presenting information that provides a less threatening appraisal of the negative implications of the threat (Lazarus and Alfert, 1964; Speisman and others, 1964).

In situations of illness or medical treatment, there are four kinds of information that can be given: (1) information about the nature of the disease or about the medical reasons for initiating particular treatments; (2) information describing in detail the medical procedures to be carried out; (3) information about particular sensations or side effects to be expected; and (4) information about coping strategies the person can use in adjusting to the upcoming threat (see also Averill, in press). Most interventions include several of these types of information and present the information in a context of support, encouragement, attention, and often implicit challenge. It is therefore difficult to determine whether supportive or informative elements are most important in aiding patients' adjustment. In addition, some interventions help patients see how they can take an active role in treatment or otherwise give them a greater sense of control. Personal control is thought to aid adjustment to stress, although the relationship is not simple or straightforward and depends on the meaning that control has for the person (Averill, 1973; Gal and Lazarus, 1975; Janis and Rodin, Chapter Nineteen in this volume).

The nature of the interaction itself could actually be more important than the specific information provided, as Meyer (1967, p. 34) has suggested: "As in all other instances of the dialogue between the surgeon and his patient, the actual verbal content of their exchange may be of relatively minor importance. Like the lullabies sung to sleeping children, with horrendous allusions to breaking branches and falling babies, the tune may prove more meaningful than the words."

Recovery from nonsurgical illness. There are very few studies that investigate the effects of psychological interventions on recovery from nonsurgical illness. The large number of studies focusing on outcome of surgery undoubtedly reflect the fact that more concrete indicators of recovery are available in the case of surgical patients. One might expect that *psychotherapy* could help patients to reduce anxiety, mobilize coping resources, and begin actively to come to terms with their illness and the constructive changes that are necessary. Psychotherapy has been found to have positive benefits for patients recovering from myocardial infarction. Hospitalized patients who received individual psychotherapy showed faster recovery and had fewer cardiac problems during hospitalization (Gruen, 1975). Rahe and others (1975) found that patients who received both information about heart disease and brief group therapy following hospitalization subsequently experienced fewer cardiac complications than did the controls.

The Simontons (1975) believe that psychological factors are central in the development of cancer and therefore can be instrumental in affecting the course of the disease. Their intervention attempts to change the belief system of the patient and to involve patients in relaxation and *visualization* exercises. Patients are taught to accept personal responsibility for the development and control of their disease and are instructed in ways to produce visual images of their cancer, treatment, and white body cells. In their visualizations, patients are told to emphasize the strength of radiation rays and bodily immunological forces bearing down on increasingly weakening and shrinking cancer cells. Although the Simontons suggest that this program, in combination with traditional radiation therapy, is extremely effective in increasing survival from cancer, to date they have presented little beyond anecdotal data to support these claims. One problem of this intervention is that more than half of the patients refuse to participate in it, which clearly limits its potential usefulness.

Recovery from surgery. The following interventions have been examined in studies of recovery from surgery: detailed accurate information about what to expect, specific instruction in postoperative coughing and deep breathing, a positive thinking approach, reassurance, systematic relaxation, hypnosis, short or lengthy psychotherapeutic interviews, intellectualizing information about the illness, and general information about hospital facilities. A more detailed discussion of this literature can be found in Cohen (1975); see also Auerbach and Kilmann (1977).

As was discussed earlier, Janis (1958) and others believe that information can benefit patients by warning them about, and thus aiding inner preparation for, the threats and discomforts of the postoperative period. However, information that conveys an accurate picture of what to expect has not consistently been related to improved recovery from surgery. *De-*

tailed, accurate information about what to expect about a forthcoming surgery was not found to reduce ratings of postoperative negative mood (Vernon and Bigelow, 1974); another study found similar preoperative information reduced the number of pain medications taken but did not influence length of hospital stay (Langer, Janis, and Wolfer, 1975). Preoperative information about sensations and procedures to be expected was effective in reducing length of hospital stay in another study; interactions with psychological questionnaire measures were also found (Wilson, 1977). Johnson and others (1977) reported that *information about sensations* was related to improved physical recovery from surgery in one study, but they were unable to replicate the results on a different operative group. Information about sensations to be expected in an endoscopic examination significantly reduced gagging during the procedure but had no clear-cut effects on other measures of behavioral adjustment (Johnson and Leventhal, 1974). Even less gagging was found when the information about sensations was combined with information about how to act when the tube was being inserted; however, those who received the combined message also required more time for tube insertion into the stomach. (See also Johnson, 1975, and Averill, in press.) Thus, accurate information about procedures or sensations to be expected does not show consistent effects in improving surgical outcomes.

Because patients are inactive postoperatively, lung problems can develop. *Postoperative coughing and deep breathing* help to expand the lungs to more normal levels and to eliminate excess mucus which might otherwise accumulate. However, those with abdominal incisions find deep breathing and coughing to be quite painful and often are reluctant to make such efforts; there are ways to instruct patients in these techniques which encourage their use, and to explain why pain may be felt and how it can be minimized. Egbert and others (1964) attempted to reduce postoperative pain in a group of patients by instruction and encouragement in moving and in the use of coughing and deep-breathing exercises. They found that these patients took less pain medication and were sent home earlier than those who did not receive such information. Healy (1968), Roe (1963), and Lindeman and Van Aernam (1971) report similar results, although their studies suffer from various methodological inadequacies, such as not randomly assigning patients to groups, using no statistical analyses or inappropriate ones, not equalizing severity of operation in experimental and control groups, and so forth. Cohen (1975) found no significant effects of information about postoperative coughing and deep breathing on psychological and physical measures of recovery; she suggested that since such procedures were now accepted as standard medical practice, specific interventions along these lines might no longer prove to have added benefit.

Being able to control negative emotions or to focus one's attention on positive events is commonly thought to improve psychological morale and aid in adjustment to unpleasant events; however, the research results are mixed in regard to surgery. Langer, Janis, and Wolfer (1975) investigated whether patients exposed to a *positive thinking* intervention, which they term a "coping device," would show faster recovery from surgery. Patients were instructed to try to control their emotions by directing their attention to the more favorable aspects of their situation—through either focusing on the secondary gains of being a patient or on the ways they would benefit from the surgery. They found patients exposed to this intervention took less pain medication but did not have a shorter hospital stay. Cohen (1975) found no significant effects on measures of psychological or physical recovery using a different positive thinking intervention strategy. Cohen also found that a *reassurance* approach did not affect indicators of recovery from surgery.

One might expect that those who know how to relax would be able to reduce postoperative anxiety and thereby have a smoother recovery from surgery, but the results are mixed regarding the effectiveness of this intervention. Wilson (1977) found that training in *systematic relaxation* improved physical indicators of recovery; interactions with psychological questionnaire measures were also found. However, other investigators have obtained equivocal results relating relaxation interventions to psychological or physical recovery measures (Aiken, 1972; Aiken and Henrichs, 1971; Smith, 1974). Various writers have suggested that *hypnosis* results in improved physical recovery from surgery (Doberneck and others, 1959, 1961; Kolouch, 1964), but no statistical analyses have been carried out to determine the significance of the findings.

Psychotherapeutic interviews are thought to help patients verbalize their fears and concerns and begin to prepare psychologically for the discomforts to be faced. Generally negative results have been found in studies of the effects of short psychotherapeutic visits on postoperative recovery (Dumas, Anderson, and Leonard, 1965; Dumas and Leonard, 1963; Lindeman and Stetzer, 1973; Solomon, 1973). However, a small preoperative group session where patients discussed their fears, received information about what to expect, and learned coughing and deep-breathing exercises did have beneficial effects on certain physical recovery measures (Schmitt and Wooldridge, 1973).

Postoperative delirium is common after open-heart surgery and is thought to be a reaction to the emotional stresses of surgery, to the physical assaults of the operative procedure, and to the sleep deprivation, immobilization, and sensory monotony of the open-heart recovery room. In-depth psychotherapeutic interviews have been found to be effective in reducing postoperative delirium after open-heart surgery (Heller and others, 1970; Kornfeld and others, 1974; Lazarus and Hagens, 1968; Layne and Yudofsky, 1971; however, Surman and others, 1974, did not confirm these results). It is extremely important in these studies to control for differences in preoperative organicity and severity of the operation; Nadelson (1976) discusses how these and other factors affect incidence of postoperative delirium.

Although most researchers have hypothesized that information or psychological preparation would benefit surgical patients, prior research has shown that information can increase anxiety for some. A few studies have investigated those personality factors that mediate the effects of preoperative

information (see also Wilson, 1977). Andrew (1967, 1970) examined the interaction between a person's general defensive style and an *intellectualizing
orientation* which discussed the etiology of hernias and what would be done
during the operation. She hypothesized that patients could use information
beneficially if it was compatible with their defensive style. She found that
avoiders had a more complicated recovery if presented with this information
before surgery, the middle group showed improved recovery if they heard
the tape preoperatively, and copers recovered well regardless of when they
received the information.

In a subsequent study (with different operative groups), DeLong
(1970) used two types of tapes—one containing specific *intellectualizing information* and the other containing *general information* about the size and
services of the hospital—but failed to confirm this pattern. She found that
rate of recovery varied only for the coper group, who showed the best recovery if they received the specific information tape and worse recovery if they
received the general information tape. Auerbach and others (1976) also used
general and specific information tapes to determine their impact on anxiety
and on behavioral adjustment during dental surgery. They found that neither
type of information presented nor the score on the Internal-External Locus
of Control scale were related to degree of anxiety during the surgery. However, they did find that internals showed better adjustment during the surgery if they viewed the specific information tape rather than the general; the
opposite was true for externals.

The only interventions that show consistent results are those that are
psychotherapeutic in nature. Psychotherapy reduces cardiac complications
after myocardial infarction; in-depth psychotherapeutic interviews reduce
postoperative delirium after open-heart surgery. It is unclear what type of
information is most beneficial to patients. The studies by Andrew (1970),
DeLong (1970), Auerbach and others (1976), and Wilson (1977) suggest that
there may be important interactions between the type of information presented and the personality characteristics of the patient. That such factors
have not been taken into account in other studies may explain why generally
negative or inconsistent results are obtained in the studies that utilize
psychological interventions. In addition, it is important to recall that the information in a particular intervention represents only a small part of the
total information that is received by patients who are ill. What physicians tell
their patients may confound or distort the intervention attempt. Thus, the
effects of an intervention on recovery may only become apparent when the
information given by physicians is systematically taken into account (Cohen,
1975).

Conclusions

In this paper, we have described a theoretical framework for understanding stress and coping issues, pointed out difficulties in assessing coping
in naturalistic settings and in evaluating coping effectiveness, outlined the
threats potential in illness and in medical treatment, emphasized the impor-

tance of individual differences in appraisal of these threats, and reviewed literature on the relationship between coping and recovery from illness. It is difficult to make any integrative statement about the research findings in this area because of the contradictory results, the few replications, the inability to make comparisons between studies because dissimilar independent and dependent measures are used, and because of lack of clarity about what are the influential components of particular psychological interventions. Despite these difficulties, the following variables were found fairly consistently to predict unfavorable medical outcomes in nonintervention studies: trait measures of depression (for nonsurgical illnesses), state measures of depression (for recovery from surgery), state measures of preoperative fear (surgery), the inhibition or expression of emotion (nonsurgery), having additional stresses or few psychological assets or an imbalance between these (nonsurgery), lack of active involvement (nonsurgery), and vigilant coping modes (surgery).

The literature on psychological interventions is inconsistent or finds interventions ineffective, making it difficult to draw any positive conclusions except to note the beneficial effects of psychotherapeutic interviews or therapy. We really do not know what types of information are most helpful to different people. Types of information may interact with personality characteristics of the patient; researchers must continue their efforts to investigate these interactions with individual difference measures. It appears that interventions that include several types of information are most beneficial, although the results are not uniform even in these cases.

Given the nature of the findings, it is important for researchers in the field to plan future studies more carefully in order to overcome some of these deficiencies and to allow us to gain greater clarity about how coping affects recovery. First, we need a wider range and more consistency in the types of outcome variables examined, so that we can understand the full impact of a coping strategy or intervention. Acquiring such information is not too difficult when hospital records are examined, since information about pain medications, minor medical complications, length of hospital stay, and so forth, is readily available. If different investigators use similar measures, this will also increase the possibility of obtaining replication of results.

Second, we must begin to try to specify which coping strategies are most effective across many illnesses and which are valuable in dealing only with certain specific illnesses. As described earlier, the expression of emotion may have different effects on the progression of disease, depending on the nature of the illness itself. Third, it may be useful to use both trait and process measures of emotional state in studying outcomes of illness, since each of these kinds of measures shows significant relationships with some medical outcomes but not with others. Severity of the illness and physical condition must be controlled for, however, since they can influence both process ratings of emotional state and outcome of surgical procedures.

Fourth, one must be careful about generalizing from results of nonintervention studies in the desire to make interventions to aid patients' coping. If those who seek information about a forthcoming surgery have more complicated recovery from surgery, that does not mean that withholding information will aid recovery efforts. It may be that those personality factors that lead an individual to seek information also influence recovery during the postoperative course. Since we do not know if the nature of the information received, the personality characteristics that cause people to seek information in the first place, or the desire to be active in a situation where passivity is required is the factor related to more complicated recovery, we do not know what intervention will be effective. We should move cautiously in applying the results of nonintervention studies until we better understand the dynamics involved.

Fifth, we must consider seriously the outcome measures to be examined. There is a sense in which it is arbitrary to say that the course of recovery is better or worse insofar as the patient goes home sooner, takes less pain medications, has fewer complications, and fewer psychological complaints. Such allegations adopt a particular set of values generated in part by practical considerations within the hospital setting. However, we know little about the determinants of each of these indexes, of the decision process related to discharging a patient or prescribing medications, or of the importance of each of these different recovery variables in reflecting the patient's return to health. Only as we know more about these processes will we be able to make more definitive statements about the effectiveness of particular coping strategies. Long-run and short-run considerations should also be made explicit, since those who show the best adjustment within the hospital environment may show worse adjustment after they return to their home situation.

Sixth, as discussed earlier, we need to broaden our assessment of coping over a longer time span so that we can determine how coping changes over time and situation. A process-oriented focus with a broad assessment of the coping strategies employed will be most useful in helping us understand how patients cope with and adjust to serious medical illnesses.

Despite all this apparent confusion, we are sanguine about the importance of coping in affecting somatic illness and recovery from it, and about its role in sustaining morale and social and occupational functioning in persons facing illness. Even if coping were shown ultimately to have relatively little effect on the physical course of disease, which we think is possible but not likely, how a person copes with illness is surely a central determinant of his or her psychological well-being and social functioning, that is, how well such a person lives, ailing or not. This was certainly the emphasis of the Hamburg group whose descriptive research and theoretical speculation we discussed earlier, and it is equally important in the writings of Engel (1977), who calls for a biopsychosocial model of thought reminiscent of the earlier writings of Adolph Meyer. As we have discussed, the case for intervention is even weaker at the moment, but here too we need not be totally pessimistic. The six concluding recommendations we have made really add up to one main theme, namely, that weaknesses of our general theory and research paradigm leave us in a state of ignorance about the central questions posed, that is, how to measure coping and how coping works to facilitate or impair adaptational outcome. In the light of such ignorance, we cannot hope to make much progress yet with intervention, be it oriented toward treatment, prevention, or education. But our present ignorance need not persist if we take to heart the theoretical, methodological, and value-related issues we have discussed here, and there is every reason to believe that we are in an early stage in the study of powerful forces that contribute to health and well-being or to illness and distress—forces that can in some measure be manipulated through intervention. The task now is to turn this conviction into increasingly sophisticated and systematic study with the aim of accurately tailoring our psychological and social interventions to the disease and its specific management requirements, the institutional setting, and the kind of person with whom we are dealing. In part through the burgeoning interest in health psychology and in the coping process, and in part as a result of growing methodological sophistication, the chances now seem good for rapid progress over the next decade.

10 ∽

Effects of Cancer
on Patients' Lives:
A Personological Approach

Norman L. Mages

Gerald A. Mendelsohn

Thoughtful researchers in the field of personality are constantly aware of a tension between the demand to produce generalizable findings and the equally pressing demand to remain true to the uniqueness of the persons being studied. The approach we will present in this paper, an approach that has guided our investigation of the psychosocial effects of cancer, attempts to resolve this tension by taking the individual patient, not a set of variables or specific behaviors, as the basic unit of analysis. We refer to

Note: This paper is based on research supported by a grant from the National Cancer Institute (Grant CA 16873). The research was conducted at the Mount Zion Hospital and Medical Center, San Francisco, with the participation of the Claire Zellerbach Saroni Tumor Institute and the Departments of Social Work and Psychiatry. This project was very much a cooperative effort; every member of the staff shares credit and responsibility for the ideas and findings that are presented in this chapter. We wish to acknowledge the indispensable contributions of Joseph Castro (principal investigator), Patricia A. Fobair, Joan S. Hall, Irene Harrison, and Abby Wolfson.

The order of the authors' names is alphabetical.

this approach as personological because it is the person conceived of as a coherent entity with enduring attributes and dispositions that constitutes our subject matter. The method of study we have chosen—the intensive analysis of a series of individual cases and the subsequent search for commonalities among them—is not the only approach that can contribute to an understanding of the psychological consequences of cancer. When one wishes to study a phenomenon as broad and multifaceted as the impact of cancer on a person's life, however, a personological approach seems both necessary and uniquely suited to the exploration of the general and the unique in patients' reactions.

In contrast to variable-centered approaches in the field of personality, personology is not primarily concerned with the prediction of behavior or the testing of hypotheses. Rather, its end product is an integrated description of a unique pattern of functioning. Thus, personology is distinguished by its ipsative character: The focus of study is on the interrelationships of variables *within* a single person, and lawfulness is derived from the coherence of an individual's behavior. It is at this point, however, that a problem arises: Though the value of case studies seems self-evident, doubts have often been raised about their capacity to yield valid, objectively verifiable generalizations. We believe they can, in fact, do so, but by inductive rather than deductive means. There is, after all, an important corollary to the fact that all individuals are unique, namely, that they also have much in common. If observations of individual cases are recorded systematically and in some standard format, it becomes possible to compare them and to detect shared patterns of functioning among individuals or subgroups of individuals. This is the essence of the natural history method and it seems to us as applicable in personality as in medicine or zoology.

In this chapter, we will be concerned with a specific application of the personological approach to the study of how cancer affects the lives of those who have been diagnosed and treated for the disease. It scarcely needs saying that these effects are both profound and widely ramified. It probably does need saying, however, that these effects unfold over a long period of time and, consequently, should be studied in a developmental perspective. We must emphasize also that the response to cancer, like all other behavior, is a function of situational, as well as personal, factors. To some extent, all cancer patients must come to grips with a common set of circumstances and resulting issues (for example, diminished life expectancy and, more concretely, the threat of recurrence). But at the same time, variations in symptomatology, personality, age, sex, social status, systems of support, and the like, make it inevitable that each patient will react in an idiosyncratic way. The dictum of Kluckhohn and Murray (1953)—that every person is in some respects like every other person, like some other persons, and like no other person—applies as meaningfully to those with cancer as to people in general.

The Psychosocial Effects of Cancer

Our discussion of the psychosocial effects of cancer will be organized around three general propositions: (1) The experience of cancer is an ongoing process that unfolds over a considerable period of time. Within that period of time, several stages of the disease, each with its own particular problems, can be delineated. (2) Cancer almost inevitably produces enduring personal change which, to be fully understood, should be viewed in the context of the individual's life stage and previous history. (3) The psychological developments at any given point in the process are integrated around the patient's need to adapt to the issues imposed by the concrete realities of the illness. The nature and the effectiveness of the adaptation are determined in large measure by the specific details of the illness and by the patient's personal characteristics and social milieu. In the material that follows, we will develop these propositions and illustrate them with empirical findings and with material drawn from individual case studies.

Time Perspective in Cancer

Cancer, like all chronic illness, evolves over an extended period of time. It has no clear onset or easily predicted course and only rarely does it have a certain end, save in death. Thus, the person with cancer is not confronted with a single stressful event, but rather with a continuing condition, with a series of threats of varying intensity and duration. Even in the absence of recurrence, patients must deal with prolonged uncertainty about the progress of the disease and often with the painful residues of treatment as well. Under these circumstances, what it means to have cancer and the problems posed by the disease necessarily change with time. The study of the psychological and social effects of cancer, then, is the study of a developmental process.

In clinical medicine, the traditional way to order such complex material is to describe the natural history of the illness, that is, the usual course or variety of courses that the illness may follow, including modifications imposed by treatment. This approach can help to define the essential elements of the illness and to delineate the most typical variations on the common theme. There is some precedent for using this method in regard to psychological phenomena as well, especially where psychological reactions are consequent to a clearly defined external event, such as grief following the loss of loved ones (Lindemann, 1944) or response to natural disaster (Rangell, 1976; Titchener and Kapp, 1976). We believe that such an approach can profitably be extended to the psychological response to cancer.

The natural history of the psychological response to cancer has not yet been investigated in a comprehensive manner and, at present, such a schema can only be partially pieced together from contributions to the literature. Though it may be obvious that cancer is a long-term and evolving condition, the most common approach to research has been to select a clinically important problem characteristic of a specific time segment of the course of cancer and to focus on its causes, complications, and therapeutic implications. There is, for example, a fairly extensive literature on such questions as: "Why do some people delay in seeking treatment for their cancer?" (Hackett, Cassem, and Raker, 1973); "Should cancer patients be told the true facts of their illness?" (McIntosh, 1974); "How do patients react to disabling or disfiguring surgery?" (Bard and Sutherland, 1955; Sutherland and others, 1952; Wirsching, Druner, and Herrmann, 1975); "How can one best help terminal patients confront death?" (Norton, 1963). Alternatively, some investigators have chosen to take a single strand of the patient's response to cancer and to trace its course through the illness—for example, Abrams' (1966) study of changes in communication patterns during cancer or Polivy's (1977) attempt to delineate variations in body image. But with a very few exceptions, it is only recently that broad-ranging, longitudinal studies of the psychosocial response to cancer have been undertaken. Thus, we know most about what happens in the acute phases of the disease—the beginning and the end of the natural history—and relatively little about the long-term adaptations made by those patients who are surviving with their disease.

It is not at all surprising that most researchers have focused on the acute phases of cancer. During initial diagnosis and primary treatment and again in the terminal stages of cancer, the physical and psychological stress on the patient is most obvious and poignant. At these times too, patients are apt to be hospitalized and accessible and their responses most dramatic and troublesome. Further, these responses often have considerable significance for treatment decisions. In recent years, there has also been increasing interest in how people cope with the prospect of impending death (Glaser and Strauss, 1965; Krant, 1974; Kübler-Ross, 1969; Weisman, 1972). Cancer patients have provided a prime source of material for these studies, since cancer is one of the few common illnesses in which the approximate time of death can be anticipated. Indeed, a substantial portion of the research on cancer patients has been concerned less with the reaction to cancer as such than with explorations of stress and coping or death and dying, for which cancer patients constitute a most appropriate population.

In our own work with cancer patients, we have been concerned from the outset with the broad question of how cancer affects the course of a person's life.* As a first step, we interviewed a group of patients who had

*This chapter is not intended to be a report of research, but, since we will often cite our findings to support or illustrate particular arguments, a short description of the samples and methods is necessary. Data were collected by means of intensive, semistructured interviews on two retrospective samples (three and six years past primary treatment, total $n = 35$) and on a prospective sample (interviewed during or just after primary treatment, $n = 31$, and then again six to twelve months later, $n = 21$). Slightly more than half the patients in both the retrospective and prospective samples were women. The patients ranged in age from eighteen to seventy-two at the time of initial diagnosis and were heterogeneous with respect to site, prognosis, race, socioeconomic background, and so forth. They were a fairly representative sample of the Mount Zion Hospital population of cancer patients. The interviews were concerned not only with cancer-related events and current functioning but also with personal history. In all but a few instances, a single interview was insufficient; typically two to four interviews were required to obtain the information we sought. In about one third of the cases, there was also a collateral interview with a spouse or a close friend. The interview protocols were quantified by means of rating scales and a specially constructed Q-sort deck designed by us for use with cancer patients. Multiple ratings were obtained on each case to assure adequate reliability and to minimize bias. In addition to the interview material, clinical observations of patients in

survived their illness for six years and then, subsequently, a group of three-year survivors. Given the emphasis in the literature on the acute phases of cancer, very little is known about this increasingly numerous group of patients who achieve long remissions or are cured, though frequently at the cost of permanent disability or body damage. We observed repeatedly that long after the trauma of diagnosis and primary treatment had been resolved or had become part of a dim past, cancer continued to affect these patients' lives in many overt and subtle ways. Certainly, those people faced with continuing disability or recurrent disease endured many changes of mood, outlook, and function as time progressed. But even people who could look forward to a good prognosis after a relatively uncomplicated course of treatment did not experience cancer as a limited episode. They frequently reported that their lives had been permanently changed by their confrontation with their own mortality and the continuing unpredictability of their future.

These kinds of observations led us to broaden our original conceptual framework and to look for ways of thinking about life change that could do justice to the data we were accumulating. A simple crisis resolution model (Parad, 1965) proved unsatisfactory. In this type of model, it is assumed that stress upsets an initial equilibrium and that the individual's task is to resolve the crisis situation so that the original equilibrium can be restored. There are several difficulties in trying to apply such a concept to the case of cancer: (1) Since people with cancer are confronted with continuing stress or a series of severe stresses over an extended period of time, it is inaccurate to speak of cancer as though it were a single event, posing a time-limited crisis that requires only immediate adaptive response. (2) As noted before, one of the major problems posed by cancer is that the patient cannot be sure for many years whether or not a cure has been effected. This problem too involves not a single event or series of events well marked in time, but rather a continuing, unremitting condition of uncertainty about potentially disastrous and poorly predictable future events. (3) The treatment of cancer usually entails irreparable physical damage which may enforce changes in patterns of activity, habits of daily living, perceptions of oneself, and the like. In such circumstances, a return to an original equilibrium is simply precluded. (4) In fact, the majority of cancer patients regard their disease as the source of a major discontinuity in their lives and report permanent changes in how they view themselves and their future existence.

Given these difficulties with a simple crisis resolution model or, for that matter, any model that fails to take the temporal aspects of chronic disease into account, we found Parkes' (1971) idea of "psychosocial transitions" a more appropriate way to conceptualize the long-term and evolving effects of cancer. It was the experience of enduring change reported by

---

discussion groups provided invaluable, though less formal data. There were two groups, one for patients thirty-five and younger ($n = 20$) and one for patients in mid-life ($n = 31$). We also conducted a group for the families of patients ($n = 25$ participants). Not surprisingly, the patients involved directly or indirectly in these groups were somewhat more seriously ill than the patients who were interviewed.

bereaved widows that led Parkes to articulate this concept, a concept he then applied to cancer patients (1975), and which Weiss (1975) has employed in discussing divorce. The common element in all of these situations is that passage through a period of crisis leads to an altered state in which values, time perspective, social roles, and self-image may be permanently changed. The person, in short, enters what can meaningfully be described as a new stage of life as a consequence of the crisis. To study the natural history of the psychosocial response to cancer, then, is to attempt to delineate the nature of these transitions and the processes by which they occur and are integrated with the past.

Naturally, there are some patients for whom cancer is an episode of limited duration, more a perturbation than a point of transition. This is most likely to happen when the malignancy is relatively benign, for example, a cervical cancer *in situ*. But as we noted earlier, the great majority of the patients we interviewed saw themselves as having undergone marked change since their cancer. For example, we asked a group of three-year survivors to describe themselves (on the Gough-Heilbrun, 1965, Adjective Check List) as they were before their illness and then as they were currently. A rather consistent picture of self-perceived change emerged. Surprisingly, patients reported relatively little alteration in the level of dysphoric affect or nervousness; however, increases in distractibility and absent-mindedness and a loss of concentration were frequent. Ambition, drive, aggressiveness, the striving for achievement and recognition were seen as having declined, while tolerance, humane concern, and understanding were reported to have increased. Overall, the impression is of lowered intensity and engagement in the external world coupled with a more benign focus on the smaller world of home, family, and friends. Associated with this is a tendency for patients in their fifties and early sixties to retire well before they were required to do so. Unexpectedly, we found significant differences between men and women in the way they perceived themselves. For the women, positive and negative changes tended to balance out and, according to their report, they were able to preserve their self-esteem relatively well over the three years. Among the men, the perceived decline in activity, assertiveness, and striving for achievement led to a much less positive self-image.

Interviews with family members confirmed the patients' own impression of how their work, family, social, and sexual lives had changed. Frequently, these changes took the form of withdrawal or a constriction of activities. A decline in sexual interest and activity was, for example, very much the rule. Situations that evoked unpleasant memories or feelings of being less attractive or desirable were avoided. Patients who felt overwhelmed by the multiple physical, emotional, and practical burdens of their illness often narrowed their interests to create a smaller and more manageable world. In some instances, patients found that they could use their illness to obtain gratification or increase their power over others, thus altering substantially patterns of interaction within the family. Interestingly, only one patient in our sample reported that no changes at all had occurred, but she did so with a fierce insistence that seemed to belie her words. Even those patients who were interviewed six years after their primary treatment and could reasonably consider themselves cured showed continuing effects of their experience, as evidenced by a chronic underlying uneasiness and feeling of vulnerability. There is, we believe, good reason to conclude that the effects of cancer typically persist indefinitely.

Situational Factors: Nature of the Illness

In our discussion thus far, we have explored some of the implications of viewing the response to cancer as a process of psychosocial transition that extends continuously through time. If one stops the process at any given point and takes a cross-sectional look at what is happening, what appears most vividly is the effort of the individual to adapt to and master the immediate stresses imposed by the illness.

There have been a number of attempts to develop concepts of adaptation and coping suitable for understanding the responses to serious disease. Janis (1958), Hamburg and Adams (1967), and Katz and others (1970) have made important contributions; more recently, Lazarus (1974), Lipowski (1970), and Moos (1977a) have been working actively in this area. In our own thinking, we have attempted to bring together psychodynamic and adaptive points of view and to extend these ideas to the specific kinds of problems that are of concern to cancer patients.

The single most important factor that determines the adjustments a cancer patient must make is the concrete nature of the disease. (Weisman and Worden, 1977, come to a similar conclusion.) To understand the adaptive efforts of a person with cancer, one must develop a clear and detailed picture of the specific realities to be faced and of how these new "facts of life" are perceived and organized by the individual. Although each patient confronts a particular situation and undergoes a unique set of experiences, we found that it was nevertheless possible to develop a sense of the commonalities among patients. We used material from individual interviews and group discussions to identify the common themes expressed by patients and found that their concerns tended to cluster around certain basic issues. For each issue, one can conceptualize an adaptive task that needs to be accomplished successfully if the patient is to function effectively. Although these issues must be faced by every cancer patient, the intensity and significance of each will vary with the individual, the character and stage of the illness, and external circumstances.

One may conveniently organize the sequence of issues and adaptive tasks around successive stages in the course of the illness: discovery and diagnosis, primary treatment, remission with return to normal activity, and—unfortunately for some—recurrence and spread, and terminal illness. (Hinton, 1973, has developed a somewhat similar sequence of issues.)

1. *Issue: Discovery of cancer.* Cancer generally begins silently and internally and often presents in innocuous and painless ways. Though occa-

sionally uncovered as part of a medical examination, more often the first presentation of a possible cancer is noted by the patient rather than a physician. Because of the intense fears associated with this possibility, there is a great temptation to ignore the earliest symptoms or to rationalize their existence as trivial.

> A young secretary discovered a lump in her breast as she turned over in bed and touched herself. She "knew inside" that it was a sign of something serious, got up, made herself a pot of coffee, and read the paper. It took her two hours to get up courage to go back to examining the lump and when she lay on her back to do self-examination the lump was no longer there. She had a temporary job to make extra money and was relieved to find she was extremely busy. Each time she had a minute between assignments she felt extremely anxious. The next morning she shared her concern with her boss, who immediately made an appointment with her gynecologist and drove her there.

Adaptive task: To appraise the significance of the discovery and initiate appropriate treatment. Usually, the patient's realistic sense of danger asserts itself and a definitive diagnosis is sought, but this is frequently the outcome of an extended process that involves much apprehension and indecision and that must be pushed along by the worsening of symptoms or the urging of others.

2. *Issue: Primary treatment.* Surgery, radiation, or chemotherapy each holds its own special terrors, and the pretreatment period is usually one of high distress. Unlike many illnesses in which one comes to the doctor feeling sick and then feels better after treatment, the reverse is often true with cancer. For many patients, the primary treatment has the characteristics of a traumatic experience: There is a sudden catastrophic event, assault on one's body, and disruption of normal life, all of which lead to a sense of being overwhelmed, with shock, numbness, an impulse to flight, outbursts of feeling, and repetitive reliving in fantasy or dream. These traumatic stigmata may still be evident years later.

> A young professional woman had suffered through several painful and mutilating surgical procedures for the treatment of vaginal cancer. After a long period of rehabilitation and counseling, she was able to resume work and eventually married. Despite some persistent urinary problems, she did not dwell much on her surgical experiences and led a full and active life. Four years after her initial treatment, she found that describing her cancer experiences in a discussion group triggered a series of nightmares in which she repetitively relived much of the pain and horror of those earlier surgeries.

Adaptive task: To be able to recognize and deal with the realities of the situation, regulate the emotional reactions, and integrate the experience of illness with the rest of one's life.

3. *Issue: Damage to one's body from the cancer and/or treatment.* Severe functional impairment or disfigurement usually produces great distress and disability and so has elicited much clinical attention (Adsett, 1963; Blacker, 1970; Schoenberg and Carr, 1970). In our samples, we have seen a number of patients in whom readily visible disfigurement led to a devastating loss of self-esteem and to reclusive behavior. More private forms of bodily injury, while not impairing one's public life to the same degree, may take their toll in diminished self-esteem and a distortion of intimate relationships. Serious impairment of body function may compel the patient to give up work, parenting, or valued leisure activities—the very pursuits that ordinarily make life seem worthwhile.

> A retired professional man in his sixties was treated for squamous cell carcinoma of the nostril and lip with radiation and surgery. After the surgical repair, he reported, "I awoke and saw a monster in the mirror." He avoided people and retired from his work. Four years later, he still remained mostly indoors, isolated, brooding about his deformity, and fearing a recurrence. To the interviewer he clearly had a moderate degree of facial scarring, but nothing like the gross deformity he experienced in himself.

Adaptive task: To mourn the loss, replace or compensate for lost parts or functions where possible, and maximize other potentials so as to maintain a sense of self-esteem and intactness.

4. *Issue: Maintaining continuity.* After the dislocations of the acute phases of the illness—the discovery and treatment of cancer—the rent fabric of one's life must, in some way, be repaired. As we noted, patients almost always report that they have been changed by the experience of cancer and have developed new attitudes toward time, mortality, work, personal relationships, and their priorities in life. In addition, they frequently find that they, in turn, are treated differently by family, friends, and employers. For some it is not easy to give up the advantages of being a patient and to return to the customary demands and responsibilities of life, especially when still feeling ill, tired, and apprehensive about the future.

> A woman in her early sixties was treated for endometrial cancer with radiation and a hysterectomy. When interviewed at home while recuperating, she was relatively cheerful and optimistic and was pleased that her rather passive and dependent husband was being more helpful and cooperative. Six months later, she had returned to her clerical job but felt tired and irritable, had some residual bladder symptoms, and was very concerned about aging. She resented the fact that her husband resumed his old pattern of leaving things to her as soon as she got back on her feet.

Adaptive task: To understand and communicate one's changed attitudes, needs, and limitations in a way that permits formation of a new balance with the environment. Ideally, this should proceed with a minimum of constriction of one's life and activities and without becoming socially excluded or assuming an identity based solely on being a "cancer patient."

5. *Issue: Possibility of recurrence and progression of disease.* In the majority of cases, primary treatment leads to the eradication of detectable disease. Though the situation may appear promising, it will be years before the cancer patient can realistically be certain that the cancer is not silently spreading and growing until it recurs in a disseminated and incurable form. The fear of recurrence tends to be most prominent after primary treatment and gradually diminishes with time, though it persists for years and may be dramatically reactivated by follow-up visits, new symptoms (whether or not related to the disease), and those many reminders of cancer so generously available in the environment. Such fear may be quite paralyzing and may influence life decisions profoundly.

> A retired man in his late sixties had apparently been treated successfully for prostatic cancer over four years previously. He seldom thought much about recurrence until his physician noted a suspicious area on a routine follow-up exam. After several days of intense fear and distress, a benign biopsy specimen proved reassuring, and he outwardly resumed his usual life. However, on being reinterviewed three months after the "scare," he was still obviously quite apprehensive and his conversation was filled with intense concerns about possible recurrence and death.

Adaptive task: In order to live with this fear, it is necessary to be able to put it out of mind most of the time and remain sufficiently aware of the realities to continue appropriate medical follow-up and to take them into consideration in making long-range plans.

6. *Issue: Persistent or recurrent disease.* If primary treatment fails or if recurrent metastatic disease is discovered, the issues posed by cancer are, of course, markedly changed. The patient is no longer a cancer "survivor"; preparation for new physical symptoms, disabling treatment, pain, progressive infirmity, and death must be undertaken. Though there can be hope for extended remission or, at least, periods of comfortable and productive life remaining, the patient's experiential world is very different from that of the disease-free survivor. One problem that patients frequently stress at this stage is the difficulty in maintaining a sense of self-sufficiency and control over their lives. The failure of their own efforts and the efforts of their physicians to stem the downward course of their disease may lead to a disturbing sense of powerlessness and it may be difficult not to succumb to fear, despair, and passivity. Helpless feelings may be further increased by an inability to control the impact of cancer on career, intimate relationships, and bodily functions.

A recently retired married professional man in his fifties had been struggling with widespread recurrent prostatic cancer for two years. He suffered from continuing bone pain, loss of energy, impotence, and gastrointestinal symptoms. For him, the shock of recurrence was a greater source of emotional distress than the original diagnosis. The doctors "were going to get it, I just knew it. . . . I had every confidence in them, and now this." He now feels that he has to try to make his existence more comfortable, retrench economically, and manage his life so that he can be around people who can care for him. He hopes for two more good years of life before he dies. "I am hopeful and I want to live, but one has to be realistic."

Adaptive task: To exercise choice where possible and to accept one's helplessness and dependence where necessary without excessive regression or turning to a magical solution in lieu of appropriate treatment.

7. *Issue: Terminal illness.* The recent proliferation of work on death and dying (for example, Hinton, 1967; Glaser and Strauss, 1965; Kübler-Ross, 1969; Schoenberg and others, 1970; Weisman, 1972; Krant, 1974) obviates any extended discussion on our part. We do find that most terminal cancer patients have at least some awareness of impending death, but the daily realities of pain and incapacity may present even more salient problems.

A young married craftsman with metastatic bone cancer entered a discussion group when he was given only a few months to live. For weeks he was unable to speak of his concerns about death but finally described a terrifying dream in which a huge black bird was pressing against his chest and draining the breath from him. Presenting the dream helped open a discussion of death, and he gradually became able to talk with great poignancy about his sadness at the prospect of separation from his wife and friends, and about the opportunities in life, such as having children, which he would never realize. He resolved to maintain close contacts with others and to make his own treatment decisions as much as possible so as to maintain some sense of control over his life. He became a central figure in the group and provided a remarkably courageous example to the other group members.

Adaptive task: The patient must prepare to leave family and friends, provide for loved ones, and learn to use medical assistance and internal resources to minimize pain and to retain as much self-sufficiency and personal dignity as possible. In brief, it is necessary to come to terms with the prospect of death so that the remainder of life can be lived as well as possible.

Modes of Handling Issues and Accomplishing Adaptive Tasks

Although many patients may entirely escape the problems raised by persistent or recurrent disease and terminal illness, the other five issues just discussed must be dealt with in some fashion or other by all cancer patients. In its most explicit form, the process of adaptation to the illness and its consequences involves appraising the issue and then deliberately acting to change one's self or circumstances, for example, by learning laryngeal speech. But the process is rarely that simple. Patients do not in actuality deal with "issues"; they deal rather with a multitude of specific problems and specific emotions that are the manifestations of those issues. Patterns of adaptation emerge from a host of individual decisions, automatic reactions, and unconscious, or barely articulated perceptions and aims. To adopt the common approach of trying to reduce these patterns to a collection of coping "mechanisms" seems to us a distortion through simplification of a very complex process. We do not mean to deny the potential utility of the concept of "coping," but if that concept is to be more than a psychologist's abstraction, modes of "coping" must be viewed in their proper contexts. These contexts include: (1) the realities of the illness, (2) the person who is acting and reacting, and (3) the interpersonal situation.

Realities of the illness. Efforts at coping do not take place in a vacuum; they are always directed toward a particular problem or circumstance. Thus, a meaningful analysis of coping must begin with a careful delineation of the problem that needs to be mastered or solved. In the case of cancer, those problems are largely reality based and the realities of the illness are often decisive in determining which modes of response are possible. For example, while an asymptomatic patient with a nonessential internal organ removed may manage to "forget" the cancer experience most of the time, this strategy cannot easily be employed by a patient who is constantly reminded of the cancer by ongoing physical symptoms or a visible deformity. Likewise, medication that dulls the senses may be the most useful way to alleviate the pain of bone metastases but it can in no way ameliorate the problem of not being able to speak after a laryngectomy. Timing, in the sense of the stage of the disease, also plays an important role. To cite one example, actively seeking information may be essential when one is faced with the problem of making decisions about initial treatment but may be largely irrelevant in dealing with the problems of the terminal stage of cancer. Under any circumstances, however, the aim and character of the information-seeking activity would be quite different in the two cases, sufficiently different that it becomes pointless to categorize both as instances of the use of the coping mechanism of "information seeking."

Historically, the analysis of coping has its roots in, and has consequently been colored by, the psychoanalytic concept of defense mechanisms. This concept of psychological defense is concerned with modes of dealing with the internal conflicts characteristic of psychopathology. It is thus worth emphasizing some of the ways in which coping with reality-based issues such as cancer differs from coping with issues of intrapsychic origin. The process of comprehending and altering the latter entails the uncovering of wishes, thoughts, and feelings and the exploration of their influences on behavior. Cancer, in contrast, though located in one's body, is in a psychological sense external to the self. It cannot be understood (or affected) by introspection; rather, it is through medical diagnostic procedures and the technical knowledge of others that a patient obtains information about the nature, seriousness, and likely progression of the problems to be faced. Furthermore, since the physical changes produced by cancer are not a product of one's thoughts or feelings, they cannot be made to go away nor can they be controlled by internal mental operations such as repression or sublimation. This does not mean that patients must remain completely passive, but it does mean that they must act through others, namely, the appropriate medical personnel. We recognize that there are theories—for example, the Simontons' (1975)—which hold that cancer cells can be directly influenced by appropriate thoughts and images, but the available evidence is unconvincing. We believe that such theories have attained popular currency precisely because they provide some hope of direct personal control of the cancer.

The "real" nature of cancer-related issues has other important consequences. Injury to one's body and the resulting deformity and loss of function cannot be repaired by wishing, fantasizing, or reforming one's behavior. Like other real losses, they can only be mourned, accepted, and compensated to some degree by developing new skills or obtaining prostheses. Such losses sometimes impair a patient's ability to perform customary adult roles and may require the aid of others in caring for one's self. "Regression," as manifest not only in greater dependence on others but also in a preoccupation with bodily complaints, increased self-absorption, and demands for attention and reassurance, has often been noted as a concomitant of illness generally and of cancer more particularly. What has been less frequently emphasized is that these "regressive" changes partly reflect shifts in needs and capacities and may be neither optional nor maladaptive. Again the pressures of reality are primary determinants of the character of the patient's adaptive response.

The arguments presented here are by no means meant to imply that for each problem there is one and only one possible mode of coping. Rather, the point we wish to emphasize is that reality sets a limit on the problem-solving strategies that may be employed. It must be noted further that within a generic mode of coping, for example, information seeking, situational factors are critical to the specific character and aim of the coping activities. In sum, a meaningful analysis of the processes of coping with cancer requires a detailing of how particular problems are managed and of how a patient adapts to the realities of the disease; it cannot be reduced to a listing and explication of "mechanisms."

Patients' reactions. Efforts to cope with cancer must also be viewed in the context of each patient's personal background and experiences, position in life, and strivings, guilts, and fears. Sutherland (1967) has emphasized that a patient's reactions can be fully understood only if one investigates the individual meaning of the illness. That meaning can be profoundly affected by past experience with cancer in a close relative or friend. Likewise, unresolved conflicts concerning dependency, sexuality, and aggression, along with their attendant guilts, may be intensified or rekindled by the disease. Indeed, we have been impressed that extreme or atypical responses to cancer are often associated with a hidden personal meaning that stirs up intense inner conflict. Thus, the general issues raised by the realities of cancer may be shared by all patients, but the idiosyncratic interpretation of those realities remains a critical determinant of a patient's immediate reactions and long-term adaptations to the disease. Although situational factors set the limits, it is individual patients who define the problems that need solution.

Personality and previous experience also have an important bearing on the available repertory and the choice and effectiveness of coping strategies. Some people have developed many ways of handling difficult issues, others are limited to a few. It appears useful in dealing with cancer to have a number of options, to be able to approach problems in more than one way. It appears also that patients tend to have characteristic styles of handling stresses and generally turn first to the methods that have worked most successfully for them in the past. It must be noted, however, that habitual modes of handling stress have typically developed in the context of a normal range of problems. For most patients, cancer presents a set of adaptive demands that are outside their previous experience. Thus, the habitual modes may prove irrelevant or ineffective, and the patient may have to develop new strategies to deal with the particularities of cancer. Consequently, past modes of handling problems do not necessarily provide a good guide to subsequent ones, and initial efforts at coping with the consequences of the disease will often differ substantially from long-term adaptations.

People differ too in how well they use a particular adaptive strategy. Discussions of "coping mechanisms" often neglect the fact that any given mode of coping with issues is not uniform but differs from person to person in the maturity and effectiveness with which it is employed. Rather than view a given type of coping strategy as "good" or "bad" in some general sense (see, for example, Weisman and Worden, 1977, pp. 29-31), it is frequently more relevant to consider how selectively and appropriately the strategy is used. Thus, for example, it is essential to distinguish between fearfully denying the meaning of a breast lump and minimizing the significance of preterminal symptoms. Both cases involve the use of denying and minimizing techniques but they differ in the detail and appropriateness of their application and, of course, in their consequences. While the former may lead to fatal delay in instituting effective treatment, the latter may enable the patient to escape the distress of unavoidable realities and so continue as satisfactory a life as possible.

Interpersonal situation. An adequate understanding of modes of coping with cancer also requires an appreciation of the social context in which these efforts take place. For the cancer patient, other people are both part of the problem and a necessary ingredient in the solution. Typically, the development of cancer entails an altered social reality. Family, friends, and employers view the patient differently, and family, social, and occupational roles may undergo marked changes (Gordon, 1966; Kassebaum and Baumann, 1965; Parsons and Fox, 1952). In some cases, the person with cancer is devalued and stigmatized (see Goffman, 1963). Other people may withdraw out of fear of contagion or their need to avoid being confronted with the unpleasantness of serious illness and death. The problem may be further compounded by the cancer patient's own negative self-image and a tendency to assume that others will share this image—will find him or her to be ugly, demanding, or pitiable. Cancer symptoms and treatment may thus seriously disrupt one's ordinary human contacts and so require a whole series of special adaptations by the patient and by those with whom the patient interacts. (Strauss, 1975, has explored these issues in several types of chronic illness.)

It can also be the case that changes in the social context of the cancer patient may present opportunities as well as drawbacks. We have seen patients use the special attention, support, and release from customary obligations, which are concomitants of chronic disease, as an opportunity to reorganize chaotic personal lives or to develop more effective ways of handling long-standing personal issues. Unfortunately, this occurs rarely in our samples (and almost always in young women), but it is important to note that transitions can be for the better as well as for the worse.

The social milieu may facilitate or discourage the use of particular styles of coping in more specific ways too. All modes of dealing with issues require the cooperation or, at least, the tolerance of those people upon whom the patient depends. This is true even for the use of such intrapsychic mechanisms as "denial." Successful avoidance of unpalatable facts is possible only if family and friends protect the patient from unwanted confrontations with those facts. At the same time, they must, to a degree, worry for the patient and ensure that the denial does not interfere with necessary treatment. Weisman and Hackett (1967) have discussed other interpersonal aspects of denial as well and have shown that mutual agreement not to discuss certain aspects of reality can serve to maintain important relationships.

Research is itself a special social context in which the method of investigation partly determines the information that can be obtained. A patient will be able to acknowledge worries, guilts, and problems fully only to those people who can be trusted to accept the truth without criticism or evaluation. Sometimes this works to the advantage of the researcher in that certain issues, such as fear of death, feelings of mutilation, or sexual concerns, may be more readily discussed with a sympathetic interviewer who is not otherwise part of the patient's life than with a spouse whom the patient fears to upset or antagonize. However, we have also seen patients conceal a problem, such as alcoholism, from an interviewer, who only learned of it later through a family member to whom it was an open issue. In general, we have been impressed by how much more readily patients will reveal their difficulties to an interested and familiar interviewer than they will on the most clever and detailed questionnaire. This may account for some of the discrepancies between clinical follow-up studies that reveal a strong continuing impact of cancer (Maguire, 1976) and questionnaire follow-ups that tend to report minimal personal problems (Craig, Comstock, and Geiser, 1974; Izsak and Medalie, 1971; Izsak, Engel, and Medalie, 1973; Schoenfield, 1972; Schottenfeld and Robbins, 1970).

Since the social context influences the patient's behavior and what is revealed or concealed about internal states, the where, when, and how of observation have particular significance for the assessment of coping. Again and again, we have found that a patient's evident modes of coping change as the social context changes. A patient who is reported to be good-natured and passively cooperative by a physician may be irritable and demanding with technicians and nursing personnel. Within the family, a brave front and a systematic avoidance of distressing issues may be observed, but an intimate friend may disclose the presence of hopeless resignation. It may appear that a patient who has delayed treatment has "denied" the potential significance of a symptom when, in fact, an interview reveals that an anxious and obsessive concern with the symptom has paralyzed action. Consequently, the implicit assumption of much research and theorizing that modes of coping are stable attributes of persons can be quite misleading. While it is true that patients do have preferred and habitual strategies of handling problems, coping is, in fact, a dynamic process closely attuned to immediate situational factors. Assessments of coping must recognize that flux is as much a part of coping activities as of other adaptive behavior.

Basic Modes of Coping with Cancer

Although fairly long lists of coping mechanisms are available in the literature (see, for example, Weisman and Worden, 1977), we believe, on conceptual and empirical grounds, that the diverse coping activities of cancer patients can be organized into three basic categories: (1) techniques to minimize distress, (2) attempts to deal with the issues, and (3) turning to others. We make no claims for the general applicability of these categories; at this point, they are meant to pertain only to the behavior of cancer patients.

Techniques to minimize distress. These include efforts to avoid, to forget, to control, and to detach oneself from disturbing thoughts and feelings. The prototype of such efforts is the erection of a barrier against painful stimuli and the "numbing" that follows and reduces the intensity of a traumatic experience (Furst, 1967; Horowitz, 1976). In the cancer patient, such adaptations are seldom massive and global but rather involve a complex variety of minimizing techniques, applied in different ways over time and usually mixed with periods of more active confrontation with the issues. The use of some variety of avoidance or denial is probably universal, and it is generally a useful and appropriate method of managing anxiety. It is well to keep in mind that the progress of the cancer itself cannot be directly affected by one's own actions or thoughts, and that control of the physical aspects of the disease is essentially in the hands of others. (This is not true of all chronic diseases; with serious heart problems, for example, the patient can take a direct role in treatment through control of diet, physical activity, and emotional states.) Consequently, an active, continuing awareness of the realities of one's situation has little utility. Indeed, an inability to rid one's self of thoughts of cancer and death after the initial phases of the disease is typically associated with a manifestly high level of chronic distress in our samples. Techniques of avoidance, then, are very much the norm. Nevertheless, the patients we interviewed were, with very few exceptions, quite careful to maintain appropriate medical follow-up and they remained alert to possible symptoms of recurrence. Thus, techniques to minimize distress rarely seem to endanger survival; rather, they represent an intentional, selective inattention to thoughts upon which it is pointless to dwell. Patients are realists—they are well aware that they have had cancer and that it can recur but they are also well aware that their psychological health depends upon being able to ignore those facts as much as circumstances will permit. Unfortunately, there are occasional exceptions where dread and pessimism may become so great that symptoms are denied and needed treatment avoided.

A more common drawback of avoidant techniques is that their use often leads to constriction of the patient's life. The need to avoid people and situations that arouse disturbing reminders of cancer may result in withdrawal from social and work situations and the giving up of potentially pleasurable activities. Our data indicate, for example, that following cancer, intimate sexual relationships usually suffer, even in well-integrated, emotionally stable people. Sexual activity seems to provide especially poignant reminders of feelings of damage, defect, and loss of attractiveness. (On occasion, we have also seen the opposite response—an increase in casual sexual contacts to gain reassurance of attractiveness.) The need to avoid talking about cancer may also lead to a marked constriction in communication with family and friends, with no one able to discuss important cancer-related issues freely.

Despite these drawbacks, the ability to minimize certain facts or to put them out of mind remains necessary for optimal functioning. Although we have emphasized the intensely practical and realistic nature of minimizing techniques, there are also times when a frank distortion of reality is useful and adaptive. This is particularly true in the terminal stage of cancer. As Weisman (1972) has described, dying patients often show a complex blend of knowing, partial knowing, and not recognizing truths, which permits a measure of equanimity in very grim circumstances.

> A retired married man in his sixties was dying of metastatic lung cancer. He was aware of his diagnosis and prospects and had gotten his affairs in order. Nevertheless, he maintained the belief that his current weakness and pain were due to radiation treatments and the stress of his efforts at rehabilitation. He avoided thinking about cancer and did not regard himself as having it. During most of his terminal illness, he persuaded himself that he was gradually getting stronger and expected to be able to resume limited work, at least for a while. He persisted in these convictions until the last few days of his life and was able

to remain impressively composed and remarkably self-sufficient throughout this period.

Active attempts to deal with the issues. These include seeking information about the illness, taking an active role in treatment decisions, attempting to compensate for or to replace lost body parts and functions, and volunteering to help others. This is a more diverse and less closely interrelated group of methods than the avoidant techniques, but they have in common an effort to confront and master cancer-related problems by active and direct means.

Insofar as a troublesome issue can actually be resolved through the patient's own efforts, it is certainly advantageous to do so. The very process of confronting problems and moving toward their solution helps to reinforce the sense of control and personal direction which cancer so typically impairs. Patients who choose this tack often report that they have learned and grown from their experiences with cancer and that this satisfaction helps to balance their losses from the illness. We have also seen a number of patients regain self-esteem and a sense of usefulness by turning from the passive role of patient to an active one of caring for and helping others.

> A young single woman with recurrent Hodgkin's disease was depressed over her apparent lack of medical progress and annoyed with her physician for his seeming indifference and his reluctance to answer her questions about an important decision regarding chemotherapy. Nevertheless, she remained passive, hesitated to assume more responsibility in making the decision, and felt too timid to confront her physician with her questions. When she discussed these problems in a patient group, she was encouraged to take a more active role, and one of the more self-confident women in the group volunteered to accompany her on her next visit to the doctor. With this support, she was able to insist on answers, make her decision, and gain some sense of control over her treatment.

Actively confronting one's problems requires a degree of optimism that something useful can be done and enough energy and confidence in one's personal resources to make the attempt. Those patients who feel defeated and depleted seldom try. As with minimizing techniques, the success of active attempts to deal with cancer-related issues often depends on the support and cooperation of family, friends, or physicians. We have found that discussion groups in which patients help each other are especially useful in providing this type of support. But it bears repeating that both the choice and effectiveness of coping activities are critically affected by the patient's social context.

Turning to others. This includes sharing concerns with others, seeking support and reassurance from family and friends, making demands on others, and using the illness to manipulate and coerce others. There is obviously a considerable range of styles and techniques here, but in our data there are strong correlations among these various modes of using other people to alleviate distress.

Because the patient's ability to meet personal needs and to influence the course of the illness are limited, the help of others is an unavoidable necessity which all but a few patients recognize and accept. Efforts to secure help may take the form of an appropriate and realistic dependence upon medical caretakers, family, and friends, but they may sometimes evolve into an exaggerated and childish dependence in which the illness is used to extort excessive care. There are also some patients who turn for rescue to "higher powers," in the form of an overly idealized physician, religious faith, or belief in a miracle cure. While a few of our patients made their physicians into gods and an occasional patient could not develop a trusting relationship with any doctor, most patients looked to their physicians for facts, understanding, and, above all, skillful treatment of their cancer. With an occasional exception, however, they did not discuss much of their personal life with their physician. They derived great support from knowing that the physician was interested, competent, and available, but rarely expected or sought anything more than a generalized sort of concern. Clearly, they distinguished between the roles of physician and of family, friends, or psychotherapist.

Both our clinical observations and more formal data analyses support the view that cancer patients handle their illness more easily if they are securely embedded in a stable social matrix. Patients tended to turn to family or friends, not to outside specialists, for ventilation of their feelings and for advice. In our samples, it was quite rare for a patient to seek professional psychological counseling, for example. Likewise, though religion was important to some patients, they seldom talked to clergy about their personal difficulties. However, those patients for whom the church represented a major social as well as religious institution were notably effective in dealing with the effects of cancer. These findings are similar to Krant's (1976) and point to the importance of various kinds of informal support systems (Caplan and Killilea, 1976). But it must be noted too that some patients who have always lived relatively isolated but stable lives find it neither comfortable nor useful to seek out close supportive relationships with others. Since their habitual autonomy continues to serve them well even in the distressing circumstances of cancer, they frequently view efforts of others to help them as intrusive. These patients, as do most other patients, often rely heavily on a type of support that is easily overlooked, namely, the important stabilizing influence of the routines of work and daily living. Indeed, one cannot exaggerate the sustaining force of those routines, accustomed obligations, and environmental regularities that can, in other circumstances, seem so tedious. The social matrix, then, must be conceptualized as including not only support systems but also the complex of social roles in which patients function.

Person Factors

We have, so far, focused primarily on how the nature of cancer determines the problems patients face and the means available to modulate or resolve those problems. At various points, however, we have also noted how individual differences affect both the significance and the mode of handling the disease and its consequences. The potential range of such factors is virtually limitless, encompassing aspects of personal history, accustomed modes of coping, sex, age, enduring attributes and dispositions, and so forth. Consequently, far more will be excluded from our discussion of person factors than can be included, but the three factors we have selected—age, sex, and personal history—seem to us representative and relatively neglected in the previous literature.

Age and stage of life. The importance of viewing psychosocial processes in the context of the human life cycle has become generally accepted (Erikson, 1950; Lidz, 1968) but, historically, the emphasis has been placed on unraveling the complexities of childhood development. It is only in recent years that adequate attention has been paid to adult development and to aging (see, for example, the reviews of Neugarten, 1968a, and Schaie and Gribbin, 1975). In similar fashion, while the developmental stage in which cancer occurs has been recognized as a significant factor in children and adolescents (Binger and others, 1969; Easson, 1968; Moore, Holton and Marten, 1969; Schowalter, 1970), a life-stage perspective has seldom been used to understand how adults deal with cancer or other life-threatening illnesses. A notable exception is the study by Rosen and Bibring (1966) which demonstrated that the manner in which men react to myocardial infarction is markedly different for different age groups. In our own research too, we have found that developmental life-stage concepts have great value, not only in helping to comprehend how adults experience cancer but also in providing an essential dimension in which to view change. In taking a long term perspective on the adaptation to cancer, some of the most important and interesting issues involve the ways cancer may hinder, distort, or even enhance aspects of the individual's development.

Adult development is not as closely tied to biological maturation as is childhood development, and so adult life stages cannot be neatly demarcated. There is wide agreement, however, that adult life may be usefully grouped into stages that differ with respect to biological functioning, social norms and expectations, time perspective, economic status, position in the family life cycle, and so forth (Neugarten, 1968b). These differences result in particular concerns and conflicts becoming uppermost at each stage of life (Erikson, 1959), concerns and conflicts that are sometimes alike and sometimes quite different for men and women (Lowenthal, Thurnher, and Chiriboga, 1975). Lowenthal and her colleagues, in their study of normative transitions that mark the entrance and exit of each life stage, found that special events, such as serious illness or impairments, may have a profound bearing on growth or regression and may thus alter normative expectations. Many of the subjects reported considerable, untimely, change in themselves, their values, and their behavioral patterns accompanying or following such events. Certainly, our data provide ample support for this generalization.

We have found it most feasible to arrange patients into the three broad stages of youth, mid-life, and old age. This is admittedly somewhat arbitrary, but this grouping by age is a first approximation to a meaningful classification, especially if one also considers other developmental landmarks, such as marriage, the presence of children at home, or retirement. The life-stage concept will be used in two ways: to provide an independent variable that partly determines the mode of experiencing cancer and the personal and social resources available for coping with it, and as a framework to help evaluate long-term outcome.

Young adults (18-35): In keeping with the findings of many observers, the young adults in our study were primarily concerned with separation from their parents and with establishing stable, intimate relationships, marriages, families, and careers. They were, that is, somewhere in the process of moving from one social context to another. The experience of cancer at this stage tended to impede the development of self-sufficiency and, for some young people, it resulted in delay and disruption of their efforts to establish independent adult roles. Their uncertain future made it difficult to embark on a commitment in any direction; the sacrifice of present satisfactions to future benefits so characteristic of this stage was rendered problematic by their cancer. The sense of soberness and altered priorities that came with facing possible death left some of the younger people feeling out of touch with their more carefree "childish" contemporaries. Resolution of "intimacy versus isolation," the conflict Erikson (1950) found most characteristic of this age group, was greatly complicated by the patient's increased needs for comfort and support. Particular pressure was placed on intimate relationships and on marriages in their beginning years. Some couples were able to grow closer in the process of dealing with these pressures, but, in other relationships, the stress of illness led to excessive clinging or to avoidance of communication and intimacy. The effect on marriages that were already in difficulty was particularly pronounced, though this is true at all stages.

Mid-life adults (36-55): In middle life (Butler, 1975a; Neugarten, 1968c), there is a gradual change in time perspective. The passage of time is clocked by career and family milestones, and life comes to be viewed in terms of time left to live. For some, this period may be experienced as the prime of life, with a maximum sense of mastery and control; but it can also be a time of considerable self-doubt. A trend toward introspection usually begins, which includes taking stock of one's accomplishments, failures, and unfinished business. Adult roles and position in life have become firmly established, for better or worse. Erikson (1950) emphasizes the need in this stage to contribute to and care for others, to be "generative" rather than "stagnant."

In the adults of this age whom we studied, the occurrence of cancer threatened disruption of the roles that they had established through so much effort and raised doubts about the completion of the important tasks they had yet to carry out. They experienced a foreshortening of the future and increased concern about their remaining time. Working men and women worried about being able to maintain their occupations, financial security, and self-sufficiency. Parents feared they would not be able to care for their children and help them grow to maturity. Husbands and wives were afraid they would no longer be adequate partners and might become unable to meet their spouse's economic, emotional, and sexual needs. Inevitably, concerns about the welfare of one's family have a special poignancy at this stage.

In our study, this age group showed the greatest variation in response; it included some patients who were best able to take their illness in stride and some who were closest to open panic. The men seemed to have an especially difficult time dealing with their illness and appeared most vulnerable to adverse emotional reactions. These impressions are in keeping with the differential age responses that Rosen and Bibring (1966) observed among men with myocardial infarctions and with the sex differences that we observed on the Adjective Check Lists. It is, perhaps, in this stage of mid-life that the sustaining effects of a stable, secure social network and of well-established routines and responsibilities are most pronounced.

Older adults (56-75): There is now a substantial and growing literature on the problems of aging (see, for example, Busse and Pfeiffer, 1969; Butler, 1975b). Many sources document the accumulation of losses faced by the older person—losses of health, vigor, friends, jobs, and social and economic status. For many an older person, the world becomes both narrower and increasingly difficult to deal with, and the tendency to withdraw into oneself, to disengage from external investments and struggles, is common. Sometimes this disengagement is a welcome choice, a simplification of life and a relief from burdens; in other situations, it may be imposed by social restrictions and personal limitations (Cumming and Henry, 1961; Havinghurst, Neugarten, and Tobin, 1968). At the same time, diminished capacities may force the older person to become more dependent on others. There also appears to be a need for the aging person to review and come to terms with the past. If pride can be taken in accomplishments, sins and limitations forgiven, and meaning found in personal experience, the future can be approached with integrity and dignity rather than despair (Butler, 1963; Erikson, 1976).

In the older adults we have observed, cancer commonly leads to an acceleration of these aging processes; it imposes new losses which result in more rapid disengagement from work, social, and leisure activities and in greater dependence on others. We have already noted, for example, that as a result of their cancer, adults in their late fifties and early sixties frequently decide to retire earlier than they had planned, even when their medical condition would permit them to continue working. Many factors appear to be involved, such as having less energy, feeling that future ambition is pointless, feeling embarrassed at facing others because of deformity, or wanting to enjoy what life remains as fully as possible. But whatever the factors involved, early retirement often has the effect of hastening the appearance of that sense of uselessness that is common in old age. In many regards, then, cancer precipitates or mimics those features of aging that have been detailed in normative studies.

Another impression gained from our data is that many of the older, already retired adults seem to face cancer with less anger than younger people. Patients at each life stage express specific kinds of anger when their hopes and wishes are thwarted: The young are angry because they may not ever have a chance to develop their lives; the mid-life adults are angry because their lives may be cut short before they can finish their tasks; the pre-retirement and retirement age group are angry because they may not be able to enjoy the leisure earned by a lifetime of work. But many of the older people, particularly those who have reviewed their past and feel they have lived their lives well, were able to deal with their illness with a greater degree of equanimity than the younger patients. They seem, by virtue of their age, to have faced their mortality and so the issue of dying per se has less intensity than it does for young and middle-aged adults. This, combined with generational differences, may well explain our finding that active modes of coping, as well as more overt and acute distress, are far more characteristic of younger than of older patients.

The crux of much of this discussion is captured in a comparison of two patients who had a testicular cancer, in both cases caught early. Both had a very favorable prognosis and had been treated without much damage to body function save that they had been made sterile by their treatment. In terms of the illness itself, the cases are remarkably similar, but their reactions differed greatly. The first, a young man in his late twenties, had begun to live with an older woman two years before his cancer and had shortly thereafter received a position in a moderately high-level technical occupation. Both the relationship and the position were secure and held much promise for the future, but were, of course, of fairly recent origin. The second, a man of forty-eight, was a very accomplished and well-regarded professional, married for about twenty-five years and with grown children. It is surely not surprising that the younger man was far more deeply distressed by his cancer than the older. His sterility was particularly painful for it meant that he could never have children of his own and, perhaps unrealistically, raised doubts about a future marriage and his sexual competence. The cancer, moreover, seemed especially disruptive and unjust to someone who had, later than most and only recently, assumed an adult role and established his independence. The older man, in contrast, was relatively little affected by his disease. Though he too had to face the issue of a potentially shortened life span, he had long since established a stable and satisfying adult existence and was securely embedded in a supportive social network. There was, of course, a degree of anxiety, but he was able to maintain the continuity of his life effectively without the uncertainties and inner turmoil that plagued the younger man. In sum, though the consequences and prognosis of the disease were virtually identical in the two cases, the psychological meaning of cancer, and thus the reaction to it, differed greatly for the two men and differed, moreover, in a way directly related to their respective stages in life.

While we have emphasized how cancer may interfere with optimal adult development, it would be misleading to leave the impression that cancer affects adult development only in negative ways. Unfortunately, the negative effects typically outweigh the positive, but we have also observed several instances in which patients whose personal affairs were in disarray used their experience with cancer to reorganize their lives by taking advantage of the new opportunities and sources of help that had become available. Less dramatic, but more frequent, is the quiet reassessment of values and goals that many patients go through, a reassessment that may lead to a keener appreciation of what is important in life and to more satisfying choices regarding the style and direction of their lives. The impact of illness leads some patients to become more constructively self-centered and more assertive in pursuing their personal goals. And for those couples and families who are able to master the stresses of cancer, the experience of surmounting crises together and perhaps communicating in ways in which they never have before may lead to a satisfying growth and deepening of relationships. We can hardly recommend cancer as a route to maturity, but, like other profound experiences, it can have the effect of clarifying the distinction between the trivial and the essential.

Sex. At various points in this chapter, we have noted differences between the sexes in their response to cancer. The Adjective Check List data for three-year survivors showed that males but not females consistently viewed themselves as having declined in effectiveness, vigor, and ambition, with a consequent loss in positive self-regard. Likewise, in both our retrospective and our prospective samples, we found clear evidence that cancer had a more negative effect on males than females irrespective of age. The men were more irritable, fearful and ill at ease than the women and were more likely to engage in self-destructive activities, for example, smoking, excessive use of alcohol, and neglecting the necessary medical follow-ups. They tended more to blame others for their distress, to be less generous, kindly, and open to others and, in general, to withdraw some from social contacts. Moreover, they kept their feelings and problems private; it was the women who turned to family and friends, as well as to professional sources, for support and reassurance. Finally, as we noted before, the few patients who used their experience with cancer in a clearly productive way were women, particularly younger women. Interestingly, these findings came as no surprise to the physicians with whom we discussed them.

It is not clear whether the sex differences just described would be found for other chronic diseases as well; it is evident, though, that the personal meaning of cancer is very much a function of sex. What factors account for the specific differences we observed is a matter for speculation at this point, but if we assume that men, more than women, define themselves and their worth in terms of striving and activity in the external world, then the decreases in vigor, physical prowess, and the capacity for sustained effort, all of which are common effects of cancer, would constitute a particular threat to men—they undermine the basic conditions on which men found their careers and their sense of masculinity. To be sure, many of the women in our samples were also employed, but it is not yet the case that work and activities outside the family are generally as central and personally salient to women as to men. We believe, further, that normally men have a bland and unthinking confidence in the smooth functioning of their bodies, whereas women, by virtue of biology, are used to bodily change and have learned better how to deal with it. Thus, men are perhaps both less well in touch with their bodies and more likely to be traumatized by breaches of its integrity. Finally, to the extent that self-reliance is seen as a masculine virtue, one important mode of handling the issues raised by cancer—turning to others—becomes problematic for many men in a way that it is not for women. We must reiterate that all of these suggestions are speculative. Nevertheless, the findings themselves are strong and coherent; they demand further pursuit.

Personal history. The influence of personal history on the psychological impact of cancer and the response to the disease is illustrated by the following case:

> A young single man with serious conflicts around sexuality developed rectal cancer a few years after his father died of this disease. Fearing the same fate, he submitted to extensive surgery that left him impotent and with a colostomy. Two weeks postoperatively he developed a transient paranoid psychosis in which his surgeon became his persecutor and he feared that he was becoming like certain of his attendants whom he believed were homosexual. Though he recovered fairly quickly from these delusions, he remained convinced that he would follow his father's fatal course. Although six months after surgery he seemed substantially better psychologically and physically, at one year he was deeply depressed, embittered, socially withdrawn, and full of foreboding about the future.

This case is unusual in its combination of factors. The site of the disease and the effects of treatment could not but activate and intensify preexisting conflicts. Further, the coincidence of the similarity of the patient's condition to that of his father, a father who was quite central to those conflicts, created a situation that even a psychologically sound person would have been hard pressed to handle successfully. Despite its unusual features, however, this case differs in degree, not in kind, from other cases, for cancer must always be seen as an event that is part of an ongoing life.

For each patient there are idiosyncratic personal factors that influence the meaning of and the adaptation to cancer; if we are to understand them, intensive individual case studies are essential. Nevertheless, it is also possible to isolate nomothetic variables that pertain to the patient's past history. Given limitations of space, two illustrations must suffice. The first variable is past psychiatric history. We have found that irrespective of the medical realities, such as prognosis or physical damage, it is those patients who have had definable psychological difficulties before their illness who are distressed and disorganized following cancer. (We have used relatively objective indicators of psychological difficulty, such as psychiatric hospitalization, psychotherapy, prolonged periods of depression or social withdrawal, drug abuse, and so forth, rather than more inferential measures.) In fact, our best single predictor of psychosocial status at all points in the disease process is the simple sum of a set of such indicators. There are, of course, exceptions. Usually, they are cases in which severe physical damage has been sustained, but, nevertheless, the absence of antedating psychological problems is a very favorable sign. This is not a surprising finding—past behavior remains the best predictor of subsequent behavior—but that makes it no less important.

The second illustrative variable from the realm of personal history is the absence or presence of experience with cancer in others. A patient's initial distress is much intensified if a close family member or friend has had cancer, particularly cancer that resulted in death. Our data indicate, however, that this relationship dissipates with time; neither in the six- to twelve-month follow-up nor in the three- and six-year retrospective samples is it a variable of discernible significance. Apparently, when uncertainty about the future is maximal, that is, at the time of diagnosis and primary treatment, the immediate and concrete example of the similar misfortune of others increases the reality of the patient's fears. But once the initial phase of the disease has been passed and long-term risks and the extent of enduring damage can be assessed, the particularities of one's own condition assume a predominant role. This finding represents one of our clearest examples of how the factors that influence the reaction to cancer change as the phase of the disease changes.

To summarize, though our discussion of person factors has necessarily been highly selective, we have focused on a subset of variables that seem to us to possess great conceptual and empirical significance for an understanding of both the immediate and long-term psychosocial effects of cancer. We believe these variables also illustrate a critical point of this chapter: Although situational factors must be the starting point of an analysis of the effects of cancer and serve to set the limits of potential response, patients define their problems in terms of who they are, what they have experienced, and what they hope for the future—in short, in individual and personal terms.

Implications for Planning and Operation of Health Systems

From a psychological viewpoint, the general goal of the health care systems that impinge on the patient should be to minimize the discontinuity between a patient's life before and after cancer and to support those transitions that maximize a patient's sense of self-determination, usefulness, satisfaction, and self-esteem. It should be apparent that the attainment of these goals requires attention to the particularities of each patient's illness, the patient's personal characteristics, and the social supports available to the patient in the everyday environment. It is doubtful that any program of intervention that fails to make such distinctions can be successful. In what follows, we will try to make these abstractions more concrete by discussing several specific implications of our approach for the planning of psychosocial services within the health system.

Identification of Times of Maximum Vulnerability in the Typical Course

Although we have stressed the fact that the response to cancer evolves over an extended period of time, it is, nevertheless, possible to identify particular points in the course of the disease when stress is likely to be most intense and the patient, consequently, most in need of special attention. These are at the time of initial diagnosis, during primary treatment, at the time recurrence or metastatic disease is discovered, and during the terminal phase. The issues to be faced at each of these points are, of course, quite different and, consequently, the character and goals of activities designed to be helpful should be attuned to the specific adaptive tasks that need to be accomplished. Thus, for example, at the time of initial diagnosis, patients should be helped to understand the character of their illness as fully as possible, both to reduce uncertainty (imaginings are often worse than actualities) and to facilitate realistic planning for the future. During the terminal phase, in contrast, the need for information will usually be secondary to the need for emotional support of patient and family.

It should be noted that at each of these specified points in the course of the disease, the patient is in direct contact with the medical system. There is, however, an additional time of vulnerability when direct contact is not the case or only infrequently the case, namely, when active treatment has ended and the patient must attempt to resume the interrupted course of life. It is during this extended period that patients come fully to grasp what has happened to them and that the course of long-term adaptation begins to take its shape. Because the events of this period, if "events" is an accurate word, are private, undramatic, and poorly marked in time, and contact with medical personnel is minimal, this is the phase in the history of the disease when patients' needs are most likely to be neglected. Consequently, provision of services for those patients who need help in planning for the future during this critical period constitutes, in our view, a particularly important challenge to the health care system.

Identification of People Who Need Special Help

If it is possible to delineate the natural history of the psychosocial response to cancer, two important consequences would follow: First, reliable predictions of future adjustments could be made, particularly from early behavior, and second, atypical responses could be identified with greater certainty than is possible now. For example, during the initial phase of cancer, patients typically experience considerable distress, but how much distress is normal and for how long should acute distress be expected to last? Is it the case that an extreme reaction at either end of the continuum—intense prolonged turmoil or an apparent absence of turmoil—foretells subsequent psychological difficulties? At this point, we simply do not have good answers to such questions, nor can we specify with any precision when in the course of the response to cancer it is reasonable to assess the effectiveness of a patient's long-term adaptation. Clearly, normative longitudinal studies are needed if we are to identify those patients who require special help before problems develop.

Our data indicate that it is also possible to identify vulnerable patients from biographical factors and from characteristics of the illness itself. It is not surprising, in regard to the latter, that serious psychological distress is reliably associated with those forms of cancer and medical treatment that lead to substantial interference with normal physical functioning or to chronic, intense discomfort. We do not think this is a matter of site per se but rather of the kind and extent of damage that is correlated with site. In regard to biographical factors, two stand out as particularly important predictors: previous psychiatric history and the degree of social isolation. Both of these factors can be assessed at the outset of illness and so, with physical damage, can form a simple and, we believe, reliable prognostic index of future psychological difficulties.

Although the identification of patients who need special help seems feasible and of manifest importance, it is not the case that such patients will necessarily seek help or respond to efforts to provide it. This is a particular problem among male patients, who, in our samples, appear loath to admit to personal difficulties and are even more loath to use those services that are available. Since the negative effects of cancer seem more pronounced in males than in females, and men are also reluctant to make use of naturally occurring support systems, the problem is all the more serious. Similarly, older patients are less likely than others to seek outside help, though their reluctance to do so seems more a result of passivity and resignation than avoidance and suppression of distressing thoughts. It may be significant, however, that members of both these groups were quite willing to participate in intensive personal interviews and were no less open than other patients in communicating their private feelings and problems. Indeed, like other patients, they frequently reported that the interviews were of value to them and they sometimes sought the interviewer's advice or support. Perhaps the research format was a critical factor in their response, for the contact was initiated by others and was not a consequence of an identified problem. If so, this may provide a clue to the kinds of procedures that can serve the needs of otherwise inaccessible patients.

Planning Interventions to Match the Problems and the Person

Most cancer patients do not require special help in dealing with the consequences of their illness; their personal resources and the support available in their everyday social milieu are strong enough to sustain an effective adaptation to cancer. To be sure, such patients also require accurate information about their condition, sympathetic treatment by medical personnel, and, in many cases, experienced advice about practical problems, for example, how to obtain a prosthesis (often, no small problem) or secure maximum insurance benefits. Though distressing exceptions can be noted, the health care system is generally prepared to provide services and support of these kinds. It is less well prepared, however, to provide for the needs of those patients who by virtue of personality or situation are unable to handle the stresses of cancer or can do so only by greatly constricting their lives. Physicians, who do have continuous, though periodic, contact with patients, rarely have the training, experience, or time to deal with psychological problems, and patients (realistically) do not expect them to be counselors or psychotherapists. Other hospital-based personnel (nurses, technicians, and medical social workers) see patients primarily during acute phases of the disease. Certainly, training programs designed to increase the understanding of the psychosocial effects of cancer and to facilitate the early identification of atypical courses and high-risk individuals would be helpful. Likewise, the availability of regular psychiatric or psychological consultation is desirable, though we are convinced that effective consultation of this kind requires extensive prior experience with cancer patients. Finally, the establishment of oncology wards and hostels where the personnel are specifically prepared to deal with the problems of cancer has much to recommend it. Such facilities, however, would, by no means, be appropriate for all patients: Many do not wish to be identified as "cancer patients," or are distressed by contact with other cancer patients, or feel a need to maintain maximum self-sufficiency and privacy, or want to spend their last days in their accustomed environment. Selectivity is essential. But having said all this, and little of it is original, we are left with a problem: How can necessary assistance be provided to those patients whose long-term adaptation to cancer is problematic, particularly at times when they are not in direct contact with the medical system?

We do not have an adequate answer to this question, but there are three alternatives that can be suggested. The first is referral to a psychotherapist. Typically, the problems raised by cancer are problems of adaptation rather than psychopathology. As noted before, however, in some cases, cancer seriously intensifies or reactivates preexisting internal conflicts. In such circumstances, psychotherapy is an appropriate alternative, but we think it should be used quite selectively and only after careful diagnosis. The second alternative derives from our observation that most patients value the opportunity to discuss their reactions to cancer and their personal problems with a disinterested, but concerned, outsider, someone who is neither a family member nor their physician. Our interviews were conducted in the context of a research project, but it might be possible to institute a program of follow-up interviews with patients that parallels their medical follow-ups. To be effective, this should be done routinely, as a standard part of follow-up procedures, rather than as a consequence of a special referral or of the identification of unusual difficulties. Despite the practical problems that would be entailed, the potential benefits of such a program are substantial enough to justify the institution of regular psychosocial follow-ups an an experimental basis. More feasible, perhaps, is the third alternative, the establishment of discussion groups in which patients can share their feelings, experience, and knowledge and provide support for each other. The advantages of groups of this kind seem obvious and, indeed, many are in operation now. How effective they are in fact is not yet known, for systematic appraisals of their utility and the factors that influence their utility are not available. Our own experience with discussion groups suggests that they are most useful for patients who lack a strong social support system and for younger patients. The latter is particularly interesting because a young person's group was instituted at the urging of the patients themselves, who saw their needs as being distinctively different from those of other patients. But these are only suggestions; evaluation research is needed to provide a sound basis for the use of this most flexible and economically viable of approaches to providing psychological assistance to cancer patients.

Summary

This chapter is a deliberate amalgam of empirical findings, case studies, conceptual analysis, and speculation designed to argue the value of a personological and developmental approach to the study of the psychosocial effects of cancer. From this perspective, cancer is construed as an event, or rather a series of events, in an individual life history whose course is, with few exceptions, substantially altered by the realities of the disease. To understand and predict these alterations, it is necessary first to delineate the natural history of the psychosocial response to cancer—to define the sequence of issues raised by the disease and the common modes of handling them. Second, it is necessary to identify the situational factors (those associated with the particularities of the disease are most important), social contexts, and individual differences that affect the course of the long-term adaptation to cancer. Third, it is necessary to get some sense of what the illness and its consequences mean to individual patients. Cancer rarely fails to affect self-conceptions as well as the conceptions of the patient by others; it also alters, to a greater or lesser degree, how a patient regards the future. In this sense, cancer represents more than a crisis to be mastered—it marks a transition point in a particular person's life. It is surely most difficult to do systematic research in this third area, for each patient has a unique developmental history, configuration of personal attributes, and set of contemporary circumstances. But these difficulties cannot alter the theoretical and practical importance of comprehending uniqueness as well as commonalities. We believe that the intensive analysis of a series of individual cases provides the best means to accomplish both objectives and thus to achieve the goal of understanding the effects of cancer on all persons, some persons, and each person.

11

Developmental Stages in Children's Conceptions of Illness

Roger Bibace

Mary E. Walsh

During a routine visit to a doctor's office, a four-year-old child explained that he had gotten "sick" (the doctor had diagnosed the illness as the flu) as a consequence of "the wind." He could offer no further explanation of how the wind caused his sickness. His nine-year-old sister laughed at his account, telling him he had really "gotten sick" because he took several licks from his friend's popsicle and swallowed the germs.

In our role as clinical psychologists in a family medicine residency training program, we have repeatedly observed how children's beliefs and assumptions about health, illness, and medical procedures differ dramatically and in unexpected ways from those of adults. Such instances have made us acutely aware that health professionals—nurses, physicians, psychologists—do not possess a general theoretical framework that would allow them to under-

Note: We wish to thank Cathleen Crider for her critical reading of the manuscript and Laureen Morrow for data collection and analysis.

stand immature conceptions of health and illness. Consequently, many professionals have no basis for understanding how children at different stages of cognitive development will construe health and illness.

That professionals sometimes operate in the dark in this area was highlighted for us when we explored the basis of young children's fears of such an innocuous instrument as the stethoscope. We have observed sensitive physicians, for instance, who try to respond to a child's fear of the stethoscope by warming the diaphragm prior to use, assuming that the cold metal against the child's skin causes some of the negative response. In fact, we found that four- and five-year-old children, when asked about the stethoscope, made no mention of the "coldness" but told us of their belief that the purpose of the stethoscope was to discover "if I have a heart," a heart, which they add, "is what makes me live." A negative finding by the physician, then, as the child sees it, could result in the child's being dead. Hence, it is not surprising that warming the diaphragm does little to console a child whose fears are based on such beliefs. An experienced, warm, and humorous pediatrician confirmed that young children often express such fears. When we asked this physician how he reacted to a child's concern that he might not have a heart, he stated, "I just laugh and tell them, 'Of course you have a heart!' " Such responses by health professionals do not take into account the child's qualitatively different way of understanding bodily functions. Hence, such responses are unlikely to serve the professional's goal of reassuring the child. These and similar experiences led us to study how children conceive of health, illness, and their causes.

Developmental Conceptions of Illness

Developmental psychologists such as Piaget (1929) and Werner (1948) have studied the causal thinking or conceptions of the child with respect to diverse phenomena. They have shown how causal thinking emerges in a developmental sequence. Both Piaget (1929) and Laurendeau and Pinard (1962), in a large-scale replication study, have elaborated stages of the development of causal thinking with respect to a number of different phenomena (life, dreams, and so on). Other researchers have investigated the causal thinking of children in diverse content areas, such as sex and birth (Bernstein and Cowan, 1975; Kreitler and Kreitler, 1966; Nagy, 1953a), psychological causality (Whiteman, 1967), internal body functioning (Gellert, 1962; Nagy, 1953b), death (Nagy, 1959), and medical procedures (Steward and Regalbuto, 1975). A number of studies have examined children's conceptions of health and/or illness (Brodie, 1974; Campbell, 1975; Mechanic, 1964; Neuhauser and others, 1978; Palmer and Lewis, 1975).

In general, these other researchers have used three methods to examine concepts held by children of different ages. Some have described the different types of explanations given by children and have tabulated the frequency of each type within each age level (Brodie, 1974; Campbell, 1975; Mechanic, 1964). Campbell (1975, p. 96), for example, in enumerating different types of themes present in children's definitions of illness, states that "older children gave relatively more attention to specific diseases or diagnoses" while "younger children were more apt to mention vague, nonlocalized feelings." These studies do not make any attempt to explain a developmental relationship between the definitions provided by younger children and those provided by older children.

Other authors, in post hoc discussions of age differences, allude to developmental theory as one possible way in which the age difference data might be understood (Gellert, 1962; Nagy, 1953a, 1953b, 1959; Palmer and Lewis, 1975). Palmer and Lewis (1975), for instance, found that young children attributed illness to such causes as "going out without a jacket and eating too much candy," whereas older children mentioned "contact with ill people and germs" as causes of illness. They suggest that such answers "exhibit the syncretic thinking identified by Piaget" (p. 2). Although these authors point out a general congruence between themes that appear in children's conceptions of disease and Piaget's stages of cognitive development, they present no comprehensive account of the child's explanations of illness at different levels of cognitive development.

A third group of authors utilizes developmental theory to make predictions about the differences in conceptions of illness to be found among different age groups (Neuhauser and others, 1978; Steward and Regalbuto, 1975; Whiteman, 1967). For example, Neuhauser and others (1978, p. 337) hypothesize that "the concrete operational child will use more internal cues for determining when they are hurt and when they are well again than will the preoperational child." Studies based on this sort of prediction provide us with data about those aspects of the concept that are of interest to the researcher. They do not systematically organize the range of constructions generated by the child with regard to a particular phenomenon. Even when attempts are made to articulate the range of constructions for a given phenomenon, as in Bernstein and Cowan's (1975) study of the concepts of sex and birth, the stages are described primarily in terms of the general stages of cognitive development. These authors do not attempt to define a novel set of categories that reflect both the general stages of cognitive development and the particular concepts children use to explain a specific phenomenon.

In brief, none of the three approaches currently used to analyze children's causal conceptions addresses the interaction between the particular content area and the general forms of cognition identified by developmental theorists. That is, there is no attempt to highlight the ways in which children assimilate a particular phenomenon to the general schemas available to them at a given point in their cognitive development. Our experience has been that we cannot predict how the *forms* of cognition outlined by Piaget and Werner will be manifested in a particular *content* area. That is, knowledge that a child is in the preoperational stage of cognitive development, as determined by performance on a variety of Piagetian tasks, does not allow one to predict on the basis of the theoretical principles that a child will believe that the physician uses the stethoscope to determine whether or not he or she has a

heart. This inability to bridge the gap between the general principles of cognitive development and their expression in a particular content area is further illustrated by Piaget's own attempts to predict children's conceptions of
birth based on his theory and findings regarding the child's conceptions of
the world. Kreitler and Kreitler (1966), who specifically studied children's
conceptions of sex and birth, criticize Piaget because they did not find any
evidence for some of his speculations regarding children's beliefs about birth.

Educators and health professionals have often experienced considerable difficulty in applying the theories of Piaget and Werner, perhaps because
they too are unable to predict the particular from the general. In order to
make these theories useful to professionals, we believe there should be efforts made to define categories that reflect the interaction between general
stages of cognitive development and particular content areas. In our own
work on children's conceptions of health and illness (Bibace and Walsh,
1977), we have attempted to address this perceived need. Our studies have
been generated within Werner's (1948) organismic developmental perspective, with its regulative principle of orthogenesis. The question Werner insisted on asking with respect to any phenomenon was: "How does it develop?" In our studies, this question becomes: "How do children's
conceptions of health and illness change as a function of changes in the developmental status of the organism?"

Both Piaget and Werner have insisted that a developmental classification of different conceptions of a given phenomenon must be based on an
analysis of the particular cognitive processes used in arriving at that conception. One cannot simply classify the contents of a conception, since the same
content may be arrived at through different cognitive processes. Researchers
in this tradition have typically relied upon a "clinical method" to achieve the
goal of articulating cognitive processes. In this method, the examiner begins
with a standard question, such as "What is a heart attack?" However, the
examiner conducts a comprehensive inquiry into the child's conception of
the formal aspects of the phenomenon (what, how, and why), following any
leads the subject offers and questioning the meaning of all terms used by the
subject. Although this method runs counter to the emphasis, found in much
of psychology, on standardizing the question, we and many other developmental psychologists in the Piagetian tradition have found an adaptation of
this type of clinical method to be the most suitable one for our goals.

Our study involved two distinct phases—a pilot phase and a testing
phase—with different subjects used for each phase. The purpose of the pilot
phase was to delineate a preliminary category system. In order to sample a
substantial developmental range of explanations initially, children aged three
to thirteen years were tested ($n = 180$). The protocol included twelve sets of
questions. Each set investigated a single content area (for example, "cold")
and probed relevant aspects of the concept, such as cause and cure of an
illness, using "how" and "why" questions. The twelve sets of questions
were: (1) What does it mean to be healthy? (2) Do you remember anyone
who was sick? What was wrong? How did he or she get sick? How did he or

she get better? (3) Were you ever sick? Why did you get sick? How did you get sick? How did you get better? (4) What is the worst sickness to have? Why? What is the best sickness to have? Why? (5) What happens to people when they are sick? What happens to people when they are very sick? (6) What is a cold? How do people get colds? Where do colds come from? What makes colds go away? (7) What are the measles? How do people get the measles? Where do measles come from? What makes the measles get better? (8) What is a heart attack? Why do people get heart attacks? (9) What is cancer? How do people get cancer? (10) What is a headache? Why do people get headaches? (11) Have you ever had a pain? Where? What is pain? Why does it come? Where does it come from? (12) What are germs? What do they look like? Can you draw germs? Where do they come from?

The data from this pilot study were readily classified in terms of Piaget's three broad stages of cognitive development: preoperational, concrete operational, and formal operational. Also consonant with Piaget, who found several subcategories for various content areas, we were able to differentiate two subcategories within the responses for each overall stage of cognitive development. Our next step was to label these categories so as to express simultaneously these six general stages of cognitive development and the contents discussed by children in their conceptions of health and illness. These categories, in their developmental sequence, were Phenomenism, Contagion, Contamination, Internalization, Physiological, and Psychophysiological.

To illustrate one of the categories, suppose that a five-year-old child told us (in response to our question, Where does a cold come from?), "From other people." (How do you get a cold from other people?) "You're just playing with them." (How does that give you a cold?) "You're just there with them, that's all." This response could be classified as preoperational in terms of Piaget's general stages of cognitive development, since the child is relying upon some immediate perceptual experience (that is, the diverse perceptual experiences implicated in the spatial priority of "there with them," that is, close to them). In addition, we can define a category for preoperational thinking in the domain of health and illness, which is a further specification of the category to which this response belongs. What we call a "contagion" concept is one in which the child attributes illness to something or someone which the child perceived in his immediate universe, that is, close to but not touching his body.

The testing phase was carried out to verify the adequacy of this category system as well as the developmental ordering of these explanations in another sample. In the testing phase, children whose chronological age would crudely be indicative of each of the three broad stages of cognitive development were sampled. Consequently, we selected children of three different age groups (four, seven, and eleven years old, evenly split between male and female, $n = 72$) to tap the range of responses characteristic of each of the three major stages of cognitive development.

The protocol used in both phases was modeled on Piaget's and Laurendeau and Pinard's questionnaires regarding causal thinking (for example, Concept of Life, Concept of Dreams) and was designed to elicit responses that revealed the quality of the child's reasoning in contrast to simple "yes/ no" responses—that is, the inquiry was designed to tap the cognitive processes on which children relied for their answers. The category system derived in the pilot study was used to categorize the concept of illness manifested by each subject. In assigning each subject's response to one of the categories of explanation, we considered the configuration of the responses as a whole, as did Piaget (1929) and Laurendeau and Pinard (1962), rather than scoring each separate response. The verbatim written protocols were scored blindly by two independent scorers with good reliability (88 percent agreement).

The results from this testing phase were consistent with the expectations of a cognitive developmental framework. In addition to the category of Incomprehension, we found two subcategories within each of the three major Piagetian stages: Phenomenism and Contagion within the preoperational stage; Contamination and Internalization within the concrete operational stage; and Physiological and Psychophysiological within the formal operational stage of cognitive development. Phenomenistic explanations represent the least mature, and Psychophysiological explanations the most mature forms of causal thinking.

We found that the type of explanation of illness varied as a function of the developmental status of our subjects. Among the four-year-olds, 12.5 percent gave a Phenomenistic explanation, 70.8 percent were categorized as giving Contagion explanations, while 16.7 percent gave Contamination explanations. Among the seven-year-olds, 16.7 percent gave Contagion explanations, while 75 percent gave Contamination explanations, and 8.3 percent gave Internalization explanations. Among the eleven-year-olds, 25 percent gave Internalization explanations, while 70.8 percent gave Physiological explanations, and 4.2 percent gave Psychophysiological explanations.

We will now describe the category system and its implications in terms of Werner's and Piaget's frames of reference.

Preoperational Explanations

Characteristic of the preoperational stage is the child's inability to differentiate between self and world. Thus, the child is swayed by the immediacy of some aspects of perceptual experience. The primary characteristics of thinking at this stage include: concreteness, or preoccupation with external perceptual events; irreversibility, or the inability to construe processes in reverse; egocentrism, or viewing the world from one's own perspective, centering or focusing on a single aspect or part of experience to the exclusion of the whole; and transductive reasoning, or thinking that proceeds from one particular to another rather than from particular to general or vice versa.

Incomprehension. The child evades the what, why, and how of the question or gives answers that appear irrelevant insofar as the child does not appear to respond in any way to the content of the question. Rather, the child's attempt to be responsive is to relate some personal or irrelevant experience.

What is a heart attack? "A heart attack is on vacation." Why is a heart attack on vacation? "Can I have the pencil?" Why do people get heart attacks? "I don't know."

Phenomenism. Within this category, illness is defined in terms of a single external symptom, usually a sensory phenomenon, that is, a sight or sound that the child has, at one time or another, associated with the illness. The child conceptualizes the cause of the illness as a source that is spatially remote and inappropriate. The causal link between this external source and the body is not articulated in terms other than co-occurrence or magic.

What is a heart attack? "A heart attack is falling on your back." Why do people get heart attacks? "A heart attack is from the sun." How does the sun cause a heart attack? "It's the sun."

Do you remember anyone who was sick? "Yup, my brother." What was wrong? "He goed to the hospital." How did he get sick? "The wind, and he went to the doctor." How did the wind make him sick? "The wind . . ." How did he get better? "Then he came home."

The specific criteria for the Phenomenistic category of explanation can be interpreted in terms of Piaget's general criteria for preoperational thought. Evident in this category is the child's centering on a concrete, single aspect of his or her own experience to define an illness. Further, egocentricity is evident in the child's identifying all illness with his or her unique experience. The lack of differentiation between self and world is apparent in his or her fusion of the source of the illness with its effect on the body, without any specification of the causal link between the source of the illness and the illness itself.

Contagion. The child describes and explains illness in terms of external persons, objects or events which, while they are within the immediate world of the ill person, are distanced from him or her either spatially or temporally. The source affects the ill person through mere proximity—temporal or spatial—and is most often characterized by the child in terms of what we call contagion.

Illness is defined in terms of a single external symptom, such as a physical activity, that is usually observed in connection with the illness and is often restricted inappropriately to a single body part. The source of the illness is usually either a person or object that is spatially near to, but not touching, the ill person, or an activity or event that is temporally prior to, but not simultaneous with, the occurrence of the illness. Significant at this level is the child's inability to articulate the causal link between the source of the illness and the illness itself. When asked how an illness is contracted, the child merely reasserts the spatial or temporal proximity, often invoking or implying some form of the general process of contagion. Similarly, the source of the cure is usually perceived as a person or object in the immediate environment, or an event or activity that occurs subsequent to the illness.

Such an activity or event often serves to remove the ill person physically from the source of illness.

While the child at this level still perceives himself or herself as the victim of illness, the universe of events to which he or she is vulnerable is now more restricted; that is, the source of the illness must be near the body in order to have an effect.

What is a heart attack? "A heart attack is falling down." Why do people get heart attacks? "You went on the bus and then you came home." How does going on the bus give someone a heart attack? "Cuz it does."

What are measles? "Measles are bumps on your arm." How do people get measles? "From other people." How do people get measles from other people? "When you walk near them." How does walking near them give you measles? "When you go near them."

What is a cold? "It's coughing a lot." How do people get colds? "Other kids." How do other kids give you a cold? "You catch it, that's all."

While this category clearly reflects preoperational thinking, the child's explanations are less vague and more articulated than in a Phenomenistic explanation. Even though he or she centers on a concrete single aspect of experience, the child can now specify an event that is more relevant to the domain of illness (for example, "bumps on your arm"). Further, the explanations are less idiosyncratic in that the child does not restrict his or her account to a single experience (for example, this child says "coughing a lot" in contrast to "I coughed at my aunt's house"). While the child still fails to distinguish explicitly between self and world, insofar as he or she still does not articulate a connection between the source of the illness (or cure) and the illness itself, the class of events invoked as the source is both spatially closer to the person and more appropriate to the domain of illness (for example, "other people" are the source of illness in contrast to "the wind").

Concrete Operational Explanations

In what Piaget has called the concrete operational stage, the major developmental shift is the accentuation of the differentiation between self and world, such that the child clearly distinguishes between what is internal and external to the self. In spite of this ability to differentiate internal and external, the focus of the child is still on external real events. At this stage, the child can only accommodate to events in the real world in contrast to hypothetical events, that is, can focus on "what is" in contrast to "what might be." Evident at this stage also is the child's ability to specify relationships among events or to classify such events. In contrast to that of the child in the preoperational stage, his or her thinking is markedly less egocentric and is not focused on a part to the exclusion of the whole. Further, the child can conceptualize the reversal of processes.

Contamination. The child at this stage does not differentiate the mind and the body. Hence, contact with either is functionally equivalent. Bad or immoral behavior, just as contact with dirt or germs, causes illness.

The definition of an illness now encompasses multiple symptoms, often including reference to bodily functions evident in external surface body parts or areas. While the source of illness is still external, the child now concretizes the causal link between the source and its effect on the body, namely, germs, dirt, or bad behavior. These sources are transmitted through physical contact, usually taking the form of direct or indirect touch or participation. Likewise, cure at this stage is conceptualized as coming into surface contact with the source of the cure, which is, again, a person, object, event, or activity in the immediate world of the child. Often, the cure involves a medicine that is rubbed on the surface of the body.

At this level, the child manifests some control over the cause and cure of the illness. For example, the child can avoid the contact with the source of the illness by not allowing his or her body to touch the contaminated source or by not allowing himself or herself to choose to engage in a contaminated or immoral activity.

What are measles? "Measles are bumps all over you, they's small and red." How do people get measles? "People get measles from someone else who has the measles." How do people get them from someone else who has them? "By rubbing up against them, they get on you and you've got them." What makes measles get better? "The doctor gives you stuff to rub on them."

What is cancer? "Cancer is when you're very sick and you got to go to the hospital and you throw up a lot, and stuff." How do people get cancer? "From smoking without their mother's permission." How does this give you cancer? "You shouldn't do that—it's bad."

What is a cold? "It's coughing and sneezing, you don't breathe so good and things." How do people get colds? "From taking your jacket off outside." How does this give you a cold? "Cause the cold air—it gets to your skin." And? "And that's how colds come—from cold air."

Evident in this category is the beginning of concrete operational thinking insofar as the child attempts to make logical sense out of all of the data of concrete reality. In defining illness, the child no longer centers on a single input of reality but mentions multiple symptoms. Further, the concrete data he or she utilizes is more directly illness related; for example, externally visible bodily processes such as breathing are mentioned. The egocentricity of the earlier stage is less apparent, as the child describes illness as a more general phenomenon ("People get measles," rather than "I got measles"; "Colds come from cold air," rather than "A cold is from the wind and I went to the doctor"). The child differentiates between self and world insofar as he or she articulates the connection between the source of the illness and the illness itself, that is, germs, dirt, badness. This is the first evidence of the child's differentiating between the source of the illness and the causal link to the body.

Internalization. Illness is described as being, in a global way, within the body. The child is not concerned with what is happening in the body but with the way in which the illness is internalized, namely, swallowing, ingestion of germs, or "bugs."

Illness is defined in terms of an internal body part that is only globally described, often using a concrete analogy, or in terms of the process of internalization. The source of the illness is perceived as an external contaminant (for example, smoke, dirt, germs) or an unhealthy body state or condition (for example, obesity, old age, high blood pressure) which the child indicates has a direct effect on internal organs. While the child's explanation of the effect is often global and undifferentiated, the process by which the source of the illness becomes internalized is generally well articulated. In a similar fashion, the source of the cure is an external agent, usually medicine, which is internalized. Concrete analogies are often used to describe the internal effects. Significantly, the child often refers to the healing power of the body and suggests that internalizing healing agents may not always be necessary.

While the child still views external agents as contributing to the cause and cure of illness, he or she now also sees the body as able to heal itself without recourse to external intervention. He or she also sees himself or herself as able to prevent illness through proper care.

What's a heart attack? "It's the heart, it stops and you stop breathing and faint." What happens to the heart? "It just shuts off, like a pump it shuts off." How do people get heart attacks? "It's lifting heavy stuff, your arms hurt and the hurt goes up your arms into your heart." Why do people get heart attacks? "From lifting stuff and working too hard."

What is a cold? "It's when your nose is stuffed up and you cough and sneeze." How do people get colds? "From germs in the air, you breathe them in." How does this give you a cold? "The germs, they get in your blood." And? "They give you a cold, I guess."

The Internalization explanations still reflect the child's thinking in terms of concrete operational thinking. While the child is able to mention an internal organ, he or she cannot articulate how it operates physiologically. Attempts to do so result in the use of concrete analogies, that is, descriptions in terms of an external perceptual object or event (the heart is a "pump"; the stomach is a "bag of food"). The primary focus of the child is not on what happens physiologically within the body but on the process of internalization which the child describes in terms of events that are visible, for example, swallowing or inhaling. It is important to note here the child's account of the healing powers of the body. A major characteristic of concrete operational thought, that is, reversibility, is manifest here in that the person who is sick can become well and vice versa.

Formal Operational Explanations

In what Piaget refers to as the formal operational stage, the child is no longer bound by concrete reality but is now able to include possibility. The child at this stage is aware of the gaps in his or her knowledge and fills these gaps with hypotheses, in contrast to the concrete constructions of the child in the prior stage. At this stage, there is the greatest amount of differentiation between the self and the world or, conversely, the child is least likely to manifest the effects of stimulus boundedness because of the compensatory character of logical thinking. In brief, what the child knows is superordinate to what he or she sees.

Physiological. While the cause of the illness may be triggered by an external event, the child describes and explains illness in terms of internal body organs and functions. Illness is defined in terms of internal physiological structures and functions whose malfunctioning manifests itself in multiple external symptoms. The explanation of internal functions is more differentiated than at the Internalization level. If knowledge of a particular function is not available to the child, he or she refers to it as "invisible" rather than constructing a concrete analogy, as in earlier levels. The cause of illness is now clearly thought to be a malfunctioning of an internal body part or process. While the child is aware of the possibility of the ultimate cause(s) being external and can describe how one or more of these causes affect the internal body parts, he or she is more concerned with describing the internal functions.

Clearly, the child now perceives himself or herself as having even more control over the onset and cure of illness insofar as he or she perceives multiple causes for any single illness and, likewise, multiple cures. The child also exhibits an increased sense that personal actions can contribute to outcome.

What is a heart attack? "A heart attack is when the heart stops pumping blood to the rest of the body. A person faints, stops breathing, and collapses." How do people get heart attacks? "The valves keep the blood from getting to the heart so the heart stops and you get a heart attack."

What is cancer? "Cancer is when there's too many cells. They're invisible but I know that they grow." How do people get cancer? "Some people think it's air pollution or chemicals; some people don't know. It causes the cells to start growing."

The child's thinking evidences a major characteristic of formal operational thought—the ability to depart in a careful manner from concrete reality. Hence, the child can now describe functions and structures that are not external or visible. Further, consistent with formal operational thinking, the child is aware of the gaps in his or her understanding (for example, referring to certain cellular processes as "invisible"). In describing illness in terms of multiple causes and symptoms, the child can make hypotheses about the relationship between the environment and the body rather than relying on a single concrete experience.

Also in this category, the child, for the first time, clearly differentiates different types of causes insofar as he or she deals with efficient causes (malfunctioning of organs) and final causes (remote agents that may trigger efficient causes). Having clearly differentiated between self and world, the child no longer bases the link between internal and external on some salient perceptual aspect of the event in a rigid one-to-one manner.

Psychophysiological. As in the Physiological explanation, the illness is described in terms of internal physiological processes, but the child now perceives an additional or alternative cause of illness, namely, psychological cause. The child is aware that a person's thoughts or feelings can affect the way the body functions. As in the Physiological level, the child still defines illness in terms of internal physiological structures and functions but now he or she includes psychological as well as physiological symptoms. While the immediate cause of illness is still malfunctioning of internal physiological structures and functions, the less immediate causes now include psychological events. Similarly, cures can now include relief of sources of psychological pressure.

What is a heart attack? "It's when your heart stops or doesn't work right." How do people get heart attacks? "A heart attack is from being all nerve racked and weary."

What is a headache? "It's pressure inside your head and it makes your head hurt." How do people get headaches? "They worry too much or think too much. It's from problems and aggravations."

Interestingly, at this most mature level, in terms of the population we have sampled, children now distinguish between the psychological and the biological and can articulate how the body is affected by the mind (for example, the cause of a headache is worry). However, the children give no evidence that the mind or the psychological events themselves are in any way controllable. When pressed, these children would revert back to biological cures for the psychological causes which they have introduced to account for the illness. For example, aggravation may be stated as cause of a heart attack, but the cure is described solely in terms of medicine, without an attempt to integrate biological, psychological, and social considerations. Psychological causes appear to be invoked earlier than psychological cures. In addition to the differentiation between the self and the world, the child is now able to distinguish the psychological from the physical domain within the self.

There are some interesting corollaries of the development of children's conceptions of illness. Of critical interest to a clinician is the change in degree of control over the illness manifested in the categories. The sequence in which the categories are ordered empirically is interesting, not only in terms of cognitive development but also in terms of the kind and extent of personal control exerted by the person over what that individual believes to be the cause of the illness. Clearly, the shift from a Phenomenistic to a Psychophysiological explanation is correlated with a sense of increasing control. The child is initially vulnerable to events which the mature adult would consider to be completely irrelevant. The child's sense of vulnerability is increased in that even events that an adult would interpret as spatially remote and irrelevant are conceived by the child as causes of illness.

The shift from Phenomenism to Contagion is primarily one of reduction in spatial distance—that is, in the Phenomenistic phase, events that are construed as remote from the individual have an effect, whereas in the Contagion phase, only events that are nearer the body can have an effect. It must be emphasized that these distinctions regarding what is near or far from the body are distinctions introduced by adults, not by the child. The child invokes these reasons precisely because he or she does not differentiate between what adults call the self and the world, or between events construed by adults as internal or external to the body. The next phase, Contamination, involves a qualitative shift. The difference now is that the event relied upon by the child as causing the illness must be located at the surface of the body. During this phase, greater control is exerted by the child in that the child believes illness can be avoided by avoiding body contact with the contaminated world of living things (animals or people) or the contaminated inanimate world of objects. Conversely, greater control is now possible because illness, once it is present, can be cured by "rubbing something on the skin," for instance.

It is only in the phase we have labeled Internalization that children perceive themselves as positively doing things to maintain health. It should be noted that earlier, in the Contamination phase, children believed they could avoid sickness, whereas now they believe they can do things to maintain health. Children's interpretation is now closer to what health professionals label "preventive medicine," in that children say that health can be maintained by certain activities, for example, by "eating the right food." The control is thus enhanced in that it is not a single event but a whole series of regularly occurring events (eating habits) which are now invoked as relevant in the children's conceptions of health and illness. In addition, children at the Internalization level believe that they are not as dependent on medicines or other external factors to make them better. Rather, children now think that the body is capable of "healing itself," so that measles, for example, "clear up by themselves." This conception is interpreted as greater control in that there is a self-curative, less-dependent-on-external-factors perception of illness.

The Physiological phase is a further differentiation of the previous Internalization phase in that children now invoke multiple causes for an illness and, further, believe that these causes are cumulative. The very multiplicity of causes enhances the children's sense of control because there are now a diversity of ways in which personal actions can contribute to health or illness.

Lastly, the Psychophysiological phase, evident in the most mature group, introduces a new realm of cause, namely, the Psychological realm. Although psychological states such as "worry" or "aggravation" are now believed to bring about physical illness, the cure is still in the realm of biological remedies, namely, medicine. Our current data do not allow us to pursue more closely the issue of control in the psychological realm. We would want to ask about the psychological procedures that children believe can alleviate illness or, even more broadly (paralleling the shift from Contamination to Internalization in the biological realm), foster psychological health.

We have tried to make clear two dimensions in the developmental sequence: the sequence of cognitive processes underlying the child's responses, and the interpersonal dimension of locus of control. However, we should emphasize that these dimensions are not isolated from each other in the child's perspective. Rather, the child's conceptions of health and illness are correlated with marked differences in degree of personal control over the cause and alleviation of illness.

Methodologically, it is often important from a cognitive-developmental perspective to carry out a series of studies that tap the ontogenesis of the concepts being investigated, that is, to determine the shifts in the concepts from early childhood through adolescence. Repeatedly, Werner and his colleagues have demonstrated how the stages of cognitive development that emerge from studies of a limited age range are indeed applicable throughout development of the life cycle (Wapner, 1969). These stages of cognitive development purport to characterize cognition for *any* content area and *all* ages.

Given this orientation, we are studying populations throughout the life cycle. For instance, we have studied college students with marked differences in educational backgrounds. To what extent does a person's educational background in biology affect his or her concepts of health, illness, and medical procedures? This study compared college students majoring in biology with a group who had not taken a single course in biology. Using the identical protocol used in the studies with children, our preliminary analysis demonstrates no significant differences in the developmental level of explanation between the two groups. (A finer analysis of content differences and meanings is in process.) It would appear, then, that the abstract and general biological principles learned as a biology major do not make themselves evident when one is asked such concrete and specific questions as: "What is a heart attack? How does one get a heart attack?" The biology majors may well be more articulate in explaining normal physiological processes; however, their explanations of particular illnesses are not markedly more mature than the explanations of nonbiology majors.

Some readers may find this unbelievable. We found, nevertheless, some biology majors whose explanation of a "cold" was formally similar to that of a seven-year-old child. These findings are entirely consistent with previous findings in other areas of causal thinking. Dennis (1953), in examining the concept of life in university and college students, found explanations that were formally similar to those given by children. Commenting on Dennis' findings, Laurendeau and Pinard (1962, p. 38) stated: "As may well be imagined, these data have been regarded with skepticism. . . . Thus Crannel (1954), Bell (1954), Lowrie (1954), Voeks (1954), Dennis (1957), and Simmons and Gross (1957) have repeated analogous experiments, always with college and university students . . . and have finally been led to the same observations." In our data, likewise, there appear to be a number of college students, irrespective of their experiences with a particular discipline, whose conceptions of illness are formally similar to those of younger children. All these studies clearly indicate the fallacy of equating stage of cognitive development with chronological age. These studies further illustrate that the concept of stage is valuable, precisely because stage transcends age in its generality.

A clinical example will further illustrate the lack of relationship between age and stage of cognitive development. On a recent visit to her family doctor, a thirty-year-old woman explained that the growing pain in her side was caused by her having accidentally touched her sister who, at the time, was under a "curse." The patient believed that the pain was transmitted through bodily contact—specifically, touch. This explanation of the source of the illness would be formally described within our sequence of stages as a "Contamination" explanation. In an ontogenetic developmental sequence, this type of response is characteristic of normal children aged five to six years.

Our intent as clinicians is to underscore the necessity for eliciting the patient's conceptions of illness as part of the data that enter into determining a course of action. In this case, the explanation offered by this woman could be, depending on other factors, interpreted as deviant or immature or as subscribing to a different, yet consensually validated system of beliefs. The fact that the patient came from a culture that makes use of the concept of curse makes this latter explanation more probable.

Implications

What are some implications for health professionals of such developmental studies? The specification of norms for such conceptions of health and illness, how these conceptions change with development, and the cognitive processes that underlie these contents and conceptions should have practical significance in a variety of ways. Such an ordering should make it easier for professionals to grasp the invariant cognitive principles that underlie what now appears to many professionals, initially, as the infinitely varied, "quaint" content character of children's conceptions. These specific categories are valuable insofar as they are consonant with the general theoretical principles of cognition and, simultaneously, reflect the specificity of the contents of interest to professionals in the health field. Thus, they constitute a bridge that will, it is hoped, facilitate appreciation and application of this general theoretical framework. Repeatedly we have found, as clinical teachers, that health professionals find it difficult to make the transition between the abstract theoretical concepts of Piaget and Werner and the concrete realities of their clinical work.

An assimilation of these categories by a clinician could be a useful adjunct to facilitate listening with empathy, providing more meaningful explanations, and changing behavior. The following clinical example illustrates the importance of eliciting and listening to the patient's conceptions of illness: A forty-year-old male with a high school education was hospitalized in an intensive care unit for a heart attack. He insisted, contrary to medical advice, on getting up to go to the bathroom, despite repeated and emphatic "reinforcement of the teaching," according to the physician and nursing personnel. A psychiatric consultation led to the conclusion that the patient demonstrated "massive denial." The behavior remained unchanged. When the clinical development psychologist* consulted with the nurse clinician, she insisted that the patient "knew" why he was being required to stay in bed. The nurse was then asked how she could be so sure that the patient understood the explanation she had given him. She replied: "Because I asked him to repeat it for me. And he had got it!" The nurse was given some illustrations from Werner and Kaplan (1963) demonstrating the interdependence of thought and diverse media other than language used to express it, namely, gesture, line drawings, and so on. The nurse was then encouraged to test her assumption that the patient had "understood" her message by asking the patient to convey to her his meaning through a drawing of what she had told him. The patient's drawing was not instructive. He drew an oval with four parts. But his interpretation of his drawing now made the problem and his behavior clear. A paraphrase of his statement to the nurse conveyed the following: "There are four chambers. I've had two heart attacks. I've got two more to go. After I've had the third attack, I'll listen to you, but not before."

Unfortunately, clinical examples do not allow for the kind of inquiry that makes the classification of a response unequivocal. Here, the ambiguity would require further inquiry to determine whether the patient's response is primarily indicative of an invalid Physiological explanation or whether the patient is relying on a Phenomenistic explanation. The latter category would be appropriate if the patient were describing the heart functions in concrete perceptual terms, that is, thinking of the heart as four separate but spatially proximate chambers. Such ambiguities underscore an important consideration. These categories are not intended to be used by health professionals in a strict Piagetian sense, as an invariant sequence of stages. Rather, our intention is that these categories are a useful heuristic device and practical clinical tool. For clinical psychologists who already elicit such data from the patient, these categories will be useful in that they systematically organize a wide variety of explanations. The limiting conditions in interpreting behavior generally recognized by clinical psychologists, such as the state of the person (stable versus regressed), and personal, cultural, intellectual, and other variables, must, of course, also be observed with respect to the use of these categories.

We have found that many members of other health professions, such as physicians and nurses, do not consider eliciting persons' own conceptions of their illness to be relevant data. For such individuals, our findings have served to stimulate them to ask patients for their ideas regarding the causes of their illness. Health professionals may, in general, be better able to explain the child's behavior by utilizing these categories. For instance, how could the pediatrician mentioned earlier have used these categories in the case of the child who felt that a stethoscope is used to find out "if I have a heart"? The

*Clinical development psychologist is the term for a clinician who is committed to a developmental approach to the entire life cycle—that is, a clinical development psychologist is not limited to childhood as is a clinical child psychologist.

health professional could have reassured both the parent and the child by recognizing such an answer as normal for young children. Such an approach would seem to be more beneficial than the appeal of some professionals to the child to "be a big boy," or the reaction of some parents who dismiss the child's fear by exhorting the child "not to be a sissy." Turiel's (1966) findings in moral development that children are most receptive to an explanation that is only one cognitive stage beyond their own could also be utilized in this context. Thus, a health professional, relying on this assumption and knowing that a child at the next stage of cognitive development does not think in such an absolutistic way, might acknowledge the child's answer as normal, yet add "I'm using this thing that I put in my ears and on your chest to hear how fast or slow your heart goes. Would you like to hear it?"

Fears that the adult professional considers irrational can, by taking into account a developmental analysis of the patient's conceptions of illness, become more understandable. Such an interpretation can have direct implications for better patient management. We have seen, for example, many five- and six-year-old children on a hospital pediatric ward become "inexplicably upset" and ask to be moved to another room. Their fear was based on their preoccupation with catching the disease of their roommate. It should be helpful for a health professional to appreciate that this is normal for children in that stage of development (Contagion). Such an appreciation will prevent the health professional's dismissing such fears as irrational and will allay the frustration caused by the child's lack of understanding. Even if the health professional is unable to make physical changes to alleviate the child's worry, he or she can at least accept and not dismiss the child's fear and hence genuinely reassure the child. Further, the health professional can better explain the reason for the child's upset to the parents and staff members.

Health professionals should use such findings flexibly, in the context of other data and variables that are available to the clinician. Our findings in the area of conceptions of illness are consistent with Piagetian stages of cognitive development. However, stages of cognitive development do not purport to take into account many psychosocial factors and individual differences that may be of crucial interest to the clinician for a particular patient. The categories in their developmental sequence will, we hope, provide useful guidelines for health professionals.

This review and the illustration of one application of developmental psychology to the health field should stimulate psychologists—within their own areas of expertise—to extend their work to include a developmental perspective. In the domain of health and illness, as in all human sciences, Werner's question remains a fruitful one: "But how does it develop?"

12 ❧

Cognition and Information Processing in Patient and Physician

Earl B. Hunt

Colin M. MacLeod

People think about their health. Practitioners think about how people's health can be maintained, and patients think about the advice they receive from the practitioners. People think about how they can keep healthy and have to keep healthy in order to think well. Cognition is both an end and a means in the quest for physical vigor. Professionals in the health care field must appreciate and use both their own and their clients' mental capacities.

A truly general definition of thinking has eluded philosophers for centuries. Pragmatically, though, we shall follow Bower (1975) and most other cognitive psychologists in equating intelligent behavior with the processing of information. This processing, in turn, has two aspects—acquiring new information and using old information. While these simple statements gloss over a number of definitional issues, they seem to capture the flavor of what we want to say. We shall discuss straightforward exchanges of information in health care, in situations in which there is no need to concern ourselves with the hidden motivations of any of the participants. This is not to deny the importance of such motivations—defenses and anxieties do create real complications in the delivery of health care (see Chapters Five, Nine, and Nineteen in this volume). At best, though, humans are restricted and biased information processors. Even when we want to face the facts, we are limited by our abilities to respond to multiple inputs, relate the past to the present, and follow complicated chains of logical reasoning. These characteristics of *homo sapiens* must be taken into account if *medicus sapiens* is to practice.

In health care, as in most other client-professional relations, practitioners exchange information with clients. From the practitioner's point of view, the client presents a problem situation that is to be classified in terms of the practitioner's previous experiences, usually in order to select some treatment. From the client's point of view, the practitioner is a source of advice about the improvement of some identified problem situation. Many of our remarks will be concerned with professional-client relationships at this level of generality and thus could as easily be applied to the legal profession or to stockbrokers as to the health sciences.

Health care does differ from other client-professional interactions in two relevant ways. First, cognitive capability itself is an important aspect of life that is to be maintained by health care. Indeed, in some cases the major purpose of a health care program is to restore lost cognitive capability (for example, in speech therapy programs following brain damage). The second difference concerns the effects of treatments upon the patient's information-processing capabilities. Sometimes, a therapy designed to combat a particular health problem may have unanticipated (and even undesirable) effects upon cognition. Although we cannot discuss all the possible psychological manipulations that might affect cognition, we shall make some remarks about the classes of mental functions that appear to be susceptible to physiological manipulation and discuss what can be done to detect and ameliorate the effects of treatments upon cognition.

One might classify our presentation as a didactic tutorial. It is didactic in that we shall first make some remarks about a general theory of cognition and then treat health care problems as a special case of the general model. The discussion is tutorial in that we shall assume that we are not addressing experts in human experimental psychology. Our goal is to present information at the level that would be provided in a seminar for practitioners, rather than at a workshop for specialists in the study of cognition. We shall try to provide pointers to key sources in the literature, although there are fewer of these than we should like. Despite the importance of the topic, investigators have given little consideration to the role of cognitive variables either in the health care system itself or in the client-professional interaction in general. These problems seem to be specific enough so that they do not attract the attention of basic researchers, yet general enough so that there is no compelling need for any one "action oriented" agency to address them. Thus, the studies that we would like to be able to cite, but which simply have not been done, have been attractive neither to the pure researcher nor to the applied scientist. Consequently, we shall be forced to speculate in these areas. We hope that these speculations are reasonable extrapolations from firm data and developed theory.

A General Theory of Cognition

Cognition is too broad a term; we shall distinguish between two rather distinct aspects of thinking. For some purposes, our model of thinking will be the activity of a scholar who attempts to bring knowledge about the past to bear on problems of the present. This sort of thinker does not operate under time pressure—the problem is simply to understand, not to understand in a few seconds. For other purposes, our model of thought will be that of the traffic cop, busy directing traffic after a football game and acutely aware of the problems of time pressures and split attention. We all like to believe that our really important thinking is done in the scholarly mode, but even scholars must resist distractions and face deadlines. Although some of our thinking may be "timeless," a great deal of it takes place under time pressure. We shall argue that this is an important point in health care.

The Scholar Mode

While we like to regard thought as uniquely human, we probably cannot defend such a proposition. Human problem solving is one of a class of information-processing situations in which past knowledge is brought to bear upon present problems. Libraries and some computer systems deal with similar situations. Let us consider some restrictions that face all problem-solving systems, be they machine or human.

A problem-solving system begins by receiving some "sensory" message about the external world. This message must be translated into an internal language and then related to internal representations of past experiences that have been stored in the same language. Since the match between present and past is never perfect, the information-processing system must possess a pattern recognition subsystem that permits matching of the present situation with records of the past to determine which are "close enough" to be relevant. Because information is cumulative, there must be some way to incorporate new information into the data base. This is just computer jargon for saying that the system must learn, but the language used emphasizes the cognitive aspects of learning. It would hardly be feasible for humans (or libraries) to make direct matches between the current situation and every piece of information stored in memory. The system must have some scheme for organizing information so that efficient searches for relevant information can be conducted.

These straightforward observations have strong implications for how human memory must be used in problem solving. Human memory has to be organized, so that certain pieces of information are tied to each other. In fact, the notion of "psychological distance" between pieces of information in memory is frequently invoked as an explanatory construct (Hutchinson and Lockhead, 1977; Smith, Shoben, and Rips, 1974). To illustrate, consider the collection of curves, straight lines, and angles that make up the *visual stimulus* CAT. These visual patterns immediately call to mind related acoustic information and perhaps even visual images. None of these bear any necessary relation to the physical form of CAT. There are other cases in which the tie is less direct, but is still present. Most of us can imagine a train of associations that runs from MARTIN LUTHER to MUNICH to BEER. The chains of associations inside our heads profoundly influence the thinking of which we are capable, a point that has been amply discussed by both philosophers and psychologists (see Anderson and Bower, 1973). At a more mundane level, advertising can be thought of as an attempt to establish associations—for instance, the association between HEADACHE and YOUR FAVORITE NOSTRUM.

Because our minds are bundles of associations, learning and remembering are but two sides of the same coin. We find information by determining associations between the present situation and our memory, or between those things that the present situation immediately brings to mind and those second-order associations to which the first recovered memory points. Now consider what this process means for learning. Information will be entered into memory not "as itself" but as it is described at the time it is presented. Subsequent recall, then, will be determined by the original interpretation of the information presented (Tulving and Thomson, 1973). How will this interplay between recall and learning affect problem solving? Classic studies in the psychology of thinking have shown that people learn to use things, and information about things, in only a few of the ways that things and information can be used. For instance, most people do not think of a hammer as a pendulum, even when they need a pendulum, because they have learned that hammers are things associated with the act of pounding nails, not the act of making strings swing through the air (Maier, 1931).

These facts lead us to an important principle: Learning is *context sensitive*. We acquire facts only in association with other facts. Thus, if learning is to be useful, we must be sure that the context cues present at acquisition time are sufficiently similar to those that will be present at retrieval time for us to remember what we need to remember when we need to remember it. We shall make frequent use of this principle in discussing medical information processing. We point out, though, that the principle is hardly new outside psychology. Advertisers have used it for years. The purveyors of tobacco and alcoholic beverages, for instance, have gone to great expense to ensure that the names of their products are associated with concepts of masculinity, sex appeal, and social confidence, rather than with thoughts of liver failure and lung cancer. These tactics are effective (Harris, in press), and the very fact of their effectiveness has produced a major health problem.

How should we describe association-based problem solving? Scholars from the psychologist Bartlett (1932) to the computer scientist Minsky (1975) have used the idea of a *schema* or *frame of reference*. We shall use the latter term. A frame of reference is a structure that we apply in order to understand events. We assume that the observer and problem solver first identifies the present situation as one of those situations for which a particular frame of reference is appropriate and then looks for those pieces of information in the situation that are crucial for understanding the situation within the adopted frame of reference. Pople (1977) has pointed out that diagnostic procedures in internal medicine are good examples of this sort of thinking. First, a general hypothesis is selected, on the basis of global impressions, and then the hypothesis is used to guide further inquiry. For instance, if a physician decides, possibly on the basis of scanty evidence, that the problem is one of liver failure, then further questions will be chosen to distinguish among types of liver failure. Questions that would be diagnostic of other situations are simply not asked. (This point is discussed further in Chapter Thirteen in this volume.)

Obviously, the use of hypotheses to guide reasoning is not confined to medicine. Neither are hypotheses used only to search for external information—hypotheses can be shown to influence our searches of our own memory. For example, recall for the details of an automobile accident can be markedly influenced by suggesting that cars *collided*, which implies one frame of reference, or suggesting that they *smashed*, which implies another (Loftus, 1975). We shall have more to say about such phenomena in our discussion of the specifics of reasoning about health care.

The Traffic Cop Mode

Now let us turn from the scholar and consider instead the officer directing traffic. More often than we would like, we must adjust our thought processes to the real time demands of the world. We must search the environment, if only to decide what is going on that is worth the scholar's attention. A superficial examination of external stimuli provides all the evidence we have when we decide to break the scholar's concentration in order to deal with a pressing problem. The reader can get a good grasp of the distinction we are trying to make by simply considering the cognitive demands of holding a conversation while driving a car.

Information in the external environment must first be changed (transduced) from its sensory form into some internal language before it can be compared to stored information. Some, but by no means all, of the information resulting from this comparison will be placed into active, or "working," memory, and some of the resulting mixture between new stimulus information and stimulus-aroused memories will be re-stored back into permanent memory so that it can be retrieved later. Psychologists interested in cognition (Atkinson and Shiffrin, 1968; Baddeley, 1977; Bower, 1975; Hunt, 1971, 1973) believe that this is accomplished by passing information through a fairly complex series of time-dependent memory stages. These are depicted in Figure 1.

The hypothesized steps in information processing will play a consider-

Figure 1. Pattern Recognition and Stimulus Transformation Activity
in Memory and Thought

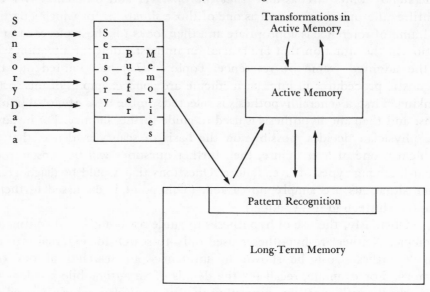

able role in our subsequent discussion, so we shall consider Figure 1 in detail. When information about the environment first impinges on the sensorium, it is transformed into a sensory-specific *buffer memory*. Buffer registers are evidently quite large but are subject to rapid fading over time. Information in visual buffers fades in less than half a second, and information in auditory buffers is retained for only one or two seconds. Nevertheless, in the short period during which information is held in buffer memory, it is subjected to a pattern-matching process that forms the basis of our recognition of the world. If a match is detected between information in a sensory buffer and some record in long-term memory, that record becomes a candidate for entry into active memory.

Active memory includes, but is almost certainly not limited to, that information of which we are consciously aware. It is likely that many more long-term memory codes are proposed for entry into active memory than are accepted, for active memory itself appears to be quite small. Some of the factors that have been shown to affect the arousal of long-term memory codes and their placement in active memory are: the closeness of the match between a prototype code in long-term memory and the contents of sensory memory (good examples are recognized more quickly), the current level of activation of the long-term memory code (codes that have been recently aroused are more easily aroused by incoming stimuli), and the priority attached to each long-term memory code (one almost always recognizes one's name).

Our conscious experience of thought appears to be limited to a subset of the information-bearing codes placed in active memory. Over time, active memory will hold a series of related codes which, taken together, form a coherent thought. For example, hearing the sound "ninety-nine" over a public address system in a hospital may first arouse the concept of the number 99, then the realization that the emergency code for cardiac arrest is 99, and then the realization that the cardiac emergency team must take action. At each step, long-term memory is used to elaborate upon the meaning of active memory. As different long-term memory codes are activated by the ever-changing contents of active memory, each code provides a cue for subsequent activations. Clearly, the pattern recognition choices that are made early in this process will constrain the probabilities of memory arousal at later stages. At the same time, as the interplay between the active and long-term memory system is taking place, long-term memory will also be receiving information from the sensory buffers. Thus, we do not see or hear information directly from our senses; what we see or hear is partly the result of sensory stimulation and partly the result of long-term memory interpretation.

As we have pointed out before, what is consolidated into long-term memory is the world as we have interpreted it. We do not remember what we have sensed, we remember what we think we sensed. This simple concept must be kept in mind in any discussion of the practical aspects of cognition. Although it is convenient to regard thinking as if it were a static process of stimulus presentation followed by elaboration, this, of course, is not so. The processes of sensation, interpretation of sensation, active memory formation and elaboration, and information consolidation in long-term memory must all go on "at once." But do they really go on at once, independently, or is it possible that each task "time shares" our mind for a few instants? The answer to this question seems to be that there is some independence and there is some sharing of resources. To explain, we now introduce two more concepts: *attention budgets* and the *automatic versus controlled process* distinction.

Certain of the cognitive functions we have described appear to be independent of each other and essentially effortless. As a rough guide, these are the processes that do not directly involve active memory. They will be called *automatic* processes. An example is the recognition of highly overlearned information, such as the meaning of common words. Such a process is so automated that one cannot easily stop it, even when suppression would be advantageous. By way of illustration, we ask the reader to count the number of words in lists A and B of Figure 2. We wager that it will be harder to count list B than to count list A.

List A is easier to count than List B because recognition of the meaning of words is an automatic process that cannot easily be suspended while conducting the controlled counting task. This simple experiment illustrates another point. Counting the second list was more of an effort than counting the first because the information that the word recognition process retrieved interfered with ongoing information processing. In general, any situation that requires the manipulation of information in active memory can be considered a *controlled* task, one which can be altered and which, when exe-

Figure 2. Lists of Words To Be Counted

List A	List B
big	three
tall	seven
red	one
apple	four
printer	six
book	two
cup	eight
friend	nine
door	five

cuted, does draw upon our limited attentional resources (Schneider and Shiffrin, 1977; Shiffrin and Schneider, 1977). Unfortunately, "attentional resources" themselves are not clearly understood. It seems best to think of them as a sort of energy budget, which may be split across several (controlled) tasks, providing that the total available resources are not exceeded by task demands. Furthermore, how well a controlled task is performed is assumed to be an increasing function of the amount of attention devoted to it.

A recent finding in our own laboratory shows both that the automatic-controlled distinction is a valid one and that, in certain contexts, it can have important implications for health. We found (MacLeod, Dekaban, and Hunt, 1978) that phenobarbital, a sedative widely used for the control of seizures in epileptic patients, had no discernible effect upon an automatic task (recognition of letters) but had a marked deleterious effect upon a controlled task (searching for information in short-term memory). Summarizing our finding in rather oversimplified terms, we believe that controlled tasks involving active memory are generally quite sensitive to transient situational effects such as the drug state of a person, whereas automatic process efficiency is more permanent and resists all but very extreme alterations.

To summarize our argument about real-time cognition, let us return to the metaphor of the traffic cop. This time, though, we will deal with the officer's task in more theoretical terms. Basically, a traffic officer responds to visual stimuli, such as lights, license plates, and even movement. Virtually everything impinging on the retina will be "seen," in the sense that it will be read into the sensory buffer. But the officer will seldom be consciously aware of more than a small subset of the stimuli seen, simply because they do not excite any long-term memory code that would then enter active memory. Normally, the officer will use his or her attentional resources to manipulate information about the state of traffic lights, the positions of automobiles, and their joint implications for action. As the traffic becomes more dense, more and more attentional resources will be required to maintain order and less will be available for daydreaming—or, for that matter, for monitoring "inessential" aspects of the environment, such as the details of passers-by. Thus, if a well-known bank robber must walk that way, the robber would be well advised to pass during rush hour. However, certain of the "ignored" stimuli will have sufficient priority to be noticed no matter what the circumstances. It is unlikely that one could drive a police officer's own car by him or her, unnoticed, on the busiest of days.

Most health care practitioners would probably like to think of their own problem solving as being at the leisurely, reasoned pace of the scholar. Similarly, we probably view the normal interchange of information between patient and client in this way. Such a view, it is hoped, is often accurate. We must remember, though, that the scholarly processes of thought are, at any instant in time, taking place in the world of the traffic cop. We must consider both the nature of the information being exchanged *and* the nature of the attentional resources that the information exchange itself requires. Both of these aspects of cognition have implications for health care delivery. In the following pages we will trace out some of them.

A Cognitive View of Health Care

We have pointed out that certain aspects of information exchange in health care and maintenance are special examples of professional-client interactions. In other situations, though, one must consider factors that are unique to the health care situation. Apart from this distinction, there are two clear-cut points of view toward the health care system—the views of those providing services and the views of those receiving them. We shall make some remarks about cognition from all these perspectives.

Communicating with a Client

In a prototype professional-client exchange, the client will wish to provide "all relevant" facts to the professional, who, in turn, has the task of relating the description of the present case to a particular body of expert knowledge. Initially, we shall also assume that the client's health care problem has not affected cognition directly. We are talking about two normal beings who have a straightforward motivation to exchange information. People do this all the time, so what can the problem be?

We begin with an example. Table 1 contains a dialogue between a physician and a patient who is evidently seeking help for a minor, noncrippling personal adjustment problem. We hazard that most readers will see this as a reasonable exchange between a client and a somewhat nondirective psychotherapist. It was not. The "doctor" in this case was a computer program written by Joseph Weizenbaum (1965). The fact that this particular "doctor" was *ex machina*, however, is not really relevant. Perhaps a computer could be programmed to contain the wisdom required to give personal guidance. That is a subtle question. What is relevant, as Weizenbaum (1976) has pointed out in detail, is that this particular program contained no such wisdom. The program contained no information whatsoever about the pro-

Table 1. Partial Text of a Conversation Between a Rogerian Therapist
(the Computer Program ELIZA) and a Female Patient

Men are all alike.
IN WHAT WAY
They're always bugging us about something or other.
CAN YOU THINK OF A SPECIFIC EXAMPLE
Well, my boyfriend made me come here.
YOUR BOYFRIEND MADE YOU COME HERE
He says I'm depressed much of the time.
I AM SORRY TO HEAR YOU ARE DEPRESSED
It's true. I am unhappy.
DO YOU THINK COMING HERE WILL HELP YOU NOT TO BE UNHAPPY
I need some help, that much seems certain.
WHAT WOULD IT MEAN TO YOU IF YOU GOT SOME HELP
Perhaps I could learn to get along with my mother.
TELL ME MORE ABOUT YOUR FAMILY
My mother takes care of me.
WHO ELSE IN YOUR FAMILY TAKES CARE OF YOU
My father.
YOUR FATHER
You are like my father in some ways.
WHAT RESEMBLANCE DO YOU SEE
You are not very aggressive, but I think you don't want me to notice that.
WHAT MAKES YOU THINK I AM NOT VERY AGGRESSIVE
You don't argue with me.
WHY DO YOU THINK I DON'T ARGUE WITH YOU
You are afraid of me.
DOES IT PLEASE YOU TO BELIEVE I AM AFRAID OF YOU
My father is afraid of everybody.
WHAT ELSE COMES TO MIND WHEN YOU THINK OF YOUR FATHER
Bullies.
DOES THAT HAVE ANYTHING TO DO WITH THE FACT THAT YOUR BOYFRIEND
MADE YOU COME HERE

Note: Upper case represents the program ELIZA; lower case represents the patient.

Source: After Weizenbaum (1965).

fessional lore of psychotherapy, nor did it store any but the most rudimentary information about the patient being interviewed. The computer's responses were solely determined by the *surface* structure of the patient's sentences. To the extent that the program "knew" anything at all, all that it
knew were some rudimentary facts about the English language. In spite of
this, the conversation in Table 1 appears natural. Why? The answer to this
question lies not in the memory of the computer but in the mind of the
client. The client, not the computer program, brought into the interview a
certain frame of reference about how things should go, and the client's frame
of reference was imposed upon the conversation, all without the client's
knowledge. The fact that the "doctor" never evidenced any understanding of
the situation passed unnoticed.

The point of introducing this example is only partly to demonstrate
that humans can talk for some time without exchanging information. A
more important point of the illustration is that in client-professional discussions, the client is inevitably in a problem-solving situation. The client will

spontaneously provide that information which he or she thinks is relevant to the situation, in accordance with the client's frame of reference for health-related problems. The health professional may approach the same situation with different schemata which require different pieces of information to complete. Thus, the client must discover the sort of information that should be volunteered in order to complete the professional's schema of the situation.

If the client is involved in problem solving, then the client must have some goals in mind. These goals will often be mixed. Many therapies are themselves discomforting, so there is a trade-off between exposing oneself to certain, immediate pain of treatment and taking one's chances on greater pain from an untreated illness in some distant future. How one reconciles the conflict will, and should, depend upon one's understanding of the nature and consequences of the alternatives. Client-professional communications can break down if the participants in the conversation do not understand each other's background knowledge and assumptions. Such breakdowns can certainly be a factor in dealing with children, who may be quite skeptical about bitter medicine. They may be just as much a factor when dealing with people who have not learned to be as much in awe of the medical professional as is the typical middle-class American. In questioning clients, the health professional must give some consideration to the extent to which the client is likely to be motivated to give direct and relevant answers. Note that we are not talking about a situation in which the client is likely to lie. We are talking about situations in which either the client has the opportunity to volunteer information or in which the client can, quite honestly and even without awareness, shade an answer to one extreme or another.

With these considerations in mind, we offer the following practical suggestions for obtaining information from a client:

1. Whenever possible, ask about specific incidents or behaviors. Such questions reduce the probability that the symptoms reported will be interpreted by the client's understanding of medical relevance. In addition, people tend to begin recalling (or reconstructing) events from "landmarks" in memory, so the more specific the incident, the better a cue it is (King and Pontious, 1969). One cautionary note: In asking specific questions, the interrogator should be careful to avoid biasing the client. If the client can guess the expected response, it should come as little surprise that he or she will often give precisely that response.

2. When a general picture of a situation is desired, it may often be useful to ask the client to report a temporal sequence of events, rather than asking a question of the "How did you feel then?" variety. For example, one might ask, "Tell me what you did between the time you got up and the time you finished breakfast" instead of "How did you feel this morning?" Such questions are specific (see point 1) and establish a temporal frame of reference that the client can use to search memory, thus reducing the client's reliance on his or her personal medical frame of reference. In effect, such questions permit the physician's frame of reference to dominate.

We point out that this technique may also be useful when it is necessary to deal with a third-person report of how a person is behaving. Again,
we are not discussing a situation in which the third person intentionally lies,
but rather the situation in which the third person's frame of reference is used
to select information. To illustrate, a prominent gerontologist once remarked
to one of us that a son's report of his elderly mother's competence will be a
mixture of the mother's behavior, the son's belief about how the aged should
act, the wording of the mother's will, and the state of the son's business. In
order to avoid the unknown biasing effects of the reporter, a temporal frame
of reference may be used.

3. People are reasonably accurate about reporting *what* they have
done, but are quite often unable to report *why* they did what they did.
Worse yet, they will often give reasons for an action which careful analysis
will show could not possibly be true (Nisbett and Wilson, 1977). Be suspicious of any report that includes with it a statement of motivation.

Our remarks so far have been directed at any interrogation. The next
two points are directed more at a person's report of his or her own cognitive
behavior, since this is often of concern in health care situations.

4. The term *cognition* covers many phenomena. If cognitive performance is an issue in health care, the professional should first try to determine whether the impairment in question falls into the "traffic cop" or
"scholarly thinker" areas of cognition. Is the concern one of being able to
solve problems, given a substantial period of time in which to do so, or is it
one of inability to respond to many stimuli in a rapidly moving situation? In
general, the scholarly aspects of thinking seem to be quite stable from mid-
adolescence until the sixth or seventh decade. (We will later qualify this
statement somewhat.) However, the traffic cop aspects of cognition, which
depend upon the allocation of attention, can vary from day to day. As a
result, they are highly susceptible to temporary shifts in health, including
such transient effects as distraction due to colds or to the side effects of
many widely used drugs.

5. Since the scholarly aspects of thinking are normally so stable, any
change in them should be viewed seriously. Unfortunately, detecting such a
change is complicated by the wide individual differences in what we would
expect from persons in "healthy" states. Whenever it is suspected that a
person has a health-related problem that affects scholarly cognition, an attempt should be made to evaluate that person's current performance with
respect to performance prior to the onset of the current problem. In doing
so, it is far better to rely on objective records than to rely on either self-
report or the reports of others, for this is precisely the sort of situation in
which perception of the present situation may bias recall of the past.

6. There are two people involved in the information interchange, and
both bring particular frames of reference to bear. We have been stressing the
fact that a client's frame of reference will distort the information that the
client volunteers. It is equally true that the health professional's frame of
reference can distort both the information that the professional seeks and

how the obtained information is interpreted. In every interview, the client should *always* have the opportunity of volunteering information. Furthermore, the opportunity should be offered in as nonthreatening a manner as possible. "Threat," here, can be as subtle as the professional's glancing at a clock, thus indicating that the time of a busy person should not be wasted. After the client has finished volunteering information, the professional should then ask whether his or her own thinking about the case ought to be reoriented.

Giving Professional Advice

At a certain point in any conversation, the emphasis will shift from the client's provision of information to the professional's provision of advice. Presumably, the professional wishes this advice to be followed. Therefore, it behooves the professional to remember a few simple rules.

The most important of these rules is that the advice will be received by the client within the client's frame of reference. For example, there are documented cases of men consuming contraceptive drugs intended for their wives. The idea may be amusing, but the fact of an unwanted child was not. And why did this situation occur? Because the professional failed to make sure that the (quite sophisticated) frame of reference about the physiology of childbearing which the professional had was shared by the client(s). More generally, professional advice is almost always tempered by the fact that the client can reject such advice. Thus, the client's understanding of the situation must be tested so that the professional is certain that the message intended was, in fact, the message received. (See Chapter Eight in this volume.)

Quite apart from being misinterpreted, instructions may simply be forgotten. To avoid this happening, the professional should try to establish connections between the information that the client is to memorize and the situation in which it is to be recalled. An unusually effective technique for recall of specific events is the *method of loci*, which has been attributed variously to Cicero, Demosthenes, and the even more ancient poet Simoneides (Reynolds and Flagg, 1977). The idea is to establish an association between the information to be recalled and the location in which recall is to take place. For instance, while in the physician's office a patient might be asked to visualize awakening, brushing teeth, and then taking medication. The formation of images, however bizarre, can enhance this process (Higbee, 1977; Paivio, 1971). For instance, one could ask the patient to balance the pillbox on the toothbrush. Such simple tricks may seem like hokum but they are very effective memory devices.

In other cases, the information that a client is to recall may be less specific. This will occur if the client is to be alert for certain symptoms, or if there are general instructions to be followed in crisis situations. In such cases, the precise context in which recall will be required is harder to predict. Therefore, the health professional should seek to establish a number of cues that could trigger recall. One of the best ways to do this is to ask the client to rehearse instructions in several different settings, such as at home and at work, as well as in the consulting room. In this way, associations will be established between the critical information and a number of cues that will potentially be available when that information is required. In fact, successful recall during the rehearsal period will itself serve as a learning trial to associate the information further with the context of the client's everyday world.

The phenomenon of *spaced learning* provides another way to ensure recall. One of the most firmly established psychological laws of learning is that it is easier to recall information that has been acquired by rehearsal over widely spaced intervals than it is to recall information that has been learned in a single burst of study, even when the total amount of study time is equated (Melton, 1970). It is easy to make use of this law. One way to do so would be to follow up any important instructions given in an office by a telephone call the following day. This would remind the client of the information after a considerable period of time, thus taking advantage of the spacing effect. It would have the added advantage of forcing the client to rehearse the instructions in the client's everyday setting, which we have already pointed out is an advantage in itself. Finally, the advantage to patient morale of such tangible evidence that "the doctor cares" and "the instructions are important" should be obvious.

We have been stressing those problems that are caused by misunderstanding or forgetting. We should not ignore confusion. Take, for example, the classic error of any bureaucracy—producing unreadable instructions. Wason and Johnson-Laird (1972) observed that the instructions for filling out a British pension application exceeded the logical complexity of problems that were beyond all but a few British university students. Similar stories can be told about the health care bureaucracy. Spriesterbach and Farrell (1977) assert that government medical insurance records are ten times as complex as equivalent private insurance carrier forms. Nor are such errors confined to the administration of medicine. We have observed prescription of a sequence of exercises in physical rehabilitation that would have taxed the memory of an Olympic gymnast. Such things can happen because, by and large, health professionals are unusually competent with and comfortable in either the written or spoken language. Not all clients are so fortunate. The problem is particularly acute when written instructions must be given to individuals who either lack understanding of key technical terms or who, in the most pessimistic situation, are close to functional illiteracy. We must face the fact that adult illiteracy is a major communication problem. Yet, some health care instructions are inherently complex. What is to be done?

Complex sequences of instructions should be broken down into manageable steps that can be learned as a single unit. Each step should be *meaningfully* rehearsed, for the client must develop a frame of reference into which each instruction can be placed. This framework cannot be achieved by parrotlike recital, as recital alone will not ensure learning (Craik and Lockhart, 1972). It is far better for the professional to insist that the client paraphrase instructions. By the act of paraphrasing, the client will show that the gist of the instructions has been captured. A considerable body of research has shown that the gist is easier to recall than precise wording (Bransford and Franks, 1971; Sachs, 1967).

No matter how well we present verbal instructions, some clients simply will not be comfortable with them. More thought should be given to visual techniques for presenting medical advice. Depending upon the client's cognitive capacities, such aids may vary from flow charts similar to those used to describe computer programs to cartoonlike sequences used in popular advertising campaigns. For example, there are several ways that one could give instructions about water safety. It would be possible to do everything verbally:

> If you can reach the victim from the shore, lie on the ground (or plant yourself firmly) and extend your hand. If you cannot reach the victim, find a pole (or rope), lie on the ground, and extend the pole to the victim. If you cannot do either of these, you may wade into the water as far as chest deep and then extend the pole to the victim. Otherwise go for aid. Do not swim to the victim unless you are an expert swimmer and trained in rescue techniques.

These same rules are presented graphically in Figure 3. The two messages are not exactly the same; indeed, the wording is more complete, so that the verbal statement is preferable if its message is received. But the message will be received more clearly, and by more people, if the figure is used. Which method of communication is preferable? It depends on the circumstances. Our point is simply that there is a choice of communication method, and that the choice is worth thinking about. What may be boring to one audience (and in particular, what may be unduly simple when considered from the view of a highly literate health professional) may be an ideal way to communicate with another audience.

Of course, when health professionals talk to clients, they do not simply give instructions. They also make predictions about what is going to happen. These messages, which are of great importance to the client, must also be fit into the client's frame of reference. Since the client's attributions of cause and effect may often influence the outcome of medical treatment, the health professional must try to adopt the client's point of view, if only to understand how a message is likely to be received. It is not possible to cover all such situations that might arise, but the following three examples will serve to show how important and varied the frame of reference is.

Unexpected side effects of either an illness or a treatment can terrify a patient. Consider the case of sexual dysfunction. Permanent male sexual impotence due to organic processes is unusual, but temporary impotence may result from a number of infectious illnesses. A patient who is not prepared for this may become quite disturbed. Indeed, the unexpected physical symptom may produce a more long-lasting psychological impotence. An

Figure 3. Cartoon Sequence for Rescue from Drowning

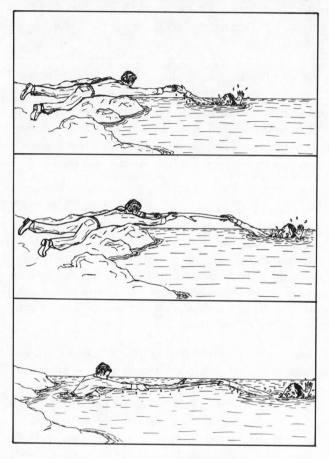

uninformed patient could require psychotherapeutic treatment that might have been avoided had there been a more careful explanation of what to expect.

Our second example of attribution was brought to our attention by a philosopher interested in medical ethics. What should a conventional practitioner do if, consistent with the client's frame of reference, treatment is being received simultaneously from reputable health care specialists and from persons who, in polite terms, are "nontraditional practitioners" and, more bluntly, may be quacks? The issue is joined if the reputable procedures effect a cure which is then attributed to the disreputable practices. This is particularly likely to occur if the patient's frame of reference includes the expectation that conventional medical practice will be ineffective. Therefore, it is consistent to believe that any relief will have arisen from the unconventional treatment. The motivation to seek such treatment and to make the resulting attribution is particularly strong if one's conventional belief is that medical science cannot help. The history of recurrent announcements of unusual cures for cancer illustrates this. Such situations produce both a psychological and an ethical dilemma. One would not want to encourage owl burning, nor lend credence to the belief that astrological signs should guide our health care practices. However, it is not ethical to withhold treatment because the therapist might not receive proper credit. The only defense that we can imagine is careful explanation of a treatment and its rationale to the client in advance and in terms that the client can understand.

Our third example of attribution involves a recently discovered fact about learning. In most training situations, the best results are achieved when the reinforcing event immediately follows the response. For instance, if you wish to train a dog to lift his paw upon hearing a bell, you should deliver a mild shock to the paw within fractions of a second after the bell is sounded. If the shock is delayed even a few minutes, the response to the bell is difficult to train. There is, however, an important exception to this general rule. Garcia and his colleagues (Garcia, Hankins, and Rusiniak, 1974) have shown that learned avoidances of foods are most easily acquired if the animal becomes sick several hours after ingesting an unusually flavored substance. The rapid response-punishment sequence that is required when sound avoidances are to be learned works very poorly with food avoidances. This sort of behavior is known as the *Garcia phenomenon*. It has been suggested that it is due to evolutionary adaptation, since the ability to learn to avoid what makes one ill would obviously increase the survival chances of an omnivore, and illness typically does not occur immediately after ingesting a poisonous substance. Bernstein (1978) has shown that the Garcia phenomenon may occur when illness is a concomitant of medical treatment. She found that patients who were receiving chemotherapy for cancer developed aversions to unusual foods that had been ingested prior to the patient's reacting to the therapeutic treatment with extreme nausea. It is important to realize that this is not a "cognitive" frame of reference effect, in the same sense that the other attributions we have discussed were. Bernstein's subjects did not consciously attribute their illness to the foods—in fact, some of them were quite aware of the effects of chemotherapy. Like laboratory rats, humans appear to have at least one inborn frame of reference, a predisposition to learn certain associations. If one were dealing with children or persons of diminished mental competence, this could become a problem in patient management.

Conversations with Clients

We began this chapter by contrasting the timeless reasoning of the scholar and the time-locked reasoning of the traffic cop. When we discuss frames of reference, we are dealing with scholarly thought. We now consider the more temporally demanding world of the traffic cop and, more generally, the problem of comprehending the world as it faces us. Patients have to do this; they must make sense out of the sometimes esoteric reasoning of the health professional and they sometimes must cope with the new and unfamiliar world of the hospital. But they have to do this at a poorly chosen time. People seek health care because they are sick, and the fact of sickness may impair their ability to reason. We shall discuss some situations in which psychological disruptions are produced as side effects but we shall ignore situations, such as brain injury, where psychological impairment is itself the major symptom.

In general, the cognitive functions most susceptible to disruption are those that require attentional resources: the manipulation of information in active memory, the maintenance of vigilance, and the ability to suppress distractions. Weakening of these simple functions of physical problems may have a disastrous effect on complex cognition because the more complex cognitive acts are built upon the simple functions. One of our own studies serves to illustrate this. We asked people to verify the truth of simple sentences such as "Plus is above star" as descriptions of simple diagrams—either a star above a plus or a plus above a star. Both the sentences and the pictures were presented visually. Thus, we produced a prototype situation in which linguistic statements are compared to conditions in the physical world. The ability to perform the task was impaired if people had to listen for a tone at the same time, even though they had to do nothing about the tone except press a button to show that they had heard it. Even this slight break in attention was enough to affect the progress of easy verbal reasoning. Our point is that physical illness itself is often a potent attention-seizing distraction. Toothaches, for instance, do not have a direct effect upon the brain but they can destroy problem solving. Furthermore, it appears that some physical illnesses reduce the "total amount of effort" one can devote to a cognitive task; the effects of alcohol and a number of sedatives appear to be partly mediated by this mechanism.

What can health professionals do with patients whose active cognitive powers are diminished? The problem is to communicate with people, but speech is so complex that it is the function most likely to be disrupted. We again offer a few guidelines:

1. Be certain that the patient's attention is captured. Conversations should take place in a quiet area with a minimum of distractions. This is particularly true when dealing with children.
2. Choose words carefully. Whenever possible, state assertions rather than negations; tell the patient what to do, rather than what not to do. It is surprisingly difficult even for healthy persons to follow the logic of negation.
3. Avoid the use of words that can be misheard as other words. A slurred "could now" can be confused with "could not." This is especially a problem if the incorrect pronunciation is meaningful. Repeating important questions or instructions with slightly different wording may also be useful.
4. As before, we urge that patients be asked to paraphrase any instructions they receive.
5. Pictorial displays are of even more use in dealing with the cognitively disabled than they are in dealing with normal individuals.

The reader will recall that we advocated spaced practice in order to ensure recall of instructions. In dealing with patients whose cognition has been impaired, spaced practice is likely to be of unusual importance for two rather special reasons. First, in learning, stimuli can be associated with internal (physiological) cues as well as with external (environmental) cues. When healthy, we probably avail ourselves more of the external context. But consider a patient in pain, for whom the physician is recommending medication. The pain cues themselves will be part of the context encoded along with the physician's instructions. As the pain diminishes with treatment, these internal cues to take the medication will also disappear. The result may be that the patient prematurely ceases taking the medication. To help prevent this, a reminder call can be made to the patient. This will help to reinstate the medication instructions in the new context, where external cues (at home or work) can become associated with the instructions. This may seem like a very common-sense sort of recommendation, but, after all, common sense is called that because it works.

Second is the related problem of state-dependent learning. Here the medication itself becomes part of the learning context and affects the associated internal cues. This effect is quite well known in the case of social drugs, such as alcohol and marijuana, but it applies to any drug with strong stimulus properties (Parker, Birnbaum, and Noble, 1976). Basically, what is learned while in the drug state is best retrieved from memory while again in the drug state. That this has to do with the role of contextual cues has been demonstrated recently by Eich and others (1975). They showed that inability to recall in a state-dependent setting diminished as better cues were provided. Enriching the associated cues is one function that spaced practice could fulfill. State dependency is not confined to drugs alone. In many situations, health care professionals must communicate with persons who are undergoing considerable physical stimulation. It is quite possible that information acquired at such a time will become associated with the transient physical cues present during learning. The only way to reverse this effect is to provide an explicit learning situation in which patients practice recalling information in a variety of contexts.

Thinking About the Client's Problems

The client is not the only person who is supposed to be thinking about health care. The professional's basic job is to acquire information about a situation, classify it, and recommend a course of action based upon that classification. (See Chapter Thirteen for some related comments.) We shall concentrate upon the psychological influences that act upon the professional during the information-gathering and classification stages. During these stages, as the decision problem is being formulated, the professional must be aware of any biases that dictate what information will be considered.

The frame of reference that a health care professional chooses will be all important, because it will guide the professional's efforts at information gathering. If a physician suspects that the patient has rubella, the patient will be examined for small red spots on the skin. If the idea of "German measles" doesn't occur, the patient's shirt may not come off. By choosing a schema, then, a professional makes a tentative diagnosis of a client as a member of a class. Logically, class membership is determined by the presence of certain defining attributes. For instance, the defining attribute of the class *mammals* is the presence of mammary glands. In deciding what class an object is "probably a member of," it appears that people do not first determine whether the defining features are present or absent, but rather they determine whether the current case resembles their understanding of a "typical" member of the class (Rosch, 1975). To continue our previous example, one's first reaction is to classify a porpoise as a fish rather than as a mammal. This appears to be because the general characteristics of porpoises are quite typical of the prototype fish. We suggest that the typical diagnosis does not proceed by the professional's saying, "On the basis of tests A, B, and C, I classify this case as an Alpha." Rather, the informal reasoning is more likely to be, "This looks like a case of Alpha, but I had better do tests A, B, and C to make sure." There is nothing wrong with such a heuristic procedure; indeed, it may be of great assistance in reducing an unmanageable set of possible tests to a set of tests that are likely to yield information.

We should be aware, however, that this decision-making method leads to characteristic errors. Chief among these is the mistake of too quickly restricting the range of hypotheses under consideration, and thus failing to make tests that would be diagnostic of the true condition. Interestingly, if one goes to a completely mechanical procedure for diagnosis, one is likely to be led into a different error—an excessive amount of time may be spent conducting nonproductive tests. For this reason, it has been suggested that the ideal diagnostic procedure would be to have a "team" evaluate each client, with the team consisting of a human and a computer-program consultant. Tests would initially be suggested by the computer, and the human would choose among them. The computer could notify the human if any line of reasoning had been overlooked completely. Prototype programs of this type have already been shown to be of considerable use in some areas of medicine (Davis, Buchanan, and Shortliffe, 1977; Feigenbaum, 1977) and will probably be in wide use by the mid 1980s.

Another characteristic human error is to treat individual cases within a class as if they were prototypical cases. People have a great deal of difficulty appreciating variability. When dealing with statistical distributions, most people will behave as if nearly all the density of the population was concentrated at the expected value. Similar stereotypic reactions occur when we deal with cognition. While it is true that the average woman in western culture has lower spatial-reasoning abilities than the average man (Maccoby and Jacklin, 1974), there are many women whose spatial-reasoning powers exceed those of many men. Cognitive functioning in the aging is an even better example. It is true that, on the average, mental powers decline in the seventh and eighth decades. It is also true that above-normal alcohol consumption is expected to accentuate such a decline, on the average. We still must be ready to accept the fact of Winston Churchill and scores of other brilliant, hard-drinking old men. The health professional should acquire a hearty respect for variation, which is a difficult thing to do, before applying statistical reasoning to individual cases.

The force of negative evidence is even harder to appreciate than the force of variation. Indeed, Sherlock Holmes demonstrated his brilliance when he observed (in "Silver Blaze") that the dog did nothing in the night, so therefore a burglar was not present. The fact that we share with Dr. Watson an inability to appreciate negative evidence can be demonstrated in experiments on reasoning with a variety of materials (Wason and Johnson-Laird, 1972). The health professional should be aware of the danger of underrating the implications of the following statement:

> If the client has disease X, test Y will be positive.
> Test Y is negative.

This observation is sufficient to determine that disease X is not present. However, if test Y were positive, then the best we could say is that disease X is still a possibility. Unfortunately, people are likely to place more weight on positive than negative evidence, even when logic dictates the opposite.

The scientific evidence that people undervalue negative information is really quite strong, so there can be little doubt about the phenomenon. We do feel, though, that a qualification should be made. The value of negative information is based on the properties of syllogistic reasoning. If X implies Y and Y is not true, then X is not true. In real life, the situation is not so straightforward. Suppose X is a disease entity and Y is a test result. Syllogistic reasoning can be applied only if Y is *known* to be true or not true. The rules of syllogistic reasoning do not allow us to say that Y is probably true or probably false. But this is often the case. Few medical tests are perfectly reliable, and many are markedly biased toward giving one result or another. The reliability of the evidence must be considered along with the implications.

At some point in the process, the health professional will make a clear-cut decision and will begin to act on it. Once this is done, there is a tendency to cut oneself off from any information that challenges the original decision. This is known to social psychologists as the phenomenon of *cognitive dissonance reduction* (Festinger, 1957). Roughly, cognitive dissonance is an unsettling condition that is produced when one is presented with information that leads one to doubt one's own rationality, and cognitive dissonance is reduced when information is obtained that confirms one's rationality. Cognitive dissonance becomes a particularly important factor in information gathering if the decision that has been made (and that may be called into question) has involved the commitment of one's prestige. Because health care practitioners, and especially physicians, have extremely high prestige in modern American society, and because they properly commit this prestige when they make diagnoses, health care experts are prime candidates for the logical errors associated with an attempt to avoid cognitive dissonance. Care must be taken to combat the human tendency to cut oneself off from any source of information that could show that one might have been wrong.

If prestige is a primary characteristic of the health-related professions, so also is harassment. Most health care professionals work hard, often under considerable pressures of time and emotion. This can have its effect on cognition. While the research is surprisingly sparse in this field, we would expect these pressures to lead, generally, to a narrowing of attention to the "most likely hypothesis" or "most relevant feature" of a case, at the expense of an examination of many alternatives. We have already noted that this is a problem in human reasoning in the best of circumstances, and we suspect that the problem is accentuated in many health care situations. Problem solving can be affected by external pressures to "get on to the next case," by fatigue, and even by diurnal variation (Folkard, 1976). If we couple all these effects with the narrowing of attention due to cognitive dissonance, how can we expect any reasonable medical decisions?

Obviously, we obtain such decisions all the time. In order to increase their frequency, there are some tricks that health care professionals can use to improve their own thinking. Our strongest piece of advice is that difficult decisions should be based partly on consultation. The ideal situation is one in which each professional makes an evaluation independently and then justifies the evaluation to a group, whose function is to evaluate ideas rather than generate them. Despite the public claims for techniques such as "brainstorming," groups are generally not efficient generators of ideas (Taylor, Berry, and Block, 1958). As we all know, the social dynamics of a group may easily control the ultimate decision-making process. Presumably, we wish to avoid this, so it may be advisable to adopt explicit rules of procedure that separate idea proposal from idea evaluation. For instance, one could always have proposals made in writing, before the meeting, and then write all proposals on the board prior to discussing any one of them. In some cases, especially when there are disparate power relationships between members of the group, it may be useful to adopt procedures that serve to equalize senior and junior members of groups. American military court-martial proceedings have an unusual and interesting way of doing this—voting is done in reverse order of seniority, so that the junior officers must express their opinion before they hear the opinion of the senior officer present. Given the marked disparity in prestige and authority in many health professional teams, this procedure could have merit in some conference situations.

The argument against group decision making is largely economic; conferences are expensive and difficult to schedule. Case conferences are routine in hospitals but may be much harder to arrange for out-patients or for patients being seen by private practitioners. There are some reasonable intermediate steps that can be taken. An individual practitioner might adopt a procedure of reviewing all decisions at least once, some time after the original decision has been made. During the second review, a conscious effort should be made to discover alternative possibilities not considered during the initial analysis. Unless the case is unusually simple, we heartily endorse the use of a formal, written decision procedure in which the practitioner justifies each step. Finally, we would urge health practitioners to keep abreast of the movement to develop computer-based consultation services, such as those referred to earlier. Table 2 presents a fragment of an interaction between a physician and one of the more successful computerized consultants, the MYCIN program for evaluating systemic infections (Davis, Buchanan, and Shortliffe, 1977). We believe that such programs will be widely available in a few years and will be an important aid in medical reasoning.

Table 2. Partial Text of a Discussion Between a Consultation Program (MYCIN) and a Physician

[*Preceding questions to determine background data.*]

(4) Have you been able to obtain positive cultures from a site at which Fred Smith has an infection?
**YES
(5) What is the infection?
**PRIMARY-BACTEREMIA
(6) Please give the data and approximate time when signs or symptoms of the primary-bacteremia (INFECTION-1) first appeared. (mo/da/yr)
**MAY 5, 1975
The most recent positive culture associated with the primary-bacteremia (INFECTION-1) will be referred to as:
------------CULTURE-1------------
(7) From what site was the specimen for CULTURE-1 taken?
**BLOOD
(8) Please give the date and time when this blood culture (CULTURE-1) was obtained. (mo/da/yr)
**MAY 9, 1975
The first significant organism from this blood culture (CULTURE-1) will be referred to as:
---------ORGANISM-1---------
(9) Enter the identity of ORGANISM-1:
**UNKNOWN
(10) Is ORGANISM-1 a rod or coccus (etc.)?
**ROD
(11) The gram stain of ORGANISM-1:
**GRAMNEG

[*Additional questions to determine identity of infecting organism(s).*]

My therapy recommendation will be based on the following probable infection(s) and potential causative organism(s):
INFECTION-1 is PRIMARY-BACTEREMIA
⟨Item 1⟩ The identity of ORGANISM-1 may be PSEUDOMONAS-AERUGINOSA
⟨Item 2⟩ The identity of ORGANISM-1 may be KLEBSIELLA-PNEUMONIAE
⟨Item 3⟩ The identity of ORGANISM-1 may be E. COLI
⟨Item 4⟩ The identity of ORGANISM-1 may be BACTEROIDES-FRAGILIS
⟨Item 5⟩ The identity of ORGANISM-1 may be ENTEROBACTER
⟨Item 6⟩ The identity of ORGANISM-1 may be PROTEUS-NON-MIRABILIS

(continued on next page)

Table 2 (continued)

---

(46) On a scale of 0 to 4, where higher numbers indicate increasing severity, how would you rate Fred Smith's degree of sickness?
**3
(47) Does Fred Smith have a clinically significant allergic reaction to any antimicrobial agent?
**NO
(48) Fred Smith's weight in kilograms (or ⟨number⟩ pounds):
**70
[Rec 1] My preferred therapy recommendation is as follows:
In order to cover for Items ⟨1 2 3 5 6⟩:
    Give: GENTAMYCIN
    Dose: 119 mg (1.7 mg/kg) q8h IV [or IM] for 10 days
    Comments: Modify dose in renal failure.
In order to cover for Item ⟨4⟩:
    Give: CLINDAMYCIN
    Dose: 595 mg (8.5 mg/kg) q6h IV [or IM] for 14 days
    Comments: If diarrhea or other GI symptoms develop, patient should be evaluated
        for possible pseudomembranous colitis.
Do you wish to see the next choice therapy?
**NO

Source: After Davis, Buchanan, and Shortliffe (1977).

Monitoring Changes in Cognition

Changes in physical state may often be associated with changes in cognitive capabilities. Such changes may be due to normal maturation or to some disease process or to the effects of a therapy provided to ameliorate a physical condition. Since cognitive capability is so much a part of our general well-being, it must be monitored as a normal part of patient management.

Assessing Cognition Through Interviews

Except in extreme cases, it is generally difficult to notice that cognition has altered, and even more difficult to be precise about how it has altered. There are very large differences in cognitive capacity within the normal range, so what is exceptionally bad performance for one person might be unusually good performance for another. Furthermore, "intelligence" does not fail, specific cognitive functions fail. If we notice that a person does not seem to be as competent as before, then saying that their intelligence is failing is no explanation at all. We have to find out specifically what it is that they no longer can do.

How do we determine whether a person is mentally competent? Both informally and in medical practice, the most common way we do this is to interview the client and form a general impression. This is a simple but dangerous tool. Face-to-face interviews are believed to be accurate by the interviewer, in spite of massive evidence that they are unreliable assessment tools (Campbell and others, 1970; Meehl, 1954). Interviews are certainly adequate for detecting gross defects associated with, say, moderate retardation or acute intoxication. We are skeptical about their utility for making finer distinctions. An interview is a social situation in which the actors are expected to play certain roles, dictated by their age, sex, social position, and the purpose of the interview. If the expected norms are violated as, for instance, they may be when a physician begins to probe about psychological rather than physical problems, the person being interviewed may become either confused or hostile. Sometimes the only defense that the client has against the perceived social threat is to refuse to communicate. Should the interviewer assume that the interviewee *cannot* give a verbal response because he or she chooses not to? Failure to answer a question is hardly evidence that one could not answer the question if one wanted to!

Particularly vexing is the problem of distinguishing between mental competence and linguistic competence. Humans are verbal animals, and much of our thought is based on language. Thus, any loss in our ability to use language as a conceptual tool is a defect in our cognitive capacity. Defects in speech production, however, can be due to purely motor problems in control of the vocal apparatus. The problem is that both the cognitive and motor defects result in overt behaviors, such as hesitant or slurred speech, that are used socially as indicators of impaired thought. In making an evaluation of a client, the health professional must be careful to distinguish between speech defects due to cognitive or motor impairment. Furthermore, the health professional should be aware of the severe psychological stress that any speech defect will place upon the client, simply because verbal facility is such an important social cue to cognitive functioning.

Mental events are private by definition, and behavior is at best an indirect way of assessing the efficiency of thought. There is a more direct way: Ask the patient how well his or her thinking is operating. People are surprisingly good at estimating their own mental capacity. The ability to estimate what one can do cognitively increases as one progresses to adulthood. In the preschool and early school years, overestimates of capacity are common, but by adolescence people should be quite accurate in knowing what they can do with their brains. This fact can be of help in assessing side effects of therapeutic measures, for the patient will be acutely aware of any diminished cognitive ability. We further suspect, although the data are less clear, that patients will be most aware of changes in their capacity for allocating attention to mental events (the "traffic cop" aspects of cognition).

There are some obvious caveats to observe in using self-reports. Since mental events are private, if the client is motivated to lie about them, lying is easy. This might occur if, for instance, any issue of legal liability arose. A second caveat is that failure to recognize one's mental capacity is itself evidence of serious disorder. The ability to monitor one's own capacities is important because this is the way we decide to deploy our attention. Mental retardates typically overestimate their capacities. We conjecture that, in certain situations wherein adults have sustained physical damage affecting mental capacity (such as senile psychoses or advanced alcoholism), the ability to evaluate one's own performance may suffer. Unfortunately, we know of no relevant studies.

Questions about cognitive capacity should be directed at what the individual can do and not at the mechanisms that are used to do it. An adult who has suffered some minor cognitive disability could, for instance, tell you whether or not he could enter a store, make a series of decisions about purchases, and complete the transaction. The same adult might be quite inaccurate in explaining how the decision to purchase a particular item was made. Furthermore, after-the-fact cognitive explanations for a particular decision are often wide of the mark (Nisbett and Wilson, 1977). The moral seems to be that people can tell you whether they will be able to muddle through but not how they will do it.

Assessing Cognition with Psychometric Tests

A psychometric intelligence test assesses mental competence through a specially designed "interview." Such tests are typically given by a trained psychologist. Depending upon the purpose of the test, a psychometric assessment may yield a "full scale" score, which assesses general mental competence (relative to some reference group) or a set of scores on subtests, each of which is supposed to measure some relatively pure aspect of mental performance. Normally, an intelligence test report will also contain a descriptive evaluation of the client. This may be more useful than the test scores themselves.

A seductively attractive aspect to psychometric testing is the provision of a single number, the famous "IQ" or something like it, as an overall assessment of the person's competence. We assert that there is no such thing as general mental competence (Hunt, 1978), so this score, unless it is very low, is apt to be misleading. Provision of separate scores for "verbal" and "nonverbal" functioning is a step in the right direction but still provides the professional with too global an evaluation. In dealing with a general psychometric test, we would first look for extreme scores, especially in the low end of the scale, as such scores usually are diagnostic of serious problems. We would then ask what sorts of scores we would have expected, given what we know about the person's background and history. We would be especially sensitive to scores that are markedly lower than a person's case history would lead us to expect, since they may be evidence of some mental disorder of recent origin. If at all possible, the health care practitioner should obtain some measure of a patient's test performance prior to illness. Change is often more interesting than the absolute level of the score.

As we have noted, general psychometric tests often provide separate scores for verbal and nonverbal mental competence. Even finer details may be given in subscale scores, which have moderate to high intercorrelations. If there is a marked disparity between subscale scores, the cause of this discrepancy should be investigated, perhaps in consultation with specialists in cognitive psychology or psychometrics.

Finally, we urge any nonpsychologists who deal with the results of general intelligence tests to read the examiner's narrative report carefully. Test scores alone cannot reflect the cognitive style of the person being examined, but style may be an important clue to the evaluation of the interplay between cognition and health care.

Cognition is not a unitary characteristic of a person in the sense that height, weight, and blood pressure are. It is better regarded as a skill, similar to athletics, that is composed from one's basic unitary mental abilities. Any physiological malfunction will affect one or more of the unitary abilities, and through them will have an effect upon cognition. For example, Turner's syndrome is a chromosomal disorder in which affected females have an XO chromosome pair. These women develop normal verbal reasoning skills but are woefully deficient in spatial reasoning (Money and Granoff, 1965). Turning to quite another etiology, it appears that disorders of the hippocampal region of the brain have a selective effect upon the ability to consolidate information from active into long-term memory (Milner, 1967). Baddeley (1977) has shown that the intake of socially acceptable amounts of alcohol can exert a marked effect upon one's ability to follow a logical line of reasoning, quite apart from any effect upon memory ability. Finally, we have already observed that phenobarbital affects one's ability to examine information in active memory but not the ability to examine information in long-term memory (MacLeod, Dekaban, and Hunt, 1978). This is true despite the apparent lack of effect of phenobarbital dosage level on the considerably more global intelligence test (Dennerll, Broeder, and Sokolov, 1964).

Results such as those just cited underline the need for procedures that assess specific cognitive functions rather than assessing general intelligence. Some medical use of such tests is being made already, especially in neurology, where the Halstead-Reitan (Halstead, 1947; Reitan, 1966) battery of cognitive tests is widely used as a means of locating specific brain injuries. We expect to see considerable development of similar, more specific tests over the next few years. Although it is often difficult to say precisely how these tests will be used for diagnosis and therapy, health science professionals should keep abreast of developments in this rapidly moving area of psychometrics.

When to Suspect Cognitive Change

In closing this section, we raise a perplexing problem. The purpose of monitoring cognitive performance in health care is to assess change relative to a person's expected performance; we are interested in *intra*-person variability. Psychometric measures of intelligence have been developed within the tradition of education rather than medicine and, as a result, are designed to measure *inter*-person variation. Imagine the case of a chronic alcoholic who was detected to have an IQ of 95, as determined by the Wechsler Adult Intelligence Scale (WAIS), a widely used measure of intelligence. This would be considered only slightly below the population norm and would not ordinarily be a cause for alarm. But suppose that the patient were a well-known lawyer who, prior to the onset of alcoholism, had a recorded WAIS score of 140? We would then be concerned. This example is a striking one. In practice, the situation is generally more subtle. Most psychometric tests are designed to be given once or twice, because practice effects can distort test scores. This is a problem that may elude a professional used to dealing with biological measures.

It is obviously not feasible to keep an extensive file of the mental performance of all potential patients. Within a few years, though, it may be normal practice to obtain profiles of mental performance for at-risk patients prior to the onset of some illness that could be accompanied by cognitive disorder. Persons in their fifties, especially where there is a record of senile psychoses in the family, persons for whom there is an indication of developing alcoholism or drug abuse, and persons about to enter a therapeutic regimen involving psychoactive drugs (including both barbiturates and stimulants) are candidates for such testing.

When there is evidence of cognitive change, one must also consider what the evidence is for permanent change. Cognitive capability, especially of the "traffic cop" variety, is labile. Efficiency in verbal tasks may vary by as much as 10 percent as a function of time of day (Folkard, 1976). Cognition is also notoriously susceptible to one's general affective mood. Thinking is work, and one of the characteristics of depression is an unwillingness to work. Informal assessment techniques, such as interviews, may be unusually prone to distortion because of transient changes in either motivation or attention.

While we would maintain that all psychological functions ultimately have a physical cause, one does not usually think of changes in attention and motivation as physical changes. There are a number of temporary physical situations that affect the "traffic cop" aspects of cognition, and these effects are most acute when the task at hand requires concentration over a substantial period of time. In addition to the drug effects previously noted, it has been suggested that extreme malnutrition can cause loss of attention and, with it, loss of many other cognitive functions. Whenever attentional deficits appear to be affecting cognition, it is well worth considering what their cause is, and determining whether or not they may be associated with a particular therapy. Assuming that some way can be found to remedy the attentional problem, the prognosis for return to normal cognitive capability is good.

Permanent cognitive defects are usually associated with structural damage to the brain, due either to mechanical injury or restriction of blood flow. There have been reports that chronic alcoholism produces damage to the hippocampal area and, with it, damage to memory consolidation functions. Similarly, there is some evidence of permanent attentional defects due to prolonged starvation, but the evidence is somewhat confusing. (The effects, if any, may occur at a level of starvation unlikely to be found in modern Western society.) Precisely what the prognosis is depends largely upon the type of functional loss. In cases of permanent disability, it may be worthwhile to expend considerable effort to determine what cognitive functions can and cannot be performed, in order to develop a mental rehabilitation program similar to a physical rehabilitation schedule.

In fact, there is now sufficient knowledge about cognition to lead to a much more elaborate technology for mental rehabilitation therapy than is now practiced. Consider, for instance, the case of a person who is reported to have "lost memory." We would first ask whether the loss is for verbal or nonverbal memory. Suppose that verbal memory has been damaged. It would be possible to train a person to use any of a number of techniques for visualizing material to be stored. A similar argument could be made for a rehabilitation program associated with virtually any cognitive defect. There are many ways in which we can execute our day-to-day cognitive tasks. A vigorous research program on mental rehabilitation, based upon a careful diagnosis of the nature of cognitive impairment, is long overdue. Such a research program could be mounted now and would have a considerable potential for payoff through its effect on medical practice.

Summary

The scholarly and traffic cop styles of thinking are both parts of thinking, but they are different parts. In a time-free analysis of a problem, the key to success is finding the right frame of reference for the current situation. We become interested in our ability to retrieve information and in our ability to recognize that the current situation is a special case of a previously observed pattern. We can only perform these functions if we have taken care to learn material in the proper way, so that it is filed properly inside our heads. When material is presented to us, it must be seen in the correct context if we are to be able to use it later.

The situation changes when we consider those aspects of cognition that allow us to react to the world around us. When we are speaking, listening, driving, or even walking and chewing gum, the key to performance is attention allocation. We do not know enough about this process, but it is reasonable to assume that within the next five years a great deal more will be known. Health professionals should watch this field for developments of value to them.

An important point for health care is that there are these separate types of cognition, and that they will be affected by different sorts of variables. Biological agents will probably have their most direct effects upon time-bound aspects of cognition. Indeed, anything that affects a person's ability to talk to others is likely to be seen as, ipso facto, something that controls cognition. However, when we give a patient information about health care, we ask that he or she play the role of scholar rather than cognitive traffic director. Thus, we must be concerned about real-time cognition as a target of therapy but more concerned about the patient's scholarly cognition as a vehicle for information reception.

As we take more notice of cognitive performance in health care and maintenance, these considerations will loom larger. We can expect that our conceptualization of health care will soon extend to maintenance of cognition; after all, most of us depend upon our wits rather than our arms and legs to make our living. Simply because the health delivery system will be forced to accept this added responsibility, we can expect to see more emphasis on tools to aid in cognitive maintenance. These will certainly include more precise procedures for testing cognitive functioning. Once these are developed, we would expect to see a rapid development in our knowledge of how specific biological manipulations, such as drug therapies, are likely to affect specific cognitive functions, such as memory for verbal material. Coupled with this increase in knowledge, we look for an increase in our knowledge about feasible methods of cognitive rehabilitation. Mental therapy will shift from the psychoanalyst's concern with abnormal personality processes to a concern with the teaching of strategies of cognition that build upon the information-processing capacities that a patient retains. Just as new methods of physical rehabilitation have made life worth living to thousands of persons who, only a few years ago, would have been doomed to live as invalids, we hope that new forms of mental therapy will lengthen the years of vigorous activity for the elderly, the recovered alcoholic, the brain injured, and the hundreds of thousands of people who, for other therapeutic reasons, must accept drugs with cognitive side effects. It may well be that, fifty years from now, psychology's contribution to health care will rest not upon its ability to ameliorate personality disorders, but rather upon its ability to rehabilitate the injured thinker.

13

Psychology
of Clinical Reasoning

Arthur S. Elstein
Georges Bordage

The rapid growth of medical knowledge and sophisticated technology has introduced new health care interventions and contributed to more intricate clinical choices. Thus, the issue inevitably raised is, which of several possible interventions should be employed in a particular case? For example, should a malignant tumor be treated by drugs, surgery, or radiation, when available evidence indicates that each is only partially effective? Should two of the treatments be combined? If drug therapy is begun, can it ethically be discontinued if the patient fails to improve? How long should we wait? Who should decide? On what basis? A host of questions concerning *how clinical decisions are made* and *how they ought to be made* arise every time a moderately complex clinical problem is examined.

At the same time, the topics of judgment, problem solving, decision making, cognition, and reasoning have become active research areas in psychology. Psychologists have sought to apply both the tools and insights of this research to problems of individual and public health (Kaplan and

Note: We are indebted to Paul Slovic, Lee Shulman, Dennis Fryback, and Sally Sprafka for their editorial comments and many helpful suggestions.

Schwartz, 1975, 1977). Clinical reasoning has been among the topics explored. Clearly, all of us have a stake in understanding how clinicians reason about the problems with which they deal and how this reasoning might be improved. The first inquiry is descriptive, the second is normative or prescriptive.

Recent reviews indicate that the psychological research on these topics is steadily increasing (Shulman and Elstein, 1975; Slovic and Lichtenstein, 1971; Slovic, Fischhoff, and Lichtenstein, 1977). These studies have been mainly carried out within one of three research paradigms: problem solving, judgment, and decision making. The problem-solving approach studies clinical reasoning from an information-processing standpoint (de Groot, 1965; Elstein, Shulman, and Sprafka, 1978; Newell and Simon, 1972). The judgment approach investigates the possibility of representing judgmental policy by means of correlational statistical models (Goldberg, 1970; Hammond and others, 1975; Hoffman, 1960). Decision making approaches clinical inference as a form of risky choice under uncertainty (Edwards, 1961; Edwards, Guttentag, and Snapper, 1975; Raiffa, 1968; Tversky and Kahneman, 1974). Each paradigm thus influences investigators to consider certain questions as more crucial than others and also conditions our view of what kind of evidence constitutes an appropriate answer.

The information-processing view of clinical reasoning aims to characterize the reasoning processes by recording and analyzing the steps and thoughts of clinicians as they attempt to solve clinical problems. The goal is to describe the process associated with the particular task and to explain it in terms of basic psychological elements and principles. Psychological research conducted within the other two frameworks has concentrated, first, on alternative mathematical representations of judgmental or decision processes and, second, on the problem of how imperfect information ought to be optimally combined. All three lead ultimately to consideration of how to improve clinical reasoning. Thus, the advantage of any single paradigm is that it provides the conceptual and methodological framework necessary to conduct an in-depth analysis of a particular aspect of clinical reasoning. However, pooling insights derived from the individual paradigms is most likely to yield an overall representation of the field.

This chapter will concentrate on a few main themes in the psychology of clinical reasoning. First, the study of clinical reasoning from an information-processing standpoint will be examined. The discussion will focus on findings derived from studies that trace the process of clinical problem solving in naturalistic settings. The second part will briefly review the judgment approach, already the best known to psychologists. The third portion of the chapter will survey decision theory, especially problems of subjective probability and utility assessment.

The goal here is not to teach clinicians how to employ these approaches to improve their reasoning, although that outcome may occur in some small percentage of readers. Our intention is to acquaint the reader with three major approaches to the analysis of clinical reasoning and to facilitate direct contact with the research literature in this field. We shall provide the reader with the conceptual background needed to understand that literature and summarize some of the salient findings. The reader will then be able to understand, analyze, and react to research using any of these approaches. We have aimed this chapter at clinicians and research psychologists who are unfamiliar with the use of these three approaches to analyze and illuminate clinical reasoning. We do not hope to make clinician-readers expert in the use of any approach, but we do hope to stimulate them to reexamine their activity in the light of the concepts and findings to be presented. For those who do or wish to do research in this field, we plan to point out areas of convergence and conflict among the three research approaches and to draw attention to places where, in our opinion, the clinical situation is least adequately represented by the research paradigms.

Information Processing

Bounded Rationality

From the standpoint of the information-processing approach, the psychological principle basic to the understanding of clinical reasoning is the concept of bounded or limited rationality (Newell and Simon, 1972). This principle emphasizes that limits exist to the human capacity for rational thought that are *not* results of unconscious motives or psychodynamic conflicts. Because of our limited information-processing capabilities, we can do some things better than others and resort to certain strategies to help overcome our inherent limitations. In considering clinical reasoning, the most relevant limit is the relatively small capacity of working memory compared to the essentially infinite size of long-term memory. This means that, in a brief time, we cannot work efficiently with all we know about a problem or all the data that could be collected. Some common features of good and poor clinical reasoning are consequences of efforts to cope with this limitation. Given the limited size of working memory, one is literally required to process data serially, to select data carefully, to represent a clinical problem in simplified ways, and to work as rationally as possible within these simplified representations. These schematized portrayals of complex situations usually do not exhaust all the possibilities but they provide some initial formulations for the problem solver. Without them it would be very difficult to make progress on solving a clinical problem of any significant magnitude. While the principles used to simplify problems are often useful, they can nevertheless lead to certain errors.

Medical Problem Solving

By representing the problem solver (the clinician) as a processor of information, "the goal of the information-processing psychologist is to define precisely the processes and states that a particular subject is using to solve a particular problem and to be able to list—for example, in the form of a computer program—the exact sequence of operations used" (Mayer, 1977, p. 133). Methodologically, the information-processing approach generally relies on direct observations of behavior combined with introspective reports to determine the thought processes used to solve a particular problem. The introspections may be obtained by having the problem solver think aloud while solving a problem or by videotaping the problem-solving session and then having the problem solver review and comment upon the performance.

A varied program of research on the psychology of medical reasoning was conducted by Elstein, Shulman, and Sprafka (1978). The core study was an in-depth descriptive analysis of the reasoning of a group of experienced internists as they performed on a number of medical and nonmedical problems. The medical problems were of varying degrees of fidelity to clinical reality. In one set, actors were trained to simulate patients, and the sequence and amount of data collection were controlled by each physician. At the other extreme, a set of paper problems was used in which both sequence and amount of data were controlled by the research team. These descriptive and comparative studies were augmented by a series of experimental investigations whose goal was to explore the role of several variables deemed to be important in medical problem solving. The use of thinking-aloud techniques and the acceptance of the problem solver's verbalizations as legitimate data place these investigations within the information-processing paradigm.

These investigators found that physicians engaged in diagnostic clinical reasoning commonly employ the strategy of generating and testing hypothetical solutions to the problem. A small set of hypotheses are generated very early in the clinical encounter, based on a very limited amount of data compared to what will eventually be collected. Often the chief complaint or the data obtained in the first few minutes of interaction with the patient are sufficient to establish this small set of working hypotheses. The clinician can then ask: "What findings would be observed if a particular hypothesis were true?" and the collection of data can be tailored to answer this question. The data collected can be used to reduce gradually the difference between the clinician's state of knowledge at any point and the knowledge needed to make a particular diagnosis.

There are four major components to this reasoning process:

1. *Cue acquisition.* Information is obtained by the clinicians by a variety of methods, including taking a history, performing a physical examination, or administering a battery of laboratory or psychological tests.
2. *Hypothesis generation.* Alternative problem formulations are retrieved from memory.
3. *Cue interpretation.* The data are interpreted in the light of the alternative hypotheses under consideration.
4. *Hypothesis evaluation.* The data are weighted and combined to determine if one of the diagnostic hypotheses already generated can be confirmed.

If not, the problem must be recycled, generating new hypotheses and collecting additional data until verification is achieved.

This reasoning process transforms the ill-defined, open-ended problem "What is wrong with the patient?" into a series of better-defined problems: "Could the abdominal pain be caused by acute appendicitis? or a twisted ovarian cyst? or pelvic inflammatory disease? or ectopic pregnancy?" This set of alternatives makes matters more manageable. By constructing a set of hypothesized end points, it becomes possible for the clinician to work backwards from the diagnostic criteria of each hypothesis to the work-up to be conducted. The search for data is simplified because only certain points will be addressed.

If a clinician proceeded purely by generating and testing hypotheses, each work-up might be totally different from its predecessors, since the set of problem formulations being evaluated would be different for each patient. But there are routine components to most, if not all, clinical work-ups. Routines are established partly as labor-saving devices. They make it easier to perform clinical work by making it unnecessary to figure out each time what will be done, thus reducing cognitive strain. Routines have other purposes as well. A problem may be so common or so important that a clinician may indeed wish to consider it for each patient, so that components of the work-up intended to explore hypotheses become routine. Routinely collected data may also suggest some additional alternatives and are thus a hedge against prematurely restricting the set of hypotheses being evaluated.

Hypothesis generation. Hypotheses are retrieved from memory, using very few cues to link up to the clinician's long-term memory store. The number of hypotheses considered simultaneously in a work-up is limited, usually around four or five. The number considered in a problem rarely exceeds six or seven. However, effective capacity can be increased by subsuming or nesting hypotheses or by substituting one for another in a reformulation so that the total number of hypotheses under consideration remains unchanged.

What principles are used to generate hypotheses? Elstein, Shulman and Sprafka (1978) found that considerations of disease incidence (frequency) were relatively more important than considerations of seriousness of disease in generating initial problem formulations. Consideration of underlying pathophysiological processes (for example, the mechanisms involved in producing jaundice in chronic progressive liver failure) was used relatively infrequently, a surprising result considering that knowledge of pathophysiology is thought to be one of the foundations of clinical medicine. It may be that the utilization of such knowledge by the experienced physician is so automatic that it is no longer in conscious awareness. Alternatively, it may be that hypotheses are generated more by consulting a network of associations in long-term memory that relate common findings to particular diseases or conditions. This network need not include much of the scientific rationale for the connections. That is, physicians could be accumulating information in the form of rough correlations between clinical findings and diseases, or conditional probabilities—statements of the probability of observing a particular finding given a particular disease. These correlations or conditional probabilities could omit statements of rationale or explanation—why a particular finding is associated with a certain condition. Such explanations would be more useful at a later stage of the diagnostic process, at the point of cue interpretation or treatment selection.

Two related strategies are used to generate most hypotheses: association from a cue or cluster of cues to a set of competing formulations and association from one formulation to additional competing formulations. The alternatives may be generated at one time based on the same set of cues or at several times using different clusters. Hypotheses are brought to mind either by a particular salient cue or by a combination of cues. As Barrows and Bennett (1972) noted in their study of neurologists, hypotheses seem to "pop" into the head of the clinician. From a psychological standpoint, strong links exist in memory between salient cues and certain hypotheses triggered by these cues.

The most salient hypotheses are identified as the most probable. But are they salient because they are subjectively probable? Or are they identified as being probable because they are experienced as vivid and salient possibilities? The work of Tversky and Kahneman (1973, 1974) on availability as a determinant of subjective probability suggests that the second explanation is likely. Errors in the subjective-probability assessments of clinicians have been found by Leaper and others (1972), a point to be elaborated in the section on decision theory. However, we wish to indicate that the theme of subjective probability in hypothesis generation is one where the information-processing and decision-making paradigms intersect.

Another useful principle in generating diagnostic alternatives is to consider deliberately competing formulations. Once a hypothesis has been generated by association from a limited number of cues, the problem solver may direct attention to thinking about competitors for this hypothesis and toward acquiring data to evaluate hypotheses. Deliberately thinking of competing formulations so as to set up the problem in the form of multiple competing hypotheses is a problem-solving strategy widely utilized by experienced physicians, apparently because it eases the burden of processing negative information, since the information that is negative for one hypothesis is positive for another. This widely recommended strategy for inference (Chamberlain, 1965; Platt, 1964) can thus be understood as an adaptation to the bounded rationality of the human information processor.

Cue interpretation. Cues are interpreted by physicians on a three-point scale: as tending to *confirm* or *disconfirm* a hypothesis or as *noncontributory*. Judgments on this scale are made spontaneously by experienced physicians. The weighting scheme is roughly equivalent to a regression equation in which only the signs of the coefficients, not their magnitudes, are important (Dawes and Corrigan, 1974). (This matter is discussed further in the next two sections.) Some clinicians feel they use a five-point scale in this inference process, but what research has been done suggests there is little difference in the predictive power of the two systems. At any rate, a three point scale and a five-point scale are both simplified ways of representing the diagnosticity of a cue that could be more formally represented by a correlation coefficient in the judgment model or by the ratio of the probability of observing this cue, given disease #1, to the probability of observing it at all in the decision theoretic model. Again, we see that the operations identified by information-processing research as those actually used in clinical reasoning are simplified approximations. The informal weighting scheme used by many clinicians is a simplified likelihood ratio that reduces the information-processing load.

Elstein, Shulman, and Sprafka (1978) found that thoroughness of cue acquisition and accuracy of cue interpretation in medicine were uncorrelated, and that diagnostic accuracy was related to both variables. Thus, inaccurate diagnosis may be due to either mistakes in data collection or in data interpretation. Further, errors in interpretation cannot necessarily be remedied by collecting additional data; indeed, the more data collected, the less likely it is that all will be used. In a related study, Gill and others (1973) reported that diagnostic error was due less to faulty data acquisition than to failure to manipulate large volumes of data correctly. However, practically any clinician can recall cases where mistakes were made because a particular item of information was omitted from the work-up. While in no way minimizing the importance of thoroughness, the point of the studies reviewed here is that greater thoroughness in acquiring data will not alone solve diagnostic problems. The data must be interpreted and integrated in the clinician's head; the difficulty of this task may be increased by adding more data, unless appropriate simplifying strategies are introduced.

Hypothesis evaluation. During a clinical work-up and especially at the conclusion of an extended sequence of data collection, the experienced clinician determines what diagnosis seems most likely *or* what actions should be taken next. In short, having interpreted individual cues or clusters of cues in terms of a set of hypotheses, the clinician must reach a diagnostic judgment. In many diagnostic problems, reasoning in this evaluation phase can be represented as a process of adding up the pros and cons for each alternative and choosing the one favored by the preponderance of the evidence. Often, the cons are ignored or discounted, as we shall see.

This simplification is another illustration of bounded rationality. We employ strategies that are satisfactory, not necessarily optimal, because to calculate the optimal strategy may be too complex a task without aids. Furthermore, the clinical work-up consists of a sequence of decisions, each made with only part of the data base. This serial data processing is, again, an adaptation to the limited size of working memory.

Potential Problems of the Clinical Method

From the information-processing standpoint, clinical reasoning is a particular form of reasoning about a specific set of problems but is governed by some principles common to all thinking. In this section, some salient features of clinical reasoning will be related to more general information-processing principles. These principles serve to explain both why clinical reasoning is ordinarily conducted as described and why certain types of errors are more common than others.

Role of hypotheses in the reasoning process. Clinical diagnostic problems are characteristically solved by formulating a small number of alternative solutions and testing them. While it is possible to reformulate the problem as one moves along and to collect some data routinely, it is nonetheless the case that these preliminary formulations help to define an area within which a solution is sought, because data collection is always selective, especially in ambulatory settings. Early formulations are essential; nevertheless, they can be misleading. They may direct attention to irrelevant features of the problem, cause the clinician to engage in a search for inconsequential cues that would otherwise be ignored, or lead the clinician to refrain from a useful search for cues that would otherwise be collected.

Barrows and others (1977, 1978) found that the number of hypotheses generated was unrelated either to successful diagnostic outcome or to level of clinical experience. They suggested that the process of hypothesis generation and testing is so characteristic of human reasoning that it occurs without encouragement or training in adults. (A similar conclusion was reached by Elstein, Shulman, and Sprafka, 1978.) Nevertheless, the most prevalent cause of incorrect diagnosis in their studies was failure to generate and consider the relevant diagnostic hypothesis. Thus, the content of the set of hypotheses being considered is crucial and is influenced by experience and expectation.

It might be simpler if clinicians were steadfastly to discipline themselves not to generate early hypotheses at all and thus avoid the biases they create. For better or worse, however, it seems practically impossible to reason without hypotheses whenever the data base is as complex as it typically is in clinical problems. People are invariably trying to make sense out of their experience as it unfolds and are always generating hypotheses to explain their observations. With experienced clinicians, these early expectations are more helpful than deceptive. Experienced clinicians also try to consider several hypotheses constructed deliberately as alternatives to those immediately suggested by the problem. Since the number that can be considered effectively is limited, it is important to work with relevant alternatives. Sheer numbers will not substitute for relevance, and massive data processing is a poor substitute for thoughtful planning.

Overemphasizing positive findings. The data in a clinical problem do not simply speak for themselves. Like all facts, they are filtered and interpreted through our expectations. The data best remembered tend to be those that fit the hypotheses generated. Where findings are distorted in recall or otherwise discounted, it is generally in the direction of making the facts more consistent with particular diagnostic pictures. The most common error in cue interpretation is to assign positive (confirmatory) weights to non-contributory findings (Elstein, Shulman, and Sprafka, 1978). Barrows and others (1977) reported that experienced physicians actively search for data to confirm hypotheses rather than to rule them out. Thus, negative findings tend to be de-emphasized. Similarly, Wallsten (1978) showed that clinical information collected in the latter portion of the work-up was systematically distorted to support prior opinions. Thus, early hypotheses tended to bias the interpretation of data collected later.

The discounting of disconfirming data is facilitated by the fact that clinical findings usually bear a probabilistic relationship to the underlying causes that produce them. As clinicians know only too well, very few signs or symptoms are pathognomonic of a particular disease. Many more are associated with several diseases, and diagnostic decisions are reached by weighing and combining evidence. One pitfall in clinical reasoning is to discount evidence that fails to confirm a favored hypothesis on the grounds that there is only a probabilistic relationship between evidence and hypotheses anyway and a perfect match is not to be expected. This error is equivalent to over-emphasizing data affirming a hypothesis and slighting data that tend to disconfirm it.

An illustration of this pitfall is found in a classic study of clinical inference (Smedslund, 1963). A group of nurses were presented with a series of cases in which the presence or absence of a particular symptom was associated equally often with the presence or absence of a particular diagnosis. Each of the four possible combinations occurred 25 percent of the time in a series of brief case descriptions, so that the correlation between symptom and disease was zero. The nurses nonetheless concluded that the correlation was positive and could, of course, point to many instances in the series to support this erroneous conclusion. Equally numerous instances of a lack of association between symptom and disease were forgotten or neglected.

Excessive data collection. Clinical decision making depends on collecting relevant data, but sometimes it is not clear what is relevant. Clinical findings are often correlated with one another, since they are effects of an underlying common cause. In this circumstance, a number of cues are, in effect, redundant and can provide little additional information on logical or statistical grounds. The clinical decision could be made just as well by a formula that used fewer variables but weighted them properly. For example, one study of the use of a battery of twelve laboratory tests (Zieve, 1966) showed that most of the meaningful information could be accounted for by a formula for weighting and combining results on just four of these tests. Positive correlations between the tests accounted for the redundancy. Similarly, Neutra and Neff (1975) showed that a very satisfactory formula for predicting high-risk pregnancy did not need to use all the information collected on a questionnaire. When redundant data are collected, they are sometimes used erroneously to bolster confidence in the judgment or decision, although the accuracy of judgment can increase but little since no new information has been provided (Oskamp, 1965).

From the clinician's viewpoint, however, there is a rationale for collecting redundant information. It is recognized that many cues have low reliabilities. For example, the reliability of many cues in physical diagnosis is not terribly high (Koran, 1975). Hence, it is reasonable to check a finding twice. However, if cues are stable and have high reliabilities, repeat observations are redundant and unnecessary. This line of argument leads to three important questions: How accurately do clinicians discriminate reliable from unreliable cues? How accurately do clinicians estimate cue reliabilities? How well do they take these into account in planning sequences of data collection? Empirical work is much needed.

When the procedures for collecting redundant information are non-invasive and relatively inexpensive, such as taking a history or performing a physical examination, the decision maker may well be uninterested in a more efficient system for information processing, for the costs of developing and maintaining it may exceed foreseeable savings or gains. But if expensive or invasive procedures are involved, careful analysis of the inference process is warranted. For example, Neuhauser and Lewicki (1975) have shown that the clinical practice of obtaining six repetitions of a particular test for colon cancer adds very little diagnostic certainty over that provided by testing twice but substantially increases the cost. Excessive numbers of tests may be ordered for another reason: limitations on the human capacity for indirect inference. A problem solver often prefers to seek direct evidence of what could be logically deduced from the data already gathered, leading to collecting more data than would be needed by a more efficient information processor (Wason and Johnson-Laird, 1972). This is yet one more consequence of the bounded rationality of the human information-processing system.

Excessive data collection may impede the process of clinical inference by overloading the system's capacity. Accurate decision making depends upon both collecting and properly interpreting clinical data. The interpretive process can be adversely affected by collecting too much data, for the sheer volume of facts may impair the clinician's ability to sort out and focus upon the relevant variables. Formal analytic techniques, or even simply drawing a decision tree or flow chart, can help to focus attention on the information that is truly relevant to the decision at hand (Sisson, Schoomaker, and Ross, 1976).

Computer Simulation and Modeling

Akin to the information-processing paradigm is the field of computer representations of psychological processes. De Groot (1966) described machine simulations as an integral part of the approach, although at that time few such realizations existed. Within the information-processing context, computer simulations are used to test out a particular theory of clinical reasoning (Bordage and others, 1977). Using analyses from Elstein, Shulman, and Sprafka (1978), the characteristic features of the clinical diagnostician have been formalized into a set of computer programs (Vinsonhaler, Wagner, and Elstein, 1977). By varying parameters in both the clinician and the task environment, the problem-solving behavior of the physician is reproduced and studied. This set of computer programs provides ways of writing computer representations of fundamental properties of both the task environment and the problem solver.

Although this first type of computer usage is intended to simulate a given psychological theory of reasoning, the computer can also be used to generate computer models of clinical reasoning processes with the aim of building a theory. In the first case, the computer simulation follows and is built from the psychological theory, whereas in the latter the computer modeling precedes and helps generate the theory. This second approach constitutes the domain of artificial intelligence (AI). The work of Myers and Pople (1977) in internal medicine and of Shortliffe (1976) in infectious diseases are two examples of the use of AI methodology in diagnostic medicine. The elaboration of heuristic strategies and the role of natural language memory structures in clinical reasoning are current avenues of psychological research where computer modeling is likely to be fruitfully employed (Epstein and Kaplan, 1977; Schoolman and Bernstein, 1978).

Information Processing as a Research Strategy

The information-processing approach to research on clinical reasoning has several strengths. First, it depends heavily on direct observation and analysis of clinical performance, even when simulated patients or problems are employed. While a psychological theory is undoubtedly employed to interpret the clinician's performance, the theory and method exercise less control over the type of data collected than is true of either judgment or decision-theoretic approaches. The researcher is thus less likely to generalize from a tightly controlled but somewhat artificial research setting to the world of clinical reality. The materials used in the research resemble closely the types of situations clinicians actually deal with, particularly when compared to the tasks typically used in the more quantitatively rigorous research pursued within the other two frameworks. For this reason, the rationale and research findings are communicated relatively easily to clinicians. Lastly, the conceptual framework used to analyze the data is closely related to the information-processing view of cognition now receiving so much attention. Research on clinical reasoning conducted from this standpoint connects naturally and directly with the active research areas of problem solving and memory. For those psychologists interested in theoretical coherence, this is a powerful reinforcement.

But the method has drawbacks too. Because the situations studied typically require a great deal of time, it is often possible to sample the subject's performance on only a limited number of problems. The use of more highly restricted task environments would make it possible to collect and analyze more instances of clinical reasoning within a given time. Since one of the major findings of research in clinical problem solving is that the strategies selected by the clinician are highly case related, concentrating on a small set of problems is a threat to generalizability at the same time that the detailed analysis of particular problems is one of the virtues of this approach. In addition, the information-processing approach yields a set of guidelines or heuristics for improving clinical reasoning, but the evidence that applying these systematically will indeed improve clinical judgment is not yet compelling. An information-processing analysis yields descriptions, understanding, and explanation of complex sequences of behavior, but these may not be the most efficient way to improve the output. Other research avenues that deliberately compare human performance to mathematical models may have greater potential in this regard.

In this connection, it may be noted that in discussing possible problems and pitfalls of clinical reasoning in this section, we drew also upon research conducted in the judgment and decision-theory traditions. We tried to show how the observed shortcomings could be understood either as consequences of or adaptations to bounded rationality, especially to the limited size of working memory. The two approaches to which we now turn have been, on the whole, more concerned with developing techniques and strategies to overcome these tendencies to error by providing a variety of aids to the reasoning clinician.

Judgment

Clinical Judgment

The central questions asked within the judgment paradigm are: How do clinicians use and weigh the information given to them to make a judgment about some criterion event, such as a diagnosis or treatment? How consistent are the judgments across judges and across similar situations? Finally, how accurate are the judgments in comparison to a criterion?

The dichotomy between the judge (person) and the criterion event (environment) led Hammond and his co-workers to elaborate a conceptual framework for judgmental studies based on Brunswik's lens model (Brunswik, 1955; Hammond, 1955, 1975, 1977; Hammond and Adelman, 1976; Hammond and others, 1975). The lens model, depicted in Figure 1, uses the analogy of a convex lens to illustrate the relation between a *judge's perception* or estimate (Y_s) and the *object of perception* or criterion (Y_e), as mediated by a set of cues $(X_{1,k})$. The cues are related probabilistically to both the judgment and the object. Thus, "judgment is a cognitive process similar to inductive inference, in which the person draws a conclusion, or an inference, Y_s, about something, Y_e, which he cannot see (or otherwise directly perceive), on the basis of data, X_k, which he can see (or otherwise directly perceive). In other words, judgments are made from palpable events and circumstances" (Hammond, 1975, p. 73). The arc, r_a, linking Y_s and Y_e, indicates the degree to which the person's judgment (Y_s) was correct (overall judgmental accuracy); that is, the extent to which the judgment made coincides with the actual event to be judged. The lens model can be used, for

Figure 1. The Lens Model

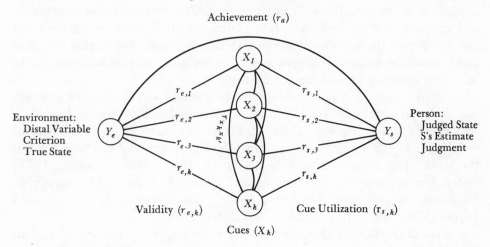

Cues (X_k)

example, to depict a clinician examining a patient with a certain number of clinical findings (X_k = symptoms, signs), such as headache and elevated blood pressure, and making a judgment (Y_s) concerning the patient's diagnosis (Y_e), such as hypertension or tension headache. Furthermore, the correlation r_a will indicate diagnostic accuracy over a series of cases (the hit rate).

Hoffman (1960), in a classic paper, suggested the use of a linear model (multiple regression equations) as a representation of clinical judges. He emphasized that the model was a *paramorphic* representation of the clinicians' policy and was to be interpreted as performing like the judges and not as describing actual information-processing strategies (Shulman and Elstein, 1975). The elements of the model include: the information given (cues, findings, attributes), their relative importance (weights), and their functional relationships (the combination rules). In the linear model, judgments are formulated as a simple weighted sum of the values of the information available. The weighted additive model can be mathematically represented as: $Y_s = C_o + w_1X_1 + w_2X_2 \ldots w_kX_k$, where Y_s represents the judgment, X the k different pieces of information available, w the relative weights, and C_o a constant.

In this approach, the investigator presents information in the form of separate cues to the judge, whose task it is to respond with a numerical or categorical classification (Cook and Stewart, 1975; Einhorn, 1974b). A regression equation is computed using these judgments as the dependent variable, and the equation is said to have captured the judge's policy (Hoffman, 1960; Slovic and Lichtenstein, 1971). For example, Moore and others (1974) asked six clinical endocrinologists to choose one of three treatments for an overactive thyroid on the basis of five pieces of clinical information. The use of the five findings was captured by a multiple regression equation in which the weights reflected each clinician's relative use of the available information. As is typical in studies of this type, analysis of the relative weights showed that the clinicians effectively used fewer than the five items in making their judgments. Overall, they tended to ignore laboratory data and concentrated on medical history. Thus, the clinicians were selective and did not use all the information given. The study implies either that the clinicians should be trained to attend more to laboratory data or that costs could be cut by omitting unused laboratory tests.

Policy capturing has been applied to a wide range of situations including: the interpretation of Minnesota Multiphasic Personality Inventory (MMPI) profiles (Goldberg, 1965, 1969; Kleinmuntz, 1963, 1968; Wiggins and Hoffman, 1968) and of x ray films (Slovic, Rorer, and Hoffman, 1971); the work of admissions committees (Dawes, 1971, 1977; Goldberg, 1977) and police departments (Hammond and Adelman, 1976); and a variety of judgments in pathology (Einhorn, 1974a), pharmacology (Hammond and Joyce, 1975), and nursing (Zedeck and Kafry, 1977).

Goldberg (1970) showed that the same regression equations used to describe a set of judgments can also generate a set of predictions that will be more accurate than the judges' unaided predictions of the same series. The use of the equation to improve judgment is termed "bootstrapping." For example, Goldberg used the regression equations that represented the judgments of twenty-nine clinical psychologists in distinguishing psychotic from neurotic patients, on the basis of their MMPI profiles, to generate predictions of undiagnosed patients. He concluded that "linear regression models of clinical judges can be more accurate diagnostic predictors than are the humans who are modeled" and that "the composite judgment of all twenty-nine clinicians, which was more accurate than that of the typical individual judge, was not improved by the modeling procedure" (1970, p. 430).

Besides the previously described correlation between true and judged states (r_a), three additional correlations are used in a lens model analysis. The second correlation, R_e (see Figure 2), indicates how well the underlying reality can be predicted by the best possible weighted linear combination of the available cues. R_e measures the predictability or uncertainty of the envi-

Figure 2. The Lens Model (Expanded Version)

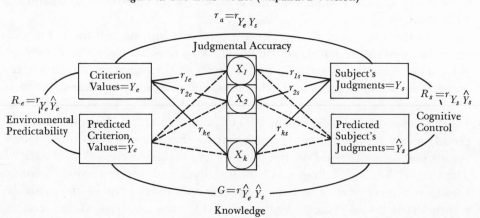

ronment (criterion) that is being judged. A third correlation, R_s, indicates how well a set of judgments can be predicted by a weighted linear combination of cue values and thus captures the judge's policy: Hammond and Summers (1972) identified this term as "cognitive control," the extent to which a subject controls the utilization of his knowledge. Knowledge of the environment, the fourth component, is represented by the correlation G between the regression predictions of reality and of the judgments. These four correlations are related (under a linear assumption) in a formula known as the lens model equation: $r_a = GR_eR_s$. The formula states that judgmental accuracy is limited first by the degree to which the task is predictable, R_e. Beyond that, accuracy is determined by knowledge of the properties of the task, G, and by cognitive control over the utilization of that knowledge, R_s. Furthermore, knowledge and cognitive control are statistically independent. Thus, to improve judgments one may either increase knowledge of the task or increase the consistency with which existing knowledge is used (Hammond and Summers, 1972).

A number of controversial issues are raised by this research paradigm. We shall consider three of these: clinical versus statistical prediction, linear versus configural models, and unit versus differential cue weighting.

Clinical Versus Statistical Prediction

Clinical refers to any artful or intuitive means used by clinicians in reaching a diagnostic or therapeutic decision. *Statistical* (or actuarial) refers to the use of any formal quantitative techniques or formulas, such as regression equations, for these same clinical tasks. The controversy regarding the merits of these two approaches includes discussions of the role and the accuracy of statistical predictions in clinical psychology (Elstein, 1976; Hoffman, 1960; Holt, 1958; Meehl, 1954). Moreover, it raises yet another fundamental issue regarding the aims of research on judgment, namely whether it should be descriptive (Kleinmuntz, 1969) or prescriptive (Goldberg, 1970). Gough (1962, p. 527) characterized the controversy in the following terms: "By its proponents the statistical method has been described as operational, objective, reliable, sound, and verifiable, whereas by its opponents it has been called atomistic, pedantic, artificial, static, and pseudoscientific. The clinical approach, on the other hand, has been called dynamic, meaningful, deep, genuine, and sophisticated by its adherents, but by its opponents vague, hazy, subjective, unscientific, and verbalistic." Goldberg (1968, 1970), Sawyer (1966), and Einhorn (1972), among others, explored optimal blends of clinical and actuarial processing. These typically involve using clinical methods to gather preliminary information or to make subtle observations, and actuarial methods to combine the data for final decisions—hence, Einhorn's apt phrase, "expert measurement and mechanical combination" (1972).

A contemporary version of this controversy centers currently around the issue of "case uniqueness" (Dawes, 1977; Einhorn and Schacht, 1977). What is the trade-off between consistently using a judgmental rule with a fixed number of cues (as obtained through a policy-capturing procedure) and the deliberate consideration of an unexpected cue that is salient but not universally distributed? Whereas clinicians may feel short-changed by using a simplified regression equation, researchers praise its accuracy and prefer to ignore incidental cues. In his study of graduate admissions committees, Dawes (1977) argued that rule-generated procedures (actuarial) are superior to case-by-case procedures (clinical). In reviewing the merits of the approach, Dawes (1977, p. 90) held that it "probably predicts graduate success better than does clinical judgment . . . it is fair and just in that it treats everyone alike . . . it supplies potential candidates with knowledge of how they are to be evaluated, it makes us publicly accountable for our decisions, and finally . . . it saves a great deal of time and effort."

Linear Versus Configural Models

This debate focuses on the form of the rules for combining data. Is the linear model an adequate representation of the judgmental process? Along with the linear model, Hoffman (1960) had also proposed a configural model that would include interaction terms to account for the possibility that a particular judge interprets one item of information as contingent upon a second: see $r_{x_k x_k'}$ in Figure 1. Subsequently, such researchers as Goldberg (1968, 1971), Hoffman (1968), and Einhorn (1970, 1972) proposed a variety of nonlinear models. In general, however, the addition of configural terms to the linear model (for example, exponential components) has failed to improve its accuracy as assessed by the proportion of variance in human judges' performance accounted for by the statistical representation (Goldberg, 1971; Dawes and Corrigan, 1974). Although clinical judges insist that they are using cues configurally, the simple linear model continues to represent judgments adequately. As previously stated, the judgment approach is paramorphic and does not intend to represent isomorphically the judge's mental process.

Unit Versus Differential Cue Weighting

How important is the calculation of exact weights to be assigned to each cue? Dawes and Corrigan (1974) and Schmidt (1971) found that by randomly assigning weights of the same sign or by assigning equal weights, the resulting linear model still did as well as (or better than) the original "captured" weights in predicting criterion values (Y_e on the left-hand side of the lens model). Dawes and Corrigan further investigated the use of unit weights (that is, +1 and −1) and found that the unit weights did extremely well in predicting the criterion. They concluded that "decision makers (insofar as they are behaving appropriately) are paramorphically well represented by linear models. . . . The whole trick is to decide what variables to look at and then to know how to add" (1974, p. 104). Accordingly, exact specification of differential weights does not appear to be critical. However, Schmitt and Levine (1977, p. 28) recently suggested that "much interesting and important research can be done on subjective weights. This conclusion is based on the fact that there are several statistical weights, and a convincing rationale for the use of one over another is unavailable." Recent research (Molidor, 1978) has shown that differential weighting models (both statistical and subjective) account for more variance on the right-hand side of the lens model than do the unit weighting models. Furthermore, additional differences were found depending on how the weighting models were computed. A unit-weighting model using raw scores yielded poorer predictions of actual judgments than did a unit-weighting model using standard scores.

The judgment paradigm intends to be both *descriptive* and *prescriptive*. It describes clinical judgments by means of multiple regression equations or similar formulas. It prescribes how to improve judgment when it points to the improvements achieved by use of a formula instead of human judgment. Studies of judgment are thus helpful to practicing clinicians in that they can explicitly describe and prescribe utilization of clinical information already available. Decision theory considers also the problem of acquiring information.

Decision Theory

Clinical Decision Analysis

A third approach to the psychological study of clinical reasoning derives from studies of decision making and the basic concepts used in these studies, collectively known as *decision theory*. Many of these concepts originated in the work of economists and applied mathematicians (Bunker, Barnes, and Mosteller, 1977; Kaufman and Thomas, 1977; Raiffa, 1968). Whereas psychologists have concentrated on the problem of understanding observed choices, decisions, and departures from rationality, these scholars are searching for models to prescribe rational choice under conditions of uncertainty. The fundamental question is: How should choices be made? Decision theory is much concerned with the costs and benefits of decisions as well as with diagnostic accuracy. The definition and measurement of costs and benefits, however, are themselves thorny problems, once we move past the basic fiscal dimensions that were of initial interest to economists.

To illustrate how this approach can be applied to research on and teaching of clinical reasoning, consider a physician dealing with a patient with acute abdominal pain (Neutra, 1977). If it were known for certain that the pain is caused by appendicitis, surgery would be indicated, but if it were known that the cause of the pain is nonsurgical, then other action—perhaps bedrest at home—would be appropriate. Unfortunately, it is impossible to be certain about the underlying state without surgery and that always has some risk. A physical examination and some laboratory tests before surgery may reduce this uncertainty but cannot eliminate it. What should be done?

To answer this question, the clinician should consider the *probability* of each possible state. Sometimes objective estimates may be available; for instance, it may be well established that 25 percent of all cases previously presented with similar abdominal pain have been found to have appendicitis, so that the prior probability of appendicitis is .25. But if quantitative data are unavailable, clinical experience can be used to provide subjective probabilities. The heart of the Bayesian position is that subjective probabilities, interpreted as *degree of belief* about states of nature, can be unhesitatingly substituted for probabilities based on counting events. As data are collected, initial differences in prior subjective probabilities will be reduced. Concluding or *posterior* probabilities will be much closer together (Phillips, 1973) than the prior opinions were. From this perspective, one function of the extensive data collection characteristic of so much clinical work is to overcome differences in subjective probability that existed prior to these extensive observations. In this way, clinicians can move toward consensus on the posterior probability of a particular diagnosis and from this consensus gain confidence that will support their action.

In addition to probabilities, however, clinician and patient must also consider the possible *outcomes* of each alternative action. The *value* or desirability of each outcome should be distinguished from the probability of its occurrence. Decision analysis (Ginsberg and Offensend, 1968; Pauker, 1976; Raiffa, 1968) is a method for systematically assessing values on a common scale (formally called *utility*) and for choosing an action that maximizes expected utility.

The usefulness of decision theory derives from some commonplace observations about clinical reasoning. What is the process of clinical reasoning? By sequentially collecting data (clinical findings) and then using these findings to revise and update opinion, the clinician moves from a state of relative uncertainty about a clinical problem to one of relative certainty. Diagnostic and therapeutic actions are available and the clinician must choose what to do. The choice of action is thus under the decision maker's control. However, the underlying condition of the patient (which may be conceptualized as possible "states of nature") is not.

Some uncertainty about either the diagnosis or the outcome of treatment is almost always present, despite the clinician's best efforts to reduce it. Consequently, "the selection of diagnostic-treatment strategies can be usefully viewed as a sequential decision problem under uncertainty" (Betaque and Gorry, 1971, p. B-422). From this standpoint, the fundamental elements in the analysis of a clinical problem are:

1. *Actions* that are available and that are controlled by the decision maker's choice.
2. *States of nature*—the different possible states that the patient could be in. In medicine, these possible states are diagnostic alternatives.
3. *Outcomes or consequences*—the results of taking particular actions. While good clinical practice tries to control these, outcomes cannot be guaranteed and so are conceptualized as chance or noncontrolled.

4. *Probabilities*—estimates, either subjective or objective, of the likelihood that each listed state of nature is in fact the case, or that each outcome will occur, or of observing a particular sign or symptom in a particular state of nature.
5. *Utilities*—assessments of the value of each possible outcome, carefully distinguished from the probability of its occurrence.

Bayes' Theorem

Decision theory is concerned with the process whereby probability estimates are obtained, revised in the light of new evidence, and then combined with assessments of value to select preferred actions. Typically, clinicians collect information in order to revise opinions about diagnosis or to select a treatment. How much impact should a particular item of information have?

Suppose a clinician is contemplating two distinct diagnoses and these are the only relevant alternatives in the problem. On the basis of information already obtained, it appears that one alternative is twice as likely as the other. In this case, $P(D_1) = .67$, and $P(D_2) = .33$. These are called the *prior probabilities*. A laboratory test is contemplated which yields a positive finding 80 percent of the time if the patient has Disease #1 and only 5 percent of the time if the patient has Disease #2. The test is performed and is positive. What are the probabilities of D_1 and D_2 now? (These are the *posterior* probabilities.)

Bayes' Theorem is the formally optimal rule for revising probabilities in the light of new evidence that is itself probabilistic. A detailed discussion of the principles is provided by Phillips (1973). Here we wish only to sketch out the approach.

The relation among the probabilities set forth in the above example is:

$$P(D_1 | \text{Test+}) = \frac{P(\text{Test+}|D_1)\, P(D_1)}{P(\text{Test+}|D_1)\, P(D_1) + P(\text{Test+}|D_2)\, P(D_2)} \tag{1}$$

The expression $P(D_1 | \text{Test+})$ is read as "the probability of the patient having Disease #1 given a positive test." Carrying out the calculations we have:

$$P(D_1 | \text{Test+}) = \frac{.80 \times .67}{(.80 \times .67) + (.05 \times .33)} = \frac{.536}{.536 + .0165} = .97 \tag{2}$$

Similarly:

$$P(D_2 | \text{Test+}) = \frac{.05 \times .33}{(.05 \times .33) + (.80 \times .67)} = \frac{.016}{.0165 + .536} = .03 \tag{3}$$

The positive test has shifted the probabilities from .67 and .33 to .97 and .03, respectively.

Since the denominator in Equations 2 and 3 is identical, it is possible to form a ratio of the numerators of the two expressions:

$$\frac{P(D_1|\text{Test}+)}{P(D_2|\text{Test}+)} = \frac{P(\text{Test}+|D_1)\,P(D_1)}{P(\text{Test}+|D_2)\,P(D_2)} \qquad (4)$$

This equation restates Bayes' Theorem on odds form: $\frac{P(D_1)}{P(D_2)}$ is the prior odds, $P(\text{Test}+|D_1)\ /\ P(\text{Test}+|D_2)$ is known as the likelihood ratio, and $P(D_1|\text{Test}+)\ /\ P(D_2|\text{Test}+)$ is known as the posterior odds. The theorem states that the posterior odds is the product of prior odds times the likelihood ratio.

Examples of clinical applications of Bayes' Theorem are provided by Lusted (1968), Fryback and Thornbury (1976), Pauker (1976), and Pliskin and Beck (1976). Significant contributions to the psychology of decision making are to be found in the work of Edwards and his collaborators (Edwards, 1961; Edwards, Lindman, and Phillips, 1965; Edwards and Tversky, 1967; Edwards, Guttentag and Snapper, 1975). Slovic and Lichtenstein (1971) and Slovic, Fischhoff, and Lichtenstein (1977) have reviewed the psychological literature on decision making extensively. Gustafson and Huber (1977) stressed the use of decision theory in health, medical, and policy problems. Rather than recapitulating and summarizing this research, we wish to expand the discussion of the fundamental concepts outlined above and to consider some of the significant psychological questions about clinical reasoning raised by decision theory.

Three major categories of questions concern: (1) subjective estimates of probability; (2) the revision of opinion in the light of new information; and (3) the assessment of the value, attractiveness, or utility of different outcomes.

Subjective Probability

Some probabilities are based upon the relative frequencies of different events and are often called "objective probabilities." If we observe that 25 percent of all patients with certain signs and symptoms turn out to have a particular disease, we can say that the probability of a patient having that disease, given the presence of these same findings, is .25 and we can write:

P (Disease|Findings) $= .25$ or $P(D|F) = .25$ (the vertical bar is read as "given")

If good statistical data are lacking, and we say that in our opinion there is a 25 percent chance of a particular patient having this disease, we may be right or wrong, but the probability statement refers to a degree of belief, not a rate of occurrence. The mathematical and philosophical arguments for using subjective or personal probabilities interchangeably with objective probabilities center around showing that both kinds of numbers obey the same laws of probability (Raiffa, 1968, especially chap. 5). The psychological problems of subjective probability are quite different. They involve the psychological processes used to generate the numbers we call subjective probabilities, how accurately these quantities can be estimated, whether different means of estimating them make a difference, and what laws govern their revision when the decision maker does not use Bayes' Theorem.

How are subjective probabilities generated? Tversky and Kahneman (1974) have identified three heuristic principles that are commonly employed to generate subjective probability estimates. These are representativeness, availability, and anchoring and adjustment. Each may lead to biased judgments under conditions of uncertainty.

The principle of *representativeness* is employed when the probability of an uncertain event is estimated by judging the degree to which the event is similar in essential properties to a larger class. It is a principle that is erroneously insensitive to sample size and to the prior probability of outcomes. Suppose the clinical picture of a particular case resembles but does not exactly match the typical picture of two alternative conditions, one more common than the other. Because the observed findings of the case fit both larger classes about equally well, many clinicians would judge both alternatives to be equally probable. In so doing, they have ignored the different prior probabilities of the two alternatives and have employed the representativeness principle. Kahneman and Tversky (1973) have shown that when no case data are provided, clinical psychologists and other judges utilize base rates and prior probabilities appropriately, but that when the clinician is given a brief case history of questionable validity, base rates tend to be ignored and probability estimation by resemblances tends to become more dominant. This phenomenon illustrates the working of representativeness.

Availability is employed when the probability of an event is judged by the ease of recalling instances or occurrences of similar events. In general, of course, it is true that more frequently occurring events are more readily remembered, but psychologists know too that meaningfulness affects recall and thus, according to this principle, judgments of probability. Observations that do not make sense tend to be forgotten, although, from a statistical point of view, they should nonetheless be tabulated in memory. Memory is also affected by salience, by how outstanding an event seems to be. In clinical work, this often means that what might be called exoticism receives undue weight: Commonplace events tend to be forgotten but unusual ones are remembered well. Every clinician can remember an unusual case whose probability is consistently overestimated despite the fact that it was seen only once. Availability is also affected by imaginability. It is easier to imagine the hazards of a disaster than it is to assess its actual likelihood, a principle widely understood by the insurance industry. The probability of a serious illness, such as a brain tumor, is overestimated every time a medical student concludes that the problem is cancer when the patient complains of headaches. Some evidence exists to suggest that this phenomenon occurs among experienced clinicians as well (Detmer, Fryback, and Gassner, 1978). Wallsten (1978) has reported another variant of the availability bias: The subjective probability of serious diseases seems to be overestimated, perhaps owing to the unwillingness of clinicians to miss a case. The cost of an error makes these alternatives more salient, and this salience, in turn, is translated into an excessively high subjective probability. Wallsten calls this a value-induced bias. This bias is contrary to one of the principles of mathematical decision theory—that estimates of probability and value must be independent of each other. (Another interpretation of these studies must be mentioned. Since the clinicians in these studies were asked only for probabilities, their responses are interpreted as overestimations. Yet it is possible that their impressions included some estimate of the cost of a false negative, and that the restrictions of the response mode obscured this element.)

In many situations where a probability estimate is required, people start from an initial value that is adjusted to yield the final answer. These adjustments are typically insufficient and are not much affected by whether the subjects are given a starting point or choose their own or by rewards of accuracy. This phenomenon is called *anchoring* (Tversky and Kahneman, 1974). The repeated demonstrations of conservatism in judgment that will be summarized later are quite likely based on the natural use of this heuristic.

These biases have all been demonstrated in tasks where very little data collection followed the initial estimation of a prior probability. Extensive data collection is a significant component of most clinical activity, however, and so, substantial opportunities exist to revise initial estimates if they are biased. How significant then are these biases in lowering the quality of clinical decisions? It is very difficult to answer this question. Presumably, both the criterion of quality and the decisions being assessed are affected by these biases. Rarely have enough good statistical data been gathered to permit extensive comparisons of decisions based on probabilities derived from different sources.

How accurate are clinical subjective probabilities? Subjective probabilities will be used in analyzing most clinical decisions since trustworthy probabilities based on good statistical data are rarely available. Thus, two questions arise: How accurate are clinical subjective probabilities? What difference do errors in these estimates make in the process of clinical decision making?

Research on the first question is not overly encouraging. One of the problems that plagues our subjective estimates of probability is overconfidence. We tend to be more confident about the accuracy of our guesses than is warranted. Fischhoff, Slovic, and Lichtenstein (1977) asked volunteer college students to respond to a questionnaire on the perceived frequency of a variety of causes of death in the United States, ranging from very rare lethal events such as measles to common causes of death such as cancer, stroke, and heart disease. The lethal events were selected because they had fairly stable death rates over the last five years for which statistics were available. Each item in the questionnaire consisted of two possible causes of death. The respondents were asked to select the cause thought to be more frequent and then to decide how confident they were about their choices. Extreme overconfidence was the predominant response. For example, on those items where the respondents gave odds of 50:1 on their preferences, they were saying they expected to be right 98 percent of the time in selecting the more frequent cause of death. Actually, only 68 percent of those choices were correct. Following a training period that included explanation of the use of odds, respondents were correct only 74 percent of the time on items where they gave 50:1 odds (1977, pp. 556-557). They should have been giving odds of about 3:1 and so were exhibiting unjustified certainty or overconfidence.

It might be argued that Fischhoff, Slovic, and Lichtenstein did not study the estimates of expert clinicians, and that experts are more accurately calibrated. There is mixed evidence for this proposition. Oskamp's (1965) study of overconfidence among clinical psychologists was discussed earlier. In a similar vein, Gilbert, McPeek, and Mosteller (1977) presented data on the relation between degree of enthusiasm for a particular surgical intervention (portacaval shunt) and degree of control of the study. They cited a review of fifty-three studies of the treatment and found that enthusiasm was greater when the study was poorly controlled or uncontrolled. Arguing for more rigorous clinical trials, they paraphrased Muench (in Bearman, Loewenson, and Gullen, 1974), who said that nothing improves the performance of an innovation as much as the lack of controls. Since degree of belief in an unproved proposition is nothing more or less than a subjective probability, the investigators in the original studies were collectively exhibiting unwarranted confidence.

A small number of studies deal with the problem of the validity of subjective probabilities in clinical medicine. Gustafson and others (1971) compared two systems for the differential diagnosis of thyroid problems. Both used prior probabilities derived from epidemiological data but differed in that one system used subjective estimates of the diagnosticity of certain laboratory tests, whereas the other system used estimates derived from statistical analysis of a large number of cases. There was little difference in the average probabilities assigned to the correct diagnosis by the subjective or the actuarial model.

Leaper and others (1972), however, found that a computer program for the diagnosis of acute abdominal pain was not more accurate than intuitive clinical judgment when subjective estimates of the probability of observing a certain symptom given a particular disease, $P(S|D)$, were entered into the program. The computer exceeded clinicians' accuracy, however, when it was given conditional probabilities derived from statistical analysis of a large sample of cases. Further analysis showed that the clinicians' subjective estimates were substantially in error in many instances. This finding is especially distressing since the estimates sought were not of the frequency of especially rare or unusual diseases, where probability estimation is known to be difficult. Rather, clinicians were asked to estimate the probabilities of certain symptoms given certain diseases, a matter about which physicians could reasonably be expected to be knowledgeable and where the probabilities estimated are not uniformly small.

The apparent discrepancy between the results of these two studies may be in their methods. Gustafson and others asked their subjects for likeli-

hood ratios, whereas the Leaper group asked directly for conditional probabilities. It may be that physicians are relatively poor at the latter task but
can do better at comparative judgment. This interpretation is consistent with
the observation (Elstein, Shulman, and Sprafka, 1978) that clinicians were
willing to rank order diagnostic hypotheses in order of likelihood but were
exceedingly reluctant to estimate probabilities more quantitatively. Selvidge
(1975) too found that people are fairly good at rank ordering events but
relatively poor at selecting absolute values to describe their probabilities.

Two other studies indicate that physicians are reasonably well calibrated. Thornbury, Fryback, and Edwards (1975) studied the use of information provided by intravenous pyelogram (IVP) on the part of six urolo-
gists. As part of the study, a questionnaire was designed to replace the usual
x ray request form. The referring physician was asked to summarize the
pertinent facts and findings of the case and the elements of the problem
about which the IVP was to provide further information, and also to make
some judgments about diagnostic certainty prior to seeing the IVP results.
One judgment was an estimate of the probability that the IVP result would
be normal. Eighty-eight questionnaires on which the question was answered
were analyzed. The investigators found that as the estimated probability of a
normal x ray increased, so did the relative frequency of a normal result.
They concluded that physicians untrained in probability estimation *can* convey usable information with numerical estimates and that these subjective
estimates *are* fairly well calibrated.

Fryback (1974) investigated the calibration of subjective probabilities
in choosing the next step in the diagnostic work-up of a renal lesion that had
been identified by excretory urography. As part of the research, six radiologists provided probability estimates both in odds form and in standard probability (percentage) form. The usefulness of these alternative forms was
assessed by evaluating average expected cost of diagnosis. Given this criterion, most of the radiologists were better able to convey their beliefs about
expected diagnoses in the form of probabilities rather than odds. Despite a
moderate amount of error in their prior probabilities, the average cost of the
decisions made by five of the radiologists could be improved by using their
probability estimates in a decision analysis, compared to the cost of their
unaided intuitive recommendations. Their judgments, however, did not
achieve the level of average cost obtained by using the estimates of the sixth
radiologist, who was the most experienced both in clinical radiology and in
decision analysis. Cost in this study excluded dollar costs, because the clinicians stated it did not matter, and included subjective costs due to time lost,
discomfort, and risk of complications.

Fryback's study suggested, as have other investigations, that a model
for medical decision making based on an expert's judgment may improve
upon the judgments of less expert physicians, even when the latter's estimates are processed systematically by the Bayesian model. The discrepancy
between this result and the findings in the study of computer-assisted diagnosis of acute abdominal pain may stem from the magnitude of the calibra-

tion errors of the two panels of physicians or from the use of different criteria for assessing the effects of the errors: Fryback used costs, whereas Leaper and others employed diagnostic accuracy.

We began by asking whether subjective probabilities provided by clinicians can be believed. This is not a simple question as the literature is conflicting. On balance, it seems that clinical experience and experience in making estimates both facilitate accuracy, and that the accuracy of those estimates may also be a function of specialty. It is unclear what is the best way to ask clinicians for estimates—probabilities, odds, or likelihood ratios. Perhaps different people use each format more effectively. Errors in probabilities may increase the costs or reduce the accuracy of diagnostic work-ups; the evidence on this question is also mixed, but it seems to be a reasonable proposition.

Can subjective estimates be improved? Subjective probabilities may not be perfectly accurate but often, in clinical medicine, they are the only ones available and have to be used because a decision must be made. What strategies are available to help the decision maker overcome the biases outlined and improve the accuracy of personal probability estimates?

One approach to this problem is the usual strategy of clinical reasoning. By systematically collecting data and revising opinions sequentially, differences in the prior probability estimates of two or more clinicians could be gradually erased. The impact of the amount of data ordinarily collected in clinical work should be such that most differences in prior probabilities would be overwhelmed by the evidence. If the data do not have this effect, one might well ask if obtaining the findings was a rational or habitual act— for if information does not cause us to change our minds, why bother to obtain it?

But there are situations where a subjective probability estimate must be carefully considered, perhaps because there is not much to go on except the clinician's opinion. How should this task be approached? Selvidge (1975) recommended breaking the problem down into smaller steps and moving gradually toward a number, instead of simply picking one out of the air. First, the uncertain event in question is thoroughly described in nonquantitative terms and related to other events more familiar to the assessor. The second step is to rank the unlikely events before grappling with tiny probability values. This part of the procedure assumes that the assessor is at least willing to say that the probability of rare event A is less than the probability of rare event B, even though he would be unwilling to say that either event has a probability of .001 or .0001 or the like. Several studies of clinical reasoning suggest that this is a reasonable assumption. After various events have been rank ordered from most likely to least likely, more specific quantitative measures can be gradually introduced. For instance, the assessor should attempt to judge how many times more likely than the least likely event is the most likely. Finally, each rare event can be compared to "standard" external events whose probabilities are known. These reference events include both naturally occurring rare events, like earthquakes, and reference processes, such as drawing a particular number in a lottery or being dealt a certain type of hand at bridge (say, an eight-card suit). The numerical expression of the probabilities of the rare events in question is a refinement of a set of these comparisons to reference events. Probability estimates are thus approached gradually via likelihood ratios. Visual aids were also recommended as a means of conveying to the decision maker the notion of very small probabilities.

Does this procedure lead to improvements in subjective probability estimates of sufficient magnitude to justify its use? So far as we are aware, no empirical studies of this question are available. The ingenious research psychologist will find this to be a challenging area of investigation.

Having heard at such length of possible defects of subjective probabilities, the reader may well wonder why we have devoted so much space to discussing an approach that so greatly depends upon such probability estimates. Our answer is that decision theory only makes explicit the fact that subjective probabilities are used in clinical reasoning all the time. They are generally the only ones available when a decision must be made and so they are used. Viewing clinical reasoning through the prism of decision theory makes this fact clear; it has not created it. There is no evidence that decisions made by formal processing of subjective probabilities are worse than decisions made by intuitive clinical judgment. In some instances, they are no better (Leaper and others, 1972), and in some instances, formally analyzed decisions have been found to be better than intuitive judgments (Fryback, 1974; Sisson, Schoomaker and Ross, 1976).

Impact of Evidence on Prior Opinion: Revising Probabilities

Psychological interest in the process of estimating subjective probabilities is fairly new. The earliest psychological research on decision making was more concerned with comparing changes in opinion (posterior probabilities or odds) with the degree of change arrived at by application of Bayes' Theorem. Attention focused not upon the adequacy of prior probabilities but on the process of opinion revision (Edwards, 1968; Slovic and Lichtenstein, 1971).

To provide the reader with some of the flavor of this research and the tenor of the major conclusions, four problems in revising probabilities follow. The reader is invited to answer each question, and then to compare answers with those provided.

1. It is estimated that about 3 percent of school-aged children in a typical American city are physically abused by their parents. It is possible to screen the children for evidence of abuse (scars, multiple fractures) with the intent of follow-up by contacting the suspected parents. While the potential damage caused by letting an abused child go undetected is great, falsely suspecting a parent is also undesirable. School health officials wish to be very confident of their suspicions before approaching the parents.

The officials believe that the screening examination used is very reliable. They claim that 95 percent of abused children will be detected, whereas only 10 percent of nonabused children will be false positives. Given these data, estimate the probability that a child is abused if the screening examination is positive. Your prior probability is .03; what is your posterior?

2. An ambulatory breast cancer screening procedure can detect 80 percent of women with undiagnosed cancer of the breast, and misclassifies only 5 percent of those without cancer. It is estimated that cancer rate in asymptomatic women who come for screening in 30 cases per 10,000 (.3 percent). Estimate the probability that a woman with a positive test actually has breast cancer.

3. Suppose that the screening test is improved and the false positive rate is reduced to 1 percent. What do you now estimate to be the probability that a woman with a positive test actually has breast cancer?

4. You enter a room containing 10,000 urns. Some of these urns (Type A) contain 7 red marbles and 3 green marbles, and the rest (Type B) contain 2 red marbles and 8 green marbles. There are 6,000 Type A urns and 4,000 Type B urns. (a) You pick an urn at random. What is the probability that it is of Type A? (b) You are allowed to sample three balls, with replacement, from the urn you selected. All three balls are red. Estimate the probability that you have selected a Type A urn.

These problems are solved by applying Bayes' Theorem. The probability of a child who is abused being picked up by the screening test is $P(\text{Test} +| \text{Child Abuse}) = .95$. The probability of a false positive, $P(\text{Test} +| \text{Normal Child}) = .10$. The prior probability of a randomly selected child being an abuse problem is the population base rate, .03. Then, according to the theorem:

$$P(\text{Child Abuse} \mid \text{Test} +) =$$
$$\frac{P(\text{Test} + \mid \text{Child Abuse})P(\text{Child Abuse})}{P(\text{Test} + \mid \text{Child Abuse})P(\text{Child Abuse}) + P(\text{Test} + \mid \text{Normal Child})P(\text{Normal Child})} =$$
$$\frac{.95 \times .03}{(.95 \times .03 + (.10 \times .97)} = \frac{.0285}{.1255} = .227$$

The problem can also be represented in a 2 × 2 table. Suppose 10,000 children are screened. The following table will be produced:

		True State		
		Abused	Not Abused	
Test	Abused	285	970	1,255
	Not Abused	15	8,730	8,745
		300	9,700	10,000

Thus, the probability of a child who is flagged by the screening test being one who is truly a problem in child abuse is 285/1255 = .227. By applying similar methods, the answers to the other problems are: (2).046; (3).206; (4a).60; (4b).9956.

Excessive opinion revision is often observed when base rates (priors) are very low. Apparently, the sensitivity of the test is weighted more than the prior probability of the condition being screened. Problems 1, 2, and 3 may give the reader some sense of the impact that a low prior probability should have when only a limited amount of data are available for processing. Problem 4 illustrates a classical phenomenon in the psychology of decision making. It is easy to estimate the probability of randomly picking a Type A urn. We know that 60 percent of the urns are Type A, and so the probability of randomly picking one is .60. It is much more difficult to assess accurately how much we should change our opinion when we know the results of even a small sampling of the contents of the urn. Nearly all decision makers underestimate the collective impact of the three red marbles. They state levels of certainty in the .70s or .80s. If you did that, you have a lot of company. The phenomenon is known as conservatism (Edwards, 1968).

Value

The last component of the decision-theoretic model requires specification of the value of each possible outcome of alternative interventions. The aim is to rate the various outcomes on a common scale of desirability and then to select that action that will maximize expected value. The common scale is frequently called "utility" (Raiffa, 1968), though one may equally want to think of the "value" or "worth" of particular outcomes.

Scaling values: Utility assessment. In the world of business, expected value can often be couched in monetary terms. How much money can a firm be expected to make if a particular venture is successful? And how much can it expect to lose if the venture fails? Even here, however, it became clear early that absolute quantities of money did not mean the same thing to everyone. It is obvious that a potential gain or loss of $100 thousand would have very different meaning to a gigantic multinational corporation than to a small neighborhood shopkeeper. Some other method of valuation was required.

Based on the classical work of von Neumann and Morgenstern (1947), the mathematical theory of decision making developed a fairly complex indirect method for estimating utilities by reference to choices between gambles or lotteries. The decision maker is asked first to rank all outcomes in order of attractiveness and then to use the best and worst as the anchoring points for a set of choices between pairs of lotteries. The aim is to find a point where the decision maker cannot choose between two lotteries or finds them equally attractive. The first lottery offers an intermediate outcome as a sure thing, and the second offers a p probability of the best alternative and a 1-p chance of the worst. This point p is then defined as the utility of the intermediate outcome, with the best and worst outcomes assigned utilities of 1.0 and 0.0 respectively. Applications of this method to the analysis of clinical decisions are to be found in Betaque and Gorry (1971), Ginsberg and Offensend (1968), Pauker (1976), and Pliskin and Beck (1976).

To illustrate the clinical application of this method of assessing values, consider the problem of an elderly patient who has suffered for years from peripheral vascular disease (poor circulation) due to diabetes. Now after a penetrating injury, a foot has become infected and appears to have developed gangrene. Prompt amputation is one possible treatment, but at this stage there is some chance that the foot may heal with proper medical care, a more conservative strategy. If surgical amputation is delayed, there is a risk that the gangrene could spread, necessitating an above-knee amputation or even resulting in death. If surgery is performed now, the amputation can be done below the knee with less resulting disability and deformity than that associated with the above-knee amputation. Limb amputation is a relatively safe procedure but there is always some risk of operative mortality. Given this description of the circumstances and of the decision problem, should below-knee surgery be performed immediately, or should one wait to see if the foot heals?

A complete decision-theoretic analysis of this problem requires specification of the probabilities of several outcomes and states. Here we wish to concentrate solely upon the evaluation of outcomes, not on the probability of any one outcome coming to pass, and so we shall not reach any definite conclusion. Four outcomes are possible. Ranking them from most to least attractive, they are: (1) cure following conservative medical therapy; (2) below-knee amputation; (3) above-knee amputation; (4) death. To assign relative values to these four outcomes using the method of basic reference lotteries, it is convenient to assign a value of 1.0 to the best outcome and 0.0 to the worst. The person whose values are being assessed is asked which of two lotteries is preferable (see Figure 3). The first lottery offers outcome B,

Figure 3. A Basic Reference Lottery

below-knee amputation, as a sure thing. The second lottery has two possible outcomes, cure and death, the best and worst alternatives. The probabilities assigned to each outcome in the second lottery are systematically varied until the decision maker cannot choose between lottery 1 and lottery 2. Suppose a decision maker finds that the two lotteries are equally attractive (or unattractive) when the probability of outcome A is .90 and the probability of outcome D is .10. This is the indifference point and consequently a value of .90 can be assigned to outcome B. Outcome C can be evaluated in similar fashion so we can arrive at a set of numbers based on probabilities that express strength of one's preference for four different outcomes.

Values or preferences calculated in this manner are called *utilities.* Assessments of more complex outcomes are possible, but discussion of this topic and of how to test these estimates for internal consistency is beyond the scope of this chapter. The reader should also note that we have temporarily set aside the question of whose values should be assessed, an important question in its own right.

A number of psychologists working in the field of behavioral decision theory have been concerned about possible sources of error in this method of eliciting preferences. When asked for value preferences by reference to lotteries, an individual is being asked to contemplate, evaluate, and assess in a novel fashion with which, very likely, he or she has had little prior experience. Even if the true preferences could be articulated, and even if subtle pressure were not being applied by the decision analyst, a lack of practice with the technique might introduce significant error into these assessments. A sense of the difficulty being discussed here can be gained by considering the problem individuals have in expressing estimates of weight, temperature, or distance in the metric system after a lifetime of use of the English system and very little practice in converting from one to the other. Even a good estimator in one system can appear to be poor indeed when asked to use an alien system. Thus, the use of lotteries might be better suited to physicians who, by repeated trials, will gradually become experienced in expressing their preferences in this way, and less useful in accurately assessing the preferences of relatively naive patients, each of whom is exposed to the procedure only once.

Alternative methods of valuation. With this difficulty in mind, several other techniques for assessing preferences have been developed, including various forms of rating scales (Kneppreth and others, 1974). These techniques are intended to be more psychologically meaningful by being more familiar and more transparent. Only those most applicable to clinical decision making are discussed here. These are methods for directly estimating magnitudes of preferences, as contrasted with the more indirect route of assessing preferences by choices between lotteries.

There are two major types of direct estimation methods. In the first, the range of the value scale is defined by the decision analyst. The outcomes or objects to be appraised are first ranked by the decision maker, just as in the choices-between-gambles approach. Then, the decision analyst assigns an arbitrary worth, say 100, to the best outcome and another value, say 1, to the worst outcome. Consequently, this method is called double-anchored direct estimation. The decision maker is then asked to indicate his or her relative preferences for all intermediate outcomes. The numbers provided are direct estimates of the decision maker's true preferences or worth ratings.

The second direct estimation method tries to eliminate the end-point problem, that is, the tendency of raters to avoid the extremes of a scale. It does this by assigning any randomly chosen outcome an arbitrary value, say

50. The decision maker then compares every other alternative to the reference alternative and is asked to specify how much more (or less) it is preferred in terms of ratios. This is one of the easiest methods for assessing preferences, but is nevertheless unpopular. It is not very sensitive to small differences in ratios, and many people feel more uncomfortable estimating in ratios than in any other mode.

In the study of radiological decision making already discussed, Fryback (1974) used a combination of double-anchored direct estimation and lotteries for obtaining utility estimates. The scales were actually scales of *dis*utility, since it was easier for the subjects to evaluate in terms of increasingly large costs. Each subject was asked to arrange four possible outcomes, typed on cards, in ascending order of perceived costs. The least costly outcome was arbitrarily rated 0 and the most costly 100. The assessor was then asked to assign a number to each intermediate outcome. These assignments were checked by the lottery method, and scale values were adjusted until they corresponded to the indifference probabilities. Very little adjustment in the assigned values was necessary.

Sources of error in valuing alternatives. Unlike subjective probabilities, values do not have an external referent to which they can be compared for accuracy. Using any of the valuation techniques described, psychologists can help people see how their values differ from one another, or how (perhaps) our values differ from what we thought they were. But we cannot, as psychologists, say that one set of preferences is wrong and another right.

The errors we are concerned about are methodological errors. Psychologists are always trying somehow to get inside someone's head and properly spend a good deal of time worrying about the extent to which the method chosen for this exploration affects the findings. So it is with valuation. All techniques for assessing the value of an alternative or a therapeutic outcome depend upon the ability of decision makers to reflect upon their feelings and then order or quantify them. Each technique, like all psychological measures, may have a degree of error of measurement associated with it. In addition to the problem of the novelty of the question, discussed earlier, three other sources of potential error may be identified.

The first source of error is the sheer instability of one's preferences. Quantitative estimates of value lend an air of permanence to what may be quite labile and shifting. This instability is not likely to be caused by evanescent shifts in taste or fashion, as might be the case with preference for automotive styles, although a case could be made for such transience in instances of cosmetic surgery. More serious, however, are radical changes in preference that may be induced when a patient is in severe pain or perceives the situation to be life threatening. A patient in severe pain or grave distress may evaluate a variety of outcomes quite differently than when pain and distress are absent. Consequently, a set of utility estimates obtained under one condition may not apply when conditions are altered. Just as we do not expect preferences to be identical from one person to another, we may find that an individual's own preferences are unstable across time. An unresolved problem, regardless of the method used to elicit utilities, is what to do with inconsistent preferences. Which set of utilities should the decision analyst accept? What weight should be given to preferences elicited when one's rational faculties are clouded by pain or pain-relieving drugs? How will the patient's true preferences be determined? What criterion should be used to determine validity?

The second source of error in valuation is that the patient as a decision maker may be ignorant of the true character of the alternatives, as when amputation of a limb must be evaluated. It is difficult to imagine what life would be like with a below-the-knee amputation, unless one has the opportunity to observe and speak with amputees. If the decision maker were better informed, the estimates obtained might be different. The patient's ignorance can be used as a powerful argument for using only experts to evaluate alternatives. But others who have identified this problem argue persuasively that the decision-theoretic model simply highlights the clinician's responsibility to inform the patient about the nature and probability of various outcomes, leaving it up to the patient to decide whose preferences should be assessed.

A third source of error operates when the person eliciting the preferences consciously or unconsciously influences the individual being assessed to respond in directions more consistent with the assessor's values than with those of the person whose opinions are ostensibly being elicited. Clinical decision making is especially prone to this bias, since physicians have great prestige in the eyes of most patients and their opinions carry much weight. Moreover, many patients wish the physician to make the difficult decisions anyway, especially when they are feeling depressed, dependent, or unable to function optimally.

Thus, techniques for making values explicit do not solve all of the problems that make clinical decisions complex and troubling. Indeed, the greatest contribution of the decision-theoretic approach to clinical issues may be that it helps to clarify where we are uncertain, why competent clinicians differ (Is it about probabilities or values?), and why certain decisions are so difficult (How many different attributes have to be considered to evaluate several alternative outcomes? What exactly are the trade-offs between longevity and quality of life?).

As always, whenever one is concerned about possible errors in estimating utilities or quantifying preferences, one can ask how great a shift in the utility estimate would be required before the decision changed. Unless one is very close to a decision boundary (the point where the choice of action changes), a relatively gross assessment of preferences may be adequate and even simple ranking may suffice. When close to a decision boundary, one may choose to assess utilities by the lottery method or by whatever method is preferred. Here, as we have seen, decision analysis often clarifies why a particular decision is difficult as much as it prescribes what to do.

The Decision-Theoretic Model as a Research Strategy

In addition to the problems and issues raised in the previous discussions of subjective probability and value, we would like to raise three more:

The use of this model is limited to situations where a specific set of alternatives is to be considered. The approach by itself cannot tell a clinician whether the set of diagnostic or therapeutic alternatives being evaluated is the best possible set, nor can it generate new alternatives. Structuring a set of alternatives is best handled by some of the principles of memory organization and reasoning that are associated with the information-processing approach. Decision theory assures that the alternatives are assessed by a method that aims to maximize the expected value of the outcome of action. That in itself should commend it to the attention of clinicians.

As we have seen, for the purpose of reaching a decision, probability estimates that may be grossly in error are acceptable to decision theory. In this sense, the theory is oriented toward selecting the perceived best available alternative rather than toward assessing the adequacy of our knowledge. Consequently, it may encourage action where continued evaluation and reflection (that is, research) is warranted (Fischhoff, 1977). This is a forceful objection and should be kept in mind. Nevertheless, the reality of clinical work is that often action must be taken in the face of insufficient information, for the patient's problem will not wait until needed research is done. For those practical situations where some decision must be made and where neither clinician nor patient is endeavoring to establish or test a general scientific proposition, decision theory can be a useful means of thinking about the alternatives. Further, the concepts of the theory direct the researcher's attention to a fruitful way of analyzing the choice of diagnostic tests or treatment strategies.

The discussion of biases in subjective probability showed that humans are not readily able to separate estimates of probability and utility. Value considerations appear regularly to influence probability estimates, contrary to the prescription of decision theory that these estimates be independent. The theory then goes on to identify this aspect of human performance as irrational and tries to offer some corrective strategies. Some psychologists might argue that a theory of decision making that demands something that humans do not do well is a poor theory, since it obviously cannot account for human behavior. This too is a powerful objection to decision theory as a description of human choice behavior. But it must be recalled that the theory never claimed to describe how people actually make decisions. Its intent rather was normative and prescriptive, and to this end it offers a set of guidelines for a decision maker who wants to be rational. Other problems that arise in medical applications of this approach are summarized in Beach (1975).

Implications for Clinical Teaching and Practice

As we reach the concluding pages of this review, let us summarize the major findings and emphases of the viewpoints surveyed. What do these research approaches tell us about clinical reasoning? And what is their import for clinical practice?

We have seen that expert clinical reasoning is a highly flexible process. The information-processing approach to clinical reasoning reveals that clinicians do exercise considerable discretion in retrieving relevant hypotheses from memory and in using them to guide the search for additional data. The rules used to reach diagnostic judgments can be adjusted to unique features of particular cases. This flexibility is subject only to a few constraints deriving from basic characteristics of the human information-processing system. The other two approaches find this flexibility to be more a source of error than a strength and are more critical of intuitive clinical reasoning. Several errors in clinical judgment documented by quantitative research within the judgment and decision-theoretic approaches may be understood as consequences of the limited human capacity for processing complex probabilistic information.

Taken as a whole, the research reviewed offers a sobering perspective on clinical reasoning. The common thread running through all of it is the notion of our limited rationality and the consequence that clinical reasoning is a more error-prone and less perfect process than we have hoped or wished it to be. Thus, we have seen that clinicians work in simplified problem spaces of limited size, do not use all the data that they collect, are too often overconfident and unaware of their true ignorance, and draw inferences imperfectly. We recognize that clinical reasoning is often effective, yet we believe that clinicians seek satisfactory rather than optimal solutions. For many problems that may be sufficient, yet it raises the prospect of somehow improving performance in this significant human activity. What can be done about this state of affairs? The first step, it appears to us, is to acknowledge it and then to set about finding appropriate correctives. We would like to suggest just some of the possibilities.

Knowing that subjective probabilities are often biased or erroneous, we can direct more of our research effort to building up bases of statistical data from which the frequencies of various events can be more accurately estimated. We can gradually become less dependent on personal clinical experience and can rely more on collective experience as recorded and analyzed in relevant clinical research.

The Bayesian approach makes it clear that more cost-effective and rational use of diagnostic tests depends upon knowledge of base rates as well as likelihood ratios. Yet clinical texts and teaching are generally weak on such matters. More effort is spent on describing diseases and their underlying mechanisms than in discussing their distribution in the population. Surely here curriculum and training can assist clinicians to acquire the knowledge needed to bring clinical intuition into greater congruence with the Bayesian model.

Ethical problems are much in the public eye at present as a burgeoning technology creates new dilemmas for clinician, patient, and society. The evaluation methods of decision theory and judgment theory cannot solve all of these problems, but we believe that talking about preferences for concrete alternatives could clarify much of the discussion now going on. In this connection, a better understanding of the effects of alternative methods of valuation upon the estimates obtained is much needed.

All three research approaches direct attention to the process of data integration and interpretation. Clinical teaching should focus on these elements. By contrast, the proliferation of laboratory tests has generally not been accompanied by growth in our capacity for processing clinical information. This discrepancy implies that more time should be spent in clinical supervision on problems of interpretation and opinion revision and that the collection of clinical data should be carefully evaluated in the light of the opinion revision that is needed.

A number of investigators have reported on the development and use of protocols and algorithms for various clinical problems. The findings summarized in this chapter surely indicate that it is proper to find means to improve clinical reasoning. These aids must be not only efficacious but also acceptable to clinicians. Finding optimal combinations of these attributes will challenge the persistence and ingenuity of many health psychologists. We take the critique of clinical reasoning offered in these pages not as a counsel of despair but as a stimulus to rethink a number of issues in clinical teaching and practice and thus to influence positively the quality of care provided.

14

Evaluating Outcomes in Health Care

Lee Sechrest
Rita Y. Cohen

The interests of psychologists in assessing the outcomes of health care intervention may arise out of the psychologist's role in planning and implementing certain types of interventions or as an expert in research design and measurement called in to assist in planning and implementing an evaluation effort. The measurement of health-related outcomes is by no means a simple matter, and much of the methodology is still at a fairly primitive level. There is a tendency for those not directly involved in a field to overestimate the level of scientific development in that field, and that may well be true of psychologists entering into health research for the first time. The aim of this chapter is to inform psychologists of both the problems of and prospects for measuring outcomes of attempts to improve health or health care. If psychologists are to contribute to an understanding of health, including its social and psychological aspects, they must do so within the context of methodologies that are sound with respect to the demands of

Note: The preparation of this chapter was supported in part by research grants funded by HS 02591-01, HS 02527-02, and HS 02702. The authors wish to thank Mary Ellen Olbrisch for her extensive comments and editorial help.

health care evaluation. Without truly adequate methodologies, we run the risks of attributing important outcomes to ineffective programs and, even more likely, of failing to detect effects of sound programs.

It is only in the last fifteen years that systematic efforts have been mounted to develop the methods for assessing quantitatively the outcomes of efforts to improve health. Previous work, while important in establishing groundwork for quantitative assessment, was scattered and mostly oriented toward evaluation of the quality of care as determined by adherence to some standard, however established (Flook and Sanazaro, 1973). An article by Donabedian (1966) was a watershed in the development of quantitative approaches to assessment of outcomes of health interventions. Donabedian's work made clear that however faithfully the principles of good medical practice might be followed, there was no guarantee that the result would be better health. His work established the necessity for independent, empirical demonstration of the phenomenon of improved health.

It is important to be able to quantify outcomes of health care—to be able to say with reasonable precision how much improvement in health is attributable to some health intervention—for the following reasons: (1) potential harm of interventions; (2) failure to develop more effective measures; (3) reduction of costs; (4) accountability; (5) verification of improvement. It is desirable to know exactly how efficacious our health interventions are in order to determine also how efficient they are. Without quantitative measures of outcomes, there is a distinct risk that ineffective or only partially effective treatment may be employed. The history of medicine is replete with instances of ineffective treatments that were regarded as standard over long periods of time, bloodletting being a notable example (Eisenberg, 1977). It is too easy for individual clinicians and individual patients to be misled about efficacy of treatments to be able to forgo the rigors of more careful quantification of outcomes. It is also likely that without quantitative estimates of treatment effects, the availability of a weakly effective treatment may divert attention from development of more effective measures. To know that a program reduces hypertension is one thing, but to know that it reduces blood pressures by an average of only four millimeters in only 30 percent of patients suggests that a search for considerably more effective programs is required.

Health interventions must also be evaluated in terms of costs to ensure that the greatest effects are obtained for the least expenditure of money, professional effort, and patient discomfort. If efficiency is to be achieved, rather precise estimates of outcomes are required. If, for example, two screening methods differ in cost, one needs to know with reasonable accuracy how they differ in results in order to determine whether the one with greater cost is worth implementing. It is possible, as another example, to spend almost limitless amounts of money in "improving" an emergency medical system by giving additional training to emergency personnel, providing more ambulances to reduce response time, equipping ambulances with telemetry to provide for monitoring of heart rhythms, and the like. Without very good data on the outcomes of such efforts, we cannot carry out with sufficient clarity the difficult task of weighing the lives thus saved against those that might be saved by different uses of the same funds.

Our health care system and those who operate it and are supported by it need to be accountable to the public they serve for the efficacy and efficiency of their efforts. That accountability can be established only by reference to carefully quantified outcomes. In health, it is no longer sufficient to claim that accountability is satisfied by professional certification. Accountability can be satisfied only in terms of demonstrable results (American Psychological Association, 1978b). Of course, the aim of all health interventions is the improvement of health, whether by prevention of disease or deterioration or by restoration of lost functions. To have the knowledge of outcomes means having ways of measuring health and changes in it.

Approaches to Assessment of Health Outcomes

There are various approaches to assessing the outcomes of health interventions, none of which is exhaustive or individually sufficient. Together they provide a comprehensive, if not yet totally satisfactory basis for decision making about health interventions. However, the approaches are differentially useful for different purposes, and only infrequently is more than one approach attempted within a single investigation. Although the expense involved often limits the approaches employed by an investigator, some inexpensive and routine sources of information are frequently overlooked.

There are several key issues in the assessment of health care regardless of the particular approach to assessment being used. One is whether the focus should be on illness or on health. Much attention is paid in writing to the concept of health in a positive sense and to the need to develop ways of assessing it and progressing toward it. In practice, however, most attempts to assess outcomes do so in terms of alleviating the symptoms of conditions or illness or disability. Most measures that have been developed assess the limitations of functioning that are the consequence of medical disabilities (Bergner and others, 1976; Fanshel and Bush, 1970; Katz and others, 1963). Health is simply taken to be the absence of any disabilities or symptoms. Something of an exception, however, is the concept of *prospective medicine* and its associated measures, as outlined by Robbins and his associates (Robbins and Hall, 1970). In prospective medicine, each person is considered to have health risks or advantages that are associated statistically with either greater or lesser risk of death than would be average for a person of that age. Each person, then, can be given a *health age* which represents the age that the person's death risk best matches. Thus, a person with a younger health age than chronological age can be viewed as, in that degree, positively healthy. The index mixes behavioral risks, which the person presumably can control to some extent, with background factors that cannot be changed. Current health status (blood pressure, for example) is not included as a risk factor. A low health age might be a reflection of not smoking, of exercising regularly, of not having a family history of coronary artery disease, and so on. The approach of prospective medicine is quite new, however, and most other work to date has been done on measures that focus on degree of illness.

The data source to be used is the second factor cutting across the various approaches to assessing health outcomes. Three major types of data are available, although not all types of data are likely to be available in every context. Clinical data may consist of objective technical data, such as laboratory results, or of less objective, often impressionistic judgments or ratings by clinically specialized personnel—ratings by a physician of a patient's condition, results of a physical examination, or a rating of degree of improvement by a nurse. A second type of data is self-report on condition by the patient. Patients may report on overall condition, on symptoms and disabilities, or on degree of improvement. The third type of data is archival—data routinely recorded, usually for administrative purposes, but which may be retrieved to make assessments of outcomes. Hospital records, mortality statistics, required reports of contagious disease, and days absent from work are all examples of archival data that have been exploited for research purposes in assessing outcomes of health interventions.

Outcome measures may also differ in that some are obtained from and applicable to individuals, and others available only for populations. For most interventions, it is highly desirable to have data for each person in the study, permitting one to relate variations in treatment to variations in outcome or to relate different outcome measures obtained from the same persons. However, the methods of epidemiology require only population data, and such data will often suffice quite well. Since the choice of individual or population measures can be critical, the advantage of obtaining outcome data from each data source will be discussed later.

The dimensionality of the outcome determination is another issue to be considered. Some interventions are intended to have a narrow range of effect and should be assessed along a single dimension, whereas others require a multidimensional assessment or a measure capable of reflecting a range of effects. For example, an intervention designed to reduce blood pressure can be assessed in terms of its effects on blood pressure—whether it has any other effects, as in reducing complaints about headaches, is not critical, even if relevant. An intervention designed to improve quality of medical care or to improve general health status would have to be assessed across a number of different medical conditions and for a wide variety of outcome indicators. If a single health status index were desired, it would have to be of such a nature as to reflect changes in all those conditions.

Still another question that must be answered when planning the assessment of any intervention is the use to which the results will be put. If a study is being conducted as a one-time evaluation of an intervention, a single outcome measure may suffice—for example, a reduction in blood pressure, a decrease in infant mortality, or a decrease in complications following surgery. However, if the outcome measure(s) will be used for continuing decision making, perhaps in the ongoing allocation of resources, there is a great risk in a single index, and even in multiple indexes, that corruption of data may occur. The corruption may take the form of misrepresentations of data, for example, systematic rounding of some blood pressure figures downward or omission of cases not considered to have "completed" a treatment. However, the index may itself corrupt the intervention by biasing it in a direction so as to produce a maximum impact on the index, whether other desirable outcomes are achieved or not. If infant mortality is the sole index of success of a program and if funding depends on the value of that index, program efforts may be distorted toward reducing infant mortality with a resultant detrimental effect on other desired program outcomes, for example, mortality rates for older children. Just such a happening has been reported for the Indian Health Service, which reduced infant mortality but left mortality rates for older children at their same distressingly high level. The program was intended to affect all children, but the use of infant mortality as the sole index seems to have altered the program (Hanft, 1978). Researchers should not be oblivious to the potential political implications of their methodological decisions.

Individual and Population Measures in Assessing Health Outcomes

Outcomes of most health interventions can be assessed at the level of the individual person, whether he or she is a patient treated for a disease or merely a member of a population exposed to some generalized health intervention. One can, for example, assess morbidity, mortality, health status, level of functioning, and other variables at this level. However, it is sometimes possible and even desirable to assess health problems at a sample or population level. One might, as an instance, determine infant mortality rates before and after the introduction of a new system of neonatal care in a catchment area for a series of neighborhood health clinics. Or one could determine venereal disease rates in two communities differing in intensity of follow-up case tracking. Population data are often easier to obtain as well as being cheaper by far, and those factors can compensate for the reduction in precision that might occur in comparison to outcome measures obtained at the individual level. The decision to use individual or population data will have advantages and disadvantages; each approach is useful, although for somewhat different purposes.

Advantages of individual assessments. The outcome focus for most treatments of specific diseases or other medical conditions must be the individual. The value of the coronary artery bypass operation, as an instance, can be effectively assessed only by examining the morbidity and mortality status of individuals who have had or might have had the operation. It would not make sense to try to determine the outcome of such surgical procedures by looking at mortality data for entire populations from which the individual surgical candidates were drawn. Similarly, the effectiveness of a mobile cardiac care unit can be assessed only in terms of success in treating individual cases who might otherwise have died (Sherman, 1977). In contrast, the effectiveness of a mass immunization program is usually better assessed by determining the number of cases of the target disease for an entire population and comparing the results with those for a similar population not inoculated, or with results expected on the basis of a historical extrapolation.

One of the advantages of assessing outcomes at the level of the individual is that it is usually possible to specify the link between the intervention being tested and the outcome, so that a more sensitive test of outcome can be devised. To assess the effectiveness of a health education effort designed to improve dietary habits of high school students, one could examine sales of different types of foods in the school cafeteria. However, by determining the level of exposure to the campaign for individual students, one might get a considerably more sensitive measure of the outcome, for example, by excluding from the study those students apparently unaware of the campaign.

When particular outcomes are rare and/or population figures are quite unreliable or unstable, assessments at the individual level are advantageous. In the evaluation of polio vaccine, for example, it was necessary to determine whether inoculated individuals did or did not get polio, because only a relative handful of cases were expected and because polio rates varied greatly from year to year (Meier, 1972). Similarly, it is improbable that the bad side effects of pediatric tetracycline could be discovered by looking at population rates for those medical problems. One has, instead, to look specifically at the medical problems of children who have been given the drug.

Advantages of population assessments. A disadvantage of assessing outcomes at the individual level is that such assessments are often quite expensive. Individual cases must be identified and then followed, often over considerable periods of time, whereas if population data are acceptable, it may suffice to take two samples at different times or perhaps even routinely to monitor epidemiological data collected for other purposes. The trade-off of cost against precision has to be weighed carefully for each problem.

Sample or population data will often answer important questions without respect to the identity of individuals. In some instances, population data have the advantage of being available when individual data are not. When assessing the effectiveness of a crisis-oriented telephone counseling service, consideration of confidentiality of client identity might preclude any evaluation based on data for individuals. One might have to depend on rates for the entire community of unsatisfactory resolutions of crises, for example, suicides, drug overdose, and runaway children. Whether such data would yield sufficiently sensitive indicators of the effectiveness of crisis counseling is open to question, but if those data were all that was available, they might merit examination.

Some health interventions, particularly those in the area of public health, can only be studied at the population level. Improvement in the sanitation system of a village (Susser, 1975) or improvement in the air-filtering system in an industrial plant can only be evaluated by epidemiological data on the incidence of target health problems for the entire group of persons at risk. In an antimalaria campaign, it is not possible to predict ahead of time who might and might not get malaria. One can only look for changes in frequency of episodes of malaria before and after the campaign.

In some cases, especially in communicable diseases and other problems that must be reported, such as automobile accident injuries, data may be more readily available for entire populations than for samples or other subsets. Since venereal diseases must be reported and since they also carry some stigma, it is easier to obtain data on their incidence for an entire community than for any subgroup within the community. Similarly, it is easier to obtain data on automobile accidents for an entire city or county than for some subgroup of the population.

Problems in using population data sampling. For assessing outcomes of health interventions, it is often desirable to make estimates of population values for some variables on the basis of samples. In such cases, methods of sampling are of paramount importance. Estimating population values from samples is not always a perfectly straightforward procedure, and it is not something that is routinely included in training programs for psychologists. There are many opportunities for error which suggest that the assistance of experts may be called for. It is by no means a simple matter to obtain a random sample of a population, and any other sort of sample requires additional statistical analysis, often of a very complex nature. When populations are quite heterogeneous with respect to variables of interest, sampling errors can easily be greatly magnified, particularly when statistical corrections must be made and when sample sizes are not large in relation to the population. If one wished, as an instance, to estimate the number of alcoholics in a population and had only a 1 percent sample, every alcoholic identified or missed in the sample would result in a change of 100 total alcoholics for the community estimate. Bruce-Briggs (1977) reports that a Census Bureau study that estimated that 20,000 U.S. children aged three to six are left unattended during the day while their mothers work was, apparently, a projection based on about twelve cases! The example given by Bruce-Briggs shows clearly the risks of projecting by multiplying small numbers of cases by large multipliers.

In health surveys, households are typically the sampling unit, with the sampling strategy based on identifying dwelling units in the community and sampling from them. However, even if the sampling plan is adequate, the troublesome question remains of who the respondent should be. It is seldom feasible to interview everyone in a household, and so usually one person becomes the respondent for the entire household or family. It may make considerable difference which member of a family is the respondent; sometimes any household member sixteen years or older is allowed to respond for the entire family, but, in most cases, someone must answer for children and for some disabled persons.

That the respondent one chooses in a survey may affect the results one obtains is widely recognized. Less well recognized is the fact that when

households are the sampling units, and most especially when one person reports for the entire household, then households should be the unit of analysis. Data obtained on individuals in the same family are likely to be correlated, even when each member answers individually, but especially when the
data on a family are all obtained from one family member. Reports of minor
illness, such as a sore throat or an earache, within the past month may be
correlated within families in part because such illnesses are contagious but
also because the reports will vary systematically with each respondent's definition of minor illness and with that respondent's memory. It would, consequently, be wrong to conclude from the survey what percentage of people in
the community had minor illnesses within the past month. The only legitimate conclusion would concern the percentage of *households* in which
minor illnesses were reported. The difference in conclusions is an important
one and might have critical implications for evaluating the outcome of a
health intervention.

    Interpretation of population data. In addition to problems of sam-
pling, population data are often difficult to interpret and can even be misleading to the unwary. For example, for a variety of reasons, there is likely
to be a positive relationship between health resources and health problems
across communities (Glazer, 1971). To some persons, such a relationship
may seem paradoxical, since we expect health to improve with the availability of health care. However, that expectation does not take into account
the fact that health resources tend to be located where they are needed and
that people in need of health care will tend to locate where the needed facilities are available. Another point to note in attributing causality is that the
more health services a person has received in a period of time, the worse the
person's health is almost certain to be. In addition, improved access to health
care by way of more facilities may generate demand that could lead to the
conclusion a year later that, despite the program, health problems were more
numerous than ever. Such errors are akin to what sociologists call the "ecological fallacy" (Robinson, 1950; Selvin, 1965).

    In order to interpret many health statistics, rates must be corrected
for, or be specific to, such statuses as age, sex, race, and socioeconomic level
(Fuchs, 1974; Klebba, Maurer, and Glass, 1973). Also, unless data were corrected for obstetrical charges, one could conclude that young women cost a
health system considerably more than do males of the same age. (It only
seems reasonable that obstetrical charges be allocated to *couples*.) Blacks and
whites differ sufficiently in prevalence of hypertension that even fairly small
race differences between groups or over time could bias conclusions about
the effectiveness of an intervention to control hypertension.

Issues in Selecting Outcome Measures

Variability in Measures

    In selecting outcome measures, one wishes to find a measure suffi-
ciently sensitive to reflect any real changes attributable to a program or

treatment and, at the same time, sufficiently stable that program-induced changes are detectable against the background of natural variability. Unfortunately, many measures are so variable over time and occasion that real change may be difficult to see. For example, blood pressure, particularly systolic pressure, can differ markedly because of anxiety level, time of day, body posture, and many other factors. In fact, blood pressure is so variable that a diagnosis of hypertension usually cannot be made on the basis of a single reading. Many other physical and physiological measures, such as blood glucose levels, are sufficiently unstable to present problems when selected for study as outcome measures.

Instability is a characteristic by no means limited to physical and physiological measures. Both mortality and morbidity rates are subject to seasonal fluctuations (Klebba, Maurer, and Glass, 1974), as are utilization rates for health services such as physician office visits (Aday and Eichhorn, 1972). Any source of change in outcome measures that is not attributable to an intervention being evaluated is a threat to our ability to detect a program effect.

Insensitivity of Measures

Measures must be not only stable but also sensitive. A measure that is slow to change or that changes only in very minute ways is unsatisfactory for evaluating effects of interventions. Mortality rates are likely to be insensitive to many types of interventions since many health problems are not lethal, and death in many other cases is long delayed. Self-reported health status may not be a particularly sensitive measure over a long period of time if, as seems likely, people make gradual adjustments in their expectations about their health to take into account their typical level of functioning (Breuer, 1974). Other measures may be insensitive because expectations lead to bias in measurement. For example, blood pressure involves sufficiently imprecise measurement operations that the clinician's expectations, built up over a series of visits, about what ought to be a patient's blood pressure may bias readings obtained. Thus, to evaluate the effects of health interventions, one must select outcome measures for which there is some chance of detecting change.

Distinction Between Symptom and Clinical Sign Outcomes

In addition to choosing measures that are reliable and sensitive, investigators must consider the sources of information used in assessing outcomes of health care programs. In particular, they must distinguish between professional and lay judgments. Traditionally, most evaluations have been based on the physician's judgment of illness status; the physician chooses a set of qualities or clinical signs to evaluate, such as blood pressure and temperature, compares the patient's standing on the measures to a set of norms that presumably reflect consensual expert beliefs about the ideal scores on those measures, and administers treatment to bring the individual close to those "ideal" norms (the idealness of which may not have any empirical justification; see Feinstein, 1974). An underlying assumption is that the service provided by the physician is the main component of health care (Blum, 1974b).

A second means of assessment is based on patients' judgments of their functional status. Patients decide that they are functioning below their usual level of ability. They may compare their current capacity to a "pre-illness" level or simply decide that a particular ability should be better than it is without reference to a premorbid capacity or in reference to others whom they perceive as similar to themselves. Initially, functional status may seem more difficult to assess, since it often includes more subjective values and perceptions than do physician-based judgments of disease status. Patients react to more aspects of the medical system than simply medical procedures, and often reactions are somewhat idiosyncratic. However, just as one can ask experts to decide upon a cluster of clinical signs that constitute illness, one may also utilize a panel of patients within a care system to delineate a cluster of functional signs of illness—that is, limitations imposed by illness. (This approach is similar to that of Kaplan, Bush, and Berry, 1976, to be described later.) Presumably, each individual's idiosyncrasies would be washed out in the group judgments, leaving adequate consensual criteria of functional status. Problems with idiosyncratic usage of health status terms may not arise if the physician notes verbatim each individual's stated dysfunction during the initial contact and compares it with stated dysfunction after clinical treatment.

To determine the utility of a particular intervention, it is necessary to consider both clinical signs and functional status, since they are not necessarily equally affected by health intervention. For example, a middle-aged man may reduce his activity level because he assumes his heart palpitations reflect some medical problem. A doctor may determine that, clinically, there is no abnormality and that the patient can continue to function as usual. Assuming the patient follows the physician's advice and returns to his or her usual level of functioning, a change has been made in functional status without an alteration in clinical sign. Similarly, patients with high blood pressure may continue to function as usual, although clinically their blood pressures are highly deviant. Because patients and physicians utilize different norms in determining health status, their estimates of the severity of a condition may be at odds. Severity for the physician is a matter of discrepancy between the population's scores and those of the individual, whereas severity in the patient's view depends on the discrepancy between present and past ability.

The choice of measures is partially dependent upon one's assumptions about medical care. A clinical sign measure focuses on illness and its eradication, whereas the functional approach considers the health status of an individual in the community. Health and illness are correlated but not identical. Health status is more of a sociological than biological variable and includes such things as psychological and economic well-being (McKinley and Dutton, 1974). Health status reflects a person's reactions to a biological condition among other conditions; therefore, the proper measure of health status is the individual's reactions, not the "clinical" state itself. Health includes not only the absence of signs but also the ability to perform as usual on a day-to-day basis.

There are some cases where neither a sign nor functional outcome offers an appropriate measure. In assessing the efficacy of health education in relation to preventive behavior, short-term outcomes are unlikely to be measurable either as clinical signs or degree of dysfunction. In this case, measures of short-term benefits must rely largely on behavior changes thought to be related to long-range outcomes.

Process, Outcome, and Impact of Health Care

It has been traditional in evaluating health care interventions to distinguish between different "levels" of effects. Donabedian (1966) drew attention to the distinctions between structure, process, and outcome of health care. By structure, he referred primarily to resources available; by process, to application of those resources; and by outcome, to the end results of the application of resources. Perhaps Donabedian's most important contribution was in calling attention to the probability that the relationships between levels were not dependable. Neither increase of resources nor more care in their application ensured that better health outcomes would be achieved. Recently, Attkisson and Hargreaves (1976) have proposed a more comprehensive model for evaluation, which has four levels: systems resource management, client utilization, outcome of intervention, and community impact. We will not discuss system resource management, since it has more to do with input than outcome variables. However, it will be helpful to consider the other three levels of evaluation.

Client Utilization

In the scheme developed by Attkisson and Hargreaves (1976), client utilization refers both to the rate of utilization of services and to the characteristics of those services, such as quality. A service cannot affect clients if it is not delivered and will affect them less well or even adversely if it is delivered at low levels of quality. One potential effect of health interventions is that more services will be utilized by more persons, an effect to be discussed subsequently. Another effect is that the presumed quality of services might be improved. Typically, studies of quality focus on the assessment of professional behavior for a particular procedure or for particular kinds of cases. One specifies the ideal or normative procedures, as determined usually by the consensus of experts, and then compares the ideal and the actual procedure followed, either through examination of records (chart review) or direct observation of daily activity. Such evaluation is relatively easy in most cases since agreement on a range of appropriate procedures for a problem is usually obtainable within a given agency, although accord is by no means universal (Brook and Davies-Avery, 1977). The maximal utility of the evaluation is probably as a training and competence rating mechanism; therefore, it is likely to be used mostly within an agency for staff evaluation. Measures chosen usually monitor treatment of acute problems; more often than not, a clinical sign approach to assessment of the patient's condition is expected of the physician. Since the evaluation approach is based on behavior of the professional, patient variables are rarely considered. For example, the physician who orders a throat culture for a sore throat and then prescribes a ten-day penicillin regimen if the culture is positive is judged as competent for the problem being studied, whether or not the patient complies with the regimen and is actually cured.

Outcome of Intervention

Quality evaluation is appropriate if one wishes to determine whether a particular procedure or program is being implemented correctly. However, it is the evaluation of outcome, that is, the effectiveness of a particular program, which is of ultimate concern for both service delivery personnel and patients. Evaluation of outcomes is usually more difficult than evaluation of quality, for two reasons. First, it is often more difficult to reach accord on the goals of a program than on the desirability of particular procedures, in part because there are often several goals. One may specify either short-term or long-term goals for a program; for instance, the aim of a particular surgical procedure may be stated merely in terms of the patient's survival of the operation or prolongation of the patient's life. The second reason that evaluation of outcomes is especially difficult is that there is often a long time lag between the implementation of a program and the appropriate time for measurement of its outcome. In the case where the goal of surgery is prolongation of life, any number of intervening variables could affect the outcome even though they might not be directly related to the procedure itself, for example, patient compliance with postoperative suggestions to cease smoking or to engage in proper self-care. Under such circumstances, it becomes of greatest importance to consider patient contributions to outcomes.

The assessment of outcomes is somewhat dependent on an adequate evaluation of process. Assessment of individual outcomes, let alone of community impact, is meaningless unless one can be assured that an intervention or treatment was actually and properly administered. Consider, for example, the ubiquitous finding that compliance with medical regimens is often quite poor (Marston, 1970; see also Chapter Eight in this volume). If patients do not take the drugs that are prescribed for them, the outcome of drug treatment cannot be adequately evaluated. Nor can a surgical procedure be adequately evaluated if performed by ill-trained physicians or if carried out in settings lacking critical support staff. Even if there is a reasonably good outcome for an intervention, evaluation of the quality of care might suggest that the outcome could have been better with a better implementation.

Community Impact

Impact evaluation, as defined by Attkisson and Hargreaves (1976), is concerned with the effects on the more broadly defined community of an intervention designed to have a favorable effect on the health status of an individual. Determination of impact involves asking questions having to do with long-run and communitywide benefits. For example, suppose some new technology were found that increased the proportion of premature infants that could be saved. At the outcome level, the evaluation would be clearly favorable from the standpoint either of the infant or the parents. However, what would be the impact, if any, on the community of having a few extra surviving babies each year? Even if heart transplants did prolong survival times of their beneficiaries, would the broader community be changed or improved in any way? Perhaps the community might be benefited if those surviving longer had unusual and important contributions to make. Impact of other interventions might be reflected in reductions in welfare costs, lowering of crime rates, increase in industrial productivity, improvement in quality of air, and the like.

It may be possible and desirable to frame questions of impact more broadly so as to encompass issues not ordinarily considered when evaluating program results. For example, Gibson (1974) has suggested that the major outcome of emergency medical interventions is to change the location of death: from the street to the emergency department or from the emergency department to a hospital bed. However correct Gibson may be, might it not be regarded as desirable that the citizens of a community die with relative dignity and privacy in a hospital rather than on the street? Might not a community have a better sense of that community if it does the very best it can for its citizens, even if that is not so much? To save the lives of a few premature infants each year might have no directly assessible impact on a community, but the indirect consequences in terms of community pride and sense of morality might be detectable.

Neither outcomes nor impacts can be assessed in terms of a single dimension; they will not even have a single valence. For any given intervention, some outcomes may be positive and some negative. A palliative treatment may, for example, reduce immediate discomfort but mask the symptoms in such a way that long-term consequences are dire. Some outcomes may be desirable, but only if the conditions producing them can be maintained; otherwise, the consequences may be worse than no treatment at all. Schultz (1976), for example, found that those residents of a long-term care facility who could control times of visitation by the student volunteers were happier and healthier than those residents visited on the same schedule but who lacked control over visitation. However, when the visitation program was stopped, those residents who had been able to control visitation suffered serious decrements in status that left them worse off than the other group. Impacts, as well as outcomes, can have different long- and short-range values.

An article in a Black Muslim newspaper attacked the treatment of sickle cell anemia on the grounds that although in the short run it would lead to a healthier community, the long-term consequence was sure to be an increase in frequency of the disease because of increased prospects for genetic transmission. Another case involving intricate trade-offs is that of eliminating addiction to heroin while creating dependence on methadone. Any sophisticated evaluation, whether at the outcome or impact level, will have to be multidimensional and alert to possibilities of unanticipated effects.

Measuring Various Aspects of Health Care

Health care is a multifaceted, complex process in which the varieties of interventions are extensive, both with respect to nature and intention. Assessing outcomes is a correspondingly complex task. There is no simple way of monitoring the myriad effects that may be the outcomes of interventions designed to maintain or improve health. Evaluations of process (quality of care) should not be mistaken for outcome evaluations, although, as will be seen, the same measure will sometimes serve for either or both. It is important, nonetheless, to be able to determine whether changes in process are occurring, since many changes in process may be necessary, if not sufficient, conditions for improvement in our health. Consequently, in the discussion that follows, we will give some consideration to the ways of assessing improvements in the processes, as well as the outcomes, of health interventions. For example, peer review has as its immediate aim the improvement of processes in the expectation that, in the long run, outcomes will be favorably affected.

Quality of Care

A prime issue in the delivery of health services today is the assurance that those services that are delivered are likely to have their intended effects. Treatments of low quality may not only fail in this respect but may even do harm, if only by making less likely the delivery of other, higher quality treatments. Unfortunately, assessing the quality of care is not a simple matter. There is not complete uniformity of opinion as to what constitutes quality of care. In addition, the problem is one of substantial technical complexity.

Assessment of the quality of health care was given impetus by Donabedian's (1966) distinction between process and outcome and by his later review (1969) of attempts to measure quality of care. Brook (1973) extended Donabedian's conceptual analysis by describing and studying the specific operational procedures by which the quality of the process of care could be measured. One of the fundamental problems in assessing quality of health care is the risk of an inadequate data base from which to make the judgment. Direct observation, even if possible, is far too expensive for routine assessments, although Peterson and others (1956) demonstrated its value. To be done on a widespread basis, quality assessment has to depend on study of medical records which are often incomplete and otherwise inadequate (Donabedian, 1969). Before quality assessment efforts begin, it is necessary to take steps to improve record keeping, mostly in the direction of more complete recording, particularly for things that were done but proved negative or unrevealing. Even if good records are available, there still must be some system for assessing the treatments and procedures recorded. Although Brook (1973) showed that physicians can agree rather well when they examine records in light of their general understanding of what constitutes good care (thus demonstrating concordant implicit standards), most efforts at quality assessment have involved the development of explicit standards—the listing of each step or procedure that should be followed for a particular medical problem (Decker and Bonner, n.d.). Clearly, the number of different medical problems precludes listing of procedures to be done for every one of them. Consequently, most investigators have relied on the concept of tracer conditions (Kessner, Kalk, and Singer, 1973) on the assumption that if such problems are properly treated, most other conditions will be similarly well managed. Tracer conditions are usually relatively common medical problems with clearly specifiable outcomes, but with some degree of complexity in terms of diagnosis and treatment.

When quality of care is assessed by application of criteria for practice, the results are likely to be expressed in terms of percentage of the providers' compliance with explicit standards, either across all criteria or separately for each one. It is assumed that adherence to criteria represents quality of health care. It is not necessarily the case, however, that percentage adherence to criteria constitutes a scale with desirable psychometric properties. For one thing, this approach assumes that all the criteria are equally important, which is unlikely to be the case for most medical problems. Ninety percent compliance may not be much better than zero percent compliance if the one thing left undone is the single absolutely essential procedure. As more knowledge is gained about the factors entering into quality assessment, measures such as percentage adherence to (weighted) criteria can be made increasingly sophisticated. As now implemented, the approach to quality assessment using explicit criteria has the advantage of being applicable to individual cases, to individual practitioners, to different medical problems, and to larger samples as well.

A rather different approach to assessment of quality of health care, one based on outcomes, has been proposed by Williamson (1975). He has defined a goal for health care as *maximum achievable benefit*, and the outcome can then be defined as the *percentage of maximum achievable benefit achieved.* For example, it would be too much to expect that a hypertension program would be 100 percent successful in reducing blood pressures of participants. However, persons responsible for the program could probably state some realistic goals for the program, perhaps as a percentage of hypertensives who should end up with diastolic pressures below 95. If it were deemed reasonable that 70 percent of program participants should have their blood pressures lowered to the criterion level, but if, in fact, only 50 percent of participants reached the desired goal, the program would be judged only about 70 percent successful. What is required for Williamson's approach to make sense is that maximum achievable benefits be set at levels low enough to be realistic and yet high enough to represent genuine goals to be achieved.

Although Williamson's approach is applicable to assessments of outcomes of health care, it is also applicable to any phenomenon that can be expressed as a goal. Thus, even improving the process of health care can be expressed as a goal and evaluated by Williamson's approach. One could, as an instance, determine that in an area served by a clinic, only 70 percent of pregnant women received prenatal care before the sixth month of pregnancy, whereas if the clinic were really serving the needs of its constituents, 95 percent of these women should have received such care. The success of an outreach program might then be judged on the basis of the amount of the gap between 70 percent and 95 percent that is closed. Williamson's approach, based on a quantitative statement of goals, can be applied to the health care of individuals (for example, reducing seizures to no more than one per month or reducing glycosuria to .5 percent or less) and is also applicable to institutions or large samples.

A third approach has been taken by the Indian Health Service on the Papago Reservation outside Tucson, Arizona. They established a set of outcome criteria for adequacy of health care by setting population limits for certain health problems. If any of the problems exceed the limits, that is considered prima facie evidence that the health care system is functioning inadequately (Indian Health Service EMCRO, 1975; see also Giancalone and Hudson, 1975). The concept of a population-based index is not a new one and is precedented in fields other than health, for example, crime rates, unemployment rates, and the like. Nonetheless, the concept and its implementation expands the meaning of quality of medical care. Thus, for example, it is perfectly possible that although a group of health practitioners might be doing all the right things, overall quality of care may be poor. It might be that too large a proportion of the population lacked interest in or access to proper care, or there might be failure of other parts of the system, such as follow-up care. One advantage of setting system goals is that it may prompt discovering where problems lie and thus where there are greatest prospects for improvement. Focusing on parts of the system separately, particularly if not all parts are evaluated, can be quite misleading.

Risks involved in using a population-based set of indicators were discussed earlier—distortion or corruption of data, choosing inappropriate measures (infant mortality in an aging population) or insensitive measures, or failing to take account of sociocultural differences (alcoholism may be of differential value as an indicator in different ethnic groups). Care should also be taken that any indicator chosen be susceptible to change as a function of interventions through the health care system (incidence of common colds, various genetic diseases, or multiple sclerosis would not be good choices), and that accurate data are likely to be available for the population or sample of the size that will be studied. Days lost from work as a result of illness is a "noisy" variable in small samples or populations. Prevalence of alcoholism may be difficult to estimate for populations of any large size, since indicators of alcoholism probably become increasingly obscure as one moves away from study of individual cases.

Still another aspect of care that needs to be assessed is the extraprocedural quality of physician performance and of physician-patient interaction, an aspect that has usually been neglected, perhaps because it is so difficult to deal with. Virtually the only way to determine whether physicians are performing adequately is to employ observers to watch them, but such methods are expensive and difficult to arrange. Nonetheless, observers have been used to study physician performance. Peterson and others (1956) showed that physician performance is often far below standard, even with an observer present. A study by Price and others (1971) showed that observers agree reasonably well in assessing physician performance, but ratings by observers do not always agree well with other measures, such as self-ratings or peer reputations. The adequacy of physician-patient interaction becomes important because so much of effective medical care clearly depends upon the degree to which a patient understands and participates in the health care processes devised for his or her case. While there is evidence suggesting that most patients are well satisfied with their physicians, so much so that it is difficult to get indications of dissatisfaction (Hulka and others, 1970; Ware, Snyder, and Wright, 1976a, b), patients often lack understanding of what is expected of them and frequently do not comply with treatment recommendations. Faulty communication has been implicated in these deficiencies (see Chapter Eight in this volume).

Distribution of Care

One of the major problems in the health care system may be more a matter of distribution than of the total quantity delivered. Some people get enough, or more than enough, health care, while others get far too little. It is tempting to suppose that if enough health care is a good thing, more than enough is even better. In fact, too much health care could be deleterious in a number of ways—in promoting hypochondriacal behavior, in diverting resources from other desirable activities, or even because of the potential harm from interventions such as excessive use of antibiotics or x rays. In any case, it has been argued that there are probably enough physicians and other health professionals in the United States but that they are maldistributed, being concentrated in urban medical centers and suburban offices (Saltzman, 1971; U.S. Department of Agriculture, 1974). The same maldistribution exists for health facilities such as hospitals, and it may even be true that there are too many hospital beds aside from their distribution. Even though certain areas may have too many health facilities, there is a widespread view that some subgroups in our population do not receive as much care as they could properly use. Therefore, one of the commonly intended outcomes of health care interventions is that more people will receive more care. Outcome measures of distribution of care include cost, convenience, utilization, and extent of underservice.

The cost of health care, as well as its convenience and availability, are outcomes of interest in assessing the effects of location of services or changes in the numbers of services available. Cost and convenience, however, are not simple to measure. It is not generally agreed just how cost is to be assessed, nor what factors should be incorporated into the cost estimates. Health care does not loom large in the expenditures of most families in those years when all that they require is a few physician's office visits and a few prescriptions to be filled. However, because there is a small, but by no means negligible, chance of a serious disease or injury that would result in major expenditures, most families prefer to have health insurance, the cost of which is much greater than they would ordinarily spend for health care in most years. Once a family is insured, there may be little incentive to keep costs down—for example, by avoiding hospitalization or costly laboratory tests—because the marginal cost to the family is quite small (Davis, 1975). Various schemes to require families to meet a certain deductible before collecting insurance or to make copayments of a certain percentage of costs, or both, have been proposed, and there is now a major experimental test under way of various combinations of deductibles and copayments (Newhouse, 1974) that may provide quite useful information for structuring the costs and benefits of a health insurance system.

Important questions also arise concerning the meaning that health care costs have for consumers. Monies spent on health care may not be regarded in the same way as, for example, monies spent on taxes or on food. People often seem willing to spend large sums of money to achieve questionable health benefits, as in cases of health fads or the prolonging of lives of individuals who seem to have no possibility for further life of acceptable quality. There are, moreover, costs that might be assessed by economists that do not necessarily figure in the reckoning of other consumers. The circumstances under which people will trade off more waiting time for lower money costs are of interest. The important point is that evaluating costs and changes of costs of health care is not a straightforward and simple matter of counting dollars and cents.

When one gets into matters such as time required to obtain health care, the issue of convenience is obviously involved. Sometimes health system interventions are made to increase convenience of care, usually on the assumption that with increased convenience there will be appropriate increases in utilization. Convenience factors include travel time and waiting time, time required to obtain an appointment, and even specific location of facilities, since location may affect availability of public transportation or parking or perceived risk in entering high-crime areas of a city. Subtle factors may make assessment of convenience problematic. For example, travel time is not necessarily a linear function of distance, and psychological distance is not a linear function of either distance or travel time (see Sechrest and Sukstorf, 1977). Geographers successfully utilize a "gravity flow" model

(Lowe and Moryadas, 1975) to account for the effects of distance on a variety of behaviors and interactions, and that model would probably apply to perceived convenience of health care. Essentially, the model relates effective psychological-behavioral distance to the logarithm of physical distance. Thus, placing a clinic 50 miles rather than 100 miles from a community might be expected to have relatively little effect on perceived convenience in comparison to the change from 50 miles to 25 miles. Similarly, complex relationships may exist for time required to obtain care: A minute spent traveling may not be equal to a minute spent waiting. Moreover, travel or time invested in seeking health care may not be viewed as totally allocable to that activity. Rural dwellers may welcome the opportunity to visit the city. One community resisted the development of a local clinic because its inhabitants did not want to be deprived of the excuse to visit the metropolis. In a well-baby clinic, the often lengthy waiting time was valued as an opportunity for visiting and as a relief from other obligations by mothers in attendance.

Utilization of health services as an objective of health care is discussed at length by Rosenstock and Kirscht in Chapter Seven. Utilization is, in some instances, a process measure, it being evident that a health care system cannot have an effect if it is not utilized. Viewed in that way, utilization becomes a focus for intervention with the aim of increasing rates. Lohr (1974) has shown that, prior to the enactment of Medicaid legislation, persons in the lowest income bracket had a lower utilization rate than persons with higher income. After Medicaid, utilization rates in the lower-income group rose to equal those at all other income levels. Equalization of utilization was taken by Lohr to be an indication of improvement in health care for the low-income group. However, high utilization may also be seen as undesirable, and the aim of some interventions is to *decrease* utilization of health services (for example, Follette and Cummings, 1967). If high utilization arises out of diverse psychopathologies, mental health interventions may be thought appropriate and potentially efficacious, a proposition afforded some empirical support (Olbrisch, 1977). There may be a group of persons whose utilization of health services is inappropriately low and another group with an inappropriately high level of utilization. Between, of course, is the bulk of the population with a level of service utilization reasonably congruent with needs.

For research and evaluation purposes, the difficult problem is to assess appropriateness of utilization. That a person sees a physician and has more laboratory studies done than most other persons cannot be taken as prima facie evidence of overutilization. Nor can failure to see a physician within a specified period of time be regarded as underutilization. Typically, appropriateness of utilization is defined normatively—in terms of the expected frequency based on all persons—but sometimes medical condition is taken into account. A good measure of appropriateness of utilization of health service would be valuable for determining whether efforts to change levels of utilization are both successful and medically desirable.

Medical Underservice

Recently, there has been a movement to develop a measure of the degree to which areas such as counties or cities are medically underserved. An Index of Medical Underservice (IMU) has been produced which identifies Medically Underserved Areas (MUA) (United States Office of the Federal Register, 1975). The IMU incorporates four readily available bits of information—ratio of primary care physicians to population, infant mortality rate, percentage of population over sixty-five, and percentage of population below poverty level—into a weighted index whose purpose is to identify areas in need of additional medical services and which, presumably, should be recipients of federal and other aid. Then, if additional medical services are obtained, the IMU should improve. There are problems with the concept of MUA, among which is the fact that a county might be classified as an MUA even though adjacent to a county with ample medical services utilized by residents of the MUA. Whether residents of MUAs actually perceive themselves to be medically underserved is open to question, and there is preliminary evidence to suggest that in at least some MUAs, residents do not necessarily think of themselves as lacking medical services (Kvis, 1976) or even show different rates of utilization of care (Kleinman and Wilson, 1977).

Patient Variables in Health Care Delivery

Increasingly in recent years, the focus in medicine and other service fields has shifted toward accountability, not only to professional organizations but also to consumers of service. Questions of allocation of resources and even of who will receive treatment for conditions for which not everyone can be treated (kidney transplants) are becoming the responsibility of consumer-run panels. Consumer evaluation and satisfaction provide input concerning the community's view of the quantity, quality, and impact of medical services.

Patient Evaluation of Care

The evaluation of the quantity and quality of health care is, to some extent, a function of patient or consumer characteristics. Unless one uses a population-based measure, such as that of the Indian Health Service described earlier, evaluation is ultimately dependent upon judgments of consumers and potential consumers about what is sufficient care either in terms of quantity or quality. Patient satisfaction with health care and the health care system is, in the long run, a potentially powerful determinant of the evolution of that system. The current growth of interest in midwifery and in extrahospital delivery of babies is a good case in point; clearly, neither trend was fostered by the medical profession and both are growing out of consumer concerns (see Ehrenreich and English, 1978).

There are various aspects of health care and its delivery that might be assessed from the patient's point of view: access, convenience, continuity, professional competence, interpersonal relations, and cost, to name but a few. Typically, a questionnaire in Likert format—generally a scale of ratings from one to five—is used for each dimension being examined (Hulka, 1975; Ware, Snyder, and Wright, 1976b). Research may focus on a target sample of patients receiving care or on a sample of community members at large, varying in their contact with the health care system. Satisfaction may be assessed in terms of general reactions to care received or to the last contact with the health care system, or even in terms of the congruence between these two aspects of satisfaction. As yet, very little is known about the effect of discrepancies between what a patient expects from the health care system and what is actually received. Those discrepancies may be more important than what is actually encountered (Brown, 1978), since the responses of patients toward the health care system are likely to be determined more by their subjective sense of satisfaction than by the care they actually receive.

The dimensionality of consumer satisfaction is still open to question, but there may be fewer independent dimensions than are suggested by the list of aspects of health care noted earlier. Zyzanski, Hulka, and Cassel (1974) have developed a scale that assesses three content areas of professional competence: personal qualities of physicians, cost of care, and convenience of care. However, Ware, Snyder, and Wright (1976b) have identified two major components of consumer satisfaction with health care, namely, satisfaction with quality of care and satisfaction with cost and convenience. Both these studies were directed toward satisfaction with care in general rather than with a specific episode of care, but the latter may be more meaningful as a quality of control measure to pinpoint problems or assets.

Patient qualities and behavior often need to be considered in interpreting findings about outcomes of health services since, as stated previously, patient compliance is an important, often critical, determinant of the outcome of a health intervention. Both short-term behaviors relevant to cure of an acute condition and long-term behaviors relevant to successful management of a chronic condition must be considered. The two sets of behaviors and the problems involved are not likely to be the same. In addition, however, still other factors relevant to patient participation in prevention of health problems must be considered. It has been found, for instance, that packaging of drugs in daily and labeled doses can produce a very substantial increase in percentage of patients taking an entire course of antibiotics (Linkewich, Catalano, and Flack, 1974). Outcome studies should not be done without ample attention to patient and system variables that influence compliance and, consequently, potential success of the intervention.

Health Status Indexes

As desirable as it would be to have an index of the health of an individual or a population (see Lerner, 1973) to appraise outcomes of health interventions, existing indexes are related to the impact of illness, and, as discussed earlier, health is usually taken to be merely the absence of illness. A common method of estimating the health of a population has been to do interviews, usually door to door, of a sample of the population, with reports being taken of days lost from work owing to illness, current medical problems, or chronic disease (Katz and others, 1973). However, even chronic conditions may not be reported accurately (Moore, 1975), and data for other problems are likely to be even more undependable (Sechrest, 1977). Consequently, a number of investigators have attempted to devise more dependable and valid indicators of the impact of illness, focusing on limitations imposed by illness or other medical conditions rather than upon disease identification or imprecise assessments of disability. There are many such indexes (for example, Berg, 1973; Kenton, 1973), but three of the more important ones will be discussed here.

One of the earlier health status indexes was the index of Activities of Daily Living (ADL) (Katz and others, 1963). The ADL attempts to assess limitations on functioning in six areas that are considered biologically primary: bathing, dressing, toileting, transfer, continence, and feeding. The overall score on the index reflects increasing levels of dependency upon others. Presumably, any positive effects of health care interventions should be reflected in lower scores, whether for individuals or populations. Katz and his associates have shown the ADL index to be useful in assessing the course of such problems as stroke and hip fracture and also in the study of the effect of provision of comprehensive health services for rheumatoid arthritis. However, the ADL is likely to have serious limitations when used for assessment of the health of unselected populations, since it does not distinguish disability attributable to chronic diseases from that of acute conditions such as viral infections. There is a lot of difference (in terms of prospect for recovery) between being bedridden because of influenza or measles and being bedridden from stroke or even being only mildly incapacitated by angina. The ADL would also change substantially with periodic changes in disability attributable to an unstable disease such as multiple sclerosis, even though the long-term prospects of the patient remained consistently morbid. Still, the ADL remains useful because of the simplicity of its application, and it can provide very useful data for assessing large samples of patients with more or less the same medical conditions.

A second index also focusing on limitations imposed by illness is the Sickness Impact Profile (SIP) (Gilson and others, 1975). The SIP consists of 235 items grouped into 14 areas of functioning. Subjects responding to the questionnaire, usually administered in an interview, are asked to indicate whether each item applies to them as it is presented. Scores are produced for each of the 14 areas and for the overall scale. The 14 areas of functioning can be weighted differentially to reflect views of different groups about the relative importance of different types of limitations. For example, some persons might be more concerned about limitations in locomotor activity, and some about social impacts of illness. One study suggested that patients place more emphasis on social and psychological impacts of illness, whereas physicians put more emphasis on immobility and confinement, locomotor restrictions, and intellectual functioning (Martin and others, 1976). Data from Bergner and others (1976) support the validity of the SIP, and both its internal consistency and test-retest reliability seem adequate (Pollard and others, 1976). A major limitation of the SIP is its length and the compounding fact that for many samples it must be administered in an interview. Consequently, its applications may tend to be limited to samples of relatively small size. Otherwise, it seems a valuable addition to the assortment of measuring instruments to assess health status.

Both the ADL and the SIP avowedly focus on the impact of illness. There is another index available that merits detailed treatment because of its conceptual and methodological complexity and the exceptional sophistication that has been displayed in its development. It gives promise of providing a means of assessing a much wider range of health statuses than the other indexes. For some years, Bush and his associates have been involved in the development of a health status index that is time specific, that is, it reflects health status at a particular moment in time (see Chen, Bush, and Patrick, 1975; Fanshel and Bush, 1970; Patrick, Bush, and Chen, 1973). The index that has been developed is known as the *Index of Well-Being* (IWB) (Kaplan, Bush, and Berry, 1976); it is part of a more comprehensive index that takes into account expected future well-being, that is, prognosis. The latter feature enables the comprehensive index to reflect the differences between acute and chronic conditions. The IWB results from data on functional limitations having to do with mobility, physical activity, and social activity plus self-care. There are five levels of functioning associated with mobility and social activity plus self care, and four with physical activity. An important feature of the IWB function levels is that no subjective judgments are called for; all responses involve reports on things that the subject did or did not do on a particular day. For example, the four levels for physical activity are: walked without physical problems, walked with physical limitations, moved own wheelchair without help, and in bed or chair.

The IWB is a single number reflecting preference ratings of large numbers of subjects for the forty-three combinations of functional statuses that seemed probable in occurrence. The main index varies from a value of 0, assigned to the least preferred status, death, to 1, which is assigned to the "best" level of every activity—"drove car and used bus or train without help, walked without physical problems, and did work, school or housework and other activities" (Kaplan, Bush, and Berry, 1976, p. 486). Values for the forty-one intervening statuses were obtained by scaling preference ratings, resulting in an interval scale that does not necessarily order the forty-three levels of functioning in an obvious way. By including death as a health status with a preference value of 0, the IWB avoids the paradox of an increase in mean level of health status of survivors when those with poorest health status die.

Bush and his colleagues recognized that at any level of functional limitation, persons still differ in health status; for example, even with no functional limitations, some persons may have various symptoms or discomforts that suggest a lower level of health than for persons lacking them. Therefore, a list of thirty-six symptom-problem "complexes" was developed, for each of which a weight was derived that could be used to adjust the IWB. The weights derived from the preference judgments for combinations of limitation and symptom-problem complex states can be either positive or negative, and it is essential to keep in mind that they are based on *preferences* for different states rather than on medical criteria. Thus, "sore throat, lips, tongue, gums, or stuffy, runny nose" (a fairly minor symptom complex) has a weight of .0933, which is added to the main index. The same level of incapacitation would have an adjusted index value .1507 *worse* if it also involved "loss of consciousness such as seizures (fits), fainting, or coma (out cold or knocked out)" (Kaplan, Bush, and Berry, 1976, p. 490). The correction associated with no symptoms or problems whatsoever is .2567; thus, the maximum IWB score is 1.2567. The adjustments to the IWB are thought by Bush and his colleagues to be important because they enable the index to discriminate between persons who are without functional limitations but who are in obviously different states of health. Presumably, that ability to discriminate should also make the IWB more sensitive to health interventions. Without the adjustment for symptom and problem complexes, nearly everyone in the general population would get a score of 1, signifying no functional limitations. As Stewart, Ware, and Brook (1977) have shown, under those conditions very large sample sizes, for example, as large as 50,000, are needed to have reasonable statistical power to detect modest program effects.

The IWB is not without its limitations. The adjustment to the IWB for symptom and problem complexes is limited to the single "most important" item on any given day, and an accumulation of problems might warrant greater adjustment. However, the limitation of ability to adjust is purely practical—a function of the difficulty in getting dependable preference ratings for large numbers of very complex conditions. Also, the IWB may not be sufficiently sensitive at the extremes of the scale. Presumably, the sensitivity of the scale is enhanced by taking symptoms into account, but it is worth noting that many of the symptom-problem complexes that are involved in adjustments are of exactly the sort that would be minimally sensitive to health interventions—hearing difficulties, ringing in ears, weak back, missing limbs, and rashes. Still, there is evidence for some degree of validity for the IWB (Kaplan, Bush, and Berry, 1976; Stewart, Ware, and Brook, 1977), and with further study and work it may be improved and demonstrated to be a valuable tool for studying outcomes of health interventions.

Evaluation of Preventive Health Interventions

With the growing interest in the prevention of illness and disability and the general maintenance of health, the health care researcher is faced with additional problems in the evaluation of outcomes. Typically, a patient in a preventive or life-style modification program is asked to modify some such behavior as smoking in the expectation that there will be an eventual effect on health. However, the time lag between the intervention, assuming it is effective, and the outcome, which is avoidance of illness, is years. The time lag is compounded by the uncertainty of interpreting an effect that consists of not becoming detectably ill. The requirement of a long-term follow-up period encumbers the investigator with problems created by subjects dropping out of treatment and of simply being lost to follow-up. Moreover, the longer the follow-up period, the larger the number of intervening events that could either enhance or mask the effects of treatment. Some problems with the construct validity of the definition of treatment might tend to arise when a long lag period occurs between original treatment and outcome measurement. For example, jogging is currently being promoted as a preventive health measure, the effects of which would surely be determinable only over a long period of time. Yet it is also suggested that joggers will almost certainly, over the long run, lose weight and smoke less. It might be a considerable mistake, then, to attribute any long-term effects to jogging directly. Sophisticated analyses will be required to separate the contributions of such associated factors. Compliance appears again as a complicating factor. It is likely to be poorer when treatments extend over time, and compliance may be especially difficult to document for problems requiring permanent alterations in behavior.

The rather general insensitivity of available measures of health status and health behavior is another problem making evaluation of preventive and life-style change programs difficult. Change in disease state is a very restricted aspect of the overall problem of assessing long-term outcome. Since there is, as yet, no satisfactory measure of positive health available, the research is thrown back upon the device of measuring no more than the absence of illness. That is a most unsatisfying state of affairs.

What is sorely needed is a measure, or set of measures, of quality of life, since the mere absence of illness conveys so very little about the totality of life experience that may result from any change in life-style. If a measure of quality of life could be developed, it could be used not only in evaluation of life-style changes but also in weighing the value of many other interventions. For example, it would be extraordinarily useful to have a quality of life measure to complement survival measures that are employed in evaluating such interventions as cardio-pulmonary resuscitation, coronary bypass surgery, and herniorraphy in elderly patients (see Neuhauser, 1977).

Implications for the Psychologist Researcher

Psychologists have methodological skills that are of great value in developing ways of assessing the effectiveness of various programs, including those in health. The research design and statistical skills of many psychologists are highly developed, and their measurement skills may be unique, unmatched by researchers trained in any other discipline. Consequently, psychologists are in a good position to contribute to the measurement of health outcomes. It is no mere happenstance that such efforts as the Sickness Impact Profile, the Index of Well-Being, and the measures of consumer satisfaction with health care by Ware and others have seen substantial involvement by psychologists. However, beyond the more purely methodological contributions of psychologists, which would be useful in virtually any measurement context, psychologists have important conceptual and theoretical contributions to make to understanding, and ultimately assessing, the experiencing of life. Even when it is possible to document change in disease state, there is very little understanding of the actual experience of health and illness. The medical severity of many diseases does not correspond in any very systematic way with the state of mind of the afflicted person. Seemingly, some people can adapt fairly readily to a quality of life that would be appalling to others. In other cases, relatively innocuous medical procedures or minor incapacities can have very devastating effects on life, effects that so far defy understanding. So much of the impact of health and illness is clearly in the domain of psychology that the discipline should be central to the development of more powerful means for assessing these impacts.

15

Psychological Perspectives on Health System Planning

Nancy E. Adler

Arnold Milstein

A widespread criticism of American health care services is that, because of their uncoordinated functioning and development, they constitute a nonsystem. Hospitals build new beds where many are already lying vacant; specialists are trained when the need for general practitioners is much more acute; and many patients lack access to needed services in spite of accelerating diversion of resources into health care. A repeatedly proposed remedy for these ills is increased health planning. Public Law 93-641, the National Health Planning and Resources Development Act, represents the latest attempt to apply this remedy. This law sets down a blueprint for health planning for the entire country and is anticipated to influence significantly the nature of the U.S. health care system. An important determinant in the success of any legislative remedy is the adequacy with which it incorporates existing knowledge from relevant disciplines. This chapter will examine the major elements of PL 93-641 from the perspective of psychology and evaluate the extent to which its

Note: Grateful thanks are due to Cliff Attkisson and Bruce Stegner for their helpful comments on an earlier draft of this chapter.

planning approach is consistent with psychological theory and research. Before turning to the specific elements of this legislation, we will consider briefly the general concept of health planning.

Health Planning

Health planning refers to a wide range of activities that vary on important dimensions such as: (1) Who is planning? (2) Toward what concept of health? (3) For whose intended benefit? (4) By what process? and (5) In what planning mode? The "who" of health planning can range from individuals making reasoned choices for themselves about a health-determining habit like smoking to the U.S. Congress developing legislation like Medicare that impacts on the health care provided to a large segment of the population. Generally, however, the term is restricted to "a deliberate intervention for change in an operating system by a source not having operating responsibility for the particular activity of the system in which change is desired. Any such source is defined as a planner" (Rosenthal, 1970, p. 293). The ends of health planning include improvement of a single dimension of a single provider's services, such as continuity of care in a community mental health center. They also encompass improving an entire society's level of wellness, as defined by a wide range of indexes such as infant mortality rate, suicide rate, or reported levels of life satisfaction. The remaining three dimensions of planning encompass a similarly broad spectrum of variables. Blum (1974a), in what is perhaps the most comprehensive exploration of health planning to date, distinguishes eight different modes of planning, including the laissez-faire, allocative, explorative, and normative approaches. These, in turn, are characterized across fifteen variables, such as planning outlook, horizon, choice of system boundaries, and cost of obtaining desired effects.

Despite the diversity and complexity of the health planning concept, some core characteristics can be identified. Arnold (1968) discerned a single commonality in all planning. Paraphrased in relation to health planning, this would be the application of scientific reasoning to health-related problem solving. Blum (1974a, pp. 56-59) condenses the wide array of purposes of societywide planning as follows: "The long-range, generally accepted purposes of planning are to define and introduce publicly intended social change which secures for society what its value systems call for."

Essential Features of Public Law 93-641

The goals of the National Health Planning and Resources Development Act are to "facilitate the development of . . . a national health planning policy, to augment areawide and state planning for health services, manpower, and facilities, and to authorize . . . development of resources to further that policy." Although this is a highly complex piece of federal legislation, the following paragraphs summarize its essential features. The law has been implemented by dividing the United States into 202 geographical areas designated as Health Service Areas. Boundaries of these areas were determined primarily by state governments, using federally prescribed factors felt to be important to the establishment of comprehensive health services delivery systems. Population minimums and maximums, referral patterns between different levels and types of health care services, and relationship to existing political and demographic boundaries were among the factors employed. Most frequently, the boundaries incorporate single counties or clusters of counties, include at least one source of each highly specialized service (such as a burn treatment or cardiac surgery center), and encompass populations ranging from 500 thousand to 2 million people.

In each Health Service Area, the federal government designated and funded an organization to be a Health Systems Agency (HSA), which is responsible for health planning for that area. Designated HSAs were formed either by ad hoc groups of citizens within the Health Service Area or by local government(s) whose borders coincided with those of the Health Service Area. Once funded, an HSA is directed by its governing body, which is composed wholly of volunteers. Though the specific processes by which governing body members were selected varied considerably from one HSA to the next, governing bodies were required to reflect the sociodemographic characteristics of the Health Service Area's population and provide for the membership of representatives of the area's health care providers and local elected officials. The legislation gives preference to the interests of consumers; at least 51 percent, though not more than 60 percent, of the governing body, as well as of the executive committee (which governs the HSA between governing body meetings), must be made up of consumers. Since everyone is potentially a consumer, the law further stipulates that consumer representatives must not themselves be or recently have been a provider, be married to a provider, or have a financial interest in a provider.

A governing body, once composed, uses its federal funds to hire a planning staff, whose work it then guides. Through its governing body, the HSA is accountable to the federal government for performing the functions specified in its designation agreement, which includes additional accountabilities to state and local government, other health or planning agencies, and the population of the health service area. In broad overview, the functions of an HSA are to develop and implement plans to improve the area's health and health care services. Every year, each HSA is required by law to develop a short-range plan, called an Annual Implementation Plan, and to update a long-range plan, called a Health Systems Plan. Both plans represent the goals for health and health care in the area and the means by which these goals will be met in the short and long term.

HSAs use their limited authorities to implement these plans, which affect both public and private health services. An HSA's authorities include approving or disapproving prospective uses of several categories of federal health services monies and granting seed money to stimulate changes in the health care system. HSAs also recommend to state governments whether existing health services are "appropriate" and whether or not states should grant certificates of need to persons or institutions proposing to alter significantly the health care system. Since no substantial tangible changes in the health care system are legally permissible without a certificate of need, this is an important influencing role. In each of these activities, an HSA uses its prospectively developed plans as its guide. For example, a hospital proposing to expand its maternity unit would submit its proposal to the HSA in its Health Service Area. The HSA would examine the proposal in relation to the maternity services component of its overall health care services plan for the area and recommend approval or disapproval to the state certificate of need agency based on their degree of congruence.

HSA Planning Processes

Federal law, regulations, and guidelines that shape an HSA's conduct of planning are very complex. While these permit a wide variety of approaches, most planning within an HSA involves the following components: (1) specifying an image of a desired health status and health care system for the population of the health services area; (2) examining the current state of the area's health and health care system in relation to the desired state; (3) developing strategies for reducing discrepancies between what exists now and what is desired; (4) implementing the strategies; and (5) evaluating implemented strategies for impact.

This sequence of steps suggests an orderliness to HSA planning that is not possible or even desirable in practice. For example, it is sometimes necessary for an HSA to implement strategies via certificate of need recommendations (step 4) before it has constructed a specific image of a desired health care system (step 1). Further, retrospective evaluation of this implemented strategy (step 5) may alter an HSA's view of the current state of the area's health care system (step 2). A specific illustration of this lack of sequential order is a case in which an HSA approves a certificate of need application from a hospital proposing to build a drug abuse treatment center before it has a detailed image of a desired system of drug abuse treatment services in the area. Later, in evaluating the impact of its certificate of need decision, the HSA may discover that several small general outpatient clinics in the neighborhood are now in jeopardy because they depended on drug abuse treatment for financial solvency. The HSA has thus gained an appreciation of a new characteristic of its area's health care system—the financial fragility of general clinics in this neighborhood. HSA planning is thus an iterative process, consisting of an ongoing interplay among each of its component parts.

In overview, then, the general HSA model whose psychological dimensions will be explored is directed by a governing body, representative of an area's sociodemographic characteristics, and assisted by a professional staff of planners. The function of this body is to discern gaps between desired status of the area's health and health care system and their current status, implement plans to close the gaps, and then evaluate its own impact.

It is difficult to present a more detailed picture of HSA planning activities because of the flexibility permitted HSAs by federal law and by the iterative nature of planning just described. However, commonalities determined by law, usual practice, or available options include the following:

First, federal guidelines for Health System Plan development recommend that HSAs consider six categories of services spanning six settings of a health care system. Services include community health promotion and protection, prevention and detection, diagnosis and treatment, habilitation and rehabilitation, maintenance, and support. Settings encompass community, home, mobile, ambulatory, short-stay, long-stay, and free-standing support facilities (such as laboratories and blood banks). For each service type, HSAs are then asked to evaluate six characteristics: cost, availability, accessibility, continuity, acceptability, and quality. This common framework for conceptualizing the current and desired status of the health care system is shared by all HSAs adhering to federal guidelines.

Second, it is the HSA governing body that is empowered to take official action on all aspects of the planning process. The members of this body determine the nature of the target status of health and health services for the area; they direct the assessment activities in which the status quo is examined and problems identified; they select strategies for improvement; they oversee their implementation; and they direct and draw conclusions from evaluation activities. Governing body activities are required by law to take place in group settings which are open to the public.

Third, there is a variety of ways that governing bodies can represent the population of the health service area. They may consider their own views to reflect the outlook of their constituency. They may solicit direct input from fellow citizens, or they may turn to the HSA's staff who may employ a variety of techniques to take the community's pulse.

Finally, HSAs relate closely to two agencies at the statewide level. A State Health Planning and Development Agency (SHPDA) primarily serves to alter the plans of HSAs in order to bring them into harmony with each other and make certificate of need decisions. The SHPDA, in turn, is monitored and directed by a consumer-majority Statewide Health Coordinating Council (SHCC), whose relationship to the SHPDA bears resemblance to the relationship between a governing body and its HSA.

In summary, though HSA planning activities vary considerably, they tend to share a common conception of the health care system, are governed in public meetings of sociodemographically determined representatives of the health service area, draw on a finite list of techniques to involve the public in the planning process, and relate to parallel agencies at the state level. The remainder of this chapter will examine the HSA approach to health planning from a psychological perspective. We will consider several assumptions of the law, focusing mainly on the question of adequate representation of the needs and desires of the population of health service areas.

Psychological Perspectives on HSA Planning Processes

As noted earlier, health planning encompasses a wide range of variables. Although most planning is at the level of general social systems, there is also concern with the understanding and prediction of individual thought, affect, and behavior. Planning decisions regarding health facilities and services are based on assumptions about the needs, values, attitudes, and actions of consumers as well as providers of health services. Further, the decision-making process is itself subject to the influence of these psychological variables. Implicit, therefore, in any planning approach is a model of human psychological functioning. Whereas some of these models and their component assumptions may be consistent with psychological theory and knowledge, others may not. We will consider some of the psychological assumptions and models implicit in the HSA approach to health planning, suggest modifications that are in line with a psychologically based analysis and identify needs and opportunities for psychological research.

Community Representation

Community representation is a key element of HSAs. Decision making rests in the hands of a governing body intended to represent the population that is to be affected by the HSA's decisions. Since, in fact, all people are affected by the health system, it becomes important to define the dimensions along which individuals' health-relevant values are most accurately represented. The present specifications of HSA governing body composition provide for representation along economic, social, and demographic lines.

Specification of economic roles permits the important differentiation between consumers and providers. Not only do patients and providers have different and potentially conflicting values in relation to the health system, but they also have different perspectives on the very basics of health and illness (Baumann, 1961; Freidson, 1970b; Kasl and Cobb, 1966). The economic distinction between consumer and provider is further differentiated by other characteristics that are assumed to account for additional variance in health-related values. Since providers differ among themselves in their position and values in relation to health and the health care system, provider representatives are subdivided into distinct functional categories designed to embody these differences: Provider-governing body membership is mandated for health professionals, health care institutions, health care insurers, health professions schools, and allied health professionals. Whether or not these functional categories ensure accurate representation of the range of health-related provider values is an empirical question. There is, at this point, no clear contrary evidence or reason to believe that important value perspectives are underrepresented. Unfortunately, this is not the case with consumer representation.

Sociodemographic approaches. According to the legislation, consumer representatives must be broadly representative of the social, economic, linguistic, and racial populations, geographic areas of the health service area, and major purchasers of health care (Federal Register, 1976). Implied in using social and demographic characteristics to obtain consumer representation are the assumptions that each of the sociodemographic characteristics is associated with different values or perspectives regarding health and health services, and that sociodemographic variables account for the major sources of variance in health-related values. From a psychological perspective, both assumptions warrant further comment.

There is empirical evidence to support the assumption that some sociodemographic variables are associated with important variance in attitudes and values toward health and the health care system. Socioeconomic status, for example, has shown consistent relationships to health-related variables. Research has demonstrated that despite lower health status among those of lower socioeconomic status, there is a negative relationship between socioeconomic status and utilization of health care service (see Chapter Seven in this volume; see also Bullough, 1972; Hyman, 1970; Muller, 1965; Pratt, 1971). Koos (1954) found class differences in the percentages of people stating that particular symptoms needed medical attention, with fewer people of lower socioeconomic status indicating a need for medical help for given symptoms. In one study of mental health services, it was found that even where ability to pay was not a factor, acceptance of therapy and clinical experience was related to the patient's social class (Myers and Schaeffer, 1954). Others have also shown that financial barriers alone do not account for the lower utilization of medical services among those of lower socioeconomic status (see, for example, Bergner and Yerley, 1968).

Other sociodemographic variables, such as ethnicity, age, and sex, have also been found to relate to a range of health values and behaviors (Bullough, 1972; Suchman, 1964; Tornstam, 1975; Zborowski, 1952; Zola, 1966). Taken together, these studies provide evidence to support the first assumption that sociodemographic variables relate to health values. A question remains, however, as to whether these variables can be wholly relied upon to account for the major sources of variance in attitudes, values, and behavior regarding health and the health care system. Ware and others (1974, p. 4) cite the suggestion of Anderson and Newman that "such individual characteristics as health values may be more useful than sociodemographic characteristics as predictors of utilization because of the intervention properties of values." Intervening variables such as attitudes toward the medical and social system have been shown to account for much of the relationship of socioeconomic status and untreated illness (Hyman, 1970). Further, Freeborn and others (1977) note that, in recent years, studies have shown a diminished relationship of socioeconomic status and health services utilization.

There is also empirical evidence suggesting that nonsociodemographic variables significantly affect health values and attitudes, casting doubt on the validity of the second assumption. Experiential variables are a case in point. Particularly important are a person's experiences in relation to health and illness and the present health care system. DiCicco and Apple (1960) found that among older people health was important only as it became poor health. Ware and others (1974) found that the value of health varied with health status among other variables. Their research examined health as a value in relation to other terminal values (Rokeach, 1973). Factor analysis of eighteen values revealed four factors. Health appeared in the first factor, which also included values of family security and salvation; an exciting life loaded negatively on this factor. Scores on this factor, which was labeled by the authors as representing "self-preservation values," were found to be related to perceptions of poor current and prior health, anxiety about health, and satisfaction with continuity of care. While sex, age, and employment status were also found to relate to the importance attached to self-preservation values, other sociodemographic variables were not.

Health experiences and aspiration level. Individuals threatened with a serious illness may be more likely to attach greater importance to health relative to other values and may support a relatively greater allocation of resources to health care than would those not facing such a threat. Since a major issue pertaining to planning health care services is cost (including opportunity costs of resources devoted to health), it would be important to assure accurate representation along the dimension of concern about health relative to other social problems. Current health status is likely to be an important variable in determining a person's position along this dimension. Chronic health problems may play a somewhat different role than more acute or short-term experiences in determining health values. Tornstam (1975) found that aspirations as to level of health were influenced by objective levels of health; individuals in better health held higher aspiration levels for health. Age influenced both objective health status and, to a lesser extent, aspiration level as to health; older people had lower levels of health and had lower aspiration levels for their health. Tornstam stressed the importance of aspiration level in determining a range of outcome variables, including satisfaction. He noted that "poor actual, objective health status can be outbalanced by a very low aspiration level" (p. 270). This phenomenon can create ethical dilemmas since satisfaction can be influenced by decreasing aspiration levels as well as by increasing services. Representation on HSAs of people with varying levels of aspiration for health would thus be important. Since age and current health status have both been found to be indicators of aspiration level, they may be logical dimensions for representation.

Is the sociodemographic approach adequate? As demonstrated in the research by Tornstam (1975), sociodemographic (in this case, age) and experiential (in this case, health status) variables are likely to be related. Lower-class individuals, certain ethnic groups, rural people, and older people may be more likely to experience ill health, be less likely to have a regular provider of health care, experience less continuity of care, and so on. However, even when statistically significant relationships between these variables are found, the absolute degree of association may be small. Lower-class people may, on average, experience poorer health than the middle class, but there is likely to be a great deal of overlap in the health status of the two groups. To take a specific example, Tornstam used path analysis to investigate relationships among the variables he was studying. While age was found to exert a direct influence on aspiration level, the path coefficient was only —.134. Thus, less than 2 percent of the variance in aspiration level was accounted for by age. Other unstudied variables account for the majority of variance in aspiration. Because of the low absolute level of association, demographic representation alone cannot be relied upon to assure experiential or value representation. One cannot assume that a lower-class representative or a representative from a rural area on an HSA board will actually have experienced poor health or lack of continuity of care.

Because of overlapping distributions, representatives of specific social groups may not embody the values "typifying" the group and which ought to be represented on HSA boards. Further, HSA representatives are, to a great extent, self-selected, which introduces an even stronger possibility for underrepresentation of certain values. Given the degree of self-selection involved in the determination of HSA governing boards, it is actually very likely that representatives of specific sociodemographic groups will *not* represent the very attributes that may differentiate those groups from others in terms of health values. Vladeck (1976, p. 49) notes that "the consumer members of the HSA are not randomly chosen individuals, not your ordinary consumers. . . . Consumers are not, indeed, going to be average patients but rather those with background experience and resources of their own." In establishing HSAs, no thought appears to have been given to psychological aspects of volunteering for governing-board representation. HSA legislation is largely silent on the question of the method by which individuals are selected to fill the governing-body positions. This silence implies that selection methods themselves pose no danger to obtaining accurate representation of the community's health values. Here again, there is reason to question this fundamental assumption in the legislation.

It is clear, for example, that there needs to be adequate representation of those who are currently underserved by the present health care system. Input from low utilizers or from those who feel alienated from the system would be particularly important in designing future service delivery systems that could serve these groups. As noted earlier, use of health services is lower among those of lower socioeconomic status and alienation is higher. However, representatives of lower socioeconomic status are not likely themselves to be alienated from the system. The very characteristics that define alienation, such as hopelessness and powerlessness (Seeman, 1959), make it unlikely that alienated individuals would be motivated to participate in HSAs. Seeman and Evans (1962) found that people high in alienation show less information-seeking behavior regarding their own disease; it is probable that they would be even less likely to seek to gain control over the future direction of the health care system.

Similar arguments could be made with regard to a range of experiential, attitudinal, and personality variables that would affect both motivation to participate in HSA governance and health-related values that could influence decisions made. Locus of control, for example, has been found to relate to health behaviors (Dabbs and Kirscht, 1971; MacDonald, 1970), especially when the concept and its measurement have been refined to measure locus of control regarding health (Wallston, Wallston, and Maides, 1976; Wallston, Maides, and Wallston, 1976). Locus of control is associated with socioeconomic status but, because of self-selection, individuals seeking to be HSA representatives from any socioeconomic class would be expected to have greater internal locus of control than those who feel more fatalistic about their health and health care and who would consequently not feel able or motivated to influence the health care delivery system.

Introversion-extroversion is an example of a characteristic that is less likely to be class linked but is pertinent to HSA participation. It is likely that individuals seeking to be HSA representatives will be more extroverted than those not seeking such positions. Introversion-extroversion could also be related to values affecting decisions about health needs and facilities. Extroverts, for example, may place relatively less stress on the importance of privacy and separation in hospital waiting rooms and patient rooms. They may consider this an irrelevant attribute of hospital design and may be unrepresentatively negative toward a proposed certificate of need for hospital modernization aimed largely at improving patient privacy.

As noted earlier, experience of health and illness would also be a likely determinant of both HSA participation and health values. If HSA boards are limited, de facto, to those who are particularly concerned about health services, the result may be continued expansion and escalation of costs beyond that which would be desired by the population as a whole. Since variables such as health status and personality attributes may substantially determine health care values and willingness to participate in HSA governance, assuring representation from persons with various experiences and attributes is important. However, this argument is speculative. Although it seems likely that health status, health care utilization, and personality characteristics would be associated with varying health values and the desire to participate in HSA activities, only the first set of relationships has been even preliminarily studied.

A useful direction for psychological research to take would be to determine the congruence between the attitudes and values of governing-board members and those of the consumers they are intended to represent. Further, psychological and experiential determinants of representative-constituency differences should be investigated. Historically, sociologists and anthropologists have been more involved in the area of health and medicine than have psychologists. Thus, more is known about differences in health values among different social and cultural groups than about differences regarding the health system among individuals varying in personality, past experience, or current behavior. There is now a body of literature on volunteering for psychological research, and we know a good deal about how volunteers differ from nonvolunteers (Rosenthal and Rosnow, 1975). This knowledge permits psychologists to establish the generalizability of the research based on volunteers and to estimate the limits of their research. Similarly, research is needed to establish whether, or to what extent, volunteers for HSA boards differ from nonvolunteers to establish whether the governing boards can be fully relied upon to represent the community's values.

Psychological representation. One outcome of the suggested research might be a plan for representation along psychological rather than, or in addition to, demographic lines. Such a psychological approach to representation is unprecedented and would be likely to generate considerable controversy. Our society has been arranged along sociodemographic and geographic lines in health as in other sectors. However, our culture has become increasingly psychologically minded and may be ready to consider such an idea. In addition to philosophical barriers, there would be practical problems in implementing such an innovative approach. However, we believe the idea has sufficient merit to warrant consideration as either an alternative or a basis for augmenting the current selection bases and procedures.

"Psychological" representation would reduce biases introduced by self-selection, since the dimensions on which representation is desired would be specified and recruited for. Practically, of course, it may be difficult or impossible to represent people along some personality dimensions such as locus of control or introversion-extroversion. In some instances, research may reveal more easily identifiable individual traits associated with health values that would be used in determining representation. Here, as in the case of demographic variables, there would have to be a very high level of association to rely on such identifying variables. Compared to representing personality dimensions, representation along attitudinal and value lines should be easier to achieve since it is easier to obtain information on the range of attitudes and values in a community than it is to obtain personality profiles.

One strength of psychological representation would be that it would force HSAs to define the relevant values and characteristics that should be represented. Problems of achieving that representation would still remain, but it would at least provide an impetus for discussing value positions. This approach would also encourage active recruitment of participants to represent particular value or attitude perspectives. In some instances, this may be difficult to do (as in the case of alienation), but better representation will result than if total self-selection is permitted. Finally, this approach would allow evaluation of the extent to which adequate representation had or had not been achieved. As it presently stands, one can get a representative of the poor or of the sick without knowing how well his or her values represent those of the group. Since it is the values that one wants to have represented, it would seem more useful to attempt representation directly along those lines.

This would be a very different approach than is presently being taken. In an analysis of the HSA approach, Vladeck (1977) argues that those on the governing boards are likely not to be true representatives of consumers but rather of specific constituencies. Thus, consumer representatives will be from interest groups such as senior citizens, retarded children, or victims of specific diseases. Provider representatives also will not represent the broad range of provider interests but rather specific interests, such as the local hospital association and medical school. This form of representation is common in our society and reflects the belief that society is made up of "groups defined by shared economic, cultural, ethnic, or geographic interests and that these are legitimate interests in public policy and policy formation" (Vladeck, 1977, p. 25). Vladeck criticized this interest-group representation since the result is often infighting and logrolling and, historically, the loser in such a process is the general public. The approach described earlier, which is aimed at obtaining an accurate representation of differing consumer values and not just sociodemographic categories, is one mechanism for promoting the frequently bypassed interests of the general public.

Fortunately, opportunities for accurate representation of consumer preference and values are not limited to governing-body composition. Consumer preference also influences the decision-making process of HSAs through the input and work of the professional planning staff. The governing body consists of volunteer members who are likely to spend only a small fraction of their time on HSA issues, and there is a full-time staff that does the background work for the board. While final decisions are made by the board, the staff has a great deal of influence in terms of their interpretation of the information provided. At least some members of the staff will be professional planners. In the next section, we will examine some of the approaches of health planners as these influence input to HSA decision making.

Professional Planners—Another Source of Consumer Input

Until recently, consumers had little true input into the planning process, and decisions were made predominantly by professional planners (B. Bloom, 1976). Even under HSAs, planners will have a great deal of influence. Perceived as experts in the field, their recommendations are likely to influence significantly consumer members who may be unsure of their own credentials regarding planning and policy (this problem will be discussed later). The structure of the HSAs also increases planners' influence, as only the planners are paid staff. As a result, they will have more time and opportunity to be fully informed than will board members, adding additional force to their recommendations.

Ideally, the process of planning is value free, and planners' own perspectives should not bias decision making. In actual practice, however, planners do have their own ideas and values which can influence their judgments. Planners may, in fact, represent their own interest groups, especially when their views and interests come into conflict with those of consumers (Kahn, 1969). Planners frequently differ in cultural and social values from clients in the area in which they are working. Planners usually hold middle-class professional values and, consequently, are more likely to share the assumptions and values of largely middle-class providers than of consumers from other socioeconomic classes. However, planners do try to measure and take into account consumer needs and preferences. As we shall see, problems arise in both the measurement of preference and in the resolution of differences between what consumers want and what planners think would be best. Psychological expertise can be useful in both areas.

Measuring Consumer Preference

Gaining an accurate assessment of needs and desires of individuals within a community is, in essence, a psychological question, and the measurement of preference involves complex psychological processes (Parker and Srinivasan, 1976). The first problem is to obtain an accurate portrayal of the population, which gets us into the familiar matter of sampling. One needs to define the relevant community and to sample a representative range of opinions from within it. Planners have often approached this problem by using "key informants" in a community to report on needs. However, such informants rarely represent a true cross-section of viewpoints, and there is not a "single statistically significant case where the rank ordering of problems was the same as between key informants and the users of services" (Delbecq, 1976, p. 219). Other approaches do involve face-to-face contact between planners and a broader cross-section of the community. This may take place at a hearing, community meeting, or meeting with individual organizations. This approach has the advantage of eliciting active involvement of affected community members and giving planners the opportunity to gauge the intensity of feeling around specific issues. The disadvantage is that participants are likely to be highly self-selected, making it difficult to determine the true distribution of concerns or feelings in the community. Further, this process can be subject to manipulation (Kahn, 1969).

To obtain a measure of the range and distribution of community views, three techniques are frequently used: telephone interviews, mail questionnaires, and cross-sectional field surveys (Warheit, 1976). Psychologists also use these techniques in conducting attitude surveys. There is a relatively sophisticated methodology associated with the use of such techniques which needs to be considered in the realm of planning as well as in psychological research. A major problem is possible bias in samples. For example, who answers telephone interviews? If such interviews are conducted in communities in which telephones are not universal, one could underrepresent the views of the poor or transient who do not have phones. If the interviews are conducted only during working hours using home phone listings, one would also obtain a biased sample of respondents. Mail surveys can potentially reach a much broader group but they are less likely to be returned. Response rates on mail questionnaires range from 10 to 40 percent (Selltiz, Wrightsman, and Cook, 1976). Those who do respond are likely to differ from those who do not, and the results may not be generalizable to the community as a whole. In addition, such questionnaires need to be evaluated in terms of reliability and validity, including whether wording is clear and neutral and whether effects of response sets, such as yea- or nay-saying, and social desirability have been controlled.

Cross-sectional interviews have fewer sampling problems. They usually elicit higher participation rates and are less likely to create biases from self-selection of respondents. However, they are more costly and may be subject to interviewer effects. Schwartz (1973, p. 25) compared responses to a phone or mail follow-up evaluation by hospital patients of their treatment. A response rate of 85 percent was obtained for the phone interview compared to 35 percent for the mail questionnaire. However, the responses in the two situations may not have been comparable. An analysis of the responses revealed differences on one out of the three outcome measures. Schwartz believed that respondents may have given more honest responses in the more anonymous mail situation than when in direct contact with an interviewer. The validity of interviews depends a great deal on the skill and training of the interviewer. The manner in which questions are asked (in addition to the actual wording of the question) and unintentional reinforcement of specific responses can influence the results obtained. Respondents may have attitudes not only toward the topic about which they are being interviewed but also toward the interviewer, the situation in which they are being interviewed, the perceived sponsor of the survey, and the uses to which results will be put. Webb and others (1969) note that respondents select from among the many "true" selves and behaviors open to them. Respondents are aware of the interview situation which forces upon them "a role-defining decision—What kind of a person should I be as I answer these questions?" (p. 16). Further, the biosocial characteristics of interviewers, such as their age, race, or status may influence responses (Benney, Riesman, and Star, 1956; Ehrlich and Riesman, 1961; Kahn and Cannell, 1957) and may interact with perceptions of the sponsor, purpose, or goals of the research. For example, studies investigating attitudes toward Jews found less expressed anti-Semitism when interviewers were either Jewish (Hyman and others, 1954) or had a Jewish name and appearance but were not necessarily Jewish (Robinson and Rhode, 1946). In surveys related to health, interviewers who are perceived as related to the medical establishment may find fewer criticisms of present services and facilities than those who are seen to be independent of the established institutions.

In recent years, in part because of growing involvement of psychologists and use of psychological knowledge, greater attention has been given to the problem of bias inherent in these techniques of assessing need and preference. Several alternatives have been suggested. An approach that has been taken on the level of general social planning has been to use "social indicators" to evaluate community needs. This approach involves nonreactive measurement and takes a detached overview of the population. An indicator should directly measure community welfare, and "if it changes in the 'right' direction, while other things remain equal, things have gotten better or people are better off" (B. Bloom, 1976, p. 159). Indicators are generally chosen inductively and a number of different indicators have been used. The specific indicators applied to a given community depend both on the particular areas of life quality that are included and the indicator chosen to represent each area. Health is one of three areas that is almost universally examined. Bloom (1976, p. 164) cites examples of some of the measures of level of health that are used: "Specific measures of life expectancy, disability, and access to medical care have been proposed. Examples of measures of life expectancy include: life expectancy at birth; life remaining at ages 30 and 50; and infant mortality rate. Examples of disability measures include: days of disability per person per year; admission rates into mental hospitals and into nursing homes; rates at which persons are limited in their major activities due to chronic conditions; and injury rate. Examples of measure of access to medical care include: extent of health insurance coverage; and personal confidence in ability to obtain good health care."

Despite the appeal of the social indicators approach, a number of problems remain. Some indicators involve subjective judgments which may create some of the same measurement problems as do other approaches to need assessment. Other indicators do lend themselves to objective measurement but their meaning may be ambiguous. Bloom (1976) gives the example of admissions to nursing homes and mental hospitals, where decreasing rates could be taken as either a good sign or bad depending on one's assumptions and point of view. The relationship between the indicator and the underlying state it is supposed to represent is not always clear. In this, as in other areas of measurement, attention needs to be paid not only to issues of reliability but also to those of validity. As a result of these problems, social indicators can be used as one input to decision making but, used alone, they cannot be wholly relied upon to guide health policy decisions accurately.

Another approach that reflects concern about psychological processes is the "nominal group approach" developed by Delbecq (1976). While the other techniques can be used in developing comprehensive plans in order to allocate resources, this approach is useful in understanding a given need in depth in order to develop innovative programs. This approach does involve measurement of consumer preference but it is focused on a very specific area rather than on a broad measurement of need or preference. The nominal group technique draws explicitly upon psychological concepts, notably those concerning group dynamics. Some of the problems in group interaction that this technique was designed to reduce will be discussed in a later section in which the dynamics of decision making in HSA governing-board meetings will be considered and essential features of the technique will be described.

Each of the techniques described thus far has its strengths and limitations. By nature of the assumptions made, measuring tools used, and scope of issue addressed, each limits the kinds of answers one can obtain. An attempted solution to this problem has been offered by Nguyen, Attkisson, and Bottino (1976). They describe the approach of convergent analysis which is based on the assumption that "no single need documentation technique and no single set of stakeholders can offer a comprehensive view of the human service needs in a particular community" (p. 37). In convergent analysis, there is an integration of information from various viewpoints and value perspectives, data are garnered using different assessment strategies, and information is gathered collectively over time. Building on these ideas originally suggested by Attkisson and his colleagues, Bell (1976) offered a convergent assessment model that employs three components: service utilization (which examines characteristics of current users and uses of facilities), social indicators, and citizen survey. Parallels can be drawn between this type of approach and attempts in psychology to attain more control over inference through triangulation of measures.

Using Consumer Preference Information

The use to which information on consumer preference is put will depend on the nature of the information and the planner's relationship to it. At one extreme, planners make decisions based on what they believe to be in the best interests of the consumers for whom they are planning. In this instance, planners may obtain consumer preference data, but the assumptions underlying the techniques chosen to assess need and the questions asked are likely to represent the planners' and not the consumers' framework and viewpoint. Lack of congruence between the views of these two groups is most likely when there is little direct contact. Techniques such as the nominal group approach were developed to minimize such instances. Delbecq (1976, p. 221) noted that it is difficult for professionals to understand the client's mind set from purely quantitative data: "I have yet to find one planning group that I have been able to convince that it is worthwhile to spend time inside the experience of the group that they are planning for, that have not come out of that experience with a whole depth of perception and sensitivity that would be missed by means of any other data-gathering mechanism."

Despite the existence of techniques that reduce potential bias, such as the nominal group approach, social indicators, and convergent analysis, an inherent conflict remains between the approach of planners, which Bloom (1976) describes as "I know what you need," versus that of consumers, which he summarizes as "I know what I want." The differentiation of need and want is important, for they may often diverge. There are problems in siding completely with one or the other. Up to now, power has resided mainly with planners. They have proceeded on the basis of what they thought was needed, and a number of problems have resulted. Problems of bias and differences in values and outlook from the clients for whom they are planning can generate planning directions that deviate significantly from public preferences. Further, planners may be working on the basis of old, incomplete, or incorrect information (Bloom, 1976). One can find a number of instances where planners' views of clients' needs differed so dramatically from the actual desires of the clients that programs broke down. An example of the problem that arises when there is conflict between experts' views of need and clients' views of wants was the program developed by military psychiatrists for returning prisoners of the Vietnam War. Psychiatrists were concerned about the reaction of ex-POWs to returning home abruptly and wanted to prevent development of severe psychological disorders. To accomplish this, they suggested that every ex-POW spend a few days in a military hospital overseas before returning home, allowing them a more gradual transition. However, neither POWs nor their families wanted a delay in their return. Following protests by them and by others, the program was scuttled (Dohrenwend, 1976).

It is not clear that a client's definition of want is necessarily the best indicator of need. In the example just given, it may well be that the planners had correctly assessed need. Following the return of the POWs, there were a number of suicides, suggesting that there may have been a need for an acclimation period or some other "unwanted" intervention at the time of their return (Dohrenwend, 1976). Frequently, advances in public good and eventual satisfaction are made by those who push beyond immediate public preference (Kahn, 1969). Demone (1976) notes that of four significant health measures, three were adopted by administrative or legislative means. He cites the case of fluoridation, where many people voted against something that most professionals viewed as "helpful, painless, and inexpensive."

The Relationship Between Want and Need

The problem of basing decisions on consumers' statements of want versus professionals' statements of need suggests a potential conflict between want and need. Want is a concept denoting current preferences among available choices. Need reflects how rewarding a selected choice will be over time. Is expressed want, in fact, the best indicator of need? Different psychological theories would take different stands on that issue, as will be seen.

Attitude and decision theory perspective. The measurement of "want" in planning decisions is frequently an attitude measure. One seeks to know what consumers' attitudes are toward the location of a new health facility or their feelings about whether such a facility is needed. Different planning questions tap different components of attitude. In some instances, it is most useful to know the cognitive, belief aspect of attitudes: What do people believe would be the consequences of building a new facility or adding new equipment? Most frequently, however, surveys are designed to tap the evaluative dimension: Do people feel positively or negatively toward option X or option Y? Of concern also is the conative, action dimension: What policy stands would people endorse and/or what actions would they be willing to take in support of their attitudes?

Inherent in all attitude measurement is the possible discrepancy between public and private attitudes. The earlier discussion of threats to validity of measurement of consumer preference reflects the belief that private attitudes are more representative of the person's "true" feelings, and thus should be more highly related to needs, than are public attitudes. One challenge, then, to adequate portrayal of need through statements of want arises from measurement problems. Even beyond the limitations of measurement techniques, there are conflicting theoretical stances toward the relationship of want and need.

The set of theories that posit the closest relationship between want and need are decision theories. There are a number of versions of such theories, including subjective expected utility theory (Edwards, 1954), cognitive-affective consistency theory (Rosenberg, 1956), and value x expectancy theory (Fishbein, 1963; Fishbein and Ajzen, 1975). These theories share the assumption that a person's attitude toward a given alternative will be a function of his or her expectations about the consequences associated with that alternative. For example, subjective expected utility theory posits that individuals act as though they were comparing the outcome of various alternatives. The alternative chosen is that in which the sum of the products of the subjective utility of each outcome multiplied by the subjective probability of its occurrence is greatest. Fishbein's model asserts that intention to perform a given act will be a function of perceived normative expectations regarding the act and beliefs about the consequences of performing the act (the sum of products of the evaluation of each outcome times the probability of its occurrence). Thus, individuals are seen to engage in cost-benefit analysis and their statement of want would be taken as the best approximation of need.

Even within a decision-making framework, there are conditions under which want may not best represent need. Simon (1957) has challenged the idea that people *maximize* value in making decisions. Rather, he argues for the idea of bounded rationality in which people "satisfice," choosing an alternative that is satisfactory but which may not necessarily be best. In situations in which there are a number of alternatives and/or outcomes (which is likely to be the case in health decisions), comparing all choices would be too complex and individuals are likely to "satisfice" rather than maximize (Mills, Meltzer, and Clark, 1977). Further, decision theories are based on subjective utilities and probabilities. These subjective values may not correspond to objective values (in those situations where objective information can be obtained). In some cases, decisions may be based on faulty, incomplete, or distorted information. Thus, while one decision may be best, given the person's knowledge and expectations, quite a different choice might be made with more accurate information.

The greatest challenge to an appropriate mesh of wants and needs from a decision-making point of view is imperfect information. Other theoretical perspectives suggest that even under conditions of accurate information (or at least information that is physically available, which some would argue does not guarantee that it is psychologically available to the person), individuals will still not necessarily make the choice that will, in the long run, bring the greatest satisfaction.

Psychoanalytic perspective. Other theoretical perspectives, such as psychoanalytic psychology, call into question the assumption that it is only imperfect information or inability to anticipate future sense of reward that might endanger using expressed want as an adequate proxy for need. Such theoretical approaches would suggest that powerful unconscious forces could lead a person to express unrewarding preferences. A few examples of how such forces may operate in the area of health planning will be discussed.

The very idea of illness and the need for health care may arouse unconscious anxiety in some individuals because of associations to ideas of helplessness, damage to self, and loss of important others. Unconscious defenses employed to reduce the anxiety may lead to expressed preferences (wants) that deviate from those choices that would, in fact, generate the most rewarding health impact for individuals. A case in point is individuals who employ denial of the true threat of health problems; for example, denial has been shown to be related to delay in seeking treatment for cancer (Shands and others, 1951) and delay in surgery (Andrew, 1972). Personality types vary in their use of denial. For example, psychoanalytic assessments have suggested that an unconsciously-based defensive sense of invulnerability is particularly likely to be shown by individuals with narcissistic personality traits. This sense of invulnerability, which is interpreted as serving as a defense against feelings of low self-esteem and physical danger, can have a direct impact on a person's health-related behavior. Kohut (1971) suggests that this explanation may underlie the health-jeopardizing behavior of racing car drivers and stunt men. On a less dramatic level, individuals with personalities in which a defensive sense of invulnerability plays a prominent role would be expected to show little regard for health hazards or support for plans to improve health care. To the degree that they would experience improved health and health services as more rewarding than less extensive services, this unconscious defense would generate wants that fall short of need.

Another illustration of how intrapsychic forces might produce divergence between wants and needs involves the defensive perception of health providers as omnipotent and omniscient parental figures. This phenomenon has been described in psychoanalytic literature as a response to the anxiety generated by the threat of serious illness (Janis, 1958). In the health planning setting, it may lead to the unconscious idea that "voting" against an option wanted by providers will become magically known to one's physician who will then exact punishment for this "disobedience" the next time one needs health care. To the degree that this defense is prevalent in a given health service area, individuals will tend to "want" a health system based on provider preferences rather than on their own real benefit. Repeated instances of successful intimidation of consumers by providers in the Comprehensive Health Planning setting may be explained, in part, by this defensive determination of consumer "want." In some cases, this defensive process may simply lead to divergence between publicly expressed and privately felt wants on the part of consumers. However, in instances where the cognition of being opposed to the interests of one's doctor is sufficiently threatening, an individual's awareness of disagreement may be totally warded off, in which case public and private wants would be consonant but potentially in conflict with need.

A final illustration of how unconscious defenses can distort the accurate expression of needs derives from the complex nature of most decisions in the health care system. These decisions usually involve substantial numbers of major factors, associated statistical data, and concepts foreign to lay members of HSA governing bodies (for example, mean waiting times for an elective hospital bed). Such complexity may provoke unconscious (and/or conscious) fears of confusion and a restitutional unconscious motivation to select the simplest option, which may or may not be associated with the greatest health payoff. Analyses of consumer preferences in relation to fluoridation (Demone, 1976) suggested that an important motivation underlying opposition was the complexity of the information supporting a change to fluoridation. Under these circumstances, some people voted against fluoridation in order to avoid interpreting complex, unfamiliar data, rather than selecting the option with the highest net health benefits.

The HSA governing-body members are faced with the task of reconciling planners' assessments of need with the public's expressed wants, as well as with members' own needs and wants. Members as individuals are themselves faced with the same threats to "rational" choice as are all other consumers. However, in this instance, choices and decisions are made in a group context, which adds a new dimension and which can either improve or impair the quality of decision making. Psychological literature on group decision making is relevant here and, once again, we find a range of theoretical perspectives and empirical findings upon which to draw.

Influence of Group Dynamics on HSA Governing Bodies

Psychoanalytic theory identifies some potential hazards to the effective workings of groups. Psychoanalyst Wilfred Bion (1961), for example, has described how fundamental task-unrelated agendas that individuals in task-oriented groups may unconsciously pursue could hinder effective group functioning. The agendas are hypothesized to serve as defenses against two unconscious fears that may be provoked by group participation: fear of ostracism from the group and fear of loss of individual identity within the group. Bion identifies three such agendas. One agenda is establishing an omnipotent leader in the group and then relating passively to that leader. An expression of this might be a governing body that tends to accept staff recommendations uncritically because the head planner is being unconsciously viewed as the omnipotent leader. The second agenda Bion proposes is the group's fleeing from or struggling with an enemy. Just as the first agenda required identification of a leader, this agenda requires selection of an enemy, which could be either inside or outside the group. This agenda could be expressed via consistent resistance to considering fully the viewpoint of a particular consumer or provider group, such as a hospital association, because they had been unconsciously chosen as "the enemy." Bion's third agenda is support for a symbolic mating intended to generate a miraculous product. Support for a merger between two hospitals because of unconscious fantasies that extraordinary (though, in fact, unrealistic) results will be produced would be a possible expression of this agenda. Some of these possibilities seem less likely than others, and it is unlikely that governing-body proceedings would be totally dominated by these agendas. Nonetheless, these processes may have some effect on decision making. The effect may be simply to distract the group from its decision-making task or it may lead to less effective decisions. However, it is also possible that some of the assumptions could improve the decision-making process, as in groups where the agenda of establishing a leader causes the group to organize around the suggestions of the most competent member.

Other theories of group behavior hypothesize potentials for deviation from task orientation but also provide evidence for the possibility of greater effectiveness in group than in individual settings. One general conclusion from research on group problem solving is that groups are more effective than individuals in solving problems in which information is needed. The more people who are involved in a decision, the greater the opportunity for someone to have access to the relevant and correct information. However, information may not be generated, presented, and evaluated in the most efficient manner in all groups. Steiner (1972) differentiates the potential from the actual productivity of a group. The former is productivity that would be achieved with maximum contribution by all members of a group, whereas the latter is what the group actually accomplishes. Actual productivity is expressed as a function of potential productivity minus losses due to faulty process. Productivity losses are likely to be greater the larger the size of the group. There is evidence that no more than eight to ten people can be directly responsive to one another in a group discussion (Hare, 1952). Steiner notes that process losses increase markedly as group size increases, and serious coordination and motivation problems are likely to arise. Given that HSA governing boards will range from ten to thirty people, it is easy to anticipate problems of communication between members and of adequate representation of all viewpoints.

In addition to problems associated with size, Steiner (1972, p. 39) identifies four conditions that contribute to faulty process: "(1) failure of status differences to parallel the quality of contributions offered by participating members, (2) the low level of confidence proficient members sometimes have in their own ability to perform the task, (3) the social pressure that an incompetent majority may exert on a competent minority, and (4) the fact that the quality of individual contributions is often very difficult to evaluate." In the HSA decision-making process, there are many opportunities for faulty process. Physician representatives may be particularly likely to dominate proceedings. Not only are they likely to be of higher social status than many of the consumer representatives but they are also likely to be viewed as experts. The physicians may also be more self-assured and may more easily dominate discussions. Further, the "magical" fear of provider retaliation discussed earlier may be a very realistic concern when decisions are made in a public setting. One consumer representative to an HSA governing body voiced private fears about the treatment she or her family would

receive in the county hospital because she had been a vocal opponent of
many of the hospital programs.

    Delbecq (1976) has noted problems of faulty process in groups and
has suggested the nominal group approach mentioned earlier as a technique
for improving outcome in such situations. He notes that interaction patterns
in groups are generally fixed within a brief time span. Individuals with more
aggressive, extroverted personalities dominate discussions, and less assertive
members generally fall into roles of merely reacting to the ideas and suggestions of the more powerful members. Other research in group decision making has also shown correlations between amount of participation in group
discussion and leadership (Fiedler, 1971). To combat this problem, Delbecq
suggests a series of structured steps. The group begins by having members
write down as many ideas as they have regarding a particular problem. Having people write their ideas, rather than simply discuss them, generates more
ideas, since members do not get caught in the frame of reference of early
speakers, and also generates ideas that are less constrained by social desirability. The second step is to have each person present an idea. This process
continues until all ideas are exhausted. This results in a list of ideas that
achieves separation of the individual (and his or her personality) from the
idea. Third, the ideas are discussed one at a time, with no more than two
minutes on any one idea. Finally, group members rank the solutions. These
are written so that they can be independent and judgments are less likely to
be swayed by the opinions of others (Deutsch and Gerard, 1955). Delbecq
suggested this approach for use in need assessment. In its full form, it may be
too cumbersome for HSA deliberations, but some of the ideas for equalizing
participation and reducing some of the dysfunctional aspects of group
process could well be applied to governing-board proceedings. Application of
other approaches to group process, such as Janis' work on group think
(Janis, 1972; see also Chapter Nineteen by Janis and Rodin in this volume),
may also yield ideas for improving the effectiveness of decision making within HSA governing boards.

Conclusions

    The overall goal of health planning is to design, implement, and eval-
uate a system of health care that is most consistent with the values of society. This is clearly a complex task that involves economic and political, as
well as psychological, considerations. However, psychology can play an important role in improving the process and outcome of health planning. This
chapter identified possible contributions to one form of health planning,
that of the HSAs. This approach, embodied in Public Law 93-641, is likely
to have a major impact on the health care system of the United States in the
coming years. The essential elements of the HSA approach were described
and a key aspect, representation of consumer values in the main decision-
making body, was examined. Potential pitfalls in the current procedures for
representation were identified. However, much of the argument presented

was based on speculation. At this point, empirical research is needed to establish whether representatives are, in fact, representative of the values of the community. If successful, research on this and on psychological correlates of health values could be used to design a plan for direct representation of health values. Such a plan might be along psychological rather than, or in addition to, demographic lines.

Regardless of the manner of selection and the representativeness of the views of the individual members, the outcome of governing-body deliberations will, in large part, be influenced by group dynamics. Since all major decisions will be made by governing bodies of ten to thirty people, there is significant risk that faulty group process could lead to suboptimal solutions. Some psychological techniques based on research on group dynamics can be used to improve the climate of decision making of HSA boards. Unfortunately, however, much of this research has been done on groups that differ from HSA governing bodies in a variety of ways. Governing bodies are groups in which (1) various values and perspectives are being represented, (2) complex issues need to be decided, and (3) there may be conflicting interests. Research is needed on factors determining the effectiveness of decision making under these conditions.

In addition to problems that arise specifically in the HSA setting, psychology can be applied to broader issues of health planning. A core task in health planning is determining individual and social values concerning health and the health care system. This task has two component questions: What do people want, and what do they need? A number of techniques are currently used by planners to determine what people want, but most of these are limited in scope and provide only a partial view. Many planning decisions are made on the basis of planners' views of what people need, but this is often based neither on empirical data nor on any theory of human behavior. As was discussed in this chapter, psychologists can help improve the solutions achieved through both theoretical and methodological contributions. On the methods side, psychological expertise in problems of attitude measurement could be particularly helpful in the area of need assessment. On the theory side, there are a number of models of human functioning that can be used to identify needs that are likely to influence health choices. These theories can suggest whether and in what ways needs can reach conscious expression in terms of a statement of desire or behavioral choice. Psychological theory can thus be used to accommodate people's needs more effectively, especially in areas where needs are not consonant with expressed wants. The application of psychological theory and methods should generate empirical data that could be used by planners and policy makers. Research could be directed at the core problem itself: What are the wants and needs of individuals regarding health and health care? How do wants and needs relate to prior experience, personality characteristics, and attitudes and values? What are the conditions under which consciously expressed desires best represent needs, and what are the conditions under which there will be some discrepancy? What are the parameters of health services and systems that individuals find most satisfying, and which are the ones that contribute most to physical and mental health? Under what conditions will these be the same, and under what conditions will they be different? In addition to research on these questions, psychologists could apply research on attitude change, acceptance of innovation, and behavior change to develop strategies for intervention in those situations in which want is, in fact, discrepant with need.

The HSA system has been heralded as an opportunity for consumers to help shape the health care system in this country. The involvement of psychologists may help to protect against threats to this latest attempt to enfranchise consumers in shaping the evolution of this system. With HSAs ride significant hopes for major improvements in health and the health care system. Psychology, through existing knowledge and skills and prospective research, offers promising opportunities for enhancing the realization of these hopes.

16

Sources and Effects of Stress in Health Careers

Lillian Kaufman Cartwright

Healing is time-honored work. Helping others and being needed by society offer important intrinsic rewards for all health professionals. For physicians, career satisfactions exist on many levels and include self-actualization, exposure to a wide range of human experiences, socially useful work, high income, and intellectually challenging pursuits. The overwhelming majority of both male and female doctors are satisfied or very satisfied with their careers (Cartwright, 1978b). At the same time that so many of the ingredients of a meaningful life are present, there is also evidence that emotional distress is an occupational hazard for some health professionals. The pressures of training and practice, the number of patients seen, the psychological drain associated with assuming responsibility for others' lives, the affective climate surrounding disease, as well as contradictory and unrealizable aspects of current roles of healers, are among the more obvious factors implicated in the search for sources of distress. Unlike the physical hazards of some work—the chemical toxins in paints, for instance—the stressors in

Note: This chapter was written while the author was engaged in a program of research on physicians, funded by the Robert Wood Johnson Foundation. The project was directed by Harrison G. Gough at the Institute of Personality Assessment and Research, University of California, Berkeley.

health careers are not unequivocal and reflect, to a greater degree, perceptual, cognitive, and affective mediating processes. Whether or not distress is
experienced largely depends upon the conscious and unconscious meanings
assigned to events by the individual (Brown, 1975; Haan, 1977; Lazarus,
1966).

This chapter provides a framework for identifying and understanding
the sources of distress in persons engaged in health careers. Because of space
limitations, research on physicians will be emphasized since doctors have
been relatively well studied compared to other health care providers. Many
general issues and inquiries are pertinent to all health professionals. Research
from dentistry, nursing, and pharmacy will be cited when available to highlight similarities and differences among the health professions. A complete
interprofessional comparison cannot be assumed here because of gaps in research and the scope of the task.

There are two urgent reasons for focusing on the problems of providers. First, to reduce suffering and to restore the capacity to enjoy life to
health professionals through selected, planned interventions is a worthwhile
and important goal in its own right. Almost five million individuals are employed in the health sector, so the number of persons involved is substantial.
The health sector of the economy has grown rapidly in the last two decades.
Between 1960 and 1970, 13 percent of all new jobs in the United States
were in the area of health (Fein, 1976, p. 656). Second, the problems of
providers can seriously interfere with the care of patients. It is easy to see
how severe malfunctioning—for example, drug abuse and alcoholism—can be
injurious to the patient. But even with less severe problems, the quality of
health care will diminish when providers are distressed. Health professionals
agree that two very important criteria for high quality care are the provider's
ability to form a good relationship with the patient and the adequacy of the
provider's knowledge and technical competency (Cartwright, 1978a; Donabedian, 1966; Parker, Walsh, and Coon, 1976). Although health experts see
the cognitive competencies as more important, consumers place greater
weight on the conduct of the provider. It is impressive that the most important factor in predicting the patient's general satisfaction with health care is
his or her perception of the adequacy of the provider's conduct (Doyle and
Ware, 1977). Yet it is the health professional's behavior that is most sensitive
and reactive to the stressors and problems encountered in practice. Anxiety
and tension impede the natural flow of communication. Stressed providers
cannot listen empathically nor can they respond sensitively. Constructive
involvement in the problems of others requires concentration, energy, and
peace of mind.

Although research is sparse, there is mounting evidence that stressed
providers suffer measurable impairment in cognitive and technical competencies and relationship skills (Artiss and Levine, 1973; Freudenberger,
1974; Hay and Oken, 1972; Maslach, 1978). Rigidity in thought processes,
inaccurate diagnosis, attribution of triviality to patients' complaints leading
to incomplete work-ups are among the deficits in the performance noted in a

broad spectrum of stressed health professionals, including nurses, doctors, social workers, and child-care aides. Research in counseling and psychotherapy offers further documentation on the importance of the provider's behavior to favorable outcomes of care. If the healer is perceived as caring and friendly, the result of treatment is more likely to be successful (Truax and Mitchell, 1971). A crucial link between the provider's behavior and the patient's satisfaction with care may reside in the patient's willingness to follow the therapeutic regime. Positive compliance—that is, taking the treatment plan seriously and putting it into action—is associated with seeing the therapist as concerned and friendly (Sackett and Haynes, 1976).

To put this chapter in perspective, remember at the outset that health professions do differ in several ways: prestige and status, income, amount of training required, and career satisfaction. For the physician, personal distress and career satisfaction may be independent dimensions (Cartwright, 1978b). However, this is probably not the case in nursing and, to a lesser extent, pharmacy, where more job dissatisfaction exists, particularly in hospital settings. In these professions, unmet needs for recognition and self-esteem and a greater disparity between career expectations and the reality of work are cited as causes of considerable dissatisfaction (Johnson, Hammel, and Heinen, 1977; Kramer, 1974; Sadler, Sadler, and Bliss, 1972).

A second reminder recognizes that having psychological problems is not tantamount to disintegration. There is challenge and excitement in meeting adaptational demands—competency and resiliency increase in much the same way that regular, strenuous exercise leads to a more flexible and stronger body. The stressful milestones of training and practice, to be described later, are successfully and creatively met by most health professionals. Selye's (1974) distinction between harmful and constructive stress— distress and "eustress"—highlights the positive factors that accompany coping with problems. He notes that self-actualization and the spice of variety, as well as simple enjoyment, follow the mastery of difficult situations. At the same time, one must bear in mind that the meanings attached to potentially stressful events rely on the person participating in the event. To a large measure, the person construes the meaning of his or her own stress. Individual differences in capacity to cope with difficulty also exist and can make the difference between those who suffer deeply and are immobilized and those who are challenged and grow (Pearlin and Schooler, 1978).

Third, although occupational intercomparisons are premature, all occupations have specific hazards and dissatisfactions. Moreover, occupations are dynamic rather than static entities. Over the years, vocations change and attract different types of individuals. For example, before the coming of the Chamberlens and their forceps to the court of England in the seventeenth century, obstetrics was in the hands of the midwives, and few disputed the belief that delivering babies was the natural work and domain of women. Now many women are reevaluating the role of the midwife in the light of changes in feminine ideology.

Both medicine and nursing are currently undergoing major transitions in many sectors, including admissions policies, curriculum, values, and roles in health care delivery. Pharmacy, in a less dramatic way, is also undergoing a process of revision. The pharmacist's identity as a health professional is itself relatively new (Knapp, 1974; Knapp, Knapp, and Edwards, 1969). Investigators find that as the pharmacist becomes more active in the clinical aspects of pharmacy, job satisfaction increases. The strong economic pressure to control rising health care costs influences the roles of all health professionals, as well as the boundaries between groups. In the future, more problems may arise as traditional lines of authority and task assignments become blurred, particularly when perceived shortages in personnel are met. Lastly, cross-cultural variations in the incidence of specific disorders, complaints, and frustrations among health providers suggest that the culture's definition of the work, its status, financing mechanisms, and customary practice characteristics influence psychological well-being and health status (Djerassi, 1971; King, 1970; Mechanic, 1972a).

The Problems—What Are They?

What evidence is there that health professionals are a particularly distressed group? Definitive documentation and exact quantification are impossible because studies examining these problems suffer from many methodological pitfalls, including inadequate socioeconomic controls, small and biased samples, uncontrolled era effects, differences in indexes used to quantify stress, and lack of replication. Moreover, the range reported for the incidence of certain symptoms, such as drug abuse and psychiatric illness, fluctuates considerably. Because social consequences can lead to revocation of license, there can be a "conspiracy of silence" among colleagues and family members to protect the stressed health professional. In the physician, patterns of denial and unrealistic feelings of superiority and omnipotence stemming from the continued exercise of authority can also lead to under-reporting of symptoms (Marmor, 1953). Within the limits of these reservations, the literature supports the view that some health professionals are under stress, that the stress expresses itself in divergent ways, and that multiple factors can be identified as contributors to disease. The causes of problems are complex and cannot be reduced to either milieu or person-centered origins. Rather, strain arises out of a transaction or adaptive commerce between a specific kind of person and a given milieu (Lazarus and Cohen, 1977).

The following section will describe a wide spectrum of health problems suffered by providers and believed to be related to occupational stressors in training and practice. Classic symptoms of emotional turmoil will be reviewed, as well as more recent, global descriptions of stress syndromes associated with work. Because this area of research is new and burgeoning, a nondoctrinaire and eclectic approach is taken toward the literature at the cost of some comforts of clarity.

Mortality, Morbidity, and Coronary Heart Disease

King's (1970) cross-cultural and cross-professional study of men provides an excellent review of the literature concerning the causes of death in doctors, lawyers, teachers, and clergymen. He synthesizes over 100 years of relevant research conducted in six countries, including the United States, the British Isles, and Denmark. King compares age-specific death rates of males under sixty-five in these professions with each other and with general population norms in the appropriate country. He concludes that physicians have lower mortality rates for infectious diseases, cancer, and accidents, while evincing a higher incidence of coronary heart disease, diabetes, strokes, and suicide than the general population. Doctors are more likely to die of heart disease than other professionals. American physicians are more prone to heart disease than medical practitioners in England and Denmark, suggesting that the professional role must be evaluated within its cultural context. Other large sample studies of doctors confirm this conclusion, finding that even though American doctors live longer, they are more prone to death from diseases of the heart (Dickinson and Martin, 1956). Research on dentists, although less extensive, suggests that they too are prone to coronary heart disease (Djerassi, 1971; Howard and others, 1976; Russek, 1962).

What are the reasons accounting for the susceptibility of doctors and dentists to coronary heart disease (CHD)? Many are implicating the role of social and psychological risk factors as major contributors to CHD (Jenkins, 1971, 1976; Russek and Russek, 1976; Syme, 1975). It has long been observed that high blood pressure, smoking, and a high cholesterol level are related to CHD. Now in addition to these classic risk factors, psychosocial precursors are cited, including specific patterns related to occupational stress, personality dispositions, precipitating life events, and sociocultural mobility. Special emphasis is assigned to the type A personality as a precursor of CHD (Rosenman, and others, 1966; see also Chapter Four in this volume). Briefly, the type A personality is characterized by a sense of time urgency, competition, and intense ambition. Jenkins, Rosenman, and Zyzanski (1974b) found type A men twice as likely to develop CHD symptoms. To bring the issue back to health providers, researchers are finding that both doctors and dentists are prone to type A orientations (Howard and others, 1976; Russek and Russek, 1976). Friedman (1978) also states that psychologists have considerably more than their share of type A personalities, particularly among those working in academic settings where a "publish or perish" ethos is most entrenched.

The demands of the work setting cannot be isolated from the person. Some believe that the pressures of work release and reinforce a coronary-prone behavior pattern in predisposed individuals through intermittent crises and disturbances in the workday. Russek (1962, 1965), the clearest spokesman of this position, sees occupational stress as the major factor in coronary heart disease and assigns it more predictive validity than diet, smoking, or heredity. In his survey of 25,000 professional men, comparing doctors, dentists, and lawyers in three age groups, he found that the relative level of stress among various specialties was predictive of coronary heart disease—CHD was two to three times more prevalent in specialties ranked as stressful by independent judges. In medicine, for example, dermatology, pathology, anesthesiology, and general practice were ranked on a gradient of stress from least to most stressful. The CHD prevalence rate of general practitioners was three times higher than that of dermatologists. In dentistry, the general dental practitioner, judged to be in the most stressful specialty, was three times as likely to suffer from CHD as the periodontist, who was perceived to be in the least stressful environment.

Summing up, doctors and dentists appear more prone to coronary heart disease than other health providers. Pressures and stresses inherent in the work itself appear important in predicting CHD. Long hours, numerous patient contacts, many and changing demands on the skills of the practitioner, and recurrent emergency calls appear salient, although the individual contribution to stress of each of these factors has not yet been determined. The personality of the doctor and the dentist is an added contributing factor. Cross-cultural differences in rates suggest that whether or not one is self-employed should also be taken into account. What happens or does not happen in nonwork hours can easily be overlooked, yet these events hold promise for better understanding of the dynamics of CHD. Stressed doctors and dentists may reject specific health and fitness patterns associated with optimal well-being (Howard, Cunningham, and Rechnitzer, 1976). Regular exercise, recreation, relaxation, and good nutrition may be slighted by tense, ambitious professionals whose outlook on life classifies such activities as "nonproductive."

Suicide

Suicide, the most drastic reaction to stress, appears more prevalent in medicine, dentistry, and pharmacy than in the general population. Some even go so far as to say that suicide is an occupational hazard for all health professionals (Rose and Rosow, 1973), although the data do not merit this generalization. Negative and ambiguous findings are present, especially in respect to suicides in male physicians. Problems of methodology and interpretation can readily be raised in this research and can account for contradictory results. For example, the reliability of the source of information concerning the death of the provider can be questioned. The obituaries of the Journal of the American Medical Association, a frequent source in suicide studies of doctors, are shown to be unreliable by Rose and Rosow (1973), who find that only half of the 1970 suicides of California physicians were correctly identified. They see this well-used source as too dependent on national newspaper obituaries and information from the family; they recommend consulting death certificates, which are more accurate. There is general agreement that suicides, especially among physicians, are underreported.

Even given this consensus, many find that medical students and doctors are still more prone to this form of death than the general population, although the magnitude of the reported difference varies considerably (Blachly, Osterud, and Josslin, 1963; King, 1970; Powell, 1972; Rose and Rosow, 1973; Simon, 1968; Steppacher and Mausner, 1974). Others find nonsignificant differences or no difference in rates (Craig and Pitts, 1968; Dickinson and Martin, 1956; Everson and Fraumeni, 1975). Because male suicide rates in American doctors appear to peak in mid-life, studies focusing solely on the young physician may be misleading. In England there appear to be more suicides among younger doctors, suggesting that the insolvable life problems facing the depressed doctor vary and should be explored within the person's cultural milieu (King, 1970).

An interesting aspect of the suicide research relates to sex differences in rates found in three studies (Craig and Pitts, 1968; Everson and Fraumeni, 1975; Steppacher and Mausner, 1974). These studies find women doctors significantly more suicide prone than men. Steppacher and Mausner (1974, p. 325) estimate that male doctors are 1.15 times as likely to kill themselves as compared to expected norms, whereas female suicides are 3.20 times greater. Negative findings come from Rose and Rosow (1973), who find no sex differences in their Californian sample; however, their sample size was small. Reports of excessive numbers of suicides among women psychologists (Mausner and Steppacher, 1973) and women chemists (Li, 1969) suggest that women in male-dominated professions are high-risk groups. Female psychologists approach the suicide rates of women doctors, with about three times as many suicides as the general female population, whereas male psychologists are not suicide prone.

The relationship between medical specialty and suicide is not clear and contradictory results exist. Although psychiatrists, anesthesiologists, and opthalmologists have been cited as more suicide prone, Rose and Rosow (1973) dispute these findings, pointing out that the differences do not exceed chance variation. Larger samples and accurately computed reference population rates are needed. Since many studies rely on samples drawn from only one state, and states themselves differ in suicide rates much the same as countries differ, national sampling is mandatory.

Contrasted to all other health professionals, pharmacists have an unusually high suicide rate. Powell (1972) reports 3.5 times as many suicides among pharmacists as compared to other professional samples. In the study by Rose and Rosow (1973), pharmacists are exceeded only by chemists in incidence of suicide. The availability of and easy access to drugs is the accepted explanation for the high rates among pharmacists and chemists: About 40 percent of the pharmacists' suicides are caused by drug ingestions, whereas only 21 percent of the general population choose this method (1973, p. 805).

Dentists appear to have similar suicide rates to physicians. Rose and Rosow (1973) report that dentists, like physicians, have higher rates than the general population. Blachly, Osterud, and Josslin (1963) also find dentists to be a group that should be considered at risk in relation to suicide. Research on suicide in nurses has not been univocal. However, the studies have generally not depicted nurses as particularly suicide prone. For example, Blachly, Osterud, and Josslin (1963) examined the suicide rate in nurses and in a population of women in general in Oregon. They found little difference in the rates between the two groups.

Some helping professions (although not necessarily those concerned with health care) have very low rates. The clergy, schoolteachers, and social workers are three such groups. King and his co-workers (King, 1970; King and Bailar, 1968; King, Zafros, and Hass, 1975), in studies contrasting the health status of the clergy with that of other occupations, including physicians, conclude that the value system of clergymen may be one factor responsible for their good health: A spiritual view of the world, combined with less emphasis on competitiveness, individuality, and materialism, may promote better psychological adaptations. Blachly, Disher, and Roduner (1968) also emphasize the excessive individualism and perfectionism in physicians who die by their own hand. At the same time, such doctors are insufficiently controlled by social regulations which govern others in society: Physicians are seldom committed to institutions; they have free access to drugs; they are rarely subjected to firm probation and control. Said another way, there may be a lack of balance or sense of proportion between their individualism and their feelings of relatedness to the community. They may not have or seek to find support groups within their milieu and may tend to devalue or avoid the healing power of others. To use Durkheim's (1951) concepts, the suicidal doctor is motivated by egoistic concerns and, at the same time, suffers from anomic feelings.

There are several critics of the methodological errors of suicide studies (Everson and Fraumeni, 1975; Rose and Rosow, 1973; von Brauchitsch, 1976). Small samples, inappropriate pooling of data, inadequate base rate controls, and inaccurate classifications of death are cited as problems. Von Brauchitsch also cites interpretations of the findings as problematic. He contends that the emotional impact of suicide causes more concern than the epidemiological facts warrant. Distinguishing between morbidity and mortality, he asserts that the availability of drugs, as well as knowledge of the human anatomy, allows the physician (and parenthetically, other health professionals) to be more successful in a suicide attempt than the general public and not necessarily to *attempt* it more often. Since attempted suicide is twice as frequent among women, and men are four times as likely to accomplish suicide, the sex difference in suicide rates may reveal only that the woman doctor and psychologist have greater competency for this form of self-destruction relative to other women. Another conclusion could readily be reached—because health professionals are stringently selected and placed in a milieu formally committed to alleviating suffering, one could reasonably expect fewer suicides in this group.

There are many gaps and unknowns in the suicide research. Being a member of a helping profession is not enough to make a person suicide prone. Nurses, social workers, teachers, and clergy are not at risk. Among the factors implicated in the search for precursors are: easy access to drugs, a value system that emphasizes individualism at the cost of a sense of community and cooperation, and a deficit in coping strategies so that suicide is perceived as the best solution to a life problem. Because the bulk of the suicide research is epidemiological, not motivational, in character, a useful future research strategy might focus on individual cases across health professions to understand better the dynamics of suicide. Such studies might explore ways in which suicides among female physicians are similar to or different from suicides among male physicians or male pharmacists. Do age-related identity crises distinguish women from men? Such an approach assumes that two groups prone to suicide may be at risk for different reasons.

Drug Abuse

Drug abuse is a frequently noted problem among health professionals. Modlin and Montes (1964) reported that the incidence of drug abuse in physicians varied from 30 to 100 times that found in the general population. The findings from the United States are confirmed in England, Germany, Holland, and France, where 30 percent of the known drug addicts are physicians, nurses, or pharmacists—this percentage far exceeds the proportion of health professionals in the general population of those countries. In states in which records have been studied, between 1 and 2 percent of all physicians come before State Boards of Medical Examiners for disciplinary action because of alcoholism, drug dependence, or mental disorders. These studies span a six- to eleven-year period (Council on Mental Health, 1973, p. 685). Often drug abuse and alcohol abuse are important symptoms in doctors who kill themselves. Blachly, Disher, and Roduner (1968, p. 14) report that in 40 percent of the suicides in their sample, drug abuse was also present. Vaillant, Sobowale, and McArthur (1972, p. 373), in a longitudinal study of highly educated men, found that 36 percent of the doctors in their sample used drugs heavily to reduce tension, in contrast to 22 percent of men matched in socioeconomic status. The easy access to narcotics for health professionals, in addition to occupational stresses that impinge on their well-being, allows addiction to be regarded as an undisputed occupational hazard.

Psychiatric Illness

In a review of studies of the prevalence of psychiatric illness among medical students, postgraduate students, and physicians, the rates of seeking professional help ranged from .5 to 46 percent (Waring, 1974, p. 520). The major reason for the wide range was that a variety of mental health facilities were surveyed, including public and private institutions. Physicians are considerably less likely to utilize public psychiatric facilities; thus, they will be underrepresented in some studies. In the Vaillant study referred to earlier, doctors resorted more frequently to psychiatric treatment than their socioeconomic controls. Vaillant acknowledges occupational stresses in these men but also posits that the vulnerable doctors had unstable childhoods and precarious adolescent adjustments which predisposed them to mental illness. In general, affective disorders (depression) appear to be among the most common presenting problems in doctors seeking psychiatric help.

Among the studies of medical students, the percentages seeking help from student psychiatric health services vary considerably, depending on the school surveyed. For example, Raskin (1972, p. 210) reports that 10 percent of the students at the University of California, San Francisco, sought aid. At McGill University in Canada, records indicate that 18 percent sought help (Hunter, Prince, and Schwartzman, 1961, p. 989). The true incidence of psychiatric disturbance is not known. Most investigators see these two figures as low estimates, since many students use informal channels for help and others deny needs. In interviews with medical school seniors at the University of Southern California, almost 57 percent said they needed psychiatric help (Woods and Natterson, 1967, p. 327). Thomas' follow-up (1976) of students and graduates of the Johns Hopkins School of Medicine found emotional disturbances and mental illness important contributors to poor academic performance, dropping out, and premature death. In general, the variation in rates of seeking treatment reflects the climate and resources of the individual school—the extent to which help is available and the degree of legitimacy attached to psychotherapeutic needs.

Marital Problems

Problems with marriage have been documented by several medical education researchers. In Vaillant's (Vaillant, Sobowale, and McArthur, 1972) sample, 47 percent of the doctors report poor marriages or divorce, compared to 32 percent of the controls. Coombs (1971) notes that studies of marital difficulty among physicians are not systematic. However, anecdotal information from a variety of sources depicts physicians as having more than their share of problems. In Coombs' research, based on interviews with medical students' wives, one out of five state that medical school adversely affected their marital relationship. The wife's role expectation for her husband is pivotal in predicting marital dissatisfaction. If the wife expects her husband to pay a good deal of attention to her, she is bound to be disappointed. The most adaptive wives are those who anticipate that they will be lonely and their sexual-affectionate relationship will be far from ideal. The wives expecting the least, suffer the least. Gerbert (1977), in a study of wives of podiatric medical students, emphasizes the ideological stance of the women: The wives assume the role of the helpmate and pacifier. Traditionally feminine in outlook, these women have put their husbands' needs first and cope with marital problems by minimizing or denying their importance. Fear of divorce after graduation from school appears to be an unspoken threat for both wives of medical and podiatric medical students.

Rose and Rosow (1972), however, doubt that doctors have especially troubled marriages. In examining initial complaint rates (including divorce, annulment, and separation) in California, they found that white male doctors had more stable marriages than some professional controls (for example, social scientists, authors, and college professors). Dentists showed similar rates to physicians. However, women physicians, black physicians, and orthopedic surgeons were more prone to divorce than other doctors. Rose and Rosow also challenge the myth that medical school marriages end in divorce by locating the peak rate of divorce among doctors at ages thirty-five to forty-four, the height of the medical career. As this study was based on a sample from one state, replication is needed.

Other Signs of Dissatisfaction and Distress

Some difficulties experienced by health professionals differ from classic symptoms but, nonetheless, are sources of distress for the professional and of potential loss to the health care system. Four special problems are: exodus from training programs and careers, burnout, role conflicts, and role ambiguities.

Attrition from training programs and career. Relative to other health professions, the national dropout rates in medicine are very low and have steadily declined (Johnson and Hutchins, 1966). Gough's finding (1976), however, that there are a high number of creative individuals among the few medical dropouts is especially alarming because of the loss of potential innovators to the profession. In addition, Thomas' (1976) study of Johns Hopkins students suggests that emotional disturbance and vulnerability to stress contributed to dropping out as well as to taking more time than customary to complete medical school.

Compared to medicine, attrition rates of other health programs are higher. Johnson and Hutchins (1966, p. 1113) estimate a 44 percent national attrition rate for nursing and 10.5 percent for dentistry. More recently, Kramer (1974) calculates rates ranging from 20.5 percent to 32.2 percent for the University of California, San Francisco, School of Nursing for the years 1968-1971 (the median percentage is 24.2 percent and the difference between years is not significant).

Exodus from the profession is another sign of career dissatisfaction which varies considerably across health careers. In nursing this is a common event, as are frequent job changes. In one study of baccalaureate nurses, almost one third left nursing practice in the two-year period following graduation. Sadler, Sadler, and Bliss (1972) report that nearly half of graduate nurses either do not practice or fail to renew their licenses. Although many see the high dropout rate in nursing as reflecting job dissatisfaction and unrealized hopes, another perspective focuses on the enduring sex role ideology of nurses. Although the faculty teaching in nursing schools are often avantgarde, women choosing to be nurses hold more traditional beliefs about the female role—their careers are less central to their identity and self-fulfillment. In this context, dropping out for reasons of marriage, childbearing, and childrearing may not represent career dissatisfaction as such but rather convey a more orthodox sex role orientation (Damrell, Lewin, and Peguillan, 1977; Davis and Olesen, 1963; Olesen and Davis, 1966).

A less severe but parallel problem relating to migration from the profession exists in pharmacy, particularly among hospital pharmacists. Job turnover is frequent, as is attrition. It has been estimated that 10 percent of the licensed pharmacists are not practicing. In one study of hospital pharmacists, two thirds of those surveyed had major doubts about their careers. Among their major dissatisfactions: lack of opportunity for advancement, little challenge in their work, and staffing practices (Johnson, Hammel, and Heinen, 1977).

Burnout. Maslach's (1976) work on burnout reveals another problem for all health professionals involved in direct patient care. Burnout is defined as a loss of concern for people—an emotional exhaustion which involves cynicism and the dehumanized perception of patients. Initial interviews were done with physicians, social welfare workers, and child care staff. From these interviews, a description of the burnout phenomenon was derived. Research in this area is in its infancy, and the degree of impairment or numbers afflicted cannot be estimated. However, Maslach believes that burnout is neither an isolated phenomenon nor a rare occurrence experienced by only a few. She hypothesizes that it is at the root of some symptoms discussed earlier, such as drug usage and job turnover. The basic causes lie in the disruptive emotional aspect of care, including demanding and unreasonable patient behaviors, illnesses that are difficult to treat, and denial of strong emotions produced in treating patients. She believes that educational institutions encourage fragmented and dehumanized perceptions of the patients so that providers are taught to split off their feelings and emotions from their intellectual approach. In this context, Lief and Fox (1963) speak of "detached concern" in the provider. They note that detached concern is idealized in professional settings and, in fact, may be seen as the prime requisite of professional behavior. Yet detached concern itself leads to discomfort because it involves erecting arbitrary walls or compartments that are difficult to maintain as well as often being counter to the patient's interests. More constructive coping mechanisms are available and include being on better terms with one's feelings and with the sources of situational stress in health care settings. Maslach (1978) also recommends other coping strategies, such as the utilization of support groups among health providers, the development of skills in humanistic humor, varying the amount of contact with severely ill patients through changes in assignments, and the institutionalized use of retreats for stressed professionals.

Role conflicts. Special problems related to sex role deserve attention as increasingly greater numbers of women are entering medical school. The percentage of women in first-year classes rose from 13.7 percent in 1971-72 to almost 24 percent in 1975-76 (Gordon and Dubé, 1976, p. 145). Many have described the difficulties women physicians have orchestrating the professional demands of a male-dominated career and the responsibilities of the female role of woman, wife, and mother (Cartwright, 1978b; Lopate, 1968; Williams, 1971). The higher suicide and divorce rates noted earlier may be indicators of difficulties. Strain comes from having too much to do, internal value conflicts, and the effects of a nonsupportive or discriminatory milieu (Epstein, 1974; Kosa and Coker, 1965).

Shuval (1970) and Linn (1971), in studies of women dentists, find certain similarities to physicians in modes of reconciling role conflicts. Through the choice of specialty and distinctive career patterns, such as part-time and salaried work, role conflicts may be reduced. However, income and status are also lessened.

Role ambiguities. Because concepts and ideals of health care are in transition, new health careers are developing. Many practitioners experience stress arising from role ambiguities in these careers. For example, nurse practitioners undergo periods of discomfort as they acquire practitioner's skills and take on decision-making competencies contrary to their previous socialization as nurses (Linn, 1975). At the same time, interviews with nurse practitioners who completed their training suggest that the new options and responsibilities increase both career satisfaction and self-esteem (White, 1977). A parallel development in pharmacy is apparent in the new role of the clinical pharmacist, which is more patient oriented and more concerned with communication and pedagogic skills. Both role enhancement and stressful ambiguities appear to be associated with new programs (Knapp, 1974).

Identifying Sources of Stress

A life-span career development model (Crites, 1976; Super, 1955a) offers a framework for better understanding factors contributing to distress. At each stage in the course of a health career, there are specified tasks and distinctive problems, as well as concomitant rewards. Variance arising from individual differences in personality, values, and needs, as well as differences in the characteristics of environmental settings such as schools, curricula, and faculty, constitute additional facets making each person's experiences unique. From the vantage point of the life span of the individual, career roles interact with other life roles (such as spouse, parent, sex, and societal roles), sometimes leading to conflict and sometimes to enrichment, harmony, and integrative complexity. Morrison (1977) posits that self-esteem and competence are a function of the individual's capacity to adapt to the requirements of changing life roles. In other words, in coping with demands from various life roles, individuals have opportunities for growth. One by-product of adaptation is stress; another is mastery and differentiation.

In addition to the challenges inherent in each stage, transitions between stages can also be problematic. Raskin (1972) refers to initiation periods—that is, going from stage to stage—as producing anxiety for medical students. The transition between school and work is particularly stressful for certain health providers, for example, nurses, owing to unrealized expectations.

In examining the medical profession from a career development model, there is a tacit assumption that all health careers can be analyzed using a stage approach, starting with the neophyte and ending with the mature professional who is adapting to the retirement or semiretirement years. The presentation of the career trajectory will often be impressionistic since the relationships that exist among a staggering number of potentially salient variables can only be suggested and not quantified because of the state of the art, the missing data, and the magnitude of the task. Despite these obvious limitations, the longitudinal model has many assets—foremost are its organizing capabilities and its heuristic value. For example, the process of viewing careers within a time perspective raises the issue of the relationship between stress experienced at one stage in the career cycle and adaptations at later stages.

Premedical Experiences

Even before entry to medical school, the potential physician is made anxious because over 60 percent of the applicant pool, despite high qualifications, will be rejected (Gordon, 1977). Hutchins and Morris' (1963) follow-up of high-ability rejected applicants found that one third eventually did enroll in a medical school and about one fourth entered a health-related field or another science. The competitiveness of premedical school is compounded by controversies over the empirical validity and fairness of admission criteria. Gough (1971) provides an excellent review, history, and critique of selection processes. He concludes that considerable progress has been made in assessing cognitive competencies but that measurement of nonintellectual qualities, such as values, personality, and motivation have lagged behind.

Professional Education

The process in which a student is transformed into a professional has been studied by many sociologists (Becker and others, 1961; Merton, Reader, and Kendall, 1957) and some psychologists (Horowitz, 1964). Professional socialization refers not only to the cognitive aspects of education where skills and knowledge are acquired but also to the acquisition of attitudes, feelings, and values. Olesen and Whittaker (1968), in a study of student nurses, emphasize the existential nature of the process. Students are not passive recipients of the professional culture but influence and choose events in their own socialization process. Said another way, Olmstead and Paget (1969) note that divergent socialization routes will be chosen by different subgroups of students in the same class.

It is well documented that the medical school experience is not easy. In discussing the vicissitudes of the training, Coombs and Vincent (1971) compare it to a rite of passage—a "refiner's fire." What are the sources of tension? Three sets of factors can be identified: the milieu, the individual personality, and patient-related experiences.

Milieu factors. The curriculum is one major source of difficulty, particularly during the first two years of medical school, owing to the historical split between basic science education and clinical training. "There is so much to learn and so little time to learn it" is a major complaint during the first year. Because the student is responsible for the vocabulary and concepts of several basic sciences (for example, biochemistry, pharmacology, anatomy, and physiology), problems of memorizing, coordinating, and integrating information arise. Lack of relevancy is another concern, since the clinical correlates of basic science information (that is, the ways in which the basic sciences affect patient care) are not uniformly presented. Most investigators (Boyle and Coombs, 1974; Edwards and Zimet, 1976; Rosenberg, 1971) agree that the primary concern of students comes from the strain of a stringent curriculum on their personal lives—not having enough time for recreation and for friends and family, feelings of loneliness, and having too much to learn. The role of student usurps time and emotional involvement from other roles. It is noteworthy that time limitations continue to be the most cited dissatisfaction in the lives of the practicing physician. A parallel problem exists in dentistry, where time pressures and scheduling problems are cited as fundamental sources of stress (Canfield, Powell, and Weinstein, 1976).

Rosenberg (1971), a pioneer in small student discussion groups organized to reduce stress, distinguishes between the manifest issues of curriculum and the dynamic or latent conflicts that undermine the self-concept of the student. She states that "the violence done to the self-image of the medical student is the most serious consequence of his educational program" (p. 214). A form of cognitive dissonance results from "double messages" from faculty when students note discrepancies between the expected idealism of the profession and the hostility and coldness of some aspects of the learning climate. Hierarchical put-downs or disrespect for patients are especially sensitive areas. Funkenstein (1971), like Rosenberg, looks beyond the curriculum for the source of difficulties but places the cause on a more molar level. He posits macrosocial changes in the values of medical schools over the last century leading to three distinct time periods: a liberal arts era (turn of the century to 1955), a graduate and research era (1955-1968), and a community era (1968 to present). Today, one source of distress resides in an implicit value conflict between faculty and students. Faculty, educated in the graduate research era, place intellectual values, research activity, and being a scientist high in their value hierarchy. Students, however, cite relevancy, pragmatism, social action, and caring as their highest values. From a social learning perspective, this conflict would result in few role models with whom students could identify. Further, the arrival of significantly more women into the profession, as well as minority members (Larson, 1976), exacerbates the problems of value conflicts and insufficient faculty role models.

In addition to psychological distress, the growth of cynicism and the relinquishment of former idealism in medical schools have been a pivotal concern because of the implications for patient care. In Eron's (1955) classic study of Yale medical students, he asks if the personality of medical students in conjunction with the school environment does not encourage a value system and defense patterning antithetical to the goals of a service occupation. In examining three attitudes—anxiety, humanitarianism, and cynicism—from a developmental vantage point, he finds seniors scoring higher on a Cynicism scale than freshmen. No class differences were evident on the other two scales. A control group of nurses show a different pattern, with seniors scoring lower on both the Cynicism and Humanitarian scales. Eron is circumspect about his results and suggests the study is exploratory at best. Still, this work has stimulated much research and controversy, since the impersonal nature of some aspects of the care process has been identified as a major problem and this research suggests that one of its sources may be in medical training. Therefore, the research on cynicism will be discussed in some detail.

Many difficulties have been encountered in interpreting the research on cynicism. The most important stumbling block lies in the meaning attributed to the concept, which often exceeds its operational basis in Eron's scales. Juan and her associates (1974) are critical of the emotional reactions to the research and believe that many have overreacted to Eron's findings, seeing implications where none exist. The concept of cynicism shares the fate of much "exotic" data—it is given "an importance far beyond its validity and farther beyond its meaning" (p. 313). In this same vein, Becker and Geer (1958) refine the notion of cynicism and idealism and avoid simplistic formulations. According to their definition, cynicism is not a generalized trait but an attitude which varies depending on the activity in question. Their observations at the University of Kansas School of Medicine suggest that the cynicism is specific to the medical school setting and that when students approach graduation, idealism reasserts itself. Essentially, they maintain that cynicism is functional in the medical school setting. Gray, Newman, and Reinhardt (1966) offer support for this hypothesis when they note differences in cynicism between specialists who are directly involved in patient care and those who are not. The "high patient interaction" doctors were less cynical than those in referral specialities. Gray and his co-workers view the doctor working in a "low patient interaction" specialty as more influenced by colleagues who may continue the competitive and evaluative atmosphere of the medical school. In this context, toughness and cynicism serve as protective devices to ward off vulnerability to peer criticism. In the light of the burnout research, it is important to note that the doctors who were involved intensively in patient care were *less* cynical, suggesting that as a group, primary care physicians are not hardened and excessively detached from compassionate feelings. This does not rule out the possibility that some primary care physicians are more prone to cynicism and detachment than others.

Changes in attitudes during training have also been shown in other health professions. Psathas (1968) documents changes in nursing students from the freshman to senior year. These shifts were in the direction of decreased idealism. However, he sees this change as reflecting vocational maturation: The neophyte idealizes the role of nurse relative to patients and physicians, whereas the senior is more realistic and task oriented. The early idealism is viewed as "functional" at the outset but will be replaced by more realistic attitudes as the student learns the role of nurse. Only to the extent that "realism" hardens into a callousness impeding patient interaction is it hazardous. In pharmacy, using different measuring instruments (semantic differential scales), Knapp and Knapp (1968) conclude that seniors are more disillusioned about professional life in general than sophomores and juniors. They indicate that this attitude may relate to increased cynicism.

Gough and Hall's (1973) study of personality changes in medical students, dentistry students, and nurses bears on the issue of cynicism. These investigators find that reserve and detachment do increase as a result of professionalization, yet there is little evidence that students become unfeeling and insensitive. My own study of changes in young women doctors (Cartwright, 1977) also supports a conservative position on cynicism and change. Although the women become more inner-directed and less reactive to social pressures than they were upon entry, they also become more aware of nurturant, loving feelings. In addition, the amount of change as measured by personality inventory scores is not great in magnitude, suggesting that deep-seated dispositions are not radically altered by professional enculturation. In my opinion, until cynicism is defined with explicit references to behaviors, beliefs, values, and feelings toward the profession, the patient, and the self, extrapolations from this research will continue to be muddied and controversial. One way to clarify the meaning of cynicism is to return to the items on the Eron scale and analyze those statements that change with time and setting. Concurrent analysis of changes in other instruments measuring values and attitudes will help distinguish what modifications occur during professional socialization. Along these lines, Perricone (1974) clarifies the distinction between social concern and cynicism. He uses students from the University of Kentucky College of Medicine as subjects and employs a battery of attitude and value scales. Perricone concludes that it is necessary to distinguish between social concern and cynicism. It is empirically possible to score high on a cynicism scale and still be very concerned with providing care for population groups who are in need. A substantial part of the impetus for special programs for disadvantaged patients—the medically indigent and economically deprived—comes from student groups, despite their alleged cynicism. Cynicism as measured by the Eron scale is viewed as only a small segment of a broader attitude, social concern, which is defined as valuing one's fellow man and engaging in relations with others that are not exploitative and manipulative.

All would agree that social concern is an extremely worthwhile attitude. How can the social concern of physicians be enhanced? One solution is to institute more humanistic programs in medical school. Yet Rezler's (1974) conclusions concerning the effects of comprehensive care programs in medical schools aimed at reinforcing humanistic and holistic attitudes among students are not encouraging. She finds the efforts of such programs to be short-lived. Basic attitude change is hard to effect and sustain. She argues, instead, for changes in selection procedures that would bring a different kind of student into medical school. The selection position is taken to its logical conclusion by Rezler. She recommends that faculty also be chosen for their attitudes, as well as for their research proclivities, to ensure appropriate role modeling. This recommendation is more readily followed by new schools than by older schools which are strongly influenced by their traditions. McMaster University Medical School in Canada is an example of a new school that has adopted a substantially different philosophy of education having implications for both selection of students and faculty. The school emphasizes small group teaching and continuous feedback to both students and faculty. Faculty are selected who are particularly interested in teaching, and the evaluation of students takes into account not only cognitive abilities but also personal qualities such as group cooperativeness and responsiveness to others (Neufeld and Barrows, 1974; Simpson, 1976).

Personality. Students bring to professional schools differences in personality. Relative differences in levels of maturity are discernible, as are variations in coping skills, ego resiliency, values, and interest patterns. Since medicine is a heterogeneous profession with many distinct facets and goals, diversity in personality is not only expected, it is desired. Only in the most general sense can one speak of a modal personality. Many investigators prefer to focus more narrowly on individual differences in specific attitudes which may influence patient care—for example, dogmatism, authoritarianism, death-anxiety, and empathy (Hornblow, Kidson, and Jones, 1977; Juan and Haley, 1970; Livingston and Zimet, 1965). Others are concerned with relating personal characteristics to career outcomes such as specialty choice, career satisfaction, and location of practice.

A wide variety of methods has been employed to examine these questions, including clinical case studies, personality inventories oriented to pathology and normal functioning, and surveys of values. Lief's (1971) influential study of the personality of medical students merits renewed attention because of its sensitivity to unconscious factors in adaptations. Utilizing a clinical approach, Lief distinguishes four different personality types among Tulane University medical students. The sixty students in his sample, from the graduating classes of 1959-1962, were interviewed in depth and tested many times during their school years. On the basis of these data, he offers the following typology: (1) The Mature student, characterized as evincing a high level of competence and ego strength (17 percent of the sample). (2) The Emergent student, portrayed as an "experience collector," whose identity diffusion is apparent in unpredictable goals and feelings (15 percent of the sample). (3) The Adjusted student, depicted as conventional and socially acceptable in behavior but who is often deficient in spontaneity, creativity, and flexibility (30 percent). (4) The Conflicted student, described as in need of formal psychotherapy, although differences in severity of pathology exist (38 percent). Lief also crosscuts this category system, reclassifies his sample according to psychiatric character types, and finds that half of the students can be grouped as obsessive-compulsive in character structure. Most of the

Mature, Adjusted, and Emergent students are obsessive-compulsive, whereas the Conflicted are predominantly paranoid in character structure.

Hunter, Prince, and Schwartzman (1961), in their study of students seeking psychiatric treatment, classify 40 percent as having major problems antedating medical school, whereas 60 percent are seen as reacting to environmental factors. It should be noted that the 40 percent correspond closely to the 38 percent in Lief's Conflicted group. These investigators, like many others concerned with the psychological problems of medical students, comment on the difficulties arising from the obsessive-compulsive character structure. The presence of such defenses and coping strategies as isolation of affect, overcontrol of feelings, suppression of aggressive and sexual interests, and intellectualization can interfere with interpersonal effectiveness and cause rigidity in outlook. Many also note that given the arduousness and complexity of medical education, a certain amount of compulsiveness is necessary to meet the demands. Inventories oriented to normal personality functioning, such as the California Psychological Inventory (Gough, 1957), depict the medical student as intellectually independent, dominant, and possessing leadership qualities (Cartwright, 1972; Gough and Hall, 1973).

There appears to be a paradox between the need for compulsivity in physicians—to be careful, responsible, conscientious—and the problems arising from compulsivity—isolation of affect and a high regard for intellectual considerations sometimes at the cost of feelings. This is not an insolvable dilemma given the reality that there is no character structure without both strengths and weaknesses. The school environment can be an important factor in enhancing and widening the scope of personality and the value perspectives of students. Students can learn to relax and can come to know their feelings when the educational milieu legitimates humanistic approaches to the self and others. Accessible faculty, a flexible curriculum, humane educational policies, and adequate student health facilities are all salient factors influencing the growth and development of students.

Patient-related experiences. There is a wide gap between the social need to help humanity and the day-to-day process of assisting individuals and their families in times of illness. Intense feelings, including fear, disgust, and anger, can be aroused in trying to reduce suffering. As noted earlier, one result of intense arousal of feelings may be burnout (Maslach, 1978). Certain practice settings pose unique problems for health professionals. For example, working in an Intensive Care Unit (ICU) has special psychological stresses. Hay and Oken (1972) describe the ICU nurses' experiences, which include facing daily affect-laden stimuli capable of arousing every human conflict area—the nurses confront screaming, blood, excreta, vomitus, and mutilation. Although the dramatic aspects of the setting startle the onlooker, the nurse complains of the continuous, unrelenting routine of monitoring tubes. In addition, interpersonal difficulties with stressed doctors and the ever present possibility of infection offer further complications. Among the suggestions for stress reduction are: finite tours of duty in the ICU, extra pay, and group discussions aimed at sharing feelings and detoxifying guilt.

Other studies concerned with the dark side of the provider-patient relationship focus on the difficulties encountered in caring for terminal patients, cancer patients, psychosomatic patients, elderly patients, and patients with sexual problems (Artiss and Levine, 1973; Kutner, 1978; Lief, 1964; Mumford, 1970). Special programs designed to increase knowledge, encourage the sharing of feelings, and foster more tolerant attitudes toward sexuality have been developed at some schools and have been well received by the participants (Coombs, 1968; Rosenberg and Chilgren, 1973).

A clearer understanding of the patient's contribution to provider stress can be gained by assessing the problems of practicing doctors. Are there attributes of contemporary Western medicine's ideology that influence the physician's sense of frustration? Reports of physicians' frustrations with patients are not new. Although anecdotal information far exceeds research, these studies shed light on problems of the patient-provider relationship. In Great Britain, Cartwright (1967) measures the proportion of unwarranted or trivial consultations in the average day of the practitioner and finds that about 20 percent of the visits were considered by the physician consulted to be trivial. Mechanic (1972a) and later Gough (1977) confirm these findings on new samples. All note considerable variation in the attribution of "triviality." Mechanic finds high reports of unwarranted consultations to be negatively related to overall satisfaction with general practice and to having a "social orientation" to medicine. In addition, the more patients seen by the doctor, the greater the proportion of trivial consultations reported.

Gough (1977), investigating psychological correlates of the attribution of triviality, finds that doctors who give higher estimates of triviality to their patients' complaints are, by no means, sour misanthropes. They are, rather, more able in scientific thinking, favoring rational over intuitive modes of thought, and more affiliative in temperament. Cartwright (1978d), studying the same cohort of doctors as did Gough, asked these doctors, "What kinds of patients would you rather not see?" The most cited patient was the one who does not assume the role of the socially desirable, motivated patient. Demanding, disruptive, and unappreciative behaviors make such patients unwelcome. Second, patients whose pathology resides in life-style maladaptations, such as addiction, psychosomatic complaints, alcoholism, and obesity, were seen as particularly burdensome. Such disorders defy simple diagnosis and/or are particularly difficult to cure.

Dentists also report that certain kinds of patients present more problems than others—demanding patients, denture patients, and patients with phobias about dental care (Kimmel, 1973; Virgilio, 1971). The research of Parsons (1951b) and his followers on the sick role is relevant. If the patient accepts or is properly "socialized" to the role of patient (that is, the patient suffers, seeks help, and is ready and willing to cooperate with the physician), the provider will find the role of expert satisfying. Essentially, he or she is allowed to help. This traditional doctor-patient relationship follows the model of guidance-cooperation. If the patient rejects or cannot follow this implicit model, the doctor may be frustrated. Blum (1974b) recommends revisions in the hierarchical model of doctor-patient relationships so that the patient has more options in choice of treatment and more responsibility for maintaining his or her health. It is hoped that the effects on the doctor in this less hierarchical relationship would be to decrease the burden of unrealistic and unmanageable professional responsibility. Increased patient independence and choice allows the physician to assume the role of consultant to an informed patient, a role that carries less stress. Since responsibility is shared, blame and demandingness—products of dependency—should be lessened.

Also pertinent to the biases of Western medicine are beliefs about the nature of illness (Freidson, 1970b). Contemporary medicine relies almost exclusively on a biological, pathophysiological model of disease. Dysfunction caused by social forces, life-style preferences, and adaptational failures may be perceived as illegitimate or carrying a stigma. The student's dislike for the "crock" or psychosomatic patient is well known (Mumford, 1970). Engel (1977), in documenting the inadequate integration of psychiatry into medicine, asserts that all medicine is in crisis. He states that the ineffectiveness of the biomedical disease model perpetuates a mind-body duality. In its stead, Engel advocates a biopsychosocial model which would accept social and psychological factors as powerful influencers of health and illness. Speculatively, what would be the consequences of such a model on the psychological well-being of the physician? One effect might be that professionals would engage in less compartmentalized thinking about their own health and become more realistic and open about problems. The stigma of emotional problems would be lessened, the relationship between illness and life events would become more obvious, and there could be increased willingness to see and explore the interrelationships among the multiple domains of life—work, family, social relations, and community—leading to insights and creative solutions to problems that are currently minimized or avoided. More tolerance for the psychological aspects of life could also have repercussions for patient care, particularly in making the patient's feelings more salient in both the diagnosis and treatment of illness.

Specialization

Among the professions, medicine is the most diversified, allowing the broadest spectrum of choice in work. The long-term trend in medical education is toward increasing specialization (Kendall, 1971; Levit, Sabshin, and Mueller, 1974). Currently, identified national needs for more primary care doctors, greater continuity of care, more comprehensive care, and greater accessibility of care have led to attempts to counteract the fragmentation inherent in specialization through federal funding of family practice residencies and the establishment of health centers in underserved areas (Rousselot, 1973).

Although some students on entry have a clear idea of what they eventually intend to do in medicine, most decide sometime during their medical school training. Specialty choice is an extremely important decision and, as noted earlier, specialization is a salient factor differentially associated with certain problems, such as coronary heart disease, suicide, and divorce. Research on specialty choice is extensive. A brief review of the literature will identify relevant issues. A unifying and comprehensive theory of choice of specialty does not exist, although Mitchell's (1975) efforts to develop a theoretical model of choice and Gough's (1975) investigations into the latent factorial structure of specialty interests provide a starting point for development of such a theory. Generally, investigators seek to determine the effects of a wide array of variables on choice. External factors such as the influence of faculty, schools, and courses have been studied (Coker and others, 1960; Geertsma and Grinols, 1972; Weinstein and Gipple, 1975). In addition, the effects of general stereotypes about specialists were significant parameters in the work of Bruhn and Parsons (1964, 1965) and of Becker and his co-workers (1961). The studies find that faculty exert more influence in recruiting students to less prestigeful and little-known specialties than to the well-known specialties. Before entrance to medical school, students already have opinions concerning surgery, medicine, psychiatry, and general practice. Stereotypes existing within the general culture portray surgeons as domineering and arrogant, psychiatrists as emotionally unstable but interested in intellectual problems, and general practitioners as very patient and concerned with people. During professional school there are changes in the stereotypes —for example, with time, internal medicine increases in attractiveness and prestige. Students see themselves as sharing the more positive traits of specialists working in areas in which they are interested.

Student characteristics such as personality, values, and academic achievements constitute another set of variables and have stimulated many studies (Livingston and Zimet, 1965; Monk and Terris, 1956; Monk and Thomas, 1973; Myers and Davis, 1964; Paiva and Haley, 1971; Schumacher, 1964). The nature of findings from these studies may be illustrated by comparing students who are attracted to psychiatry with those attracted to surgery—those planning to enter psychiatry are less authoritarian and have higher anxiety about death. Social and esthetic values are held in greater esteem by the psychiatry group, whereas economic values are more important to the surgery group. The interpersonal aspects of health care are more interesting to potential psychiatrists, whereas the would-be surgeons prefer diagnosis, treatment, or research problems. Both surgery and psychiatry attract students who were already interested in the specialty before the start of medical school—faculty influence per se is not as important as it may be for other specialties.

Broad demographic and biographic factors have also merited attention in the specialization literature. For example, socioeconomic status, parental occupation, place of birth, sex, ethnicity, and religion are salient variables, influencing choice as well as location of practice (Coker and others, 1960; Gough and Ducker, 1977; Gough and Hall, 1977a; Kehrer, 1974; Kritzer and Zimet, 1967; Lieberson, 1958). A sampling of results from a multitude of findings shows the following: Students from low status backgrounds are less

likely to specialize and more often choose general practice and family medicine—prior debts are probably a salient factor influencing choice. Students
from medical families, by way of contrast, are more likely to select certain
specialties over others—they will gravitate to opthalmology, dermatology,
and surgery and are less likely to choose psychiatry, pediatrics, and obstetrics. Jewish doctors are more likely to specialize than Catholics of Irish,
Polish, and Italian extraction. Jews are more likely to choose internal medicine and psychiatry than surgery or obstetrics. Women also gravitate to certain specialties—psychiatry, pediatrics, and anesthesiology—and have in the
past avoided others, such as surgery and radiology.

To return to the topic of stress, the issue of the resolving powers and
integrative potential of the specialty for a specific individual is most important in mitigating day-to-day tension. A good choice is one in which the individual finds his or her niche within the profession based on self-knowledge
and awareness of the satisfactions and limitations of various occupational
options. Not every specialty is equally knowable; often stereotypes are inaccurate and, as Wheelis (1958) states in his commentary on the hazards of
psychoanalysis for the analyst, some vocations are knowable only from within and may be misleading to the novice who seeks to find something that is
not there.

What are the characteristics of a good choice of specialty for the professional? Yufit, Pollack, and Wasserman (1969) see a conflict-free choice in
specialty as satisfying a number of conscious and unconscious needs, including the utilization and actualization of talents and abilities, neutralization
and sublimation of impulses (such as looking, touching), fulfillment of ego-
ideals, establishment of self-stabilizing processes through increased competencies, and, perhaps most important, avoidance of areas of difficulty and
deficiency. Yufit selects the polarity of intimacy-isolation as pivotal in
understanding choice. Some individuals want close and reciprocal relations
and others need more distance. Many specialties, such as internal medicine
and psychiatry, entail continual and intense contact with patients, whereas
others, such as surgery, are episodic and oriented to special techniques and
methods. Gray, Newman, and Reinhardt (1966) also note that the specialties
demanding much interaction with patients are characterized by total responsibility for care, a lay referral system, and lower levels of visibility for peer
review and evaluation. A particularly stressful occupational integration might
be one in which an isolate-prone person elects a specialty demanding intimacy. Within a longitudinal model, there will also be times in a given person's life when intense contact with patients will be more difficult owing to
life cycle changes and concomitant increased demands from lateral roles. For
example, women physicians often take less demanding jobs during the early
childbearing years.

Practice

Further channeling of careers occurs after completion of training. For
example, choices must be made concerning the location of practice and prac-

tice settings, such as hospital, university, or private office. The organization of practice—solo, group, pre-paid—is an additional issue for physicians and dentists.

As was stated earlier, physicians as a group are well satisfied with their careers and, although they acknowledge defects in their education, the gaps between their training and professional life are not felt to be great (Gough and Hall, 1977b). However, for some health providers, there are marked incongruities between training and work. These disappointments have been termed "role-training incongruities" and "inconsistent or inadequate socializations." Baccalaureate nursing training has been criticized as not preparing nurses for the reality of hospital work. Ideals and objectives taught in school have little relevance for hospital nursing. Kramer (1974) identifies "reality shock" as the primary cause of migration from the nursing profession. Shock, resulting from the disparity between professional values and norms learned in school and the bureaucratic norms of the hospital setting, is also accompanied by role deprivation. Lack of social reinforcement for attitudes and work habits previously held in high esteem produces the deprivation. In this vein, Sadler, Sadler, and Bliss (1972, p. 39) refer to the paradoxical schism between nursing education and nursing services. They point out that out of 700,000 practicing nurses, only 20,000 (about 3 percent) hold a master's degree or higher. These small numbers of educators determine the educational policy for the 97 percent providing services. Closer communication and linkages between educators and diploma nurses are advocated by many.

To a lesser extent, pharmacists also suffer from role deprivation. Professional values are not always realized in the work settings: Some pharmacists lack opportunities to advance and develop their talents. Drug manufacturers have been accused of usurping the role of the "real" pharmacist (Johnson, Hammel, and Heinen, 1977). The marginality of the profession, stemming from conflict between business and professional goals, has also been cited as a problem. When the clinical and patient-oriented aspects of pharmacy are enhanced, as is the case in the new role of clinical pharmacist, career satisfactions increase.

The patient-related problems discussed earlier continue to be a source of stress throughout practice. In my research, doctors were asked to discuss dissatisfactions and limitations within their careers (Cartwright, 1978c). Over half believe that they do not have enough time for other pursuits—family, hobbies, and interests. An interesting subtle limitation is the belief that medicine binds the doctor emotionally to patients beyond actual time requirements. Almost 13 percent of the sample comment that they cannot put medicine aside, that it intrudes on their private lives, that they often wake up with recurring dreams of diagnoses they should have made. In addition, the threat of legal difficulties involving malpractice adds a financial and emotional burden to the careers of physicians and dentists. Problems arising from the business aspects of management of practice are other sources of stress.

Women doctors have special problems. Synchronizing the timetable of career and the timetable of family life is an ever-present challenge. Since the peak of a professional career is also the most demanding time for meeting the responsibilities of familial roles, many women find the integrative tasks stressful. However, individual differences do exist. In the University of California sample (Cartwright, 1978b), women who were especially tolerant and who set clear priorities, either by putting career or family first, achieved harmonious role integrations and experienced little stress while still maintaining a high level of career satisfaction. Interestingly, personality traits, visible upon entry to medical school, forecast successful role integrations.

As is the case with most research on occupations, considerably more attention has been paid to the early stages of career development than to the later stages involving establishment, maintenance, and retirement. The later stages represent an important area of needed research. Among the salient topics warranting investigation are the nature and relationship between stress experienced at the early stages of career development and problems in the later stages. Vaillant, Sobowale, and McArthur's (1972) longitudinal study of professionals suggests early predisposition to psychological vulnerability among those in the sample. We need to know more about the continuity and discontinuity of distress in the careers of health professionals, and about those successful individuals who deal with life and career crises with innovative strategies, furthering their own development and resiliency. In addition to focusing on individuals, we should study specialty differences relative to the life cycle. Are mid-life career problems more apt to be associated with membership in certain specialties and practice conditions? What role can interventions, such as occupational counseling, play in the lives of health professionals who are well into their careers? Can lateral moves, such as transferring from a high patient ratio practice to a lower one, influence psychological well-being? What support groups, both within the profession and the community, can be utilized to assist in later career adaptations?

Conclusions

The assessment of the psychological problems of health professionals is a new area and there is still much to be learned. More systematic approaches to the occupational hazards of different health careers and the satisfactions inherent in the work are needed. A longitudinal perspective of the career trajectory offers an organizing framework for such studies. There are many tasks to be accomplished, including a compendium of the sources of stress, accurate statistics recording the incidence of stress syndromes for different professional and age groups, and cross-cultural comparisons that take into account variations in the definitions of occupations. In addition, the relationship between stress experienced at one stage of a health career and a range of variables—health status, emotional stability, career success, career satisfaction—at a later stage represents a crucial, but often overlooked, aspect of the research agenda.

Fruitful directions are suggested by prior studies. Specialty differences within a given profession appear to be related to the formation of stress symptoms, with individuals involved in high interaction specialties under more tension. More clarity is needed in identifying the agents of stress in these specialties. Among the variables meriting attention are: the number of patients seen, the nature of the patient's complaint, the number of emergency calls, the personality and value system of the professional, and characteristics of the practice setting itself. Special attention might also be given to those individuals who cope creatively with specialties acknowledged to be stressful. What strategies do they use to reduce stress?

A holistic approach to work, acknowledging the relationship between the occupational sector of life and other domains—personal, family, and community—offers promise for better understanding of the mechanisms of good health. Each occupation has unique life-style aspects, some of which have a bearing on health status. A clearer picture of the enhancing and depriving aspects of work will emerge if we examine the habits of those in a given occupation that are relevant to health and disease—habits affecting nutrition, exercise, smoking, drinking, drug usage, relaxation, and recreation. Behavioral settings such as Intensive Care Units, Free Clinics, and Ambulatory Outpatient Clinics, acknowledged to be stressful, might also be studied with particular emphasis on the interaction among health providers, since there is evidence that friction exists (see Hay and Oken, 1972). The effects of planned interventions—group discussions, change in task assignments, retreats—might also be systematically investigated to determine their respective roles in stress reduction.

Broad macrosocial changes in concepts and ideals of health care have implications for the training and practice conditions of future health professionals. Galdston (1959), a medical historian, notes the shift toward more holistic and ecological concepts of care. He distinguishes between the "gnosis" of medicine, which emphasizes knowledge and understanding of humans as organisms dwelling in multiple realities, and the "techné" of medicine, where operational modalities and episodic approaches predominate. Although macrosocial changes take place over long time periods, changes in curriculum and admission policies occurring during the last decade appear to have had modest impact on the values of doctors, so that recent graduates are more alert to the gnosis of medicine than their predecessors (Cartwright, 1978a). At the same time that education continues to change, the increased participation of the government and other third parties in health care serves to reinforce orientations and concepts relating to public health and preventive medicine as a major means of reducing the costs of care. This greater emphasis on the gnosis of medicine will place increased importance on the individual's responsibility for maintaining and enhancing his or her own health, as well as identifying the need for institutional support systems that reinforce healthy life-styles. These changes have implications for both patient care and for the life-style of health providers. As the ethos and ideology of training depart from a strict pathophysiological model of disease, the health professional's awareness of the staggering number of variables influencing his or her well-being will also increase. In addition to these salutary predictions, some adverse trends can be forecast. New sources of stress may arise because of economic pressures and changes within the professions themselves. Interprofessional problems associated with new careers may increase. In addition, bureaucratic controls relating to the cost of care, number of patients seen, and intraprofessional regulation may create new difficulties for some providers.

Alterations in the roles of provider and consumer also presage change. Consumer education, leading to greater awareness of the patient's contributions to provider stress, is important for the reductions of tension in the professional. Provider education directed toward better understanding of the biases and myths concerning patient care is also necessary. More general acceptance of the legitimacy of the care-taking aspects of medicine, in contrast to the curative components of care, can lead to greater tolerance for socioemotional problems in both provider and consumer.

17

Clinical Psychologists as Health Professionals

William Schofield

Clinical psychology is the application of psychological science to adjustment problems of individuals (Sundberg and Tyler, 1962). As a field of professional psychology, its present status and visibility mark a stage in a steady evolution that was set in motion at the end of World War II. In 1945, the Veterans Administration asked the American Psychological Association for a list of universities with satisfactory graduate training programs in clinical psychology. A similar request was made in 1946 by the United States Public Health Service (Schofield, 1964). These requests were made in response to the increased demands for skilled mental health personnel to assist the great number of emotional casualties, both military and civilian, arising out of the war. Both of the federal agencies soon mounted programs in conjunction with university departments of psychology to support the training of clinical psychologists. These programs involved a core academic curriculum and a related clinical internship experience designed to prepare the trainee to work in psychiatric hospitals and mental health clinics and to provide diagnostic and therapeutic services to individuals with emotional disorders (Blank, 1964). The thoughtful, collaborative, and continuous planning of the Veterans Administration, the Public Health Service, and the university psychology departments created a new mental health professional —the clinical psychologist.

In addition to their technical skills of assessment and intervention, clinical psychologists differ from other mental health professionals in that they are trained in research methodology and are expected to contribute research expertise as special input to the interdisciplinary team. A major portion of the improvement in diagnostic procedures and of the evaluation of therapies for mental patients accomplished in the past thirty years reflects in significant part the scientific contribution of the clinical psychologist. The clinical psychologist is a well-established and recognized mental health scientist. In this sense then, as a specialty, clinical psychology can be perceived as one of the health sciences.

Can clinical psychology be viewed as a health science in broader perspective? This query may be pursued in two ways, logically and empirically. For the former, it serves to note that psychology is one of the life sciences, concerned with the processes and principles that determine and predict the adaptive behavior of organisms. "In the study of the normal growth and decline of the 'psychological person' there is a possibility of discovery at every stage with potential relevance for the prevention of disorder, the promotion of health" (Schofield, 1969, p. 567). In brief, the behaviors of individuals have import for their physical as well as mental health, and psychology as the science of behavior is thus, at least potentially, a general health science.

Clinical psychologists' special competencies equip them to make diagnostic, therapeutic, and research contributions over the full range of problems manifested by persons whose primary source of help is a mental health agency or mental health professional. However, many of the fears and frustrations experienced by the patients of general hospitals and outpatient medical clinics give rise to emotional or psychological disturbances that may be not only very distressing in and of themselves but may also impair significantly the patient's capacity to understand and cooperate in the plan for treatment. Also, the persistence of emotional stresses arising from a person's general life situation may contribute to the total complex of causal factors that culminate in a physical ailment. Clinical psychologists are skilled in techniques to detect and assay the presence of such psychological factors (especially, anxiety and depression) but they are also prepared to select and apply intervention techniques designed to ease or remove them.

How many clinical psychologists work primarily in a *general* medical setting, that is, a nonpsychiatric clinic or hospital, and are devoting their assessment and intervention skills primarily to patients with nonpsychiatric health problems? No comprehensive data are available. The great majority of clinical psychologists, either in private practice or institutional service, specialize in evaluation and management of psychosocial or psychiatric disorders. However, clinical psychology has had a growing impact, albeit indirect, on the general health care arena through its role in medical education. Twenty-five years ago there were only 252 psychologists with medical school appointments (Mensh, 1953). A few years later, Matarazzo and Daniel (1957) found that three fourths of existing medical schools had at least one psychologist on their faculties, with an average of four psychologists per school. In all, this survey identified 346 psychologists with medical school appointments. Even in this early period, the teaching activities of these psychologists were directed not only at undergraduate medical students but also at physicians in psychiatric and other medical residencies, nurses, occupational and physical therapy students, and social workers. By 1964, the number of medical school psychologists was 993 (Wagner and Stegeman, 1964) and by 1972, the number had reached 1,300 (Witkin, Mensh, and Cates, 1972). This represents a significant growth phenomenon. Between 1972 and 1977, the number of medical school psychologists doubled (Matarazzo, Lubin, and Nathan, 1978). Part of this increase may be attributed to the founding of new medical schools; between 1969 and 1977, the number of medical schools had increased from 97 to 115. However, the 18 new medical schools could hardly account for the increase of over 1,000 psychologists with new medical school appointments in that interval. Rather, the growth must be attributed in large measure to the growing awareness of medical school faculties of the contributions that psychologists could make to clinical psychiatric services and, even more importantly, in providing core teaching programs in behavioral science for undergraduate medical students.

The pioneers among medical school psychologists were frequently individuals with particular research interests in physiology or neurology. As they pursued their research in university-affiliated teaching hospitals, they frequently were consulted on clinical problems, especially by their colleagues in psychiatry, and were among the first to exemplify the role of the medical psychologist (Hathaway, 1958; Watson, 1953). In the current development of the field of health care psychology, there is an interesting reversal of this evolution, as many clinical psychologists are finding themselves drawn toward basic and applied research on general medical problems outside of psychiatry.

Beginning in the 1970s, psychologists in detectable numbers began to show interest in bringing their skills to bear on behavioral and emotional problems associated with physical illness or with programs to reduce susceptibility to certain diseases (Cummings, 1975; Dörken and Whiting, 1974; McAllister and Philip, 1975). In 1973, the Task Force on Health Research established by the American Psychological Association (APA) compiled a roster of some 500 educators, scientists, and health administrators, mostly psychologists, who were interested or directly involved in health-related research *outside* of the psychiatric realm (American Psychological Association, 1974a). Ten percent of the psychologists on the roster had clinical backgrounds. A survey of the activities of this special-interest group revealed that typically some 75 percent of their time was spent in health-illness research and that their most important research collaborators were specialists in medicine, not psychiatry. Many of their research contributions are published in medical and health journals. The number of health-related papers reported in *Psychological Abstracts* in 1971-1973, inclusive, totaled 14,427. Over 40 percent of these papers related to nonpsychiatric topics and were concerned with such general health-illness areas as nonmedical hospitalization, cardiac problems, surgery, pain, and psychosomatics (American Psychological Association, 1974b). The Task Force found that most of the major units in the National Institutes of Health were interested in providing for the investigation of the role of behavioral factors in the major disease categories.

The involvement of psychologists of all specialties, but especially those with clinical background, in the nation's health and illness problems has paralleled the growing concern for a national health program. Psychologists have played prominent roles in conferences on health behavior and behavioral medicine (S. Weiss, 1975). The founding of a Section on Health Research in APA's Division of Psychologists in Public Service is further evidence that an increasing number of psychologists are identifying themselves as health scientists who are interested in applying the methods of psychology to the study of health-illness behavior. Landmarks in the development of this new field of endeavor for clinical psychologists—namely, medical psychology (Asken, 1975)—are the founding of the Society of Pediatric Psychologists in 1968 (Gardner, 1969) and the Conference on Behavioral Medicine in 1977 (Schwartz and Weiss, 1978). Of the seventeen participants in this conference, ten were psychologists.

To the extent that psychologists are defined as "students of the mind," the appropriateness of their involvement in the diagnosis and treatment of mental illness has been self-evident and unquestioned. Their role in study and management of physical illness, by contrast, seems to require an explicit rationale. This is afforded by recognition that the hoary mind-body dualism is a conceptual convention that has facilitated scientific inquiry more than it has encouraged a truly comprehensive medicine. Within a reductionist philosophy of physical monism, the focus of the basic medical sciences on the physical structure and function of organs has made possible increasing precision of theory and prediction and increasingly refined understanding of cause, prevention, and treatment of physical illness. Similarly, the general focus of psychology, and especially the clinical specialty on macromolecular aspects of cognitive and affective behaviors, has brought increasing awareness of the working of the "mind." Specialization and focus on body *or* mind has made for effective and progressive programmatic research. A small number of illnesses have been viewed as "psychosomatic," and only a very few physicians or psychologists have been attracted to the complex interface of the physical and the mental. Recent years have seen an increasing appreciation for the need to study the reciprocity between psyche and soma, as there has been growing awareness that the individual's health status is a personal gestalt to which situational/environmental and mental/emotional conditions contribute in a complex interactive fashion (Engel, 1977; Moss, 1973). This growing awareness is reflected in the introduction of behavioral sciences, including a large measure of psychology, into the curricula of our medical schools and the related inclusion of a section on behavioral science in the National Board Examinations (Part I) for medical students (Fletcher, 1974). Clinical psychologists are playing an important role in curriculum design and instruction in the behavioral sciences for medical students and for residents in the recently established medical school departments of family practice.

The human being is an organismic, holistic, integrated, interactive, unified field of continuous energy exchange between the poles of the psyche and the soma. It has been well documented that physical illness can give rise to emotional disturbance, personality disruption, and impaired psychological functioning (Silverman, 1968). It is only relatively more difficult to establish solid evidence that psychological factors (personality type, life-style, current situational or cumulative stress) can be stimuli to a physical illness response (Dohrenwend and Dohrenwend, 1974b; Engel, 1977; Jenkins, 1972). All illnesses can be classified with equal meaning as either psychosomatic or somatopsychic (Wright, 1977). No discipline is better equipped than psychology to discover, delineate, and demonstrate the organismic nature of humans and to encourage an ever-broadening realization that the individual's total functional health is threatened whenever either component of the interactive mind $\longleftrightarrow$ body equation is impaired (American Psychological Association, 1976).

The Clinical Psychologist in a Medical Setting

Assessment

With basic training in techniques for assessment of intelligence, personality, and special perceptual or learning disabilities, the clinical psychologist brings to the general medical setting a professional armamentarium which, with selective, individualized modification, can be applied to the clinic or hospital patient to facilitate the understanding of the patient by other professional health staff, sharpen their delineation of functional and organic components in the patient's complaint, and contribute to the design and implementation of a therapeutic or preventive regimen with greatest likelihood of eliciting an optimal "therapeutic alliance." In this assessment function, psychologists utilize their knowledge of the general principles of psychometric methodology and their awareness of the indications for and data yield of particular instruments.

The clinical psychologist's assessment activities most often are directed to three major domains of the patient's functioning: intelligence, or cognitive processes; current affective state, or mood level, for example, arousal or lethargy; and temperament, or personality. In most instances of general practice, the psychologist can directly make use of the "instrument of choice," using the standard procedures of administration. However, in working with the physically ill or handicapped, the psychologist must be knowledgeable about suitably validated and normed alternative forms that permit reliable measurements despite peculiarities of the patient (for example, loss of voice, loss of sight, physical weakness or easy fatigability) that prevent use of customary procedures. In other instances, the psychologist must use ingenuity and clinical sensitivity in preparing suitable adaptations of standard procedures; in these cases, experienced judgment must be used in appraising the patient's performance, since the standard norms will be inappropriate. In the following section, the rationale for assessment in each of the domains of cognition, affect, and temperament is discussed in relation to implications for optimal treatment of the medical patient.

The psychologist may apply clinical judgment to assay whether the patient shows signs of a cognitive deficit which would call for individual intelligence testing, with such determination critical only if the patient must be taught a complex medical regimen and its rationale. Also, the psychologist can determine whether the patient's level of comprehension is sufficient to produce valid responses to a medical procedure that entails moderately complex instructions (Duché and others, 1971; Rice, McDaniel, and Denny, 1968). Where a group education program is indicated, only a quick screening inventory for intelligence level may suffice to afford development of homogeneous groups for a training program pitched at an appropriate level of comprehension (Kulcar, Seso, and Majnaric, 1966). Suggestion of serious cognitive limitation may indicate a careful individual appraisal of intelligence to support the prescription of extended, personal nursing care.

The patients coming to a general medical facility may have significant perceptual deficiencies (of sight or hearing, especially in those of advanced age), and the psychologist must be proficient with those psychological instruments designed especially for assessment of such handicapped persons. In large urban clinics with a sizable complement of foreign-speaking or foreign-reading clients, the psychologist must be cognizant of foreign language instruments or skilled in the training of foreign-speaking aides to help in the assessment process.

The psychologist can make clinical appraisals of the sensorium of hospitalized patients to detect elements of clouding of consciousness which may impair comprehension of instructions and increase disorientation, especially for place (Wells and Ruesch, 1969). Such deficits, in turn, may raise the patient's anxiety. Appropriate assessment of mental status and communication about impairment with staff can encourage individual orientation procedures as well as provide a basis for arranging environmental elements. An example might be color coding of room doors and hallways to reduce the patient's possible confusion and loss of independence and to prevent undesirable episodes of panic.

The tension experienced by many patients in the earliest phases of medical examination may be of a different quality than that associated with the intellectual appraisal that goes on in educational or occupational settings. Such anxiety may not only constitute a hazard to accurate estimation of a patient's cognitive capacities but may also impair his or her ability to give a lucid account of the complaint and its history and/or cause faulty data (for example, elevated blood pressure). Thoughtful preparation of the patient by ancillary staff may reduce anxiety to levels that are consonant with good appraisals. Clinical psychologists can use their knowledge of assessment techniques to assist medical, nursing, and other staff in creating an examination environment that will enhance the reliability of diagnostic procedures.

Factors of personality, temperament, and emotional reactivity (anxiety proneness) are as important as cognitive variables as sources of undesirable complications in the diagnostic-therapeutic endeavor. Individuals differ in their tolerance for frustration and for ambiguity. Those who have very low tolerance for invasion of privacy, for delay in receiving attention, or for lack of information find these frequent characteristics of hospital life particularly stressful. Such stress can contribute to a state of mind that may worsen already distressful physical symptoms or even contribute to physical collapse (for example, with the hypertensive patient). At best, these tolerance deficiencies may arouse hostile, resentful attitudes which reduce the patient's readiness to cooperate with prescribed procedures and medication. Also, patients may adopt a general mode of response to their medical situation that causes impairment of personal and social adjustment (Goldstein, 1976; Huggan, 1968).

The appraisal of tolerance deficiencies may not only suggest procedures to improve the patient's adjustment to the treatment regimen but, by providing further diagnostic understanding, may also mitigate the effect of the patient's hostility on attitudes of the treatment staff. The psychologist has skills in clinical interviewing and in application of specific measures designed to minimize frustration and to enhance the patient's understanding of and cooperation with hospital procedures or outpatient treatment.

For patients who are not deviant on such variables as resentment of authority and tolerance for ambiguity, there may still be significant emotional complications. All major illnesses have an emotional component of some degree. Most frequently, this may be depression or anxiety, or a mixture of the two. In many patients, such effects are normal, appropriate emotional responses to discomfort, loss of independence, and uncertainty. In some patients, however, particularly those with conditions that are life threatening or imply a demand for a significant change in the patient's living patterns, the emotional response may reach pathologic levels (Pearson and Steinhilber, 1971). Also, there is evidence that major affective disturbance may play a causal role in the etiology of physical illness (Weiner, 1977). The psychologist can employ screening procedures to detect the presence and magnitude of emotional disturbance (Lucente and Fleck, 1972; Vetter and others, 1977). Whether the emotional symptomatology is reactive to a physical illness or possibly a part of its etiology, the psychologist can alert the health care staff to its presence and to the possible need for remediation of the psychological state of the patient as well as therapy for the somatic problem.

In addition to the cognitive, temperamental, and affective dimensions which characterize the unique "psychological surround" of every patient, the domain of attitudes is important. Broadly, attitudes or predispositional "sets" may operate either to enhance or impair the patient's response to treatment. Most focally, each individual has attitudes toward his or her body and toward pain, medication, and physicians. These important attitudes have their origins in early life experiences, in family modeling, and in education or lack thereof. In their content, these attitudes constitute a general receptivity or resistance to the idea of seeking medical opinion to begin with and acting positively upon it when it is received (Becker, Drachman, and Kirscht, 1972b; Becker and Maiman, 1975; Sexton, 1974). Programs designed to influence attitudes in the proper direction are appropriate for those patients whose biases, prejudices, and mind sets are most countertherapeutic (Leventhal, 1973). Measurement of attitudes and evaluation of modes of achieving attitude change are generally in the domain of social psychologists; these psychologists are chiefly identified with group research and rarely apply their instruments to appraisal and management of individuals in a clinical context. The clinical psychologist, however, possesses the technical knowledge to select or construct attitude measures that reliably identify prime targets for educational endeavors aimed at increasing the patient's readiness for diagnostic and therapeutic procedures (Bultz, 1975; Shaw and Wright, 1967).

In some settings, many of the assessment needs outlined might be satisfied by sensitive, individual interviewing by an appropriately trained medical specialist, the psychiatrist. However, at least three considerations reduce the feasibility of this approach to an assay of the medical patient's psychology: (1) it is extremely expensive; (2) it is subject to the very modest reliability of personality diagnosis by interview (Sundberg, 1977); and (3) it entails the potentially counterproductive resistance of the patient to the notion that he or she is "crazy." Additionally, the use of psychiatric or psychological consultation requires a preliminary clinical judgment by medical staff as to whether a patient probably is manifesting a significant personality configuration that may hamper the treatment program.

The clinical psychologist has access to a variety of well-researched objective screening measures—the Cornell Medical Index (Brodman and others, 1952a, 1952b), the Minnesota Multiphasic Personality Inventory or MMPI (Guthrie, 1949; Newmark and Raft, 1976; Tsushima, 1975), and the Jenkins Activity Survey (Jenkins, 1971)—which have the advantages of reliability as well as economy of time and expense. They can be used in routine fashion for preliminary screening of all clinic patients or of patients newly admitted to a specialty service. In addition, the psychologist knows how to construct screening measures useful for a particular setting, such as a pediatric clinic or ward (Ireton and Thwing, 1976).

In general, the purpose of such screening procedures is to determine whether the applicant for medical attention, whose presenting complaint consists of one or several physical symptoms, is also experiencing a significant degree of emotional disturbance. Marked aberration of psychological functioning (especially in the affective domain) may play a causal role in the patient's physical status or may reflect inadequacies of the patient's effort to cope with the discomfort and threat of the somatic ailment. In either case, it is important for the physician to be alerted when the patient's psychological state is clearly deviant so that attention may be given, directly or by referral, to that aspect of the patient's gestalt and a comprehensive program of health care designed. It has been estimated that not less than one third and possibly as many as three fourths of the patients of general physicians have a significant psychological component in their presenting complaint. Use of appropriate psychometric screening instruments can reliably identify those patients whose psychosocial conditions warrant attention. Most questionnaires are well received by patients and can be administered, scored, and profiled by paraprofessional psychological assistants working under the supervision of the doctoral psychologist who is responsible for the selection of appropriate instruments and their interpretation. (A widely used instrument, the MMPI, is available in well-studied, shortened versions when necessary.) Such an arrangement provides an efficient and cost-effective approach to provision of the diagnostic foundation required in any effort to provide a truly comprehensive program of health care.

As part of the growing concern to improve our health care system, there has been much interest in providing periodic health examinations that are comprehensive and economically feasible, taking advantage of computerized laboratory procedures. Opinion of the medical community is divided as to whether automated health screening for medical problems is cost effective in providing early detection of abnormalities that require physician attention (Collen, 1971; Gordon, 1971; Howe, 1972; Olsen, 1976). There is evidence, however, that such multiphasic health screening should include appraisal of the individual's mental health (Fowler, 1969). Health care delivery systems which have provided such screening and which, when indicated, have provided mental health services have found that patients who, upon postscreening referral, receive psychotherapy make significantly reduced use of medical services. For example, patients with discernible emotional difficulties were found to make higher than average utilization of both inpatient and outpatient medical facilities. When such patients received psychotherapy, their subsequent use of medical facilities showed a significant decrease which was maintained over a five-year period, in contrast to a control group of emotionally distressed patients who did not receive therapy (Follette and Cummings, 1967).

With the recognition that our delivery of health care services, both preventive and therapeutic, lags behind the potential of our medical technology, there is increased desire to design a health care system that will be both comprehensive and integrated. Such a system must provide for adequate appraisal of both the somatic and psychological components that are interactive in the person as a functional unit. The assessment of the psychological status of the patient constitutes a primary area for application of the special skills, techniques, and knowledge of clinical psychology and a basic element of its role as a health care profession.

Intervention Techniques

The individual is always, to a greater or lesser degree, a potential host to the variety of pathogenic agents (bacteria, toxins, viruses, and neoplasms)

that are necessary causes of physical illness. Moreover, he or she is a potential victim of trauma or premature physical deterioration. Both one's susceptibility as host and one's probability as victim are thought to be significantly
influenced by behavior and recent life experiences (Holmes and Masuda,
1974). When an individual does succumb to illness or trauma, the course of
the disease and recovery or rehabilitation is determined in part by specific
behaviors. This relationship is particularly notable for illnesses of a chronic
nature in which the patient may achieve either an almost normal life-style or
succumb to a progressively debilitated condition, depending in part, at least,
upon the extent to which the patient conscientiously and consistently carries
out those behaviors that are medically prescribed (Kaplan-de Nour and
Czaczkes, 1972; Moos, 1977a).

As a student of behavior and as an expert in the management of those
variables that determine the direction and strengths of behavioral adjustments, the psychologist can play a role in both preventive and therapeutic
medicine. Because of the nature of their basic training and skills, most clinical psychologists are unlikely to find their major work assignment to be one
in which they contribute directly to programs designed for primary prevention of major illnesses. However, by integrating both their diagnostic and
intervention skills with the special skills of physicians, nurses, social workers,
and other health care professionals, they can have significant input into the
design of secondary prevention programs. With respect to a major emphasis
on prevention in the Forward Plan for Health, and with particular awareness
of those major sources of illness that appear to be influenced by life-styles
and health-related behaviors, it will behoove psychologists who wish to expand their contributions to the nation's health care system to be particularly
alert to opportunities for preventive intervention (U.S. Department of
Health, Education, and Welfare, 1976).

In preventive programs, the insights of the clinical psychologist, especially with respect to hidden motivation, can contribute to the expertise of
the educational psychologist in the design of programs that have optimal appeal and elicit responsive motivation (Evans and others, 1970). The individual's activities are a function of information (understanding), motivation,
risk-taking stance, and attitudes. These factors are viewed in the context of
models that must provide both for the relationship of life events (situations)
to illness susceptibility (Cobb, 1974) and for the individual's "cost-benefit"
perspectives (Becker and Maiman, 1975; Gochman, 1971; Rosenstock,
1966).

Particular expertise in psychotherapy has broad relevance to a role
either as consultant or as a primary therapist in the management of behaviors
related to health and illness. For the individual who is physically ill, the clinical psychologist can intervene directly to alter those emotional responses
that significantly compound the illness or detract from the patient's motivation to cooperate in his or her treatment and to get well. This may entail
psychotherapy to reduce anxiety or alter attitudes (Gruen, 1975; Leon,
1976; Olbrisch, 1977). In general, a psychologist performing this function

will require skill in brief therapy, which utilizes major elements of suggestion and persuasion in a broadly rational-emotive context. Where concrete behavioral patterns are involved, the psychologist may be called upon to design a contingency program to shape the patient's behavior. Systemic desensitization, hypnosis, conditioning, and the general techniques of behavior modification may also be used (Kristt and Engel, 1975; Price, 1974; Wright, 1976).

Intervention activities of the clinical psychologist with the medical patient are likely to focus on problems of motivation (depression), of cognitive difficulties in learning self-treatment techniques (colostomy care in patients of borderline intelligence), anxiety reduction (phobias in preoperative patients; Lloyd and Deakin, 1975), attitude (patients who reject prostheses: Weiss, Fishman, and Krause, 1970), and teaching techniques of tension reduction (hypertension: Stone and DeLeo, 1976). For the most part, the psychologist must effect a therapy program within a brief time span, limited by the urgency of the clinical condition, the brevity of hospitalization, or the limited access of the patient for outpatient consultation. Within those constraints, nearly all of the psychologist's techniques of intervention will be differentially applicable, depending on the nature of the problem. Because of those constraints, only long-term, insight-oriented, or dynamic therapy will be generally inappropriate in contributing to the overall management of the acutely ill medical patient. However, psychotherapeutic efforts to assist the patient toward more healthful behavior patterns, a change in values, and a new perspective on goals (as for the cardiac patient) may require a moderately extended course of counseling after the acute phase of medical intervention has restored physiological balance (Rahe and others, 1975).

While significant elements of personality aberration or emotional hyperreactivity may occupy a prominent role in a patient's illness and adjustment to it, it is usually not the case that the patient presents a full-blown psychiatric syndrome or a need for psychiatric intervention. The psychiatrist can, in some instances, provide valuable consultation regarding the use of ataractic medication to ameliorate anxiety or depression and enhance the patient's accessibility to psychological approaches to psychological problems. Since psychotherapy is generally associated with severe neurotic and characterological disturbances, it is probably wiser to think of the psychologist's role in direct intervention in terms of counseling rather than psychotherapy (Hodges, 1977; see also Chapter Eighteen in this volume). The psychologist can help medical colleagues to develop mutually acceptable modes for achieving the successful referral of the patient for such counseling. For example, following informal contact or a more formal consultation, the psychologist might encourage the physician to make use, either routinely or selectively, of an appropriate questionnaire to screen new patients for the presence of psychological disturbance. An instrument such as the MMPI has generally good acceptance in the offices of physicians because it includes, in addition to more "psychological" items, a large number of inquiries about physical symptoms and complaints. The psychologist can help the physician in developing an approach to interpreting the questionnaire results to the patient, using the findings as a bridge to the suggestion of a referral for psychological counseling. An advantage of this procedure is that it provides the psychologist with some initial diagnostic information which, together with the physician's statement as to the patient's medical problem, enables the psychologist to get under way more quickly with psychological counseling.

Strategies of Involvement

The psychologist working as a clinician in a medical setting needs to be aware of the full range of opportunities for contribution to the general goal of the health care system—that is, the efficient treatment of ailments, the prevention of recurrences, and the encouragement of health-maintaining behaviors. In contributing to these goals, the clinical psychologist, in some instances, can contribute most effectively through a one-to-one contact with the patient—for example, establishing and maintaining an appropriate set of eating behaviors in the diabetic (Cohen, 1976). In other instances (for example, assuring proper administration of antibiotics in childhood infections), it may be more effective for the psychologist to provide advice and management programs to the mother (Becker, Drachman, and Kirscht, 1972b). In still other cases, where there is a long-standing and close relationship with the patient, the physician may be able to utilize the psychologist as a consultant in preparing to deal directly with the patient's psychological problem (for example, in achieving successful referral to a therapy group such as Alcoholics Anonymous).

Whether attention to the patient's psychological needs will be provided best by emotional support and counsel by the physician or by referral to a psychologist will depend on: the nature of those needs; the interest, inclination, and skills of the physician; and the particular skills of the psychologist (for example, in biofeedback techniques, marriage counseling, brief psychotherapy, and so forth). With the developing residency programs in family practice and the expanding role of primary care physicians (and the contributions of psychologists to the related training programs!), it is to be hoped that there will be an increasing number of physicians who have both a willingness to attend to the emotional-situational problems of their patients and a sensitive awareness of the need for and timing of psychological consultation (Hodges, 1977; Pope and Lisansky, 1969).

In a proper consultative relationship, the physician will not "dump" the patient, and the psychologist will not "kidnap" the patient. In good referral practice, the professional participants maintain focus on the ongoing total status of the patient. Good professional relationships and appropriate referrals are fostered when the psychologist keeps the referring physician informed of the patient's progress and sees to it that the patient maintains contact with the physician as indicated by the medical problem.

While important contributions can be made in these ways to the provision of comprehensive health care for the individual patient, overall impact is enhanced when the psychologist takes advantage of opportunities, formal (in-service training seminars) or informal (at coffee breaks and over the lunch table), to discuss the impact of psychosocial variables on susceptibility to physical illness and their role in the patient's mode of coping with illness. A prime example is the development of programs to change the medication-dependent and socially constricted behaviors of patients whose pain has not been responsive to the usual medical anodynes. Psychologists play crucial roles in such programs as the designers of individualized programs for the gradual freeing of the patient's behavior from the demand characteristics of his or her pain (Fordyce, 1976).

Clinical psychologists have expertise in the design of behaviorally oriented programs to enhance health maintenance behaviors (weight control) or to extinguish health-threatening behaviors (smoking). Moreover, their education and basic orientation toward measurement of psychological variables equip them to be the professionals who are both skilled and motivated to evaluate the effectiveness of such programs in many health care settings (Hunt and Matarazzo, 1973; Leon and Roth, 1977; see also Chapter Six in this volume). Working in collaboration with other health professionals and statisticians, clinical psychologists have played a prominent role in developing techniques that are designed to yield objective, replicable outcome measures tailored to the goals of particular programs of health services (Hodgkin and others, 1975; Kiresuk and Sherman, 1968; Linn and Linn, 1975).

In a broader way, the psychologist has opportunities to influence the quality of medical service as a teacher to undergraduate medical students. Recent years have witnessed a general increase in provision in the undergraduate medical curriculum of courses in behavioral science, social science, and "psychological medicine." In general, these courses, while highly varied in content and emphasis, share the common goal of seeking to influence the future physician to be person-oriented—to be sensitive to the total environmental, social, and psychological situation in which the patient's complaint has arisen. They are an attempt to balance the exclusive organ pathology focus of the older generation of physician and the impersonal orientation of the medical specialist. Psychologists can play key roles in these courses which afford them a forum for educating physicians as to the role of the psyche in total health.

The summative impact of traditional medical education, with its necessary focus on physical disease and pathology of cells and organs, heads the medical students toward a practice embedded in the ubiquitous dualism of the Dark Ages. The problem for the medical student is to keep an *organism* orientation while studying organs. The physician must acquire constant awareness that the patient with pathology in any of his or her bodily functions is a *person* who is *dis-eased*. In his lectures while Regents' Professor Emeritus of Philosophy at the University of Minnesota, Herbert Feigl stated the general problem succinctly when he cautioned that we must avoid entrapment by either the seductive fallacies of "either-or" or the reductive fallacies of "nothing but" arguments.

Professional Problems of the Psychologist in Medical Settings

As indicated earlier, clinical psychology as a field of applied professional psychology was created in the years immediately after World War II in response to social need. In the beginning, it was designed exclusively as a mental health profession and its members were expected to be employed primarily in mental health clinics and psychiatric hospitals where they would contribute chiefly as diagnosticians and researchers. The very nature of their graduate study (personality, learning theory, and the like), however, prepared them also to become psychotherapists. The seeking of roles as therapists brought clinical psychologists into direct competition with and resistance from organized psychiatry. For some years, the two professions were engaged in more or less continuous debate, with clinical psychology seeking to establish itself as an independent mental health profession and psychiatry seeking to restrict psychology to an ancillary paraprofession whose members should be allowed to function as therapists only under medical supervision (Grinker and others, 1971).

Part of the early strife between clinical psychology and psychiatry, and part of the frustrations experienced in the treatment of mental illness, gave rise to a rejection of the diagnostic function as part of the equally rejected "medical model" of mental illness. Quasi-logical exhortation against the so-called medical model generated a philosophical antipathy to medicine and to physicians which still affects a number of psychologists (Balance, Hirschfield, and Bringman, 1970). With this attitudinal set, with their legitimacy as independent practitioners of psychotherapy established, and with their limited exposure during training to general medical problems, clinical psychologists have rarely, until very recently, developed roles in nonpsychiatric medical settings.

The controversy over psychotherapy has been resolved in large measure by social developments. At present, all fifty states have statutory legislation that recognizes the practice of psychology as a legitimate, independent health profession. The state licensing laws generally recognize the practice of psychotherapy to be a legitimate aspect of psychological practice. With gradual increase in the number of states that certify or license psychologists, the major underwriters of comprehensive health insurance have become increasingly more willing to provide for the reimbursement of psychological services, especially if these services are prescribed by a physician. A growing number of states have passed "freedom of choice" legislation which eliminates the previous requirement of a medical referral in order for the patient to have psychological services reimbursed. With statutory regulation by all states, with the provision of specialty, postgraduate examination by the American Board of Professional Psychology (1974), and with the publication of the *National Register of Health Service Providers in Psychology* (1976), clinical psychology has been firmly established as one of the health care professions (Schofield, 1975).

New opportunities and new settings in which clinical psychologists can contribute their skills and knowledge toward a truly comprehensive medicine (Schofield, 1976) are taking shape. Because residents training in primary care and family practice are being exposed to the techniques and expertise of the psychologist, especially in the evaluation of emotional components of illness, it is expected that these future practitioners will be more ready to turn to the psychologist for consultation. Growing national concern for improved delivery of health services has led to the emergence of family practice and the concept of the primary care physician (community medicine) as a medical specialty and to federal support for the establishment of Health Maintenance Organizations.

Medical psychology, viewed as the extension of clinical psychology into the arena of physical health and illness, is in its infancy. Its visibility is presently limited. Physicians who are generally aware of the clinical signs that justify a psychiatric consultation are not yet aware, in general, of the applicable skills of the psychologist. Development of such awareness is impeded because, as yet, there are only a small number of psychologists who have been drawn to the general medical setting. Those who have developed an abiding interest have usually found their introduction through a chance consultation or through a research interest (especially of psychophysiological nature) into a topic with medical import. A research interest may lead to consultation on clinical problems, or a clinical consultation may stimulate a research program.

The recognition of the clinical psychologist as a health professional in a broad sense has been delayed partly because of cultural lag. Most senior physicians, to the extent that they have any awareness of the field of clinical psychology, perceive it as a specialty closely identified with psychiatry. If they are aware of those clinical psychologists who are in independent practice, they are likely to view them as primarily "junior psychiatrists" who specialize in intensive psychotherapy of mental patients. This view is encouraged by those psychologists whose appointments in hospitals and clinics are usually as members of a psychiatric staff. If the psychiatric service is in a general medical setting, the psychologist has the opportunity to become acquainted with a range of medical specialists and to learn informally of recurrent psychological (nonpsychiatric) problems in specific medical clinics or wards. A diplomatic expression of interest and tentative suggestions of possible psychological interventions or programs are likely to be well received.

If there is to be sound growth in the new specialty of medical psychology, there must be provision for innovations in the standard graduate training for clinical psychologists. "While much of the current training of the scientist-practitioner clinician is appropriate, the education of the health psychologist will require greater emphasis on the biological sciences, on public health, and health administration. The pattern of internship training must be different, with deemphasis of psychiatric services and greater time spent in medical, pediatric, and surgical clinics. Of prime importance will be the interns' introduction to the special problems and methodologies for research in the area of health" (Schofield, 1976).

A positive development in the training of psychologists for work in general medical settings may be seen in the increasing number of psychology doctorates offered by medical schools and university health centers. As of 1977, there were nine such programs, with an additional thirteen in various stages of development (L. Cohen, 1977). Five of the established doctoral programs and six of the thirteen being planned are clinically oriented and designed to train psychologists for work in medical settings.

Research Frontiers

Just as psychology's role in research in the field of mental health and illness has been consistently recognized and supported, the research potential for psychology in the domain of physical health and illness will be readily recognized as more and more psychologists are drawn to this arena by an awareness of rich research opportunity (Kahana, 1972). The behavior of the individual plays a contributing role in susceptibility to a variety of illnesses (Garrity, Somes, and Marx, 1977; Jenkins, 1972); response to illness is not only biological but also includes psychological and behavioral elements; accessibility to medical counsel and therapeutics and the quality of the patient's role in the sought-for "therapeutic alliance" are heavily influenced by psychological elements (Becker, Drachman, and Kirscht, 1972b; Greenberg and others, 1975); and the patient's adaptation to serious limitation in physical capacity or to life-threatening or terminal illness is clearly as much a function of personality as of medical status (Moos, 1977a). The behavior of the ill person is a function of the same complex of psychological variables that motivates and directs the behavior of the well person. This means that there are few, if any, branches of psychological science that do not have potential application in working toward a better understanding (research) and more effective management (intervention) of physical illness. An example of basic research is study of the elements that determine successful communication (reception and retention by the patients) of medical information (Ley, 1972a, 1972b). The clinic and hospital provide special field-type laboratories for the study of adaptive (or nonadaptive) behaviors and for real-life investigations of attitudes and affect, frustration tolerance and cognitive functioning under stress, personality correlates (for example, inner versus outer control orientation), resistance to or compliance with a therapeutic regimen, and motivational elements of injurious behaviors.

Most of the specialty fields of psychology hold the possibility of contribution to an increased understanding of those behavioral, affective, and cognitive variables that are determining influences in susceptibility to physical illness, adaptation to illness, and cooperation with or resistance to corrective or prophylactic programs (American Psychological Association, 1976). By virtue of historical evolution as the first field of applied psychology to make significant impact on a major health area—that of mental health—and by virtue of its established role as a health profession in clinics and hospitals, clinical psychology is in a preeminent position to break new ground, to extend the application of psychological science and technology to the area of physical illness, and to lead the way in bringing other fields of psychology into the health care enterprise.

What are the predominant patterns of individual psychology (predisposing and reactive) associated with specific physical illnesses? Which are the most effective and efficient methods for the detection of significant psychological complications of physical illness? What modes of intervention are most effective for alleviating the emotional upheaval associated with acute physical illness? What are the psychological variables that optimize or reduce the effectiveness of medication? What psychological characteristics identify the patient with special susceptibility to side effects of drugs? Which patients are able most readily to learn biofeedback mechanisms in gaining control of symptoms?

These questions illustrate something of the range of possibilities for the application of psychological principles and methods in research to improve the treatment and recovery of medical patients. Support for research on the behavioral dimensions of major health problems has been increasing. In particular, various federal agencies are funding the work of behavioral scientists in exploring the psychological precursors and consequences of acute and chronic illness. These include the National Heart, Lung, and Blood Institute, National Institute of Dental Research, National Institute of Neurological Diseases, National Cancer Institute, National Institute of General Medical Sciences, National Institute of Alcohol Abuse and Alcoholism, and National Institute of Occupational Safety and Health (American Psychological Association, 1974b).

As indicated earlier, with modest modifications in the core graduate curriculum and an internship planned to provide exposure to a variety of medical settings and problems, the clinical psychologist can be prepared for a career in health care psychology (University of Minnesota, 1975). Funding agencies, especially those of the federal government, provide support for graduate training in the behavioral aspects of medical illness and care ("Guidelines," 1977). Medical students and graduate physicians in the medical specialties (especially pediatrics, neurology, and family practice) are being increasingly exposed to demonstrations of the relevance of psychological science and its methods for the maintenance of health and the treatment of illness. It is a reasonable expectation that in the not too distant future every major health care agency (hospital, extended care facility, or clinic) will include a health care psychologist on its resident or consultant staff and that this psychologist will be appropriately prepared by education, training, and experience to provide clinical, consultative, and research skills to the care of its patients.

18

Counseling Psychology, Interpersonal Skills, and Health Care

Norman Kagan

Counseling psychology grew out of a need to meet the mental health needs of those who are ambulatory but want to function better—people who know they could work more effectively, love more fully, and feel healthier and happier. Counseling psychologists share with psychology's other disciplines a generic core of knowledge and skill, but counseling psychology's unique mission is mass application. The counselor seeks an efficient balance between offering trace amounts of help to an overwhelming number of people, and the opposite extreme, giving massive doses of attention to a select few. In many ways, counselors are mental health's primary care workers, broadly skilled generalists. They work as vocational specialists and personal counselors in a wide variety of settings: community agencies, primary and secondary schools and colleges, and private practice. Most doctoral programs in counseling psychology follow guidelines established by the American Psychological Association and include supervised practicum, internship, field and laboratory training, and instruction in scientific and professional ethics and standards, research design and methodology, statistics and psychometrics, as well as core training in such substantive content areas as biological, social, and cognitive-affective bases of behavior. In addition, counseling psychologists receive didactic and experiential training specifically geared toward preparing them to influence large numbers of adequately functioning people. Many programs offer courses in improving skills in interpersonal relationships and learning to teach such skills to others. Self-study and self-improvement techniques are included in many programs (Fretz, 1977).

Counseling psychologists' particular training qualifies them to fill a need in an area traditionally independent of psychology—the field of medical health care. To understand the role of counseling psychology in health care, it is necessary to look at its development and potential and at the health care system's growing need for outside assistance. After examining the history of the union between counseling psychology and health care, I will offer a model for the introduction of counseling skills into the health care fields. The specific issue of counselor involvement in areas such as health care has been the subject of my own research for the past fifteen years, and the model, called Interpersonal Process Recall, is the product of that research. This chapter, then, will contain my own point of view, rather than an objective survey of the field.

History of Counseling Psychology

The history of counseling psychology has been an odyssey in search of theories and methods that would offer optimum personal enhancement to the greatest number of people. In the earliest years of the counseling movement, around the turn of the century, counselors concerned themselves exclusively with finding jobs for people. Burgeoning immigration aggravated a chaotic urbanization, creating demand for professional efforts to provide occupational information. Guidance workers combined basic trait and factor theory with test administration and interpretation (which was given impetus by the Army's testing programs during World War I). Along with a little common sense, this training served the counselor sufficiently for working in a job-placement capacity (Super, 1955b).

As mass education was forced upon schools, and educators were frustrated by academically disadvantaged youth, schools began employing counselors to develop guidance programs. The new emphasis was on steering clients into appropriate educational and training programs. Counselors became the champions of individual development and student need. They helped translate between teacher and student, often walking a tightwire between teacher demand that students "adjust" and student demands that they be allowed to grow and actualize. As the complexities of vocational planning and career development became evident, vocational development theorists emerged within the movement. Some derived their ideas from psychoanalytic concepts, others from self-concept, trait and factor, and behavioral theories (Aubrey, 1977).

Personality traits, self-concept, and underlying, often nebulous motivations confounded what had been seen as a simple process of matching people and work. To make an occupational choice, much less plan a career, clients needed to "think clearly" and appraise themselves "realistically." Job success was discovered to be only partially attributable to aptitude and interest; the ability to get along with co-workers was found to be another essential ingredient (Hoppock, 1957). Vocational counseling therefore had to be expanded to include "personal" counseling. Interested counselors found a great client demand for group and individual counseling; participants wished to improve their interpersonal behavior first as an adjunct to vocational counseling and then as a worthwhile activity in its own right. An increasingly affluent society helped stimulate the shift in emphasis from occupational to interpersonal counseling; employment became less of a concern to people than improving the quality of their lives.

In seeking the new skills required to do personal counseling, guidance workers were confronted by a body of research and theory that had most often grown out of work with severely troubled client populations. Freudian, Adlerian, and Sullivanian concepts and techniques were incorporated, sometimes haphazardly, in the counseling psychologist's repertoire. Fragments were extracted that seemed applicable to large numbers of clients and were used in an eclectic, intuitively integrated fashion. Ultimately, counseling psychologists developed better integrated theories and created new technologies. Williamson (1965) formulated a logical system designed to help clients with educational, social, and occupational decision making and problem solving. Because the model described an active, trait-and-factor-based role for the counselor, it came to be known as the "directive" approach (Stefflre, 1965). Rogers' (1942) early work advocated a client-centered process in which clients were helped to verbalize their perceptions and come to know themselves in greater depth. The early model was usually referred to as the "nondirective" approach. Rogers' later work led to the definition of qualities that were found to characterize effective therapists. These so-called core conditions included empathy for the client, unconditional positive regard for the client, and congruence with oneself (Rogers, 1957). Truax and Carkhuff developed scales that raters could reliably use to evaluate counselors on the presence or absence of these core conditions. The next logical step was to determine if neophytes could be trained to exhibit the core conditions. Research findings indicated that they could, and the interpersonal skills or "empathy training" movement began (Carkhuff, 1969). Interpersonal skills originally referred to those specific behaviors identified by Rogers. Ivey (Ivey and Authier, 1978) later identified other basic skills that were derived from studies of effective therapists. Ivey's skills included such specific behaviors as eye contact, paraphrasing, and verbal following. Using videotapes to enable students to compare their efforts to emulate the behaviors, Ivey found that the skills he had defined could reliably be taught to neophytes in relatively few hours. About the same time, Kagan, Krathwohl, and Miller (1963) developed a technology for students to study their own behavior in ways that reliably resulted in improved interpersonal skills. Kagan's approach is based on the assumption that major process dynamics are involved in interpersonal skills, including communicating one's involvement and interest as well as using the ongoing process as content (this model will be elaborated on later in the chapter). The Gestalt and other encounter approaches to problem solving also had an impact on counseling psychology (Zimpfer, 1976). Behavioral counseling programs and texts are the most recent systems to have an impact on the field of counseling psychology (Krumboltz, 1966). Film and videotape materials, along with student and instructor manuals, have been produced to facilitate the teaching of the basic skills of these various models (Brammer, 1973).

By the early 1960s, counseling psychology had become a recognized discipline. When the USSR leaped ahead in space exploration, the United States, as part of a national response, spent millions of dollars developing counseling and guidance programs with the aim of maximizing the identification and deployment of talented youth. In a time of epidemic drug abuse, counselors were again called upon to help meet the crisis. As the medical profession becomes increasingly interested in patient counseling and patient education, counselor educators and counseling psychologists are often turned to for instruction and consultation.

Today the demand for services of counseling psychologists is greater than ever. So-called normal people are no longer content to seek help only for vocational uncertainties and emotional crises, or when their sexual interest or functioning wanes. The mass media have been a powerful force for enlightenment, as has economic prosperity. People do not wait until their marriages and careers are a shambles to seek professional help. They want prevention and enrichment. They want to possess the interpersonal skills necessary to anticipate and deal with the major events of living. They want to maintain and repair their own human relations when they do not run well. People have begun to turn to each other. They have discovered, at last, that one human being is the most perfect, most complete source of sensory stimulation for another human being. But people have also begun to realize how woefully unprepared they are to interact meaningfully. We have been taught to fear intimacy. Although people do not express the fear explicitly, they know that they want more from human relations than "normal" development in our society has prepared them for. This need has resulted in new demands for special psychological services which counselors were eager to provide alone or as part of an interdisciplinary effort, or to teach to other professionals. For instance, counselors are now employed to work on health teams with other professionals and to teach counseling courses in medical, law, and nursing school programs. Family counseling is now a routine part of termination of long-term hospital care or prison confinement in some communities.

Increasing demand necessitated the incorporation of extant psychological knowledge into the counseling profession. The need for new techniques and knowledge to help people achieve improved interpersonal relations led counselors increasingly to identify themselves with psychology in general and with either the research, academic, or practitioner model in the psychology profession. Because counseling psychology is devoted to helping that great mass of people who are not ordinarily considered chronically disturbed, counseling has many of the same characteristics as general practice or primary care in medicine and dentistry. From the perspective of primary care, certain theoretical positions proved especially attractive to counseling psychologists.

Probably the single most important contribution to the development of counseling theory came from the works of Carl Rogers and his colleagues (Rogers, 1942, 1951, 1957). Rogers' attempt to identify the core qualities of effective therapeutic relationship led to a simplification and demystification of the therapeutic process. The "client-centered" approach afforded consistent theoretical constructs and therapeutic techniques that emphasized client self-determination and growth rather than personality change or treatment and so seemed to speak more directly to the needs of the clientele served by counseling psychologists. Moreover, the techniques appeared able to be mastered with far less training than that required to learn other models such as psychoanalytic theories and methods. This was an important attribute from the perspective of primary care workers who need to be proficient in so many areas that they are eager consumers of models and techniques that appear to promise quick mastery. But Rogers' greatest contribution to the mental health profession was neither his "streamlined, uncluttered" theories nor his "demystification" of the counseling process. Rather, it was that his work stimulated a whole generation of research and evaluation in mental health. From the beginning of his client-centered movement, Rogers made extensive use of audio recordings and independent raters. His early use of Q-sort methodology to evaluate changes in self-concept resulted directly in such major breakthroughs as the discovery that there were specific teachable behaviors that differentiated effective psychotherapists from similarly educated ineffective ones. The skills of the effective counselor, however artistic, are no longer seen as outside the possibility of analysis, identification, and communication to others (Carkhuff, 1969; Danish and Hauer, 1973; Ivey and Authier, 1978; Kagan, 1973).

Behavioral approaches to counseling derived from operant conditioning and social-learning theories were also well received by a sizable portion of the counseling force. These "nothing-but" theories and skills, like the early work of Rogers, were especially attractive at least in part because they appeared to be quickly learned approaches to influencing human behavior. The peak of the behavioral influence came in the late sixties and early seventies (Krumboltz, 1966; Thoresen and Mahoney, 1974; Wolpe and Lazarus, 1966). In the final analysis, behaviorism's major contribution to counseling is probably its impact on traditional analytic and humanistic approaches. Behaviorism challenged those of us who are committed to a dynamic view of human behavior, who perceive behavior as part of a complex interpersonal and intrapersonal process. It compelled us to define our terms, further demystify our art, conduct more controlled studies, evaluate our training procedures, and determine precisely the nature of the effects of our interventions on client populations (Archer and Kagan, 1973).

The pressure caused by behaviorism's popularity, combined with the model presented by Rogers and the accessibility of modern educational technologies, has resulted in the formulation of techniques for the efficient instruction of larger numbers of mental health workers than was conceived of twenty years ago. Clearly delineated instructional methods and materials have simplified the task of the instructor and have increased the percentage of effective counselors in each graduating class. The methods that have proved effective in the education of professional counselors have also been applied to paraprofessionals with equal success. Our progress during the past ten to fifteen years has made it feasible to "give psychology away"—to teach basic human interaction and counseling skills to paraprofessional peer counselors on college campuses, to community volunteers in crisis centers, and directly to client populations such as prison inmates. The development of efficient methods has offered greatly expanded opportunities to provide skills to groups that have long been interested. Teachers, supervisors, nurses, dentists, and physicians all can be provided with skills at influencing human interaction within a minimum amount of time, usually no more than fifty or sixty total hours of commitment to training.

Counseling Skills for Health Care Professionals

Physicians and medical educators want more from psychology than lectures on psychosomatic illness or brief courses in developmental and abnormal psychology. They want to learn to relate to patients more effectively. Although counseling psychology has much to offer other professions in the area of vocational and educational counseling, it is the teaching of interpersonal skills that has been of greatest interest to the health care professions. Why are health care providers now so interested in learning the basic interpersonal skills of the counseling psychologist? The reasons are central to the traditional practice of good medicine (Engel, 1973, 1977). First, physicians are beginning to realize that because of poor interviewing skills they often miss receiving information from a patient that could alter their diagnosis. That is, physicians' inability to communicate may keep vital information from them. The most important information needed for an accurate diagnosis is often that which the patient has and needs to report to the doctor, such as an accurate history of the illness, current and previous emotional stress, history of medication, additional symptoms, and successful and unsuccessful prior treatments. Second, patients are often frightened of physicians, who are seen as holding the power to cure or not, to prescribe painful treatments, or even to pronounce the patient incurably ill. Patients are frequently ashamed of their illness and embarrassed by the medical examination. Patients are in a vulnerable position and are easily intimidated and frightened. Physicians want to learn counseling skills so that they do not inadvertently exacerbate the patient's illness, adding stress by their own statements and manner. Third, physicians want to learn to relate to patients in such a way as to invite cooperation, so that the patients will follow treatment plans effectively and reliably, something they often fail to do at present. In addition, physicians want to be able to reduce the likelihood that patients will become so suspicious and hostile that they seek every opportunity to bring legal suit against their doctor. Finally, physicians want to improve relations with their colleagues in order to enjoy their practice, so that their own professional lives will be both effective and satisfying.

Ever increasing numbers of physicians, medical students, and medical educators want more than these minimum goals. More and more, patient education and patient counseling are seen as basic parts of medical treatment (Stephens, 1978). For some time, science watchers and medical ecological researchers have told us that there are years of life to be gained for patients by helping them not to smoke, drink excessively, overeat, or create life-styles in which they are under constant emotional stress. Increasingly, physicians see as a central part of their medical treatment helping patients to understand their bodies, any chronic medical conditions they may have, and the importance of a balanced diet, exercise, and the elimination of destructive behaviors and habits (Engel, 1973, 1977). Physicians want to enable patients to discuss concerns about their health, misinformation they harbor, and shame they may feel about their body image and function—problems the physician could help alleviate. Recent writings about death and dying indicate another area in which physicians can and want to have an important role in alleviating unnecessary pain (Simon and Paredes, 1977).

There are physicians who are very much concerned by the startling statistics on physician longevity, alcoholism, drug abuse, and suicide rate (Bowden and Burstein, 1974; see also Chapter Sixteen in this volume). Many physicians, medical students, and medical educators want to understand their own interpersonal and intrapersonal functioning, to establish support groups in their work so they are less lonely as professionals and have an opportunity to "let off steam" and help each other with stresses in their own lives.

The patient too is interested in change. The consumer rights movement has stimulated patients' interest in becoming more equal participants in all phases of their own health care. People are less and less willing to be passive recipients of an all-powerful health care system. They insist upon being involved in the major decisions affecting their lives. This patient demand should be viewed as a positive force by the medical profession because it could facilitate effective health care delivery.

One of the ways the health care system has responded to these recent interests is to involve social workers and clinical and counseling psychologists in patient care. Counseling psychologists have been employed by hospitals and medical groups to provide direct vocational, developmental, crisis, and rehabilitation counseling to patients as an adjunct to medical treatment. The health care system has also begun to seek ways of teaching physicians, nurses, and all others involved in health care to take an active role in patient counseling (Allen, 1977).

As the medical profession begins to examine environmental stress as a factor in causing disease, and recognizes patient counseling as an important function of the practicing physician, criteria for selecting medical students on the basis of ability for learning this role must be added to the other criteria that have traditionally been a part of the screening process. Counseling psychologists have been active in designing ways of reliably rating helper behavior in interviews (Carkhuff, 1969; Kagan, 1976a, 1976b). These techniques can be used to rate applicants. My colleagues and I (Campbell, Kagan, and Krathwohl, 1971; Danish and Kagan, 1971; Schneider, Werner, and Kagan, 1977) have developed objective, multiple-choice scales that purport to measure a person's sensitivity to the feelings of others. The same programs used to teach counseling skills to medical students and residents (Werner and Schneider, 1974) have been used to teach medical school admission committees to improve their interviewing skills and abilities to evaluate an applicant's interpersonal behavior.

Which Skills Are Useful to the Physician?

What do we mean by "interpersonal" or "counseling" skills? In what skills are health care providers really interested? Core conditions (Carkhuff, 1969) and basic helping and relating skills (Ivey and Authier, 1978) have already been mentioned. Danish and Hauer (1973) and Froelich and Bishop (1972) have also developed definitions and training manuals. Most writers have limited their definitions to specific behaviors that can be reliably measured and reliably taught. The finding that elements could be identified that were a part of the repertoire of effective therapists was a major breakthrough. Previously, it had been assumed that the art of the skillful therapist, much like the bedside manner of the trusted physician or the warmth and concern of the dedicated teacher, was a quality that one either had or developed slowly after years of experience. It was believed that such art could not possibly be learned in a training program. When it was established that some of these qualities could be taught to neophytes (Carkhuff, 1969), the necessary first step in developing technologies for reliably teaching interpersonal helping skills was achieved. But need we continue to limit ourselves to the most narrow of definitions for the sake of precise measurement and high replicability of training effects? Is it possible to expand the concept of interpersonal skills to include more of the qualities of effective therapists and yet not abandon the essential criterion that the skills be reliably teachable? My colleagues and I have devoted the past sixteen years to that task. In the pages that follow, I will present a brief history of the Interpersonal Process Recall methods and then the definition of interpersonal skills that grew out of our earlier experiences and determined the shape of the final model. The definition that emerged is elaborated under the headings of *response modes, knowing, patient feedback, understanding, the process as content,* and *continuing education and external review.* That section is followed by a description of how the IPR methods are then used to teach each of the major components included in the definition of interpersonal skills presented.

Introduction of a Counseling Model: Interpersonal Process Recall

For my colleagues and me, the past sixteen years have represented a concentrated effort to research and develop reliable, valid methods for teaching interpersonal skills to large numbers of people. The central and unique feature of the model we have developed is the recall process. A participant, let us use a physician for this example, interviews a patient, and the two are videorecorded or audiorecorded while they interact. Afterward, the physician reviews the tape with the help of a third person. We have labeled the task of the third person the "inquirer" role since that term seemed most reflective of the helper's attitude and approach in assisting with the recall.

In 1961 I discovered that viewing a videotape playback with the help of a probing, nonevaluative inquirer provided a powerful stimulus for self-examination and growth. The realization came quite serendipitously. A National Defense Education Act Guidance and Counseling Institute that I directed provided funds to bring distinguished psychologists, some of them my former professors, to campus. Michigan State University freely lent its professional videotape equipment to faculty members (a very uncommon provision at that time) and I used the opportunity to create a videotape library for future students of the presentations made by these visitors. Curious about videorecording, then a new process, the visitors and I would often go to the taping room to see a replay of the lecture. We were permitted to stop and start the equipment whenever we chose. The psychologists, fascinated by seeing themselves on tape, often stopped the playback to discuss reactions they had to their own images. I was shocked to hear them describe themselves in terms we had often used, as their students, in discussing them behind their backs. "I come across as a stuffed shirt, I'm talking down to the audience." As a beginning assistant professor, I could not criticize without appearing disrespectful. My only option was to inquire politely: "Do you think your audience saw you that way?" or "Do you recall what you were thinking at the time?" Recalling thoughts and feelings they had had during the lecture seemed even more productive than self-criticism. "I remember that there was some movement in the control room, I looked up and lost my place. I wanted it to appear that I was not relying on my notes as heavily as I was. All sorts of thoughts went through my head like 'Now everyone will know I'm not as competent as I appear to be.'" One early recall statement that impressed me with the potential power of the technique was: "Notice at that point I said 'now obviously.' That's the weakest part of my theory and what's going through my head is if I say 'obviously,' people won't challenge me." Since there was no way I could, as a new psychologist, critique, advise, or use any traditional supervisory approach, I found myself in the role of precocious listener and active inquirer. Under the conditions of immediate videotape playback and probes rather than interpretations, the guests often went on to say things that suggested they were studying themselves in depth and learning about themselves. Most of them later mentioned that the experience had been exciting and informative.

When we tested the process with professional psychologists and found that they too could learn rapidly during recall, critique themselves openly, and label many of the subtle messages they had perceived but not acknowledged during the interview, we realized we had, in fact, hit upon a strong technique for stimulating learning-by-discovery. We recognized that the inquirer role was central to the potency of the technique.

The inquirer does not critique or offer suggestions, nor does the inquirer encourage the person to engage in self-confrontation or self-critique; rather, the person is encouraged to use the video or audio playback as a stimulus for *memory*. The person is given control of the recorder and is asked to stop the playback whenever any underlying thought or feeling is recalled. Whenever the person stops the tape, the inquirer's role is to listen and to respond with noninterpretive probes. The inquirer assumes that the person knows better than anyone else the meaning the recorded experience had for that person, and the inquirer's task is to help elucidate those meanings. This assumption, based on experience with hundreds of recall sessions, is that people sense all manner of subtle meanings and underlying emotions in each other but usually acknowledge only a very limited range of what they actually perceive. The inquirer asks such questions as: "Can you tell me what you felt at that point? Can you recall more of the details of your feelings? Where did you feel those things? What parts of your body responded? What did you think the other thought? Felt? How had you hoped the other would respond? Were you thinking of saying anything which you then decided not to say? Did the age, sex, or physical appearance of the other affect you in any way? What did you think the other wanted from you? Were you aware of any risks to you or the other?" The list of possible inquirer leads can be quite extensive. They cover the inevitable or highly probable areas of content in human interactions. That is, when two people interact they are bound to have thoughts and feelings, impressions of the other, impressions they want the other to have of them, and so on. The inquirer asks the person to find words to make explicit the previously perceived, but not labeled, information.

Our initial use of the method to teach interpersonal skills to students proved to be a failure. The experimental group performed no better on final interviews and on measurement of affective sensitivity than did the control group that received traditional supervision (Kagan and Krathwohl, 1967). We had used a single format of the Interpersonal Process Recall (IPR) process. In our early experiments using each other as subjects, we found that client recall was a particularly exciting and informative experience. A colleague interviewed a client, the colleague then left, and the videotape recording of the interaction was reviewed by an inquirer. The colleague listened to the client's recall. What we failed to take into account was that this experience as the first and only application of IPR was too threatening for many neophytes. In retrospect, we realized that we were so enamored of the apparent potency of the techniques that we had failed to develop first a definition of interpersonal skills and then fashion learning experiences to accomplish the learning of those skills. We had used a technique without a theory and it simply did not work.

The history of the development of the definition that follows is beyond the scope of this chapter, but here is what we eventually concluded as our definition of interpersonal skills.

Response Modes

There are specific kinds of responses a physician may offer to statements by patients that will encourage them to elaborate upon their concerns. Certain ways of reacting demonstrate to patients that the doctor cares about their problems and is a trustworthy listener. Effective response modes promote honest communication of important medical information and of personal issues in the patient's life. There are numerous ways of conceptualizing response modes. My colleagues and I have identified four as a useful base for instruction:

1. *Exploratory responses* elicit further discussion of an issue. They are open-ended questions encouraging elaboration. For example, the question "Can you tell me more about that?" invites the patient to expand on the subject, whereas a true-false type question, such as "Did it come on slowly or suddenly?" limits the patient's answer to a single word or idea. The exploratory response also acts as an equalizer between doctor and patient; the patient is allowed to play an active role in the examination process.
2. *Listening responses* clarify and paraphrase. The physician communicates back to the patient an understanding of what the patient has said. Patients then can correct any misunderstandings and are aware that they have been heard. This mode may include the physician's admission of failing to hear or understand, of needing clarification. For example, "I'm sorry. I was thinking about something you mentioned earlier and missed what you just said. Could you repeat it?" A patient can see that this reflects a genuine effort on the physician's part to listen carefully and understand each point.
3. *Feeling responses* focus on the emotional tone, the physiological state, the general affect of the patient. They examine the mood behind the story, invite the patient to label feelings about the issue. For example, "As you think about your condition, what feelings come to you?" Often this involves the physician's offering perceptions about what the patient appears to be experiencing. For example, "You seem tense as you tell me this."
4. *Honest labeling* is a communicative behavior in which the physician re-

veals honest thoughts about the patient's behavior or attitude, ideas sometimes considered to be "better left unsaid." When the physician opens such ideas for discussion in a gentle, caring way, obstacles preventing a good doctor-patient relationship can often be removed. A doctor might say, for example, "I sense you have some doubts about my competence in the area of your illness." Or, "You say you're not concerned, but I notice you're very tense which makes me think you are, indeed, quite worried."

These skills, although complex, are easily identified and can be learned with just a few hours' practice (Spivack and Kagan, 1972). They are useful with individuals, families, or groups, and appear to be a small, but statistically significant, factor in relating effectively. People usually increase their scores after training (Boltuch, 1975; Spivack and Kagan, 1972; Werner and Schneider, 1974), and advanced graduate students score higher than beginners (Kagan and Krathwohl, 1967).

Interpersonal Allergies

In listening to a person's concerns, we react physiologically as well as emotionally and intellectually and exhibit nonverbal behaviors, usually without even being aware of them. In this way, a physician communicates the degree of willingness to relate to a patient's most intimate concerns. The physician brings to interaction a host of stereotypes and prejudices about age, sex, body size and shape, and even about "good" and "bad" defenses. Physicians must examine and understand their own unique "interpersonal allergies" and learn to overcome them in order to be genuinely open to the patient's concerns.

Knowing

Counseling skills should include theoretical constructs affording the physician a cognitive understanding of the *value* of exploring personal material and patient concerns. The physician needs a well-considered framework for understanding how patient counseling can accomplish important medical goals. For instance, he or she needs to understand the value to the patient of identifying and labeling previous unnamed doubts and feelings and the importance to the patient of knowing that the doctor is really listening and cares.

Self-Study

An important aspect of counseling skills is the ability to examine oneself and the part one plays in an interaction. Through self-exploration comes the possibility of clarifying one's own goals and confusion and improving behaviors in interaction. Training in counseling skills must therefore include the opportunity for "stepping outside oneself" during or after an interview and examining the session.

Patient Feedback

Another essential ingredient in effective doctor-patient counseling is the physician's ability to accept patient feedback, demonstrated by a willingness to learn from the patient's perceptions. This can occur through direct questions—"Did that make sense to you?" or "Do you think you'll really be able to follow this diet?"—or the invitation for feedback may be evident in the physician's manner and tone of voice. Interpersonal skills include *communicating* this interest in patient feedback.

Understanding

Physicians should be more than technicians at interpersonal skills; they need theoretical constructs for understanding how patients defend and distort as well as how they can improve their own interpersonal behavior. Although the physician need not become an expert on personality theory, without some additional cognitive framework for understanding ways in which patients have learned inappropriate and ineffective behaviors and beliefs, the physician's ability to help patients change may be limited. (This component of our definition of interpersonal skills may seem all too obvious to the reader, but, surprisingly, most definitions and the training programs derived from these definitions are typically atheoretical. Later in this chapter, the theoretical constructs taught in the IPR methods will be presented. What is important, however, is not *which* theories are taught but that *some* relevant theory is provided the student of interpersonal skills.)

The Process as Content

Interpersonal skills include the ability to use the interaction itself as content—that is, not only to recognize important messages communicated in the interaction between doctor and patient but also to discuss these observations directly with the patient. There is usually evidence of at least some of this behavior in the recordings of effective interviewers. Discussing these perceptions may range from the obvious—"I'm not sure you understood my question" or "I sense that my last comment troubles you"—to more subtle and complex themes—"As you tell me these things you seem to be concerned that I might misunderstand you" or "You seem to hope that somehow I'll be able to reassure you, to put your worries to rest."

Continuing Education and External Review

Interpersonal skills should also include seeking, giving, and learning from peer review and other ongoing procedures for improving the physician's interpersonal behaviors. A model could provide a natural avenue for such an ongoing appraisal if physicians come together to share recorded interactions with each other and with their patients.

The extent to which a physician chooses to serve as patient counselor will determine the degree of competence he or she needs to acquire in the foregoing interpersonal skills. After having defined these skills, my colleagues and I then spent several years investigating and developing methods. The final model proved reliable and valid. In comparison with students given equal hours of intensive traditional supervision, the students in the IPR groups scored higher on a scale of affective sensitivity, on judge evaluation of recorded interviews, and on evaluation by the client (Kagan and Krathwohl, 1967). In other studies, IPR training resulted in counselor changes that persisted over time (Boltuch, 1975) and had an impact on client level of self-exploration (Kingdon, 1975) and on student attitude toward teachers (Burke and Kagan, 1976).

Our approach is based on a strategy of counselor developmental tasks specific enough to enable the neophyte to grasp the concepts and understand the skills but not so limited as to be of questionable value in practice. No assumption is made about the student's previous experience or knowledge of personality theory. Thirty to fifty hours is an ideal training period, although statistically significant differences between the IPR model and traditional supervision have been obtained in as few as eight to ten hours. The entire program is packaged in eight hours of film which is coordinated with a program of instruction (Kagan, 1976a). I will present first an overview of our teaching model, followed by a detailed description of the ways in which each of the components of interpersonal skills is addressed.

The task sequence begins with a didactic presentation of concepts, followed by simulation exercises giving participants a chance to practice the skills presented. The next step in training involves viewing a series of filmed vignettes that are designed to elicit emotional reactions of various types. The experience of watching these films and sharing reactions with other group members serves both to help students explore their emotional reactions to different kinds of people and messages and as a warm-up to dealing in an introspective manner later in the training. It is useful, when possible, to make videorecordings and physiological reaction recordings of the participants as they view the films. Medical students are particularly interested in the physiological recordings of their reactions to interpersonal messages. Following the stimulus films is the study-of-self-in-action, in the form of IPR video playback. Next the student listens to patient feedback as the patient too goes through recall sessions. In these sessions, patients are either people who have chronic illnesses and have been willing to share their concerns with medical students or else they are the students themselves who have been asked to share a personal concern (preferably health related) with a fellow student. Finally, a block of time is devoted to getting an understanding of and skill at dealing with the complex interactions between patient and student. This is achieved through mutual recall sessions. In mutual recall, an inquirer asks student and patient to share recalled thoughts and feelings directly with each other. This mutual recall is the last stage of the learning process. Let us now consider, how these processes actually teach the component skills that were listed earlier in our definition.

Elements of Facilitating Communication

This first phase is designed to teach students the four specific response modes discussed earlier (exploratory, listening, feeling, and honest labeling). These are taught by means of a film presentation. The student watches vignettes of a patient (dramatization) making a statement and an interviewer responding to one facet of the statement. In the next vignette, the patient repeats the statement, but now the interviewer responds to the affective component. Several patient types and interviewer types are presented for each of the four sets of concepts. The film narrator points out that cognitive, nonexploratory, nonlistening, and avoiding response modes are usually used in social conversation, whereas these new response modes in the model are frequently adopted for counseling and therapeutic communication. Students practice the new modes by responding to filmed patients who "address them" with statements of varying complexity and intensity.

Overcoming Interpersonal Allergies

In the course of learning interpersonal skills, it is imperative that students learn to deal with those types of patient messages that they find especially threatening and difficult. To this end, affect simulation or "stimulus" vignettes were developed. The idea for such vignettes grew out of our experience conducting recall sessions with students and with experienced physicians and counselors (Danish and Brodsky, 1970; Kagan and Krathwohl, 1967; Kagan and Schauble, 1969). Time and time again we observed that people feared from each other behaviors which, in all likelihood, they would never encounter. Medical students often feared being discredited or even mocked by patients because of their youth and fallibility. Some older physicians feared being seduced, even when there was no reason to believe this would occur. The students' fears could be categorized under four general rubrics: (1) fear of facing the other's hostility—"If I drop my guard, if I get too close I'll get hurt." (2) fear of loss of control of their own aggressive impulses—"If I drop my guard I may hurt others." (3) fear that the other would become too intimate, too seductive—"If I'm not careful others will get too close, too intimate. They may engulf me." and (4) fear of their own potential for seductiveness—"If I don't protect myself from my own impulses, my need for affection, my sexual interest, I may engulf them."

We hoped to help people face these interpersonal fears by filming actors directly addressing the viewer and portraying one of the more universal nightmares. It seemed that it might even be possible to use such vignettes to help students discuss and understand their resistances to interpersonal involvement. A series of vignettes were created; the method worked. There are now more than seventy vignettes depicting numerous interpersonal concerns presented by people of different ages, sexes, and races. For example, an older woman looks directly at the student and says, "Oh, are you the doctor? You're so young. Could I see someone a little older?" Students are asked to imagine that the actor is talking privately to them. Then they are asked such questions as: "Did you have any feelings? What did you think? Has anything like that ever happened to you? Have you ever been concerned that something like that might happen to you? When people treat you that way how do you usually respond? How do you wish you could bring yourself to respond?" Students usually have no difficulty getting involved in the vignettes. Students share reactions in various formats: total class discussion, small group interaction, or working in pairs. In one format already mentioned, students are videorecorded as they watch the vignettes, while electrodes on the hand, chest, and around the waist record specific physiological parameters. The videotape is played back to the students so they can see what they looked like and what their heart rate, skin conductance, and other physiological processes had been as they viewed a particular vignette.

Knowing

The instructor presents a film dealing with the general nature of interpersonal fears associated with involvement and aloneness. The four basic fears of interpersonal involvement—"I will hurt you." "You will hurt me." "I will engulf you." "You will engulf me."—are presented as general statements of peoples' fears of each other. In general, when people become too involved for their own comfort level, they experience fear and anxiety. When they are too distant from human contact, they experience boredom, loneliness, and the pain of sensory deprivation. People establish a distance sufficient to receive some level of sensory stimulation from other human beings and yet feel safe. The more fully functioning people appear to be capable of both extreme intimacy and aloneness. Interpersonal flexibility is thus presented as a characteristic of more fully functioning people. These concepts were derived by my colleagues and me on the basis of speculations about the meaning of recall data gathered through the years.

Next the film defines the value of helping patients to verbalize their own experiences of interpersonal stress. "Finding labels, finding words for what had been vague thoughts, finding words for what had been pre-language feelings helps us know ourselves in language. We may be literally informing one part of the brain about the content of another . . . having a language, having words makes our fears more manageable, less frightening. It's almost as if the ferocious wolf, on close examination, is found to be very old and toothless" (Kagan, 1975). At several points, the narrator asks questions encouraging student discussion.

Self-Study

Next the student conducts an interview session with a person who seeks help. The person may be a fellow student, an actor, or a patient who has recently had extensive medical care. The interaction is recorded on videotape or audiotape. Immediately after the interview, the student is joined by a staff person or another student who has already been through the IPR course. The tape is reviewed with an emphasis on remembering and describing covert processes. The visual or audio playback is used to help the student remember goals, plans, assumptions, fears, and difficulties, as well as feelings of achievement and satisfaction. The student is encouraged through the playback and the inquirer's probing, nonjudgmental questions to verbalize moment-by-moment thoughts and feelings and to express things he or she was tempted to say during the interview but was afraid to try out. The recall thus provides an opportunity for students not only to come to know themselves better but also to experiment vicariously with new behaviors.

Accepting Patient Feedback

The next phase of the model requires that all students be taught the inquirer role. This is done through a series of exercises and film presentations. Once students have learned the inquirer role, they engage in exercises geared toward learning more about patient interviewing and counseling through a process called "patient recall." The instruction comes not from texts or lecture but directly from the patients themselves. Students pair up, and one of the pair conducts an interview. At the end of the session, the interviewer introduces the patient to his or her colleague, leaves the room, and the partner then conducts a recall session with the patient. Later the students reverse roles. Each student thus learns about the other's interactions. During class sessions, students are encouraged to share what they have learned about each other's patients. Patient recall sessions are not only informative but also give students practice at receiving direct patient feedback.

Understanding

At this point, the experiential learning is supplemented by filmed material describing interpersonal defense styles.

> The attitudes a person anticipates another person has about him or her are the most influential factors in determining how we will behave and our degree of interpersonal comfort. That is, we anticipate reactions by other people, and this fosters a self-fulfilling prophecy. . . . That is, we make our nightmares happen. We expect to be reacted to in certain ways and so we search for proof that indeed we are being reacted to in the ways we expected or feared. It's as if someone painted a picture and

then moved himself or herself in. The position we find ourselves in interpersonally is the position we have carefully maneuvered ourselves into, sometimes with much difficulty and cunning.

Are there an infinite number of ways in which we can respond to other people? Karen Horney suggested that there were only a limited number of basic possibilities. And I find that her idea is extremely useful and helps explain a lot of what we have seen in recall sessions. But we find we need to modify and expand her ideas quite a bit. Here's what I've observed (Kagan, 1975).

The film then proceeds to describe a typology based on interpersonal styles—*attack, withdraw,* and *conform.* The instructor encourages discussion of interpersonal effectiveness, again in terms of an expanded repertoire of ways of behaving. That is, the more fully functional people are conceptualized as those who are capable of a wide range of behaviors to meet their needs.

Learning to Use the Process as Content

We have found that students do not "naturally" discuss with a patient their mutual relationship. Even when given direct instruction in the skill, students seldom are able to use it. A learning experience was designed that has resulted in increased use of the process by medical students (Kagan and Krathwohl, 1967). In the last stage of the IPR Model, a student and a patient together review the videotape while a second student serves as inquirer. With the encouragement of the inquirer, the student and patient share feedback on how they interpreted each other's behaviors and what each had expected from the other. Such mutual recall sessions typically enable students to improve communication with patients about the here-and-now of their interaction. The immediacy of the feedback, the opportunity to test statements one had ruled out as too risky during the interaction, and the satisfaction of sharing thoughts and feelings with another person make the mutual recall sessions the most exciting part of the entire IPR course for most students.

Continuing Education and External Review

Throughout the IPR Model, students are actively involved in one another's instruction—reviewing tapes for one another rather than depending on the instructor to conduct all review sessions. The students thus have considerable experience at giving and receiving help from their colleagues. Not only does this make the model efficient, but also the peer-to-peer communication serves as preparation for future openness to exchanging help with professional colleagues.

In this way, the IPR Model that was originally designed to answer a critical need in counselor education also proved a useful tool for filling an important need in medical education. As mentioned before, the model just described is not the only one that has grown out of counseling psychology

(Carkhuff, 1969; Danish and Hauer, 1973; Ivey and Authier, 1978) but it is the one that has been most widely adopted in medical schools and medical residency programs. We have obtained data indicating that medical students learn to increase their affective sensitivity to others and improve their interviewing skills through the IPR Model in much the same way that counseling and psychology students do (Werner and Schneider, 1974). There are currently studies in progress to determine the long-term impact of IPR training on residents in medical specialties, including family practice and internal medicine. One study completed with Duke University's family practice residents indicated that the residents could learn and would then use interpersonal skills with patients after IPR training (Novik, 1978). A three-year evaluation is currently under way with residents in several specialty areas at the University of California at Los Angeles.

Opposition to the Teaching of Interpersonal Skills

Even though we have been successful in introducing IPR materials in more than forty programs in six different countries, we have encountered many medical settings in which the teaching of physician-counseling skills has not been welcomed. Our experience may offer some guidance in identifying some obstacles to successful introduction of such teaching and in meeting those obstacles. At this time, there has been no systematic study of the reasons. In some cases, there is a clear-cut healthy skepticism on the part of program directors: "Prove to me that this will make a difference over time and then I'll look into it." One can respond by pointing out that the data already available to support the teaching of interpersonal skills, some of which have been cited earlier in this chapter, are probably equal to the data supporting several of the other course offerings in medical and residency programs. Other arguments are more difficult to overcome. Physicians fear that if they open a Pandora's box full of patients' emotional stresses, they will be consumed by the huge amount of time required: "There isn't time in a busy physician's schedule to be a patient counselor." It is true that the physician who becomes interested in the emotional stresses of patients may want to spend more time talking with them. However, as my colleagues and I videotape actual medical interactions in private practice and clinical settings as a part of physician continuing education projects, we find that oftentimes physicians are already spending several minutes talking with patients about issues unrelated to medicine *or* counseling. Time is often spent on "pseudomedical" practice. By that unkind term I mean asking medical questions the physician knows are irrelevant to the patient's physical or emotional life or else going through a routine physical examination with the knowledge that nothing will be found. That is not to say that all physician questions or all routine physical examinations are irrelevant, but time and again we hear physicians on recall say: "I knew it was a waste of time but a good doctor is supposed to ask those questions" or "I knew I wouldn't see anything by looking into his throat, but I was concerned that he would feel he hadn't

gotten good medical treatment if I didn't do doctor-type things like that."
Ironically, patients rarely praised physicians for such behaviors during their
own recall sessions. Most often, when patients were very satisfied with their
medical session, we heard: "The doctor's great—I really felt *understood*." We
were surprised, in the course of conducting recall sessions with neurologists
known among their peers as outstanding diagnosticians, to find that even
these experienced specialists described much of their behavior as unnecessary
(Elstein and others, 1972). If physicians used their time more efficiently, if
they had the skills and were convinced of the legitimacy of using these skills,
could they deal with some of the more pressing issues influencing the patient's life within the realities of the average patient visit? When lengthier,
critical issues emerge, could physicians invite patients to return for another
interview and could a fee structure be established so that the physician's
time spent at additional counseling would be properly remunerated? These
are important questions to be researched.

Another issue is a concern of physicians that they are incapable of
psychotherapeutic influence on a patient without extensive training as
psychotherapists. The concern extends beyond the use by physicians of
psychotherapeutic techniques and applies to the broader issue of paraprofessional mental health workers as well. One might argue that the majority of
patients do not need, and would refuse, a referral for long-term psychotherapy and, since most function adequately and are reasonably productive, *any*
help they get with emotional stress is likely to be better than no help at all.
Another argument is that a physician has long-term contact with patients in
primary care and will have numerous opportunities to understand and have
an impact on the patient, probably at critical life stages when patients may
be especially receptive to help. From the other point of view, one might
argue that most people do not need extensive or esoteric *medical* procedures
either, when they see a physician, but only those who are very well trained
would know when such procedures are needed. Here too, the issues seem to
beg for research efforts.

However realistic the concerns about validity, time constraints, and
skill level, the physician has certain advantages which possibly could compensate for time and skill limitations. The physician comes closer to being a
powerful, omniscient figure than most other people in the patient's life. Consider the basic psychological tenet that low self-esteem and insecurity come,
at least in part, from messages we wanted but never got from our parents
when we were small children. No one now in our lives is as godlike as our
parents appeared to us when we were small. We are unable, in most cases, to
give ourselves the approval we need. In our minds, we are simply not as big
as our parents were. But the physician has immense power. A physician telling a patient that his or her body is perfectly adequate, or that sexual fantasies are not only normal but important, probably is more likely to be believed than any other person in the patient's life who offers similar messages.
Indeed, the physician's words, respect, and understanding probably have
more impact in the adult patient's life than would the words of the very

parents of those adult patients at present. It is my belief that physicians can have a major counseling impact on their patients within the time limitations of medical practice and the skill level which one could reasonably expect physicians to achieve, given their many other responsibilities.

Summary

Counseling psychologists define their mission as bringing the benefits of the mental health movement to the average person. To do so, they must find ways to improve people's ability to face the kinds of life stresses they probably would survive on their own, but often at great expense. Physicians too need to accomplish the same task with patients, and the methods developed for educating counseling psychologists are appropriate for improving physicians' interviewing and counseling skills. In addition, counseling psychologists serve as members of health teams and clinic staffs providing direct counseling help for patients individually, in groups, and in family units. Their increasing involvement has paralleled an increasing awareness on the part of the medical profession that environmental stress and interpersonal and intrapersonal behaviors pose medical problems that cannot be ignored by the health care system. Simultaneously, patient expectations of the health care system have changed from that of simply receiving treatment for disease to one of enhancement of their health.

Through medicine, counseling psychology has been able to further its professional objectives. For health care providers, an important void is filled. For patients, better medical care is available and health can come to mean more than merely the absence of disease.

19

Attribution, Control, and Decision Making: Social Psychology and Health Care

Irving L. Janis

Judith Rodin

Recent developments in theory and research in social psychology have an important bearing on health problems. This chapter focuses on four such developments pertaining to the causes and consequences of (1) attributions of causality for desirable and undesirable events; (2) perceived control versus helplessness; (3) social power of authority figures; and (4) commitment and adherence to difficult decisions. Each of the four topics has significant implications for the crucial problems of inducing people to make decisions that are conducive to good health and to adhere to difficult decisions that entail a temporary increase in deprivations or physical suffering.

These topics pertain equally to healthy and ill persons. However, we have sometimes given more focus to the patient because the patient role has often been defined as a passive one in middle-class America and Europe. Ill

persons are supposed to put themselves into the hands of medical authorities
and do whatever they say without complaining very much. But, in fact, patients are active decision makers. First they must decide whether to seek
medical treatment and from whom. Then they must decide whether to
accept the treatment the doctor recommends. After that, they must make a
series of decisions, sometimes every day, as to how conscientiously they are
going to follow all of the rules laid down for them in the recommended
medical regimen.

All four topics also bear on the closely related problems of inducing
healthy people to adhere to public health recommendations in order to prevent illnesses and injuries. As Dr. Robert R. Whalen, Commissioner of the
New York State Department of Health, points out: "Many of our most difficult contemporary health problems, such as cancer, heart disease, and accidental injury, have a built-in behavioral component: We eat, drink, worry
and smoke too much, and we drive too fast." He cites a long-term study
done in California that indicates that women and men at age forty-five have
an average life expectancy that is seven and eleven years longer respectively
if they follow six or seven of the following health practices (as compared
with those who follow fewer than four of these practices): "getting seven or
eight hours of sleep a night, eating breakfast, eating regularly and not between meals, keeping a normal weight in relation to height, refraining from
smoking, exercising regularly, and drinking moderately." Whalen concludes
that "unless we assume such individual and moral responsibility for our own
health, we will soon learn what a cruel and expensive hoax we have worked
upon ourselves through our belief that more money spent on health care is
the way to better health" (Whalen, 1977).

Each of the four topics also has something to say about how physicians, nurses, and other health care personnel might become more effective
in carrying out their primary tasks. At a more basic level, some of the topics
provide concepts to help explain how certain illnesses or unhealthy subclini-
cal conditions are mediated.

Attributing the Causes of Illness and Health

A person's health-seeking behavior is, to a great extent, based on his or
her *perception* of a bodily state, rather than on the body's true, physical
condition.* Several factors support this tendency. First, real feedback from
physiological processes is not monitored at the conscious level when everything is working smoothly (Rodin, 1978). Even when we do feel some physical perturbation or illness, we first try to interpret the events and information surrounding this condition in order to arrive at an appropriate
explanation for what we are feeling (Schachter and Singer, 1962). All such
attributions have the result of placing information in a cause-and-effect con-

*This section is based on an article by Judith Rodin, "Somatopsychics and Attri-
bution" (Rodin, 1978).

text. Our assumptions and expectations further shape the attribution process by filling in gaps in our information and redistributing attention. Because attributions go beyond the cues actually available at the moment and because much of the information from physical cues is ambiguous, a person's causal attributions may often be in error.

Analysis of attributional processes takes on special importance in health behavior for several reasons. First, it appears that people are especially motivated to seek causal attributions under periods of high uncertainty (Gerard and Rabbie, 1961). When symptoms are unfamiliar or difficult to evaluate objectively, they lead to highly speculative inferences, which make for erroneous attributions.

Second, most illnesses can be expected to produce some degree of fear and distress. To suspect or actually learn that one is ill can be profoundly unsettling. As a result of the high level of emotionality surrounding most health-relevant problems, some people are likely to draw inaccurate or distressing inferences about what is wrong. These misattributions, in turn, lead to inappropriate action or inaction.

Third, people may put off seeking proper medical attention while engaging in a search for explanation and causation. People often seek out others for purposes of social comparison, reassurance, or advice when doubts arise about their own experience (Schachter, 1959). This is especially likely when someone is concerned about possible symptoms of illness, about the effects of medical treatments, or about the consequences of inaction. However, if individuals feel ashamed about their physical sensations, they may show the opposite tendency, that is, staying away from others and not talking about and appraising what is bothersome (Sarnoff and Zimbardo, 1961). In either case, delay of treatment results.

Reattribution and Stress Reduction

Under certain conditions, emotional arousal in response to physical symptoms or other signs of threat can be reduced, rather than enhanced, by attributional processes. There is now considerable evidence showing that the degree of pain and the level of distress that people experience depend in large part on the labels and cognitions that are applied to physical state and are not intrinsic properties of the state itself (Beecher, 1959; Nisbett and Valins, 1971; Schachter and Singer, 1962). These labels, in turn, can further influence perceptions regarding both the source and the level of arousal.

Nisbett and Schachter (1966) were the first to show that if subjects attribute their fear arousal state to the side effects of a placebo pill, they actually rate electric shock as less painful and take more painful stimulation than if they have no alternative label except fear for their emotional state. Following this study, Ross, Rodin, and Zimbardo (1969) observed similar effects when they induced high levels of physiological arousal by threatening subjects with electric shock. When subjects were given unsolvable problems that they thought needed to be solved in order to avoid shock, those who were encouraged to attribute their arousal symptoms to a loud noise showed less perseveration than those who were left to attribute their symptoms of fear to the threat of shock alone. The authors suggested that a version of this reattribution technique might be used to reduce excessive fears in people who display phobic reactions. For example, a hospitalized patient who tries to avoid being given intravenous feedings because of a phobic type of reaction to needles might be told about various neutral features of the treatment that contribute to autonomic arousal in many people—the momentary prick from inserting the needle, the restriction of the arm's movement, and so on. When arousal symptoms occur, a fearful patient who has been given this information would have a ready explanation in circumstantial, nonfearful terms. In attempting to produce reattributions, it is essential to highlight relatively innocuous elements of the situation that are potential sources of arousal. If deception were necessary, however, this would not be a viable clinical technique and would pose serious ethical issues.

A variant of the reattribution device was employed with therapeutic results by Storms and Nisbett (1970). Some of their subjects, all of whom were insomniacs, were given placebos described as drugs capable of producing the arousal symptoms accompanying insomnia—alertness, heart rate increase, and sensations of excessive body heat. They reasoned that subjects taking the pills would be able to attribute their arousal to the drug (in other words, to some externally imposed circumstance) instead of to the self-generated emotional thoughts that intensified their insomnia. This external attribution would be expected to result in lowered emotionality and quicker onset of sleep. The subjects did, in fact, report getting to sleep about twelve minutes sooner on the night they took the placebo pills than on the nights without the pills.

Obviously, this same kind of reattribution might be applicable to other emotional reactions that interfere with health, but the major deterrent is that patients would have to be given false information. In addition to ethical constraints, there is a strong possibility of extremely unfavorable consequences in the long run whenever patients discover that they have been deliberately misinformed, even though the purpose was to try to help them. Furthermore, the misinformation contained in the reattribution procedure designed to reduce perception of pain and emotional stress could lead some patients to fail to take essential steps for preserving their physical or mental health. In our opinion, reattribution techniques requiring deception do not have much promise as a psychological therapy. But the research results from reattribution experiments can nevertheless prove to be a valuable source of evidence bearing on explanatory hypotheses to account for some of the well-known placebo effects that have been repeatedly observed among people suffering from a wide variety of physical disabilities and illnesses.

Stress Reduction from Nonattributional Sources in Attribution Studies

Recent evidence suggests that reattribution regarding the locus or level of arousal has not been the only source of stress reduction in attribution studies. Rodin (1976b) found that other aspects of the attribution process can also produce arousal-reducing effects. Typically, reattribution treatments give subjects false information about an alleged nonemotional cause of their arousal but they give correct information about how subjects can expect to feel when they are exposed to the emotion-arousing situation. In contrast, the subjects in the base-line control group are given either false information about how they will feel or no information at all. Since subjects given the re-attribution treatment differ from the controls in that they receive correct information about how they are likely to feel, this information could have a reassuring effect; they might perceive their emotional reactions as appro-priate since they were told that this is what most subjects report in a similar situation. Such reassurance could, in itself, lessen emotional arousal without involving reattributions of the causes of the emotional reactions.

Rodin showed that performance and emotional responsiveness were benefited even when attributions correctly linked the arousal state to the emotional source, so long as subjects were given correct information that led them to expect the feelings they would have, along with information provid-ing a normative standard against which they could compare their reactions. An essential feature of this experiment is that the subjects' expectations were confirmed by their actual experience. This experiment suggests that health practitioners can reduce their patients' physical and psychological stress by providing correct information and normative standards that allow them to evaluate their emotional arousal as a normal reaction.

There is some evidence that reattribution techniques also reduce emo-tional arousal if, shortly after their initial successful trial, the procedure is explained to the subjects in a way that convinces them of their own capabili-ties for tolerating pain. Davison and Valins (1969) induced subjects to be-lieve that a placebo pill reduced their skin sensitivity, enabling them to take twice as much electric shock as they had previously taken and to find it less painful. In actuality, the experimenters had surreptitiously changed the meter on the shock apparatus to make it appear that stronger shocks were being given. Half the subjects were then told that the pill was wearing off, and the other half learned that the pill had actually been a placebo. The latter subjects, who had been led to believe that they had been responsible for their improvement on the second shock series, took significantly more shock on a third series than they had on the first. Drug subjects, who pre-sumably believed that a drug had been responsible for their improvement on the second series, took even less shock on the third series than they had on the first. Thus, subjects who were led to believe that their pain-enduring be-havior was a reflection of their own ability to withstand pain rather than due to a drug subsequently were able to tolerate more painful stimulation.

Presumably, in some circumstances, people can tolerate pain better if they attribute their pain reactions to themselves, whereas in other circum-stances, their pain tolerance is higher if they attribute their pain reactions to extrinsic or circumstantial causes. So far, however, there is little evidence from experimental or clinical investigations of pain specifying the conditions under which one or the other reaction will occur. This problem, in our opinion, should be high on the research agenda of psychologists who are studying attribution effects.

Attribution Errors Arising from Chronic Physical Changes

Errors can also arise when people are inattentive to chronic physical states as sources of attribution, such as the physiological changes that occur gradually with aging, metabolic changes that result from overeating, and cardiovascular changes that arise from stress. These internal changes often are incorrectly attributed to external, situational causes. For example, when people overeat for longer than a few days and undergo a period of active weight gain, several hormonal and metabolic changes occur and there is enhanced lipolytic activity. Also associated with overeating and obesity are: decreased glucose tolerance; elevated triglyceride, blood cholesterol, and insulin levels; increased cortisol secretion rate; and blunted growth hormone secretions (Bortz, 1969; Forsham, 1974; Rabinowitz, 1970). The hyperinsulinemia is significant because elevated levels of insulin increase the experience of hunger and thus could lead to more eating. They also promote greater storage of what is eaten as fat. The higher the basal levels of insulin, the more insulin is released at the sight, thought, and smell of highly appealing food (Rodin, 1977). Thus, some overweight people may become more physically primed to be tempted by tasty foods as a result of overeating, especially those who were already most responsive to environmental food cues. Not being aware of these physiological changes, however, but experiencing their effects, people often attribute the causes of overeating and increased hunger to erroneous and demoralizing sources, such as gluttony or depression.

Rodin also has preliminary data suggesting that some of the emotional reactivity typically found in overweight people may be a consequence of obesity-caused irregularities in the circadian rhythms of certain hormones, such as cortisol. The ambiguity of arousal produced by disturbances in these rhythms could generate anxiety and lead obese persons to search the external environment for an explanation for their arousal. Similar attributional processes may occur in response to other ambiguous arousal states produced by shifts in metabolic and endocrine processes that are associated with overeating and overweight (Horton and others, 1975). Consequently, obese people may attribute their ambiguous and variable symptoms, which are actually caused primarily by internal physiological changes, to family quarrels or other external events happening in the environment.

By contrast, under certain conditions, people make too many attributions to internal physical processes rather than to the environment. This often happens among the elderly. Although biological changes obviously do occur with aging, the debilitating label of "senility," which is applied by the older person and health care providers alike to memory disturbances and other internal changes, may greatly exaggerate the defects. Kahn and others (1975), for example, have shown that there was only a small amount of real memory loss in their elderly sample, but a high degree of perceived memory loss by the patients, which was significantly correlated with depression. The attributional process can create two types of problems for older people. First, there is a tendency to overattribute all negative changes in health and mood to aging per se, especially to the presumed physical decline with which aging is associated. Biological attributions may incorrectly focus the person away from situational and social factors, such as separation from loved ones, that are stress inducing and affect health. Second, when events are attributed to inevitable aging processes, remedial steps, which could be extremely beneficial, are not undertaken.

The health-relevant issues of obesity and aging are suggested as examples of the complex way that a particular physical state and one's attributions—either correct or incorrect—can influence subsequent behavior. The labels given to symptoms may also directly affect the severity of the physical condition itself. For example, when the elderly are given explicit means of focusing on environmental attributions for their perceived distress, they show greatly improved behavior, including an actual increase in memory and intellectual performance, relative to those who continue to focus on the perceived physical decline that they associate with aging per se (Rodin and Langer, 1978). Thus, debilitating and often excessive attribution to physical states can be refocused with beneficial effects to more easily changed sources in the environment.

Actor-Observer Biases

A third type of attribution error emerges frequently because actors and observers tend to make divergent inferences about behavioral causes (Jones and Nisbett, 1971). Actors usually see their behavior primarily as a response to the situation in which they find themselves. Observers, however, typically attribute the same behavior to the actor's dispositional characteristics—in other words, to his or her personality. Jones and Nisbett suggest some reasons why this actor-observer divergence might occur. To start with, the observer is typically ignorant about details of the actor's history and is likely to take a cross-sectional or normative view, asking how this person's reactions differ from those expected from others, from the average, from the norm. Thus, the observer's orientation is individuating. He or she seeks out and exaggerates differences among people and thereby often fails to see provocations in the situation as a sufficient cause of the behavior observed. In short, the observer typically is handicapped by a relative poverty of information about what the observed person is responding to. But other factors also enter in because the same information will be processed differently by an observer than by an actor. For the observer, another person's action is changing and unpredictable and therefore more salient than the environmental context. Because the observer is not focusing as much on the environment, he or she typically attributes the actions of other people to their motives or abilities. Actors, however, tend to focus on changes in their environment, which they then assume are the causes of their behavior.

In hospitals, clinics, and other health care settings, the differences between the actors' biases and the observers' biases in attribution could sow seeds for misunderstanding between patients and staff. Health professionals, like any other observers, would be expected to show a strong tendency to make dispositional interpretations because of attributional biases, in addition to the need to protect their self-esteem (see Davis, 1966). Thus, a patient not taking his or her medicine is viewed as recalcitrant and uncooperative. Patients, however, as actors would be inclined to attribute their reactions to environmental events. Thus, they would know that they had stopped the medication because it made them overwhelmingly sick, for example. Clearly, physician and patients may therefore see the same event from two different perspectives as each attends to a different set of cues. Some of the cues available to one may be unavailable to the other. Also, their interpretive frameworks are different. The consequence of these differing perspectives may have both positive and negative effects on patients.

Possible negative outcomes arise because physicians and nurses are typically exposed to patients' complaints, not to their feelings of well-being. As an observer of these behaviors, the physician may attribute complaints or nonadherence to the patient's type of personality rather than to his or her stress reactions to illness and fear. On the positive side of the ledger, the physician's focus on physical disease can provide a beneficial corrective perspective for patients who form maladaptive or incorrect causal attributions to account for their illness. For example, a patient who blames burning genital sensations on illicit sexual behavior and feels guilty may be much relieved when the physician attributes the response to a local irritation caused by medication.

Refocusing attention may also be a way to avoid initial misunderstanding between health care professionals and their patients. Long-term health care settings, such as nursing homes and mental institutions, have begun to broaden the perspectives of the caretakers by having them play the patient role through role-playing techniques. This procedure can be thought of as an empathy-inducing device—to make health care deliverers conscious of what it feels like to be a patient. From an attributional standpoint this technique has added value in that it focuses the attention of health care personnel on the situational variables surrounding the illness, once they take the perspective of the patient.

Although there is a bias among actors toward giving situational explanations for their own behavior, they sometimes overlook real situational causes (Nisbett and Wilson, 1977). They base their judgments about the effects of stimuli on implicit a priori theories about a causal connection between stimulus and response, and these theories are systematically biased by the processes of availability and representativeness (Kahneman and Tversky, 1972, 1973).

When a person uses the availability heuristic, his or her estimates of the frequency or probability of events are based on how easy it is to imagine or remember those events. Availability is often poorly correlated with actual frequency or probability and thus leads to systematic errors. For example, in our daily lives, we seldom encounter persons suffering from severe respiratory diseases such as emphysema or lung cancer and, consequently, vivid images of those diseases are not available to our imagination when we hear about the health consequences of smoking. We are likely, therefore, to underestimate the likelihood that those illnesses could befall us and to ignore the recommended preventive action of cutting down on smoking. But when an illness is close to home or publicized by the mass media—as when both Mrs. Ford and Mrs. Rockefeller had mastectomies because of breast cancer—the tendency is to increase one's estimate of the likelihood of becoming a victim of such a disease. According to the availability hypothesis, judgments about the probability of being afflicted by any disease depend partly on the extent to which vivid images of that disease are available when people think about it. An implication of this hypothesis is that public health communications could sometimes prove to be more effective if, instead of being restricted to solely verbal warnings and information, they provide, along with factual evidence, a series of concrete images that increase the "availability" of the unfavorable consequences that the warnings are intended to prevent (see, however, the discussion below of problems of excessive fear arousal).

Incorrect attributions based on availability or observational biases can be difficult to reverse, even with new information that completely negates the original misleading evidence. This was shown in studies by Ross, Lepper, and Hubbard (1975). In their experiments, subjects first received continuous false feedback about their performance as they worked on a novel discrimination task, distinguishing authentic suicide notes from fictitious ones. The experimenter then completely discredited the "evidence" upon which the false feedback had been based in a standard debriefing session in which he explained the purpose of the experimental deception. Following this, a questionnaire was completed dealing with the subject's performance and ability to judge the suicide notes. On virtually every measure, the discredited initial information produced significant residual effects upon subjects' self assessments. In subsequent experiments, Ross, Lepper, and their colleagues have pursued the perseveration phenomenon using a variety of experimental settings and personal abilities. Although much of this research is still in progress, it is already apparent that the phenomenon is not restricted to the debriefing paradigm and could help to explain certain health-relevant behaviors.

The perseveration effect apparently occurs because evidence, once coded, becomes autonomous from the coding scheme, so that its influence may no longer depend upon the validity of that scheme. Consider, for example, a female patient who is given misleading information about her recovery from a serious illness. Suppose an acquaintance tells her that her reflexes are obviously slow, which means that she is very weak and needs to restrict her activities. The patient attempts to place this information in an already existing coding schema relevant to her judgments of her own physical health and abilities. Because everyone has some negative concepts about his or her own physical weaknesses, a coding schema is already available that allows any such new negative information to be readily assimilated. Even when the information is subsequently contradicted by new information from a physician, who tells her that her reflexes and all other physiological functions are quite normal, the person may have found new signs from her self-observations that bolster the negative judgment originally based on the incorrect information. The availability heuristic may work against the individual in this instance, because she has accessible information that allows her to confirm the negative input that she has already received.

Clearly, self-attributions of the type under discussion can have a very strong influence on patients' beliefs and actions. The information they receive regarding their physical symptoms, including the way they are treated initially when the illness is being diagnosed, provides the basis for a general schema which patients then use to interpret whatever happens during the rest of the illness. Change may be harder to induce once the initial information calls forth an inappropriate cognitive schema. If ill persons are treated as helpless and begin to view themselves in that way, actual improvement may not be sufficient to change their initial passive attitudes and behaviors. Moreover, the explanations that individuals receive for their illness and for their treatment profoundly affect their expectations of successful recovery, which may determine the degree to which they take appropriate actions that contribute to their own improvement.

Victimization and Self-Blame

In recent years, social psychologists have started to take a new look at reactions to victimization. Studies of how victims of serious accidents or illnesses cope with their misfortunes suggest that their reactions are affected by three motives: (1) to maintain a belief in a just world (Lerner, 1965, 1971; Lerner and Matthews, 1967; Lerner and Simmons, 1966); (2) to perceive themselves as having control over their environment (Kelley, 1971; Walster, 1966); and (3) to protect themselves from blame (Shaver, 1975).

According to the "just world" hypothesis, all of us have a need to believe that people get what they deserve and deserve what they get. In a series of intriguing experiments, Lerner and his colleagues found that when subjects observe misfortunes in others, they either blame or derogate the victims. Lerner argues: "It seems obvious that most people cannot afford for the sake of their own sanity to believe in a world governed by a schedule of random reinforcement. To maintain the belief that there is an appropriate fit between effort and outcome, the person who sees suffering or misfortune will be motivated to believe that the unfortunate victim in some sense merited his fate" (Lerner and Simmons, 1966, p. 203).

Another motivational bias for derogating victims emphasizes a desire for control. According to Walster (1966), assigning blame to the victim for a severe accident or illness reassures observers that they will be able to avoid similar disasters. If causality were assigned to an unpredictable and uncontrollable set of circumstances, people would be forced to concede that such an event might happen to them at any time.

The third hypothesis relevant to the issue of victimization, advanced by Shaver (1975), pertains to "defensive attribution." Shaver uses this term to suggest that people assign causality in order to maintain or enhance their self-esteem. He postulates that observers' reactions to victims are affected by their desire to avoid blame for their own future accidents. Victims would be less likely to be blamed for misfortunes if the observers believed that they could find themselves in the same circumstances as the victims.

The three hypotheses dealing with victimization have direct implications for how individuals react to unfortunate experiences of others. On the one hand, if they see themselves as similar to the victim, their defensive attributions incline them to play down the victim's own role in bringing about the misfortune—for example, denying that a friend's lung cancer could be the result of heavy cigarette smoking, especially if they smoke too. On the other hand, if they see a victim as different from themselves, they tend to blame the victim and treat him or her as deserving of suffering.

"Just world" effects could lead the family and friends of a person with a chronic illness to derogate the victim, which protects them from acknowledging that a similar illness or misfortune could befall them. The victim would either undergo a loss of support and comfort from these friends and relatives or receive excessive indulgence if they feel guilty about their lack of sympathy. In either case, there would be a breakdown in the support network for the ill patient just at the time when he or she needs it most. Health care deliverers are also subject to these same motivated biases. Patients are sometimes viewed as deserving of their problems and are blamed for their own victimization (Ryan, 1971). As a consequence, they may receive less than adequate care.

How do the patients themselves react when they are victimized by acute or chronic illness? Although Lerner and his colleagues have not dealt directly with this issue, it seems to follow from their "just world" hypothesis that people should be motivated to believe that they deserve the outcomes that they receive. If so, people who are victimized will either blame themselves or will reevaluate the outcome as desirable. It also appears likely that if environmental factors are believed to be within the victims' own control, they will blame themselves for their suffering. Attribution might rarely be made to chance since, according to Walster's analysis, it is the most elusive and uncontrollable of all explanatory factors.

So far there is little evidence bearing on the attributions of victims themselves. In one of the few relevant studies, Bulman and Wortman (1977) investigated victims of common life-threatening events, such as auto accidents and injurious falls. In interviews, the accident victims were asked whether they had asked themselves the question "Why me?", and if so, how they answered it. Every respondent stated that he or she had asked that question and all except one had come up with a specific answer, such as "predetermination," "chance," "God had a reason," "it was deserved," or "it was a blessing in disguise." Every type of attribution was evident, but over 50 percent showed self-blame. Bulman and Wortman found that individuals were most predisposed to blame themselves if they were alone at the time of the accident and had voluntarily chosen the activity in which they were engaged. Similarly, a study by Sogin and Pallak (1976) showed that people are more likely to assume responsibility after making a choice if negative consequences occur that were foreseeable. In this study, forewarned subjects made stronger internal attributions of causality for negative consequences than did control subjects who had received no forewarnings.

In the Bulman and Wortman study, those patients who blamed another for the accident showed the greatest difficulty in coping. This may seem surprising since blaming another allows one to avoid the lowering of self-esteem that results from blaming the accident on one's own shortcomings. But self-blame may be beneficial under conditions where the person believes he or she can do something about subsequently averting the kind of disaster just undergone.

In another study (Chodoff, Friedman, and Hamburg, 1964), dealing with the coping behavior of families of children who were diagnosed as having leukemia, personal blame for negative outcomes also appeared to facilitate coping. The authors suggest that parents' self-blame often serves a defensive purpose of denying the intolerable conclusion that no one is responsible and that nothing could affect this malignant disease, whose causes are completely unknown. The same defensive tendency can be seen in older victims themselves. Physicians might be able to deal more effectively with their patients' naive, unscientific theories if they recognized that their causal attributions may be serving defensive needs that facilitate coping.

Personal attributions for uncontrollable negative outcomes have also been found to impair coping. Abrams and Finesinger (1953) showed that this occurs when attributions of self-blame lead to debilitating feelings of guilt and inferiority. They reported that many cancer patients say that some past experience is responsible for their illness. Feelings of guilt caused patients to deny symptoms and frequently led to delay in obtaining medical treatment. Self-blame also stimulated attitudes of inferiority, dependency, and feelings of rejection. Abrams and Finesinger suggested that unless patients were able to talk about how they felt about being stricken by cancer, they were inhibited from discussing their concern and unable to form helpful relationships with doctors, social workers, or members of the family. When the patients' attitude of self-blame was counteracted by realistic information designed to correct misattributions of personal responsibility, they were less likely to delay treatments and felt more adequate and less dependent. In this instance, self-blame impaired effective coping because it prevented realistic appraisal of action that could be taken. We believe that a crucial problem for current research is to determine precisely when self-blame facilitates and when it impairs coping.

Deindividuation

Another perceptual bias, more extreme than derogation of the victim, is deindividuation (Zimbardo, 1970). This refers to the tendency of people to view mutilated, ill, or defective persons in terms of stereotyped categories rather than as individual human beings. When patients attribute those same traits to themselves, they may experience a loss of personal identity. One major condition for deindividuation to occur is anonymity, which results when people in a group are seen as an aggregate rather than as individuals. Other conditions that foster loss of personal identity include circumstances where a high degree of emotional arousal is evoked and where a change in time perspective is induced such that the past and the future are contracted or the present is expanded to become of primary significance for the individual.

It is easy to see how precisely these situational factors are sometimes unintentionally created by health care systems. We assume that as greater numbers of people require treatment, their names often become replaced by ID numbers and codes. While this is especially true in hospitals and clinics, many private physicians now have group practices and a patient may see a different doctor on each visit. Thus, close personal relationships with one's own doctor are minimized and patients are often treated as medical problems rather than as unique individuals. Since most problems related to health arouse some degree of fear and uncertainty in patients, their contacts with health care professionals often occur in an emotionally charged context. Furthermore, they may have a distorted sense of the present if their severe illness makes the future look bleak and the past seem no longer relevant. The potential for increased feelings of depersonalization becomes greater as emotional arousal and the distortions of time perspective increase.

When situational features of the hospital or clinic contribute to a loss of personal identity on the part of the patient, psychological stress is added to that which is experienced as a direct result of the medical problem itself. Distressing feelings of depersonalization make patients less willing to follow health-relevant recommendations or to return for subsequent visits. Thus, adherence or nonadherence to medical recommendations should not be viewed solely in the context of types of people or types of information given. Deliverers of health care may achieve better results if they correct for the dehumanizing features intrinsic to their health care delivery system (Finnerty, Mattie, and Finnerty, 1973).

Perceived Control

The assertion that human beings are not merely interested in avoiding pain and seeking pleasure but are motivated to achieve mastery is hardly new. The point has been made emphatically by eminent psychologists in the past—by Adler (1929), Erikson (1950), Piaget (1952), and White (1959). Now it is being taken up again by social psychologists with a slight twist and with much renewed vigor.

As defined by Baron and Rodin (1979), control is the ability to regulate or influence intended outcomes through selective responding. *Perceived* control refers to expectations of having the power to participate in making decisions in order to obtain desirable consequences. One aspect of perceived control involves a sense of freedom of choice, being aware of opportunities to select preferred goals and means. Another aspect—perceived control over outcomes—refers to the person's belief in a causal link between his or her own actions or action capabilities and the consequences that will ensue. The crucial component is the assumption, held with varying degrees of conviction by different people and in different situations, that they are responsible for the outcomes that accrue to them through their own efforts.

Issues of control are especially relevant to health-related attitudes and behaviors because sometimes strong social constraints as well as physical restrictions increase psychological stress. Increases in perceived control presumably lead to improvements in coping with stress. Thus, control becomes relevant to understanding how patients may prepare for threat and how they cope when they encounter physical stressors. Control processes are also important in dealing with choice of and commitment to health-relevant behaviors in general. Here the processes of dissonance reduction and reactance may also play a significant role.

There is now a sizable literature indicating that both actual and perceived control over present or impending harm plays an important role in coping with stress (Bowers, 1968; Houston, 1972; Pervin, 1963; Pranulis, Dabbs, and Johnson, 1975; Staub, Tursky, and Schwartz, 1971). At present there are two dominant views about how control results in stress reduction. One is that self-regulated administration, which allows for actual control, is positively reinforcing and may sometimes decrease the effects of the painful stimulus (Averill, 1973; Kanfer and Seider, 1973; Seligman, 1975). The second holds that increased sense of control in the face of uncertain threats leads to increased predictability, which is stress reducing (Ball and Vogler, 1971; Klemp and Rodin, 1976; Pervin, 1963; Weiss, 1970). Both could be true, depending on the type of control that is provided.

Some control interventions give patients a great deal of preparatory information, including precise descriptions of expected reactions, medical procedures, and the like, as in Johnson's (1975) work on gastroendoscopy. These interventions enable patients to make plans for coping with the predicted stress, which can enhance feelings of control. Johnson argues that preparatory information not only increases expectancies about likely sensations but also decreases expectancies about unlikely ones. The consequences of such preparation are to reduce significantly the degree of pain experienced, the need for medication following surgery, and the time needed for postoperative recovery (Johnson, 1975). Focusing attention on the task at hand may also increase predictability and control in other ways. Pranulis, Dabbs, and Johnson (1975), for example, found that patients showed better reactions to anesthesia and surgery when their focus of attention was directed away from their own emotional reactions as passive recipients of treatments to specific tasks that made them feel more in control as active collaborators with the staff. In a laboratory study, Klemp and Rodin (1976) showed that subjects found shock more painful and had lower pain tolerance when they were instructed to focus on their emotional reactions to the shock than when they were asked to focus their attention on the sensory properties of the shock stimuli. The value of directing the patient's attentional focus has been directly tested in a study of effectiveness of a cognitive reappraisal technique with surgical patients by Langer, Janis, and Wolfer (1975). Without encouraging denial of realistic threats, their technique encouraged each patient to' feel confident about being able to deal effectively with whatever pains, discomforts, and setbacks were subsequently encountered.

Other studies have had similar beneficial outcomes by actually providing patients the opportunity to have some degree of control. Work with breast cancer patients has shown that patients do better, as measured by rate of recovery from surgery, when they have had a two-stage surgical procedure (Taylor and Levin, 1977), as compared with those who have undergone a one-stage procedure. The two-stage procedure allows time for orderly planning and evaluation prior to surgery or therapy and often includes active participation of the patient in the decision to resort to surgery. The patient's knowledge that she has a malignancy and her psychological preparation in advance for the removal of the breast, as well as her participation in the relevant planning and decision making, are likely to enhance her feelings of personal control.

In a field study, Langer and Rodin (1976) assessed the effects of an intervention designed to encourage elderly nursing home residents to make a greater number of choices and to feel more in control of day-to-day events. The study was intended to determine whether the decline in health, alertness, and activity that generally occurs among the aged in nursing home settings could be slowed or reversed by giving them more responsibility for making daily decisions. The results indicated that residents in the group given more responsibility became more active and reported feeling less unhappy than the comparison group of residents who were encouraged to feel that the staff would care for them and try to satisfy their needs. Patients given responsibility for making their own decisions also showed significant improvement in alertness along with increased involvement in many different kinds of activities, such as attending movies, participating in contests, actively socializing with staff, and seeking out friends. From a physician's blind evaluations of the patients' medical records, it was found that during the six-month period following the intervention the "responsible" patients showed a significantly greater improvement in health than the comparable patients in the control group. The most striking follow-up data were obtained in death rate differences between the treatment groups assessed eighteen months after the original intervention: Only 15 percent in the intervention group died, whereas 30 percent in the comparison group died. These findings are in line with Ferrare's (1962) original correlational observation that aged people who were relocated in a new nursing home of their own choice lived longer than those who were sent there without being given any choice.

We are not suggesting that it is universally beneficial for patients to feel increased personal control. Feelings of control may be stress inducing, especially when the individual believes that there are actions that he or she ought to be taking but is not (Averill, 1973). Similarly, futile attempts to control health-relevant processes that are uncontrollable may be stress inducing. And of course, if patients' decisions turn out to have been wrong, they are likely to blame themselves, which could have further debilitating effects. Nonetheless, it seems clear that in most aspects of health care, there can be potential benefits from increasing the patients' opportunities to exercise control.

The studies we have described of the ill and the elderly are compelling because the dependent variables are clear health indicators—that is, improvement rates, amount of narcotics taken to counteract pain, and death rates. Adherence to preventive health measures might also be benefited through increasing perceived control if people were encouraged to be more active in making choices and in implementing their own decisions. Consider, for example, adherence to a long-term treatment program for hypertension, which includes keeping appointments for medical checkups, taking prescribed medication, and restricting activities like smoking and eating. In many cases, it is possible and desirable to afford the patient some degree of behavioral control. Preventive health behavior such as breast self-examination and rehabilitation measures such as postcoronary exercise plans are other areas where this may be essential. Feelings of personal responsibility and self-initiation appear to be especially important for sustaining behavior changes whenever the recommended medical regimen cannot be readily monitored.

Methods to induce feelings of increased responsibility and commitment obviously must be used judiciously, lest they boomerang and further reduce the person's sense of control. Brehm (1966) has suggested that a restriction of feelings of choice produces a negative motivation state, which he calls "reactance." When this occurs, the person is motivated to restore his lost freedom and to regain his sense of control. This type of reaction might help to explain why patients sometimes act against what appears to be their own best interests by leaving the hospital or quitting treatment against medical advice. These patients may be attempting to restore freedoms that they perceive as having been taken away from them by the health care professionals, especially when they are told to eliminate sexual activities, favorite foods, or drugs that they feel are an important part of their lives. The general position of reactance theory in regard to any communication to the patient is that if it threatens the recipient's freedom, reactance will result. This suggests that if health care professionals use words like "must," "should," and "have to," they may arouse reactance in their patients and therefore reduce acceptance. Nonverbal cues that convey the same meaning can have the same effect. Less obvious is the possibility that if the physician reinforces the patient's own decision too strongly (for example, "Yes, you really *must* do that"), freedom of choice is minimized and reactance may be aroused to such an extent that the patient fails to adhere in order to restore a sense of freedom (Brehm, 1976). Thus, lack of adherence may sometimes be an active coping strategy on the part of the patient to restore a lost sense of control. But the conditions under which such reactions are most likely to occur have yet to be investigated.

As Wortman and Brehm (1975) suggest, reactance is but the first step in dealing with threats to personal control. If all efforts to restore control fail, the final step in the process is perceived helplessness (Seligman, 1975). An individual experiencing helplessness no longer believes that his or her actions and their outcomes are related. In other words, helpless people feel that no matter what response they make or do not make, they will suffer consequences over which they have no control.

Feelings of loss of control that contribute to helplessness can derive from the context of illness itself. From the patients' standpoint, symptoms are generally ambiguous and novel, with clear implications of threat, making them hard to evaluate objectively. All too often patients feel that they are getting incomplete information from health care professionals about illnesses that afflict them but that they cannot understand. All of these factors contribute to feelings of helplessness, which may be linked to a variety of negative health outcomes, including depression, duration of somatic illness, and death (Seligman, 1975). Thus, it is not only the happiness of the patient that is at issue; his or her biological state may be affected when lack of perceived control is so extreme that it creates feelings of helplessness. As Rodin and Langer (1977) showed in their nursing home study, changes in control on the social and situational level can also have profound physiological effects. These findings reiterate an important theme that must be emphasized in viewing the social psychology of health behavior. The problems facing any person in regard to health cannot be understood solely from the perspective of the biological disease process, or personal psychology, or the social situation. The physical state and the behavior of a person, whether healthy, injured, or ill, is a product of the interaction of factors from all three domains.

Social Power of Authority Figures

Many medical practitioners experience considerable dissatisfaction with their professional life because they are unable to influence their patients to do what they recommend (Kasl, 1975a).* Studies from the patients' perspective, however, suggest that nonadherence derives from their physician's inability to *motivate* them even when adequately communicating all the crucial information about what patients are supposed to do (Kasl, 1975a). Among the sources of patients' deficient motivation is their dissatisfaction with the physician for failing to give them expected reassurances and explanations. Patients' disappointment in the physician during the initial visit—which sometimes might be avoided if the physician simply were to be a bit more attentive to what is really worrying them, without expending much

*This section is based on a chapter by Irving Janis, "Helping Relationships" (Janis, in press).

additional time—has been found to lead to their not keeping subsequent appointments or breaking off the treatment entirely (Davis and Von der Lippe, 1967; Vincent, 1971; Zola, 1973).

When physicians do not provide the social reinforcement necessary for building and maintaining a strong affiliative bond, they are losing a major source of social power, called referent power (derived from the concept of "reference group"). A person has referent power for those who perceive him or her as likable, benevolent, admirable, and accepting. It should be relatively easy for physicians to build up their referent power because patients in a stressful dilemma may have greater need for affiliation (Schachter, 1959). The question of whether or not patients who are longing to develop strong affiliative ties with a professional helper will, in fact, do so depends partly on the degree to which they receive positive social reinforcement (see Berscheid and Walster, 1969).

According to social psychological research, there are several different ways that physicians or any other professional persons can build the type of relationship that results in their becoming significant reference persons for the patients or clients with whom they deal (Berscheid and Walster, 1969; Byrne, 1971; Levinger and Breedlove, 1966; Tedeschi, 1974). One way is to make salient the *similarities* between oneself and the patient, particularly with regard to beliefs, attitudes, and values. Another way is to give *contingent praises* for specific accomplishments, actions, or intentions that are in line with the goals of the treatment. A third way is to talk and act in a manner that conveys a *benevolent attitude* toward the client, an unselfish willingness to provide help out of a genuine sense of caring about the client's welfare. Still another, which may overlap somewhat with the third way, is to give *acceptance* statements, which convey to the client that he or she is held in high regard as a worthwhile person despite whatever weaknesses and shortcomings might be apparent. Such statements enhance the patient's self-esteem.

Social psychological research has identified four other sources of social power in addition to referent power (French and Raven, 1959): coercive power, reward power, legitimate power, and expert power. The most productive social psychological research on this topic pertains to differential effects of the various sources of power. The research has suggested several plausible hypotheses that can be applied to the physician-patient relationship. One important hypothesis is that when patients comply because of the coercive or reward power of the physician, the patients attribute their compliance to the external incentives and are less likely to perceive themselves as having personal responsibility for their own health. By contrast, the use of referent power by the physician is most likely to produce internalization of the authority's recommendations. For any treatment, medical regimen, or daily health practice that requires voluntary action by the patient without constant surveillance by the physician, internalization is essential.

There are, of course, marked individual differences among physicians and other practitioners in the degree to which they use one or another means of building up their referent power and also in the extent to which they rely upon the other sources of social power. Years ago, many family physicians developed their referent power to such a high degree that their patients would strive to get well partly because they did not want to disappoint their lovable "old Doc." This component is often missing in present-day treatment by specialists. Some health professionals fail to do anything at all to build up their power as reference persons. These are to be found among physicians and nurses who conscientiously concentrate on their professional tasks and tell their patients exactly what they ought to do without paying much attention to patients' psychological resistances. Some are so businesslike that they do not express any concern about the patients' current plight or future welfare. These practitioners, in effect, appear to rely heavily on their coercive, reward, legitimate, and expert power but neglect the potential increase in their ability to influence patients that could come from acquiring referent power as well.

Even if businesslike physicians or nurses are using the other four sources of power to the very limit, their effectiveness would be expected to increase if they were to adopt one or another of the means for acquiring social power as a significant reference person in the life of each patient. By adding referent power to the other bases of social power, according to the foregoing analysis, a physician or nurse would become a model with whom the patients identify. Then his or her health-promoting recommendations would not only meet with less initial psychological resistance but would also be more conscientiously adhered to long after the consultations have come to an end.

Critical Phases in Helping Relationships

A theoretical analysis of critical phases in helping relationships by Janis (1975a; in press) attempts to answer the following question: What else does it take, besides the factors already discussed, for a physician or any other professional helper to build up and use effectively his or her power as a significant reference person? The analysis, which is based on clinical observations and systematic field studies of helping relationships, can be applied whenever people have to decide whether or not to accept and adhere to a course of action recommended by health care practitioners, such as taking medications, dieting, or carrying out any prescribed regimen. Three critical phases are postulated that are surmounted successfully when a person becomes motivated to carry out a recommended course of action even though he or she may be initially deterred by the threat of pain or other short-term losses:

1. In the first critical phase, the practitioner dissipates the patient's wariness and acquires motivating power as a significant "reference person." The patient develops an attitude of reliance upon the practitioner for enhancing and maintaining his or her self-esteem if the practitioner encourages

the person to disclose personal feelings, troubles, or weaknesses and responds to the self-disclosures with noncontingent acceptance statements. The patient's image of the practitioner then becomes that of a warm, understanding parental figure who can be counted on to accept personal weaknesses and defects.

2. In the second critical phase, the practitioner begins to use his or her motivating power. However, the relationship built up during the first phase is impaired as the practitioner begins to function as a norm-sending communicator by encouraging or urging the patient to carry out a necessary but stressful course of action. If the practitioner makes no such demands, either explicitly or implicitly, the relationship will continue in a warm, friendly way but will be totally ineffective in achieving the objectives of helping the person carry out a difficult decision. The crisis arising when the practitioner recommends a new course of action probably can be successfully surmounted if he or she makes it clear that the demands being made are very limited in scope and that occasional failures to live up to those demands following a sincere attempt to do so will not change his or her basic attitude of acceptance toward the patient. A norm-sending practitioner is most likely to retain motivating power if he or she uses a *selective pattern of social reinforcement* whereby criticism is given in a nonthreatening way for counternorm assertions by the patient and positive regard is expressed the rest of the time, including when the patient admits to personal weaknesses or shortcomings that are irrelevant to the task at hand. By expressing noncontingent acceptance most of the time and restricting contingent acceptance to the agreed-upon task, a practitioner can build an authentic image of himself or herself in the patient's mind as a quasi-dependable source of self-esteem enhancement, which greatly facilitates the practitioner's effectiveness. It may also be helpful for the practitioner to attribute the norms that are being endorsed to a respected secondary group and to negotiate an agreement with the patient so that he or she becomes committed to those norms.

3. In the third critical phase, the influence of the supportive norm-sending practitioner is threatened by the patient's disappointment and resentment about the termination of direct contact. The practitioner's goal is to promote internalization of his or her recommended changes. However, once the sessions with the practitioner have ended, the patient may fail to internalize the norms the practitioner has been advocating if he or she interprets the termination of contact as a sign of rejection or indifference. Patients whose chronic diabetes has been stabilized, for example, may stop following the prescribed medical regimen after a period of several months when they no longer have any appointments to see the physician. Adverse reactions to separation may be minimized if the practitioner gives *assurances of continuing positive regard* and arranges for *gradual rather than abrupt termination* of contact. In order to prevent backsliding and other adverse effects when contact with the practitioner is terminated, the patient must internalize the norms sponsored by the practi-

tioner by somehow converting other-directed approval motivation into self-directed approval motivation. Little is known as yet about the determinants of this process, but it seems plausible to expect that internalization might be facilitated by communications and training procedures that build up appropriate self-attributions and a sense of personal responsibility.

Part of the art of effective health care may require dealing with each of the three critical phases in a way that minimizes adverse reactions. Perhaps only a very small proportion of practitioners have the talents and acquired interpersonal skills that enable them to function with consummate artistry in dealing successfully with all three phases when treating the majority of their patients. Nevertheless, practitioners with modest amounts of talent and skill in dealing with people in trouble may be able to improve their percentage of successful cases by taking account of the prescriptive hypotheses that follow from the analysis of the three stages.

The main hypotheses appear to be plausible in the light of the clinical and social psychological literature on helping relationships and are consistent with findings from systematic studies indicating that social support from a significant person or group can have markedly positive effects when two main conditions are met: (1) the relationship is characterized by a high degree of *cohesiveness*, which is determined by the participants' anticipations of socioemotional gains (such as esteem) as well as utilitarian gains (such as improved health) resulting from the relationship with the significant person or group; and (2) the relationship entails being exposed to *norm-setting* communications, which convey the behavioral standards that the significant person or group expects one to live up to (Cartwright and Zander, 1968; Hare, 1976; Shaw, 1971).

There are bits and pieces of empirical evidence from systematic investigations that support most of the hypotheses derived from the analysis of the three hypothesized stages, although all the theoretical assumptions concerning the positive effects of self-esteem enhancement have not yet been adequately tested. These views concerning what is necessary in order to build up, use, and retain motivating power can be stated as testable hypotheses: (1) encouraging substantial self-disclosure and giving positive feedback will build up the practitioner's motivating power; (2) making directive statements or endorsing specific recommendations regarding actions the patient should carry out, eliciting commitment to the recommended course of action, and giving selective feedback will facilitate the practitioner's using his or her motivating power; and (3) giving reassurances that the practitioner will continue to maintain an attitude of positive regard, making arrangements for phone calls and other forms of communication that foster hope for future contact (real or symbolic) at the time of terminating face-to-face meetings will facilitate the practitioner's retaining motivating power and will promote internalization after termination of contact.

Evidence from controlled field experiments by Janis and his co-workers carried out in antismoking clinics, weight-reduction clinics, and other health-care settings, indicates that the forgoing variables affect the degree to which a professional helper is perceived as a source of self-esteem enhancement and functions as an effective norm-setter (Janis, 1975a, b; in press). There is also evidence in some of these studies, however, indicating that authority figures who remain detached and demanding can be effective even though they do not enhance self-esteem, provided that they are seen by the clients as benign protectors. Thus, legitimate and expert power are also useful in motivating patients.

Studies by other investigators also provide some evidence that appears to be consistent with hypotheses about the effects of the variables specified in the foregoing theoretical analysis. In a study of mothers in a rheumatic fever prophylaxis program, for example, adherence to medical recommendations for their children was found to be twice as great among those mothers who thought their pediatricians had favorable regard for them than among those who did not (Elling, Whittemore, and Green, 1960). Self-esteem enhancement may be especially relevant in pediatric practice inasmuch as a high percentage of the mothers of ill children have been found to blame themselves and to feel guilty about their children's illnesses—40 percent is the figure reported in a study of 800 mothers by Korsch, Gozzi, and Francis (1968). Another study showed that mothers who openly disclosed their fears and emotional tension (other than anger) to the pediatrician subsequently tended to show more adherence to the medical recommendations (Freeman, 1971).

Several studies of adult patients also supply evidence that is consistent with the theoretical analysis of Phase 1 (acquiring motivating power). Adherence to the physician's recommendations was found to be greater when the tone of the physician's comments to his or her patients was positive (Francis, Korsch, and Morris, 1969). In the same study adherence was found to be significantly lower when the physician gave essentially neutral feedback after asking the patients to disclose personal information or made no reference to the disclosed information.

A major deterrent to giving noncontingent acceptance is that the practitioner must take account of the patients' point of view, or empathize with their feelings, in order for his or her positive comments to be impressive and believable. But this is difficult for anyone, no matter how well trained, when a patient is weak, miserable, and lacking in self-control. Yet this is the way that many patients appear to be. Aside from the problem of empathy, considerable skill is needed to avoid the pitfalls of using noncontingent acceptance. Patients are just as aware of the norms of social equity as practitioners and they are likely to be suspicious when given unearned praise or compliments. Practitioners' attempts to use noncontingent acceptance can have boomerang effects if they give so much praise that they are presumed to be either habitually insincere or attempting to be ingratiating with a hidden manipulative intent (see Jones, 1964).

Decision Making

Acting in accordance with information about how to restore one's health or how to avoid illness can be viewed as the outcome of a process of decision making. As with most decisions, there is typically some conflict when a decision concerns a person's health. For example, when we examine the decisions that must be made by physically afflicted patients, we discover that many of them require the acceptance of short-term losses, such as the physical discomforts of orthopedic exercises, nauseating medicines, or surgery, in order to attain the long-term goals of counteracting a structural defect or a disease that might get worse but has not yet created much suffering. All such choices entail a high degree of decisional conflict about what to do. The more severe the anticipated losses for each of the available alternatives, the greater the stress engendered by the decisional conflict.

Coping with Threats

Janis and Mann (1977) describe five basic patterns of coping with realistic threats, each of which is assumed to be associated with a specific set of antecedent conditions and a characteristic level of stress. These patterns were derived from an analysis of the research literature on how people react to emergency warnings and public health messages that urge protective action. The five coping patterns are:

1. *Unconflicted persistence.* The decision maker complacently decides to continue whatever he or she has been doing, ignoring information about the risk of losses.
2. *Unconflicted change.* The decision maker uncritically adopts whichever new course of action is most salient or most strongly recommended.
3. *Defensive avoidance.* The decision maker evades the conflict by procrastinating, shifting responsibility to someone else, or constructing wishful rationalizations that bolster the least objectionable alternative, remaining selectively inattentive to corrective information.
4. *Hypervigilance.* The decision maker searches frantically for a way out of the dilemma and impulsively seizes upon a hastily contrived solution that seems to promise immediate relief, overlooking the full range of consequences of his or her choice because of emotional excitement, repetitive thinking, and cognitive constriction (manifested by reduction in immediate memory span and by simplistic ideas). In its most extreme form, hypervigilance is referred to as "panic."
5. *Vigilance.* The decision maker searches painstakingly for relevant information, assimilates it in an unbiased manner, and appraises alternatives carefully before making a choice.

While the first two patterns are occasionally adaptive in saving time,

effort, and emotional wear and tear, especially for routine or minor decisions, they often lead to defective decision making if the person must make a
vital choice. Similarly, defensive avoidance and hypervigilance may occasionally be adaptive but they generally reduce one's chances of averting serious
losses. Consequently, all four are regarded as defective patterns of decision
making. The fifth pattern, vigilance, although occasionally maladaptive if
danger is imminent and a split-second response is required, generally leads to
decisions of the best quality.

   According to Janis and Mann's (1977) analysis of research on psychological stress, the coping pattern selected is determined by the presence or
absence of three conditions: (1) awareness of serious risks for whichever
alternative is chosen (that is, arousal of conflict); (2) hope of finding a better
alternative; and (3) belief that there is adequate time to search and deliberate
before a decision is required. Janis and Mann assume that the vigilance pattern occurs only when all three of these conditions are met. They assume
further that if the first condition is not met, unconflicted adherence or unconflicted change is to be expected; if the second condition is not met,
defensive avoidance will be the dominant coping pattern; if the third condition is the only one that is not met, hypervigilance will be the dominant
coping pattern.

   The three conditions that make for vigilant decision making appear to
be essential for the psychological preparation needed to deal with postdecisional stress in cases where adherence to a decision entails some degree of
suffering or loss. Later on, when we discuss the effects of preparatory information, it will be apparent that many different psychological processes are
involved in preparation for stress, including correcting faulty beliefs, recon-
ceptualizing the threat as a problem that can be solved, engaging in realistic
self-persuasion about the value of protective action, and developing concepts
and self-instructions that enable the person to cope more effectively with
setbacks (Janis, 1971; Meichenbaum, 1977; Meichenbaum, Turk, and Burstein, 1975; Taylor and Levin, 1977). All these processes are more likely to
occur when a person engages in the vigilant type of cognitive activity required for a well-conceived decision. Vigilant activity includes intensively
searching for the best available information about the consequences of all
known alternatives, carefully appraising the negative as well as the positive
consequences that could flow from the chosen course of action, and making
detailed contingency plans that might be required if known risks were to
materialize (see Janis and Mann, 1977). But very few people can carry out all
the high-level procedures required without help from advisors, especially
when the costs and risks that need to be appraised pertain to the personal
threats of physical suffering, body damage, or death.

   What kind of help from health care advisors will motivate patients to
make and adhere to difficult decisions? The first type of assistance may
simply be in the form of realistic warnings regarding health problems with
which the person may be confronted currently or in the future.

Effective Warnings

When physicians become concerned that patients may fail to follow regimens that they regard as essential and urgent, they often give these patients a brief fear-arousing warning about the dangers of noncompliance. If their verbal warnings prove to have little or no sustained effect, they sometimes resort to more elaborate fear-arousing information that is intended to "scare the hell out of the patient." An extreme example is furnished by a specialist in the treatment of diseases of the liver. He was perturbed that many of his patients in the early stages of cirrhosis were not abstaining from alcohol despite his verbal warnings (some claiming that a cocktail or two a day cannot do much harm and is essential for business contacts or for relaxation). He arranged for them to be hospitalized for medical tests and deliberately placed them in a ward where they inescapably perceived the agony of advanced cases dying of the same disease. The physician told them to take a good look because that is what they would be like if they did not stop drinking. He reported that most of the patients treated this way promptly converted. We do not know as yet, however, exactly under what conditions strong arousal of fear succeeds in inducing prescribed changes and under what conditions it fails or has boomerang effects. We shall return to this problem shortly.

Personalized warnings from one's private physician, as well as all public health warnings, are conceptualized by Janis and Mann (1977) as challenges to inadequate courses of action. Until people are challenged by some disturbing information or event that calls attention to a real loss soon to be expected, they will retain an attitude of complacency about whatever course of action (or inaction) they have been pursuing. Being exposed to information that effectively challenges a current course of action marks the beginning of the decision-making process. The challenging information produces a temporary personal crisis if the person starts thinking that there could be serious risks unless he or she changes; the person then proceeds to search for alternatives.

The challenging information can be of two kinds:

1. A challenge may be generated by impressive *communications* that argue in favor of a new course of action. News stories about the Surgeon General's report on smoking and lung cancer in 1964 made many smokers begin to take seriously the risks posed by smoking. Cigarette consumption throughout the United States declined by a substantial percentage during the year immediately following publication of that report, although subsequently many people regressed and consumption resumed its upward trend (Wagner, 1971).
2. An *event* may disturb the person's equanimity because a particular threat can no longer be ignored. A man who smokes cigarettes, for example, may notice that he has developed a chronic cough that gets worse each

time he smokes. This is a powerful form of negative feedback and is capable of inducing a smoker to reconsider his or her habitual course of smoking a pack or more of cigarettes each day. Effective challenges are a necessary, but not a sufficient condition for inducing people to make a pro-health decision to which they will adhere. Some threatening challenges may be only temporarily effective and may even have boomerang effects in the long run.

Specialists in research on compliance of medical patients have suggested that the extensive investigations on the effects of warnings and fear appeals by social psychologists might furnish useful guidelines for physicians and other practitioners about what constitutes an effective challenge (Harper, 1971; Korsch, Gozzi, and Francis, 1968). Although a large number of relevant experiments have been reported, we cannot yet formulate any definitive rule about the intensity of emotional arousal that is most likely to be effective (see Janis, 1967, 1971; McGuire, 1968; Rogers and Mewborn, 1976). Some, but not all, attitude-change experiments show less acceptance of precautionary health recommendations when very strong fear appeals are used in warning messages than when milder ones are used. In the initial experiment on this problem, Janis and Feshbach (1953) gave equivalent groups of high school students three different fear-evoking versions of a dental hygiene communication, all of them containing the same set of recommendations about when and how to brush their teeth. The results showed that there were diminishing returns as the level of fear increased. A number of subsequent studies have supported the conclusion that when fear is strongly aroused by a persuasive communication but is not fully relieved by reassurances, the recipients will be motivated to ignore, minimize, or even deny the importance of the threat (for example, Janis and Terwilliger, 1962; Rogers and Thistlethwaite, 1970).

There have been similar experiments, however, that show a gain in effectiveness when strong threat appeals are used, and these experiments point to the facilitating effects of fear arousal (for example, Insko, Arkoff, and Insko, 1965; Leventhal, Singer, and Jones, 1965). Changes in feelings of vulnerability to a threat and in subsequent adoption of a recommended course of action apparently depend upon the *relative* strength of facilitating and interfering reactions, both of which are likely to be evoked whenever a warning by an authority arouses fear. Consequently, we cannot expect to discover any simple generalization applicable to all warnings about health that will tell us whether strong fear-arousing presentations that vividly depict the expected dangers or milder versions that merely allude to the threats will be more effective in general. Rather, we must expect the optimal level of fear arousal to vary for different types of threat, for different types of recommended action, and for different personalities. Optimal level of fear arousal refers to the point on the fear continuum at which the facilitating effects of fear arousal evoked by a warning most strongly outweigh the interfering effects. Once the level of fear arousal exceeds the optimal level, interference begins to get the upper hand and responsiveness to the warning will decrease.

Warnings may be rendered ineffective because people who are exposed to authoritative predictions about the undesirable consequences of continuing to do what they have been doing try to alleviate their unpleasant emotional arousal. One way they accomplish this is by scrutinizing the communicator's arguments carefully to discover loopholes that can serve as excuses for dismissing the warnings, which would otherwise require costly or unpleasant protective actions. Such discounting is reduced when the person cannot deny the personal relevance of what is being said. This is sometimes accomplished by introducing impressive new considerations that arouse vivid images of personal vulnerability along with arguments about the efficacy of the recommended action. To be effective, a challenging event or communication must be powerful enough to induce an image of oneself as headed for serious setbacks and as ultimately failing to attain one's main objectives unless one adopts a new course of action that is perceived as a successful means for counteracting a threat. Such a challenge usually generates not only images of suffering tangible losses but also anticipations of losing the esteem of friends and relatives, as well as losing self-esteem, which leads the person to consider adopting an effective alternative to the present course of action or inaction.

Counteracting Cognitive Defenses

Janis and Mann (1977) point out that many persons who claim that they want to go on a diet, give up smoking, or carry out some other desired form of self-improvement are clinging to rather flimsy rationalizations that exaggerate the withdrawal symptoms and other difficulties involved in changing their habits. Thus, they respond to repeated verbal warnings and other challenges at well below the optimal level of arousal necessary for behavior change. If these cognitive defenses can somehow be undermined or bypassed, only threadbare support remains for their current course of action; they will then be more likely actually to carry out a decision to change, instead of merely continuing to say they would like to. For example, in a group of very heavy smokers undergoing treatment at the Yale antismoking clinic, one man showed a sudden transformation after seven weekly meetings at which he, like most of the others, had consistently used the rationalization that he was hopelessly addicted to cigarette smoking. At the eighth meeting, he reported a dramatic "conversion" experience. He told the group that a few days earlier he had visited in the hospital a close friend who was dying of lung cancer. After leaving the hospital, he had thrown away his cigarettes and had not touched one since. He offered to try to arrange for others in the group to visit his dying friend. But just his description of that visit and the effect it had on him was sufficient to convince two other members of the group of the falsity of the "addiction" rationalization, both of whom promptly followed his example. One month later, all three of these supposedly hopeless cases were still not smoking.

Such observations led to a search for effective forms of intervention that would embody the essential components of those successful challenges that occasionally occur spontaneously. Two such interventions, which will be described, appear to be promising means for transforming mere talk about good intentions into action. One is the "awareness-of-rationalizations" technique, which involves inducing *cognitive confrontations* designed to counteract the rationalizations that are typically used to bolster outworn decisions (Reed and Janis, 1974). The other is the "emotional role playing" technique, a form of *emotional confrontation* that was devised for the purpose of undermining and bypassing the cognitive defenses that function as a protective facade for an outworn decision (Janis and Mann, 1965, 1977). Both techniques could be used by medical or paramedical personnel with a variety of patients in clinics and hospitals.

Cognitive confrontations may be useful for overcoming some resistances to change (see Katz, Sarnoff, and McClintock, 1956; Rokeach, 1971). Reed and Janis (1974) developed the "awareness-of-rationalizations" technique for heavy smokers, to eliminate some of the main rationalizations that serve to bolster their decision to continue smoking. This, in turn, was expected to make them more responsive to challenging information that they typically discount or ignore. The effectiveness of the new technique was tested by Reed and Janis in a controlled field experiment. In their study, each of the heavy smokers given the special treatment was presented with a list of eight statements (referred to as "excuses") and was asked if he or she was aware of any personal tendencies to use each of the excuses. The list consisted of typical rationalizations made by heavy smokers (for example, "It hasn't really been proved that cigarette smoking is a cause of lung cancer"; "If I stop smoking I will gain too much weight"). Next the subject was given a recorded lecture that refuted the eight rationalizations, followed by two dramatic antismoking films, and then reactions were measured on questionnaires. The same lecture, films, and questionnaires were presented to the control group. Reed and Janis found that smokers who had received the awareness-of-rationalizations treatment before the lecture and films expressed greater feelings of susceptibility to lung cancer and emphysema, a stronger belief in the harmfulness of smoking, and a more complete endorsement of the antismoking films. Follow-up interviews two to three months later revealed that, so far as the reported amount of smoking was concerned, the treatment had a significant effect when given by one psychologist but not by the other. Hence, the technique cannot be regarded as an adequate cure for smoking. But the procedure of inducing a decision maker to acknowledge and explore his or her own tendencies to rationalize appears to have considerable promise for reducing resistance to realistic warning messages.

Another type of intervention for overcoming defensive avoidance of health-relevant information is the psychodramatic technique known as "emotional role playing" (Janis and Mann, 1965; Mann and Janis, 1968). In the initial laboratory experiments, the investigators asked heavy smokers to play the role of a lung cancer patient who receives bad news from a physician. They found that this disquieting psychodramatic experience could be so realistic that heavy smokers would, for the first time, acknowledge their personal vulnerability to the threat of lung disease. The typical cognitive defense, "It can't happen to me," can be undermined by this technique. Sufficient research has been done on emotional role playing in antismoking clinics to show that it is capable of producing long-term changes in attitudes of personal vulnerability and in cigarette consumption among heavy smokers (see Janis and Mann, 1977; Mausner and Platt, 1971). One study, for example, showed that after eighteen months a group of female college students who had engaged in emotional role playing had cut their cigarette consumption almost in half and showed significantly less cigarette consumption than a control group (Mann and Janis, 1968). Additional studies suggest that the technique may prove effective for other types of decisions as well—for example, inducing heavy users of alcohol to stop drinking (Toomey, 1972).

Preparatory Information

In addition to providing warnings that increase motivation for decision making and behavior change, relevant information about illness and medical treatments may fill a second function, that of realistically preparing the person for what lies ahead. Much research bears on the conditions under which forewarnings and other attempts at psychological preparation for subsequent stress are most likely to be effective. But in order to apply this knowledge in health care settings, it is necessary for physicians and others on the staff to overcome their own resistances to presenting forewarnings to their clients. For example, some physicians display the well-known MUM effect (Tesser and Rosen, 1975), the tendency to avoid transmitting bad news (Snyder, 1977). Others sometimes show the opposite tendency when dealing with a risky treatment for seriously ill patients—emphasizing the bad news and all its potentially dire ramifications in such a way that if the treatment works out badly no one can deny that fully informed consent was obtained, whereas if the treatment works out well, the patients and their families will be grateful. If health professionals avoid these extremes, they may find the use of preparatory information extremely effective.

Field experiments repeatedly indicate that preparatory communications containing forewarnings combined with realistic reassurances can function as stress inoculation to increase patients' adherence to difficult decisions (see Girodo, 1977; Janis, 1958; Janis and Mann, 1977; Meichenbaum, 1977). Preparatory information functions as a form of stress inoculation if it enables a person to increase his or her tolerance for postdecisional stress by developing effective reassurances and coping mechanisms. The process is called stress inoculation because it may be analogous to what happens when antibodies are induced by injections of attenuated strains of virulent or pathogenic viruses.

Stress inoculation is usually administered shortly after a decision is made but before it is implemented. The underlying principle is that accurate preparatory information about an impending crisis gives a person the opportunity to anticipate the loss, to start working through anxiety or grief, and to make plans that might enable him or her to cope more adequately (see Janis, 1971). The person also needs such information to gain a sense of control over the threatening environmental events, as was suggested earlier. We would expect stress inoculation to be effective for any decision that entails undergoing painful treatments and deprivations before physical well-being improves. Much of the evidence on the effectiveness of stress inoculation comes from studies of such decisions—voluntarily undergoing abdominal surgery, painful medical treatments, and the like.

Janis's (1958) correlational evidence from a study of surgical patients indicates that those patients who receive information about the unpleasant consequences beforehand are less likely than those given little information to overreact to setbacks during the postoperative period. Supporting evidence for the effectiveness of stress inoculation comes from a variety of controlled field experiments with people who decided to undergo surgery (Egbert and others, 1964; Johnson, 1966; Schmidt, 1966; Schmitt and Wooldridge, 1973; Vernon and Bigelow, 1974). These studies indicate that when physicians or nurses give preoperative information about the stresses of surgery and ways of coping with those stresses, adult patients show less postoperative distress and sometimes better recovery from surgery. Positive results on the value of stress inoculation have also been found in studies of childbirth (Breen, 1975; Levy and McGee, 1975) and noxious medical examinations requiring patients to swallow tubes (Johnson and Leventhal, 1974). Field experiments by Moran (1963) and Wolfer and Visintainer (1975) with children on pediatric surgery wards yielded similar results.

Although the evidence so far comes from only a few types of decisions, it seems probable that stress inoculation can be applied to all consequential decisions. There is some additional evidence to support this assumption from social psychological experiments: A number of laboratory studies indicate that people are less likely to display strong emotional reactions or extreme changes in attitude when confronted with a disagreeable experience if they have already been made aware of the unpleasant event beforehand (for example, Epstein and Clarke, 1970; Lazarus and Alfert, 1964; Staub and Kellett, 1972). We expect, therefore, that giving realistic preparatory information about the potential threats that are likely to materialize will likewise have positive effects, enabling the inoculated person to cope more effectively with whatever predicted setbacks occur.

Meichenbaum (1977) has developed a stress-inoculation training program that involves three main steps: (1) discussing the general nature of stress reactions with clients in order to provide them with a conceptual framework and also to motivate them to acquire new coping skills; (2) teaching and inducing rehearsal of specific coping skills, such as collecting information about what is likely to happen and arranging for ways to deal effectively with anxiety-engendering events; and (3) encouraging clients to practice and apply the newly acquired coping skills to stressful conditions, either by means of role playing in imagined stress situations or actual exposures to real-life stresses. This type of stress-inoculation training has been found to be at least partially successful for a number of anxiety-arousing situations (Meichenbaum and Cameron, 1973) and experimentally induced pain (Turk, 1975). Some negative results, however, are reported by Girodo and Roehl (1976) for fear-of-flying among college women. After reviewing the positive and negative outcomes of studies employing stress-inoculation training, Girodo (1977) suggests that the successful components are those that induce the person to reconceptualize the threat into nonthreatening terms and that all other self-statements merely serve as attention-diversion mechanisms. Any such generalization, however, gives undue weight to a limited set of findings and would be premature until we have well-replicated results from a variety of investigations that carefully test the effectiveness of each component of stress inoculation.

It remains for the next phase of research to determine which components are the necessary and sufficient ingredients for promoting effective coping in stressful situations like those that beset people undergoing treatment for serious illness or injury. This type of research is especially relevant for adherence to a distressing course of treatment, such as radiation therapy, and to a variety of health-related regimens involving deprivations, because a frequent source of breaking off a treatment or regimen is the patient's inability to tolerate the stresses it entails.

Other psychological interventions to supplement stress inoculation also need to be developed in order to help patients cope more effectively with subsequent stress. For example, an effective coping device developed by Langer, Janis, and Wolfer (1975) involves encouraging an optimistic reappraisal of anxiety-provoking events. These investigators gave surgical patients several examples of the positive or compensatory consequences of their decision to undergo surgery (for example, improvement in health, extra care and attention in the hospital, temporary vacation from outside pressure). Each patient was invited to think up additional examples that pertained to his or her individual case. Then the patient was given the recommendation to rehearse these compensatory consequences whenever he or she started to feel upset about the unpleasant aspects of the surgical experience. Patients were urged to be as realistic as possible about the compensatory features, to emphasize that what was being recommended was not equivalent to trying to deceive oneself. The instructions were designed to promote warranted optimism and awareness of anticipated gains that outweighed the losses to be expected from the chosen course of action. The findings supported the hypothesis that cognitive reappraisal serve to reduce stress both before and after an operation, as measured by nurses' blind ratings of pre-operative stress and by unobtrusive postoperative measures of the number of times pain-relieving drugs and sedatives were requested.

Adherence to Difficult Decisions

Why do so many people who decide to do what physicians or public health authorities tell them break off before completing the prescribed regimen? Obviously, a major factor is the actual suffering or deprivation imposed, which is especially hard to take over a long period of time. But psychological factors affect a person's tolerance for pain, frustration, and unpleasant experiences. Stress inoculation and cognitive reappraisal are two such factors. Additional variables also directly affect adherence. It is well known, for example, that deprivations are more difficult to tolerate when the person is constantly exposed to temptations and reminders of what he or she is missing. Stunkard (1977b) has suggested that institutional changes could reduce the salience of temptations that interfere with efforts made by large numbers of people to adhere to public health recommendations, such as those pertaining to good nutrition and avoidance of overeating. He emphasizes the disruptive role of TV, magazines, and other mass media, food producers, distributors, and other food advertisers, restaurants, and institutional cafeterias, all of which could facilitate rather than interfere with adherence to healthy diets.

Additional factors that influence adherence are suggested by social psychological research on commitment and cognitive coping devices. Research on commitment, for example, indicates that if a person is induced to announce his or her intention to an esteemed other, such as a physician, the person is anchored to the decision not just by anticipated social disapproval but also by anticipated self-disapproval (Janis and Mann, 1977). A study by McFall and Hammen (1971) indicates that commitment followed by reminders of the commitment and self-monitoring is sufficient to enable many heavy smokers to cut down and is as effective as several more elaborate therapeutic procedures commonly used in antismoking clinics.

The stabilizing effect of commitment, according to Kiesler's (1971) research, is enhanced by exposure to a mild challenging attack, such as counterpropaganda that is easy to refute. Another pertinent finding is that forewarnings designed to prevent backsliding are likely to be effective if the person has already committed himself or herself, but ineffective and even detrimental if the person has not. These findings could be applied by health care personnel in many different types of clinics, where people can be asked to sign a pledge card to carry out a recommended health practice, such as to cut down on alcohol or smoking, and can then be given a mild dose of stress inoculation that calls attention to the unpleasant consequences to be expected.

Adherence might also be enhanced by using intervention procedures that attempt to bring about the conditions necessary for vigilance, described by Janis and Mann (1977) as generally being the most effective coping strategy. The "balance-sheet" procedure, for example, is a predecisional exercise that requires a decision maker to confront and answer questions about potential risks and gains he or she had not previously contemplated. Without a systematic procedure, even the most alert and well-motivated person may overlook vital aspects of the alternatives, remaining unaware of some of the losses that will ensue from the preferred course and maintaining false expectations about potential gains.

The balance-sheet procedure has been used with some success in studies of health-related decisions, as well as career decisions (Janis and Mann, 1977, pp. 149-155). For example, Colten and Janis (in press), on a random basis, gave 80 women who had come to a diet clinic either a high or a low self-disclosure interview, and then either a balance-sheet procedure dealing with the pros and cons of going on a recommended 1,200-calorie diet or a control interview that gave the clients essentially the same information but without inducing them to consider the pros and cons of the alternative courses of action. The women who underwent both the high self-disclosure interview and the balance-sheet procedure showed significantly more adherence to the recommended plan than the others. They sent in more weekly reports concerning their dieting and, most important, were more successful in losing weight.

Further evidence of the effectiveness of the balance-sheet procedure comes from a field experiment by Hoyt and Janis (1975) with women who had signed up for an early-morning exercise class. Twenty women, assigned on a random basis to the relevant balance-sheet condition, were induced to consider carefully all the advantages and disadvantages of regular participation in the exercise class. Twenty others, randomly assigned to the irrelevant balance-sheet condition, were asked to consider all the pros and cons involved in another health-oriented decision—abstaining from cigarette smoking. Records of attendance in the exercise class for a seven-week period were used to obtain an unobtrusive behavioral measure of the effect of these treatments. As predicted, the women given the relevant balance sheet attended significantly more classes than those in the comparison group.

Preliminary evidence of the effectiveness of these new types of interventions, together with the much more extensive research bearing on the effectiveness of stress inoculation cited earlier, is consistent with a major assumption of conflict theory: A decision maker is much more likely to display and adhere to adaptive behavior when making a difficult decision if his or her dominant coping pattern is vigilance rather than defensive avoidance or hypervigilance. When the vigilance pattern is dominant, the decision maker engages in careful search and appraisal before implementing a new course of action and thereafter remains relatively unshaken by setbacks that challenge the decision.

The analysis of interventions for promoting vigilance are applicable not just to patients but also to physicians, hospital administrators, and other health care personnel who make professional or policy decisions. They are subject to the stresses of decisional conflict, just as the rest of humanity is. Of course, physicians are trained to be vigilant and to be aware of the pitfalls both of wishful thinking and of impulsive paniclike actions in emergency situations. Nevertheless, there are probably occasions in every physician's career when vigilance is not the dominant coping pattern in dealing with an important professional decision, however rare such deviations may be.

Preventing Groupthink in Medical Teams

Physicians' errors arising from the temporary blind spots created by defensive avoidance or hypervigilance will sometimes be promptly corrected if they are members of a medical team. But colleagues in a professional group cannot always be counted on to make independent judgments and to communicate their disagreements with a fellow member's erroneous decision (see Cartwright and Zander, 1968; Janis, 1972; Shaw, 1971). For one thing, there is a tendency for everyone, including persons with high status and considerable expertise, to conform with group norms and to avoid challenging the judgment of someone else in a policy-making group out of fear of recriminations. This type of compliance is least likely when the would-be challengers have confidence that they are members in good standing and will be valued by the group whether or not they disagree about the issues under discussion. When members of a professional or executive group develop bonds of friendship and esprit de corps, they trust each other to tolerate disagreements and are unlikely to play it safe by dancing around the issues with vapid or conventional comments. We can expect that the more cohesive a group of physicians or other health care personnel becomes, the less the members will deliberately censor what they say because of fear of being socially punished for antagonizing anyone else in the group.

The effects of group cohesiveness are complicated, however, because the more cohesive a group becomes, the more likely the members are to censor their disagreements because of their strong motivation to preserve the unity of the group (see Janis, 1972). Thus, although the members of a cohesive, well-functioning team may feel freer to deviate from the group norms, their desire for genuine concurrence on all important issues may incline them not to use this freedom. When the concurrence-seeking tendency is dominant, the members collectively develop rationalizations supporting shared illusions about the wisdom and invulnerability of their team and display a collective pattern of defensive avoidance referred to as the "groupthink" syndrome (Janis, 1972; Janis and Mann, 1977, pp. 129-133 and 398-407). Although medical teams have not yet been studied with regard to concurrence-seeking tendencies, there is no reason to believe that groups of medical decision makers—such as partners in private medical practice, staffs on hospital wards, boards of directors of medical organizations, and public health executive committees—are somehow immune to groupthink.

There appear to be four main conditions that promote this source of defective decision making in moderately or highly cohesive groups: insulation of the group; lack of methodical procedures for search and appraisal; directive leadership; and high stress with a low degree of hope for finding a better solution than the one favored by the team leader or other influential persons in the group (see Janis, 1972; Janis and Mann, 1977). Procedures suggested by Janis (1972) to eliminate these conditions might have a number of beneficial effects on decision-making groups in clinics, hospitals, and other health organizations. The suggested procedures might also help counteract initial biases of the members and avoid other sources of error that can arise independently of groupthink (see Elms, 1976). Their primary purpose, however, would be to prevent a collusive form of defensive avoidance among health care professionals, which would greatly decrease the chances for avoidable errors resulting from defective search and appraisal when group decisions are made in life-and-death matters.

Summary

In this chapter, we have suggested how social psychological processes relate to health-relevant behavior. In taking preventive measures while healthy, as well as in taking a patient role when ill, the individual is seen as an active decision maker. He or she seeks causes and explanations for illness and health, then acts according to these attributions. We discussed a number of hypotheses for which there is some important evidence that specifies when attributions increase or decrease stress and how errors in attribution may arise for both recipients and providers of health care.

Preparatory information and warnings serve as effective challenges to action and enhance an individual's sense of control over health-relevant events. Feelings of control increase commitment to difficult decisions, tolerance of physical pain, and rate of recovery. The type of social power used by communicators of medical information further influences the extent of acceptance and continued adherence to recommended courses of action. The kind of coping pattern a person uses in arriving at a decision also influences degree of commitment and adherence to prescribed regimens. We discussed the advantages and disadvantages of vigilant and nonvigilant coping patterns that determine decision-making processes and that influence postdecisional behavior. The theory and research reviewed in this chapter provide a few significant examples of the potential contributions of social psychology in analyzing health problems.

20 ⸙

Social-Ecological Perspectives on Health

Rudolf H. Moos

∾ Speculation about the relationship between environmental factors and health has been the central focus of public health and epidemiology for more than a century. Except for a concern with the social-environmental aspects of the onset and treatment of mental illness, however, psychologists have not been deeply involved in these areas. My thesis here is that health psychology and environmental psychology, two recently emerged fields that have developed somewhat separately, can mutually enhance each other's growth and increase our knowledge of the relationship between the social-ecological environment and health-related outcomes. The four sections of this chapter develop support for this thesis.

The Development of Environmentally Oriented Approaches to Health

Early Public Health and Epidemiologic Approaches

The notion that the physical and social environment influences health and disease has a long and varied history. For example, the Book of Proverbs tells us: "A merry heart doeth good like medicine, but a broken spirit drieth

Note: Preparation of this chapter was supported by NIMH Grant MH28177, Veterans Administration Health Services Research and Development Service funds, and NIAAA Grant AA02863. Deborah Leiderman's help in searching and abstracting the literature facilitated this work.

the bones" (17: 22) and "A sound heart is the life of the flesh, but envy is the rottenness of the bones" (14: 30). These and similar quotations indicate that the ancients believed that emotional factors play an important role in disease processes (Macht, 1945). Presumably, these emotions were aroused by the physical and social context in which an individual lived.

The idea that various diseases and plagues occur more frequently in densely settled cities, partly through the "corruption of the air" (climate) and through rapid population growth, was prevalent in the Middle Ages. More specific studies, which began about 150 years ago, dealt with the physical geography and natural history of particular areas. Nutrition, housing, poverty, social class, and other variables were related to the occurrence of disease and were shown to have an impact on growth and physique. For example, as far back as 1847, Rudolf Virchow concluded that social, economic, and political factors had as much to do with causing a typhus epidemic as did biological and physical factors. The fields of public health and social medicine, which grew out of these notions, were based on the idea that a society has an obligation to protect and enhance the health of its members (Rosen, 1972).

There is an important contrast between the "disease specific" orientation of much of modern medicine and the "holistic-ecological" orientation of public health. Although, as we have seen, this latter orientation antedates the disease orientation, it has been thought of as a "third revolution" in medicine: "The major crowd diseases have been effectively controlled. What we face now as the great challenge are the disorders of bad hygiene, of insalubrious environments, of a malign physical and moral ecology. These are not to be dealt with as were the infectious, epidemic diseases. They are disorders engendered by malign environments and man's corrupt relations to his immediate world and his individual existence. These disorders are not to be remedied by sterilization, vaccines, immune serums, nor by medicinal specifics. They are, in the broadest sense of the term, *ecological disorders*" (Galdston, 1968, pp. 8-9).

Many agents of disease are thought to be ubiquitous in the environment of modern society (Dubos, 1965), yet the majority of people are relatively healthy most of the time. This suggests that a full understanding of the distribution and determinants of disease requires knowledge of the prevalence and toxicity of disease agents *and* of the factors that change the relationship between the host and these agents (Cassell, 1976). These factors can transform an innocuous, possibly symbiotic, relationship into one in which clinical disease is the outcome. This line of thinking supports the notion that a social-ecological perspective needs to underlie epidemiological thinking.

Psychosomatic Approaches

The psychosomatic perspective classically asserts that emotional experiences can affect bodily functions, health status, and the onset and course of disease. Much of the initial research in this field in the 1930s and 1940s developed out of a psychodynamic perspective and focused on personality traits or conflicts thought to be characteristic of individuals with particular types of disorders (see Wittkower, 1974, for a brief historical overview). Harold Wolff and his colleagues (see, for example, Wolff and Goodell, 1968) studied the physiological effects of experimental stress situations and evolved a theory that psychosomatic illness is an *adaptive* response to "life stress." This focus subsequently led to attempts to relate aspects of the physical and social environment to the onset and course of diseases such as diabetes, peptic ulcer, rheumatoid arthritis, and the like (Backus and Dudley, 1974).

A new ecological perspective, which integrates and extends prior approaches, has recently been developed in psychosomatic medicine. Lipowski (1973a, 1973b) suggests that the social and physical environment influences psychosomatic relationships in four overlapping ways. He calls for a combined ecological and psychosomatic approach, one that views people as psychobiological entities in dynamic interaction with their environment. First, according to Lipowski, the environment can be seen as a source of symbolic stimuli. Specifically, pollution of the physical environment may result in social communications that alert individuals to its noxious aspects. Thus alerted, they may notice and interpret certain sensory cues, such as the color of the water or the smell of the air, as subjectively meaningful danger signals. These may make them view their physical environment as alien and potentially lethal, and lead to the formation of values, norms, and problem-solving actions related to the quality of the environment. Second, noxious biological, chemical, or physical pollutants can also cause tissue changes, which may result in altered somatic perceptions (for example, of impaired breathing or diarrhea). Third, environmental factors can directly affect the biological substrate of psychic processes and change a person's habitual modes of perceiving, thinking, and feeling. Specifically, some pollutants may bring about changes in the physical-chemical milieu of the brain and alter its functioning.

Fourth, Lipowski emphasizes information or stimulus overload as another class of variables conceptually linking people's social and physical environment to their psychophysiological functioning. Information is seen as a useful concept for formulating research on the impact of social events and change on the psychological and physiological processes codetermining health and illness. Although Lipowski focuses on the fact that an affluent society subjects its members to an overload of attractive stimuli, thereby causing stress and necessitating coping behavior, others (for example, Cohen, 1978) have focused specifically on the role of unattractive stimuli such as those involved in noise and crowding.

Environmental and Ecological Psychology Approaches

Environmental psychologists have been primarily concerned with the physical and architectural environment. The recent reemergence of interest in this area began with research programs on the influence of ward design on psychiatric patients. For example, there were attempts to encourage social interaction by rearranging chairs around small square tables, to equip a solarium with comfortable and attractive furniture placed to facilitate conversation, and to formulate and test ideas about how physically remodeling wards could effect changes in patients' behavior. Interest in these areas led to studies of how urban dwellers used the space of a city to form images, of the anthropology of space or proxemics, of how certain arrangements of space (defensible space) might affect the crime rate and security in urban housing projects, and so forth (see Proshansky and O'Hanlon, 1977, for more details regarding the emergence and growth of this area).

Developments in ecological psychology, pioneered by Roger Barker, emerged out of the intellectual tradition fostered by Kurt Lewin and Egon Brunswick. Barker's theory includes elements of Lewin's concern with the psychological environment and of Brunswick's emphasis on the ecological setting of behavior. Lewin felt that it was impossible to make predictions about behavior directly from knowledge about the nonpsychological environment (that is, the preperceptual environment). Although he evolved a system of psychological constructs, Lewin had no adequate conceptual bridge to link psychology and ecology.

Kurt Lewin's psychology was a postperceptual psychology, in that he focused on the environment as perceived by the person. Lewin coined the term "foreign hull" to represent the outside preperceptual environment and suggested the phrase "ecological psychology" for the study of influences from the foreign hull on the person (Cartwright, 1951). These influences could stem from aspects of both the physical and the social setting, and, in this respect, the concerns of ecological psychology were formulated somewhat more broadly than those of environmental psychology. Lewin's framework rested primarily on whether the environmental influences were preperceptual (as seen by an "objective" observer) or postperceptual (as seen by the person whose behavior was being studied), rather than on the type of environmental influence involved (physical or social).

Roger Barker and his colleagues have worked in this area for more than three decades. They defined ecological psychology as dealing with naturalistic studies of a person's everyday behavior and his or her psychological situation. They focused on children in a small Midwestern community and evaluated the "psychological situation" using observers' descriptions of the influences parents, teachers, and other children attempted to exert on the specific child they were studying. Primary focus was later shifted from the person (that is, from ecological psychology) to extraindividual behavior-milieu units called behavior settings (that is, to "eco-behavioral science"), which are defined by their environmental characteristics (both physical and social) and by the patterns of behavior that occur in them.

Barker and his colleagues have found that the characteristics of behavior settings (for example, a classroom, a student committee meeting, a school play) may influence the amount of pressure students feel to perform and the extent to which they report being satisfied, developing confidence, being challenged, engaging in important actions, gaining moral and cultural values, and so forth (see Barker and Associates, 1978, and Barker and Schoggen, 1973, for an overview of this line of research). Barker sees behavior settings as composed of three major classes of variables: physical properties, human components, and programs. Environmental psychology focuses primarily on the physical properties of settings and, in a sense, can be conceptualized as one aspect of eco-behavioral science.

Willems has recently illustrated an eco-behavioral approach to problems of health status and health care by focusing on naturalistic studies of the process of rehabilitation from spinal cord injuries. He and his colleagues (Willems, 1976, 1977; Willems and Halstead, 1978) have found that the degree of independence shown by patients varies dramatically among hospital behavior settings; that, contrary to expectations, patients show more independence and active initiation of behavior in the cafeteria and hallways of a rehabilitation ward than in physical or recreational therapy; and that there are substantial variations among settings in the changes patients display, sometimes leading to disagreements among staff members about the degree of patient progress. This work represents an excellent example of the utility of naturalistic observations, in conjunction with a coherent conceptualization of the environment, for monitoring patient behavior and providing clinically useful feedback to staff.

Current interest in public health and environmental psychology derived further impetus from societal concern with environmental factors and their influence on our style of life. For example, crime and physical and mental illness in the slums of industrial cities contributed to the growth of a massive public housing program, in which thousands of families were rehoused in sanitary, modern, and frequently high-rise facilities. Problems of disease and crime were not alleviated by this program. In fact, many new difficulties, which were directly attributable to the poor design of the new projects, particularly the massive high-rise structures, emerged. Social scientists became increasingly interested in the consequences of the design of physical spaces when they were asked to evaluate the effects of public housing programs and the reasons for the failure of these programs.

An Integrative Conceptual Framework

The foregoing overview indicates that a social-ecological perspective has developed somewhat independently in public health and epidemiology, in psychosomatic medicine, and in environmental psychology. A social-ecological perspective provides a distinctive framework by which the transactions between people and their environments, and the impacts of these transactions on human functioning, can be conceptualized. This perspective is being integrated into clinical and community psychology (Holahan, 1978), developmental psychology (Bronfenbrenner, 1977) and gerontology (Lawton and Nahemow, 1973). It is also relevant to many of the concerns of health psychologists.

Figure 1 presents a simplified conceptual framework designed to illustrate the major sets of factors mediating the relationship between environmental and personal variables and health status. I call this framework social-ecological to emphasize the inclusion of social-environmental (for example, social climate) and physical-environmental (that is, ecological) variables, which I believe need to be conceptualized and studied together (Moos, 1976a, chap. 1). The framework is "simplified" because it primarily depicts a unidirectional causal flow, even though there are feedback mechanisms by which the different sets of factors can mutually influence each other. The point is to represent and illustrate the major sets of variables involved in the development of a social-ecological perspective on health.

The Environmental System

Although there is an infinite number of relevant environmental variables, they can be conceptualized in four major groups. Each of the four sets of variables can influence health outcomes directly, as well as indirectly through the other sets; for example, the physical environment's influence on health may be mediated through its effect on the social environment. (See Moos, 1979, chap. 4, for a discussion of the relationships among these sets of environmental variables.)

Physical setting. Relevant variables include geographic and meteorological characteristics (such as temperature, rainfall, topography) of an environment, as well as its architectural and physical design characteristics. There has been extensive work attempting to relate these categories of variables to health. For example, Lynn (1971) has linked high alcoholism and suicide rates, as mediated by an anxiety factor, to climatic variations such as summer heat, storminess, and solar radiation. Hollander and Yeostros (1963) used a climatron (a controlled experimental climate chamber) to study pain sensations of arthritic patients and found that successive occurrence of a "stormlike pressure and humidity" variation had a cumulative deteriorating effect on patients' symptom reports. Moos (1964) found that accident rates in Zurich, Switzerland, were related to the onset of the Foehn (a warm, dry, descending wind found in several regions near the Alps in Europe), and that there was an anticipatory effect, with accident rates being significantly higher during the four hours preceding the onset of the Foehn.

Schuman (1972) found an increase in mortality associated with heat waves in several American cities and noted that this increase was related to certain sociodemographic and other personal characteristics. The poor, the elderly, the physically handicapped, and those with circulatory problems had especially high increases in death rates, up to 140 percent for nonwhite females in St. Louis. Persons with higher income, better medical care, fewer handicapping physical conditions, and access to air conditioning or to the cooler suburbs were less likely to fall into the excess mortality group. Climate variables have also been related to the pattern of admissions to mental hospitals, to suicide, homicide, and accident rates, to physical symptoms, and so on (Moos, 1976a, chap. 3).

Figure 1. A Simplified Model of the Relationship Between Environmental and Personal Variables and Health

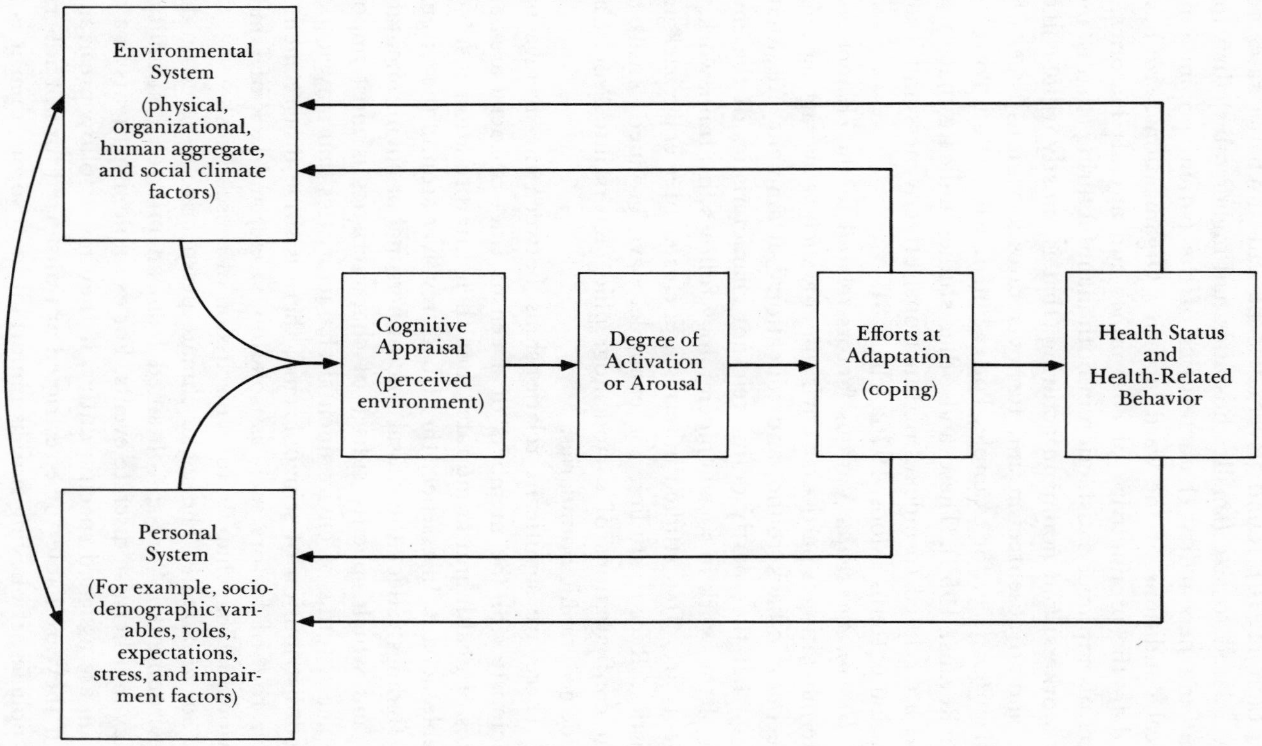

Organizational factors. Organizations such as factories and work plants, colleges and universities, and hospitals and correctional facilities have been extensively studied in relation to their impact on health-related variables. Linn (1970) found psychiatric patient discharge rates to be more highly related to size (smaller hospitals had higher rates) than to the background and personality characteristics of the patient population or to the physical conditions of the ward facilities. Organizational size has also been related to the productivity of coal mines and aircraft factories, to various indexes of employee satisfaction in both manufacturing (that is, mostly blue-collar workers) and nonmanufacturing (that is, mostly white-collar workers) firms, and to absenteeism and turnover rates in various types of industrial organizations (see, for example, Porter and Lawler, 1965; Porter and Steers, 1973; Revans, 1958). These and other studies indicate that organizational factors are related to indexes of functional effectiveness and health services utilization patterns (Moos, 1976a, chap. 8).

Human aggregate. Various factors related to the characteristics of the people inhabiting a particular environment, such as average age, ability level, socioeconomic background, and educational attainment, are situational variables in that they partly define relevant characteristics of the environment. Much of the work in social epidemiology follows this framework, since environments are often studied in terms of a cluster of average background characteristics. Recent studies, for example, have grouped census tracts with similar configurations of sociodemographic factors into "social areas" that override geographic boundaries.

There are significant relationships between the average background characteristics of the members of a census tract or social area and various indexes of health and crime rates, but their interpretation is subject to considerable debate. In essence, the debate revolves around the extent to which these findings reflect the causal role of personal or environmental characteristics and which specific subset of characteristics is most important. For example, in terms of environmental characteristics that may account for the skewed distribution of schizophrenia, there is some disagreement about the relative role of factors such as isolation, stress, and lack of family support (see Moos, 1976a, chap. 9, for a discussion of these issues).

Social climate. The social climate perspective is based on descriptions of environmental "press," obtained from an inferred continuity and consistency in otherwise discrete events. For example, if patients in a psychiatric program are assigned specific duties, if they must follow prearranged schedules, if they are liable to be restricted or transferred for not adhering to program policies, if obeying staff is important, and so on, then it is likely that the program emphasizes staff control and the development of submissive responses on the part of patients. It is these conditions that establish the climate or atmosphere of a setting.

On the basis of extensive work in a variety of social environments, I have conceptualized the basic dimensions in this area in three broad categories (Moos, 1974a, chap. 12; 1976a, chap. 10). *Relationship* dimensions assess the extent to which people are involved in the environment, the extent to which they support one another, and the extent to which they express themselves freely and openly. *Personal growth or goal orientation* dimensions assess the basic directions along which personal development and self-enhancement tend to occur in a particular setting. *System maintenance and system change* dimensions deal with the extent to which the environment is orderly, is clear in its expectations, maintains control, and is responsive to change.

Social climate variables drawn from these categories have been related to important health variables such as complaints of physical symptoms, absenteeism and sick-call rates, and the outcome of psychiatric treatment. For example, classes that are high in competition and teacher control, and low in teacher support, have high student absenteeism rates. University student living groups that are competitive and lack involvement and student influence are characterized by high student complaints of physical symptoms. Military basic training companies that emphasize strict organization and officer control and de-emphasize the enlisted man's personal status tend to have high sick-call rates. Psychiatric wards with few social activities, little emphasis on involving patients in programs, poor planning of patient activities, and staff who discourage criticism from patients and are unwilling to act on patients' suggestions tend to have high dropout rates (see Moos, 1974a, chap. 7; 1975, chap. 12; Moos and Moos, 1978; Moos and Van Dort, in press).

The Personal System

Many sets of personal variables can help to explain individual differences in response to different environmental contexts. Since others have focused on these variables (for example, see Chapters Four and Ten in this volume), I deal with them only briefly here. Background and personal characteristics include age, socioeconomic status, sex, intelligence, cognitive and emotional development, ego strength and self-esteem, and previous coping experiences. These factors influence the meaning that an environment carries for an individual (see Figure 1) and affect the psychological and intellectual resources available to handle the situation. For example, intelligence and the level of cognitive development may play a role in determining an individual's ability to seek or use information to counteract uncertainty or a sense of powerlessness.

Other categories of personal variables include attitudes, values and traits, expectations, roles and role concomitants, and illness-related factors. For example, the roles and role concomitants of an individual affect the way an environment is perceived. People who have more responsible organizational roles (such as managers, staff, and teachers as opposed to employees, patients, and students) tend to perceive organizational environments more positively. Expectations of what environments will be like can also influence both an individual's choice and later perception of those environments. Illness-related factors, which include the type and location of symptoms—

whether painful, disfiguring, disabling, or in a body region vested with special importance, like the heart or reproductive organs—can define the way in which various components of the environment are perceived, the exact nature of the tasks patients and others face, and consequently their adaptive responses.

Mediating Factors: Appraisal, Activation and Adaptation

The role of cognitive appraisal has been heavily emphasized by others, most notably Lazarus (1966), who uses it as a central construct in his formulation of the coping process (see also Chapter Nine in this volume). The main point is that one cannot usually directly relate an "objective" environmental variable to a "dependent" health-related variable. The individual's cognitive appraisal, that is, how the environment is perceived, is usually (though not always) a critical mediating factor. Both the environmental system (for example, through air pollution or carcinogenic agents) and the personal system (through genetic or constitutional predisposition) can affect health status directly—that is, their effects are not necessarily mediated through cognitive appraisal. However, cognitive appraisal is an important mediating factor in the majority of problems to which health psychology is addressed.

Activation or arousal usually occurs when the environment is appraised as necessitating a response. This gives rise to efforts at adaptation and coping, which may change the environmental system (for example, an individual with a mild hearing loss reschedules a conference in a quiet room) or the personal system (for example, a person seeks and obtains information that changes his or her attitudes and expectations). There is a growing literature on coping and adaptation (Haan, 1977), and some sets of coping skills of particular importance in health-related behavior have been identified, for example: denying or minimizing the seriousness of a crisis, seeking relevant information, requesting reassurance and emotional support, learning specific illness-related procedures, setting concrete limited goals, rehearsing alternative outcomes, and finding a general purpose or pattern of meaning in the course of events (Moos, 1977a).

Health Status and Health-Related Behavior

Somewhat different categorizations of the most relevant sets of "dependent" variables have been used to relate these variables to health status (Hinkle, 1977; Kasl, 1977), although the broad types of variables tend to be relatively similar. I choose to categorize these variables into five sets of indexes related to: (1) the onset and development of illness, (2) the course of illness and outcome of treatment, (3) the utilization of health services and compliance with treatment, (4) functional effectiveness, and (5) satisfaction and well-being.

Environmental conditions may also constrain behavior (for example, airport noise may interfere with sleep or conversation, or induce fatigue) and have effects on growth and development not directly linked to an individual's health status. Constant train or airplane noise may retard the development of verbal communication and thus impair reading ability and school performance (Cohen, Glass, and Singer, 1973). Although this is not specifically a "health effect," it is likely to have an impact on a child's self-esteem and competence and to relate to later health status.

Each of the four sets of environmental variables I have described has been related to one or more categories of health status or health-related behavior. However, few if any studies have related dimensions of the environment and personal variables and mediating coping factors to health. To illustrate the utility of the foregoing conceptual framework, we turn now to an overview of research on the health correlates of population density and crowding. The framework helps to organize and comprehend existing research, to formulate and guide future research, and to suggest alternative strategies for practical intervention.

Health Correlates of Population Density and Crowding

In this section, research relating physical and architectural factors to health is discussed, with a focus on studies that include perceptual measures of the physical factors, studies that provide evidence on the mediating impact of social-environmental and personal factors, and studies that detail the adaptive and coping mechanisms involved. My overview of the research is necessarily selective and the reader may wish to consult recent reviews for more information (Baum and Valins, 1977; Hinkle and Loring, 1977; Stokols, 1977).

Physical and Architectural Factors and Health

Demographic studies of population density and crowding. Demographic studies have generally used the number of people per unit of space both as a definition of density and a measure of crowding. In this review, I use the term *population density* to refer to measures of outside density (such as the population per acre in a census tract) and the term *crowding* to refer to inside density (such as the number of people per unit of living space).

Studies of the pattern of physical and mental illness, mortality and accident rates, psychosomatic complaints, and utilization of mental health services have shown that these indexes are higher in urban than in rural areas and highest in the crowded downtown sections of cities (Collins, Kasap, and Holland, 1971; Marsella, Escudero, and Gordon, 1970; Moos, 1976a, chap. 5).

For example, Levy and Herzog (1974) found positive associations between population density in the Netherlands and overall age-adjusted death rate, age-adjusted male death rate for heart disease, admissions to general and mental hospitals, illegitimate births, and divorce. Since the effects of density were adjusted for social class and population heterogeneity, the authors concluded that higher morbidity and mortality rates were associated with living in densely populated areas. Crowding was not highly related to social pathology (in fact, some of the relationships were negative); however, there is little or no overcrowding in the Netherlands.

Galle, Gove, and McPherson (1972) studied four components of population density and crowding in Chicago: the number of persons per room, the number of rooms per housing unit, the number of housing units per structure, and the number of residential structures per acre. They examined the combined influences of the four components and found a relationship with each of five health-related indexes (for example, fertility, delinquency, and mental hospital admission rates) that remained significant even when social class and ethnicity were controlled. They also considered the combined influences of social class and ethnicity on each pathology, uncovering significant relationships; however, these relationships were markedly reduced when the four components of density were controlled, indicating that population density significantly influenced each relationship.

The few studies that have focused on "captive populations," in which the groups living under different conditions of density are comparable on sociodemographic characteristics, have found relationships between crowding and health indexes. Dean, Pugh, and Gunderson (1975) studied naval enlisted men aboard thirteen ships and found that the amount of space available and the social density in specific areas (such as the mess hall, berths, work areas, and sanitary facilities) were related to dispensary visits and accident rates. Studies in correctional institutions have found more frequent complaints of physical symptoms and higher mean blood pressure readings for inmates in crowded dormitory settings than for their counterparts in single or two-person cell settings (D'Atri, 1975; McCain, Cox, and Paulus, 1976).

The evidence indicates that measures of density and crowding are related to health indexes, but the fact that population characteristics (such as social class and ethnicity) and environmental characteristics (density) are inextricably related (that is, they share a considerable portion of the explainable variance in the outcome measures) makes it difficult to draw unequivocal causal implications.

Studies focusing on dwelling units or "primary" environments. The importance of detailed studies of the family living situation, and of including subjective measures of crowding both at the dwelling unit and the neighborhood level, was noted in a recent study of thirteen census tracts in Toronto. Booth and Edwards (1976) found that indexes of household crowding were related to the extent to which parents hit children, to the number of quarrels reported by mothers, and to the quality of the relationship between the spouses. They also noted that subjective household crowding was related to reports that lack of privacy interfered with sexual intercourse, that people living in objectively crowded neighborhoods were more likely to report having engaged in extramarital relations, and that some of the crowding measures were related to the frequency of reports of homosexual experiences and incestuous behavior (Edwards and Booth, 1977). Although these results generally held up when sociodemographic factors were controlled, the crowding variables only accounted for increments of between 1 and 8 percent of the variance in the dependent variables.

A study done in Hong Kong related inside density to measures of stress, entertainment patterns, emotional health, and parental supervision (Mitchell, 1971). People in higher-density dwelling units rated themselves as less happy and more worried than people in lower-density units. High dwelling unit density discouraged friendship practices among neighbors and nonfamily members. Mitchell also found that people in multiple-family dwelling units, who were located on the upper floors of buildings, were more likely to complain of symptoms such as headaches, nervousness, and insomnia. He theorized that crowded interaction with nonrelatives (strangers) is more stressful than crowded interaction with family members. In addition, the adaptive response of going out into the street for more space allows lower-floor dwellers to cope better with crowded multifamily conditions (see also McCarthy and Saegert, 1978).

Two studies have focused on the mediating mechanisms by which dwelling unit density may facilitate the occurrence of respiratory illnesses. Monto and Johnson (1968) found the intrafamilial transmission rates for three actively transmitted rhinoviruses to be significantly related to dwelling unit density, leading them to conclude that crowded sleeping conditions contribute to virus spread. These results were supported by Ota and Bang (1972) in a one-year longitudinal case study of the epidemiology of respiratory virus infections in members of six families living in a crowded section of Calcutta. There was a close relation between dwelling unit density and the frequency of virus isolation from the upper respiratory tract found among the members of the six families, indicating that closeness of contact is a definite contributing factor. Taken as a whole, this set of studies illustrates that crowded conditions can affect health directly (through interpersonal contact) and indirectly (through their effect on emotional resources and coping abilities).

The Interaction of Environmental Factors

Architectural and physical design. Relevant characteristics that may mitigate the effects of density include the presence of gardens and open space, the provision of balconies, light-colored rather than dark-colored rooms, quiet rather than noisy surroundings, the presence of sunlight, and so forth (Rapoport, 1975; Schiffenbauer and others, 1977). In addition, the visual complexity, the presence of pictures, the existence of partitions, the number of doors in a room, and the shape of the room (rectangular versus square) may influence the perceptual and behavioral effects of crowding (Baum and Davis, 1976; Worchel and Teddlie, 1976).

Organizational structure and functioning. The size or number of people in a group (that is, the social density) and the amount of social interaction and level of interpersonal proximity are important factors mediating the effects of crowding. Paulus and his colleagues (1975, 1976) found that higher social density led to less tolerance of overcrowding, more negative affective responses to the physical environment, and decrements in task performance. Other studies have found that the type of activity or task involved and expectations regarding the degree of social structure are important mediators (Baum and Koman, 1976; Cozby, 1973; Stokols, 1976). Kasl (1977) suggests that dwelling unit density is not as important as organizational variables such as the way in which space at home is used; for example, it is possible to set aside times when a particular room is devoted only to quiet pursuits such as studying.

Human aggregate. Several investigators have suggested that greater social heterogeneity should give rise to more experience of crowding (Rapoport, 1975). This notion is supported by Mitchell's (1971) finding of more adverse effects of dwelling unit density when unrelated people shared the same housing unit. Fisher (1974) found that subjects who interacted with a similar, as opposed to those who interacted with a dissimilar, confederate judged the environment to be of higher esthetic quality, perceived themselves to be less crowded, and felt affectively more positive. Saegert (1977) reasons that friends have coordinated habitual patterns of interaction, whereas strangers are often perceived as unpredictable and potentially uncontrollable. They thus require close monitoring, which demands attentional capacity otherwise available for high information processing needs, such as those in complex task performance.

Social climate. Although this area represents a particularly important set of mediating variables, it has received relatively little study. Some studies have focused on the role of cohesion and support in mediating the crowding experience (Levy and Herzog, 1974). Baum, Harpin, and Valins (1975) note that cohesive student groups are less likely to form in crowded dormitory environments, but that the experience of crowding and stress is markedly reduced when they do form. Bickman and his colleagues (1973) found less evidence of helping behavior (support) in larger high-rise than in smaller low-rise dormitories. Students also felt that lower-density buildings tended to have more cheerful, friendly, relaxing, and "warm" social environments.

In other relevant work, Wilcox and Holahan (1976) have shown that high-rise dormitories develop social environments that are less involving, supportive, organized, and permissive of student input and more encouraging of independence than low-rise dormitories. In comparing upper (seven to ten) and lower (one to five) floors of high-rise units, they found that the social climates on the upper floors emphasized less commitment and concern for others and less student input and innovation than that on lower floors. These results suggest that the social environment may be an important mediator of the effects of density and other housing-related characteristics on health. The basic notion is that socially cohesive groups have the capacity to mitigate harmful or aversive effects of high density. The social channels and spatial conventions established by cohesive groups may provide protection for group members from unwanted outside stimulation and interference.

Overall context. The overall context in which environmental stressors occur can play a central mediating role. The importance of the "life setting" context is illustrated by Michelson (1977), who found that families living in high-rise apartments, which were perceived to have grave inadequacies in a wide range of attributes, nonetheless professed to be satisfied. These families thought of the high-rise apartments as interim accommodations, and this assumption of future mobility allowed them to focus on those criteria of the housing that were fulfilled, rather than on the many that were not.

Kasl (1977) emphasizes the broader context and the time dimension, that is, the duration and the expected duration of the stressor. For example, it is probably more difficult to cope with high density under conditions of economic change and high unemployment, which may themselves be related to less cohesion and more conflict (Catalano and Dooley, 1977). There may also be a relationship between overall social change and disorganization and a feeling that one cannot control the environment (Cassel, 1977).

These results indicate that the variables of architectural and physical design, organizational structure and functioning, the human aggregate, and social climate each have mediating effects on the relation between density, crowding, and health. The social context or "life setting" in which an environmental stressor occurs is also important. In general, the evidence suggests that various "environmental resources" (such as cohesion, structure, some open space, and social stability) act as buffers that reduce or totally vitiate the potential adverse effects of density and crowding.

Person-Related Factors

Various authors have underscored the importance of person-related factors in mediating the perception and impact of environmental factors (Stokols, 1976). There is some evidence on the mediating role of three relevant sets of variables: sociodemographic variables, stress and impairment factors, and biological risk factors.

Sociodemographic variables. Age, sex, and socioeconomic status have been studied most extensively. Housewives and young children are more strongly influenced than working husbands and fathers by crowding in households, whether for better (Wilner and others, 1962) or for worse (Fanning, 1967; Kasl, 1977). Recent evidence suggests that variables such as household composition, child supervision, amount of confinement to the dwelling unit, and degree of social isolation do not account for these effects, although feelings of physical insecurity and vulnerability, sex differences regarding the esthetics of living settings, and the fact that "it may be difficult for women who occupy a traditional wife-mother status to perform their roles in man-made environments" may be important (Gillis, 1977, p. 420).

A "vulnerability" explanation is supported by the finding that the effect of population density on age-adjusted heart disease deaths is especially high among men and older age groups (Levy and Herzog, 1974) and by speculations that people with lower education and income are more affected by population density and other environmental stressors (Kasl, 1977; Mitchell, 1971). In addition, McCarthy and Saegert (1978) suggest that findings relating high residential density to social overload and withdrawal in low socioeconomic status tenants may not apply to middle- and upper-income adults, who have more opportunities to choose their residential environments and to live with people with whom they already have social ties.

   Stress and impairment factors. Booth and Edwards (1976) and Edwards and Booth (1977) found that stress, as measured by complaints of psychophysiological symptoms, intensified the problems in family relationships associated with dwelling unit density and increased the frequency with which men engaged in extramarital intercourse. Density is also more likely to affect people who are in an unfamiliar setting, such as migrants or those without prior urban residential experience who move to urban settings (Cassel, 1977).

   In related work, several studies have suggested that prior experience with crowding exacerbates its later effects (Booth and Edwards, 1976; Edwards and Booth, 1977). This supports the notion that a person's expectations of being crowded may be as stressful as or more stressful than actual levels of density. Expectations of being crowded can cause subjects to feel crowded and to take actions aimed at coping with crowding even before a setting actually becomes crowded (Baum and Greenberg, 1975). These and other studies suggest that people who are under stress (such as those who have experienced crowding, who expect to be crowded, who are impaired or subordinated in society, and who are unfamiliar with their setting) are more likely to experience the negative effects of further environmental stressors.

   Biological risk factors. Biological risk factors are an important set of person-related mediating variables but they remain largely unexplored in relation to population density and crowding. In one relevant study, household crowding (people per room) acted as a risk factor for myocardial infarction among women only when biological risk factors (a history of hypertension, angina pectoris, or diabetes) were present (Szklo, Tonascia, and Gordis, 1976). The earlier cited finding that density is more highly associated with age-adjusted male than female death rates for heart disease may also reflect the influence of biological risk factors (Levy and Herzog, 1974).

   McLean and Tarnopolsky (1977) review evidence suggesting that certain groups are at high risk in relation to negative impacts of noise. They conclude that some people fail to habituate to repeated noise, that there are identifiable subgroups of noise-sensitive people, and that hypertensive patients are especially susceptible to noise. For example, they note one community survey in which more people were found under medical treatment for hypertension and heart conditions, and more women were taking cardiovascular drugs, in areas of high aircraft noise exposure. Effects like this have not been documented for crowding, but it is logical to assume that people with high blood pressure, for example, may react with greater pressor responses to crowding than do their normotensive counterparts.

   The evidence on person-related factors is consistent with the *environmental docility hypothesis,* which proposes that people who are disabled, impaired, or under stress are more likely to be influenced by environmental conditions (Lawton and Nahemow, 1973). Other recent reviews also conclude that certain susceptible population groups, such as the very young or old, those with low income or education, and those under stress, are more likely to be affected by population density and crowding, as well as other environmental stressors (Cohen, Glass, and Phillips, 1977; Hinkle, 1977; Kasl, 1977). The notion that certain groups of individuals are more responsive to their environment suggests the hypothesis that greater positive effects of environmental change might be manifested in these groups. One study that bears on this point found that women and young children were somewhat more positively affected by a move to new housing than were other groups (Wilner and others, 1962).

The Role of Cognitive Appraisal of the Environment

Recent investigators have emphasized the intervening processes by which people appraise and cope with the environment, their preventive and reactive responses, and the ways in which they regulate their interaction with one another. Two major models of crowding phenomena—overload and behavioral constraint models—have been formulated.

Cohen (1978) has described an overload or "capacity" model of attention, based on the notion that a person has a limited amount of attention to be allocated at any one time (see also Kahneman, 1973). Information overload occurs when this capacity is exceeded, that is, when there are too many inputs for the system to cope with, or when successive inputs come too quickly. He believes that a person who is exposed to unpredictable environmental stimulation has less attentional capacity available for task performance than would be the case under normal environmental conditions. Stressors such as crowding and noise are viewed in terms of the uncertainty they arouse. Those that occur in a predictable sequence, eliciting little uncertainty, can be monitored at an attenuated level with a small but not substantial demand on attentional capacity, whereas those that occur unpredictably (eliciting high levels of uncertainty) demand a continual monitoring and evaluation process.

Consistent with this model are the findings by MacKintosh, West, and Saegert (1975) that greater social density leads to information overload, an inability to gain a clear image of the environment, and performance decrements and negative affect in people required to complete tasks necessitating understanding and manipulation of the environment. Saegert (1977) distinguishes among three distinct kinds of overload: stimulus overload (such as meaningless noise), information overload (such as crowding or a surfeit of signs on a highway), and decisional overload (such as attempting to construct social relationships in a high density environment, or to respond effectively to complex unpredictable task demands). She suggests that stimulus overload may be ameliorated by adaptation, but that the pressures presented by information or decisional overload result in continuing arousal and stress.

A second promising model, the behavioral constraint model, focuses primarily on the reduced freedom of choice and the loss of behavioral options in crowded settings. Altman's (1977) theory emphasizes personal control in relation to the social and physical environment. The basic notion involves the regulation of interpersonal interaction through a boundary control process. One type of breakdown, "crowding," occurs when there is more interaction than desired. Stokols (1976) believes that crowding involves a perception of insufficient control over events and an assessment of the direction and intentionality of thwarting. Some recent studies strongly support these formulations. For example, one mediator between the type of activity and density preference is whether the presence of other people facilitates (as in parties) or inhibits (as in studying) an individual's goals (Cozby, 1973). Sundstrom (1975) found stress responses to interactions in which confederates introduced intrusion (by leaning forward, touching the subjects, and attempting eye contact as they talked) and goal blocking (which involved inattention and interruptions as subjects talked). Heller, Groff, and Solomon (1977) theorized that both demands placed on attentional mechanisms and the goal blocking created by other subjects mediated performance decrements in a high-density, high physical interaction setting. Several other investigators have also focused on the role of behavioral constraints or goal blocking in mediating the effects of crowding (Galle, Gove, and McPherson, 1972; Loring, 1977) and noise (McLean and Tarnopolsky, 1977).

Although there has been considerable speculation about the role of physiological mediating mechanisms (D'Atri, 1975), very little research has been done in this area. One recent study investigated commuters to Stockholm under different levels of crowding, before (trip 1) and after (trip 2) a period of gas rationing during the oil crisis in 1974 (Lundberg, 1976). Two groups of subjects, one boarding the train at its first stop and the other boarding it midway on its route, were studied. Feelings of discomfort grew more intense as the train approached Stockholm and the number of passengers increased. During both trips, the subjects who made the longer trip had a lower rate of epinephrine and norepinephrine excretion than those who made the shorter trip. The rate of epinephrine excretion was higher for both groups during trip 2 when the train was more crowded. These results indicate that the stress involved in traveling by train varied more with the social and ecological conditions of the trip than with its length or duration. Lundberg speculated that the degree of control over the situation on the train (such as the possibility of choosing seats and company) was the relevant factor in reducing the stress involved and noted that very small changes within a relatively comfortable situation (almost everyone had a seat even in the crowded condition) were associated with changes in physiological arousal. (See Frankenhaeuser and Gardell, 1976, for a review of other studies relating high environmental demand and lack of control over the environment to physiological arousal.)

Adaptation and Coping in Crowding-Related Stress

The foregoing studies, which show that cognitive appraisal—particularly the perception of the degree of predictability and controllability of the environment—is an important mediator of environmental stressors, have also identified a range of cognitive and behavioral mechanisms by which people adapt to crowding stress. Cohen (1978) points out that a typical strategy for dealing with information overload is to use available attention on inputs that are most relevant to the task at hand. Attentional overload may thus result in focusing attention on environmental inputs relevant to a person's own goals and neglecting other social and nonsocial cues, such as those that carry information concerning the moods and subtly expressed needs of others. The neglect of such cues may lower the probability of helping behavior, of expressing sympathy, or of reacting appropriately to another's needs (Korte, Ypma, and Toppen, 1975).

Several investigators have focused on behavioral coping methods linked to withdrawal and isolation. Baum and Greenberg (1975) found that subjects coped with the anticipation of crowding by choosing more socially isolated seat positions and avoiding contact with others (see also Baum and Koman, 1976; Sundstrom, 1975). Crowded parents attempt to bring about order and reduce interaction by using more physical punishment and encouraging their children to go outside (Booth and Edwards, 1976; Mitchell, 1971). Kutner (1973) has noted the importance of visual "overexposure" in mediating reactions to crowding and suggests that people adapt by conforming and reducing the spontaneity of their behavior to gain relative privacy through anonymity.

A greater degree of passivity and helplessness may constitute one form of adaptation to environmental stressors. Rodin (1976a) indicates that chronic density limits prediction and control in the home environment and consequently leads to the development of decreased expectancies for contingency between response and outcome. Thus, as a consequence of high-density living, people may come to feel that they are at the mercy of their environment. Helplessness has been implicated as a precursor of various types of physical and psychological illnesses (Huesmann, 1978; Seligman, 1975). This type of response may be related to the development of chronic heart disease in "Type A" people who initially strive to control their environment but who are awkward and insecure in social settings and may tend to feel helpless and to "give up" in unpredictable and uncontrollable situations (Glass, 1977; Jenkins and others, 1977).

Saegert (1977) notes other related coping mechanisms, such as: (1) reducing the number of decisions made, (2) engaging in more habitual or routine activities, (3) avoiding novel situations, (4) relying on more easily available and interpretable cues, (5) organizing the environment into larger meaningful subunits or "chunks" to facilitate information processing, and (6) relying on external sources, such as religious or political groups, for information. Most of these mechanisms point to a simplification of behavior patterns and a greater dependence on authority or inflexible routines to reduce cognitive complexity.

Focusing on the mediating mechanisms of cognitive appraisal and behavioral adaptation provides further understanding of some of the findings regarding person-related and environmental factors. For example, attentional capacity may be less and social overload greater for the elderly, the disabled, those who are strangers in a new environment, and so forth. Further, the relevance of cohesion and support as "buffering" factors may depend on the fact that friends and acquaintances already have information about each other and have coordinated habitual patterns of interaction that reduce demands on their attentional and decision-making capacities. Recent evidence that women, the less well educated, and the poor are less likely to use efficacious coping mechanisms supports the notion that these "vulnerable" groups are more likely to be exposed to environmental stressors (such as population density and crowding) and, at the same time, have fewer personal resources to handle the resulting stress effectively (Pearlin and Schooler, 1978).

I have tried to illustrate how the research in one area can be understood with the aid of a conceptual model. The work points to the additive or synergistic role of different environmental stimuli, sociodemographic and other personal characteristics, and less effective coping abilities in influencing a generalized susceptibility to disease. My interpretation of the results is that social-environmental and human aggregate variables tend to be more important than physical-environmental or organizational variables in understanding the types of health effects reviewed here. This conclusion is limited, however, by the mutual interrelationships among the four sets of environmental variables (see Moos, 1979, chap. 4), and by their limited variation (this applies particularly to physical and organizational factors) in modern well-developed countries, in which almost all of the relevant studies have been conducted. Regardless of the relative importance of the four sets of environmental factors, it is clear that cognitive and coping variables are essential to an understanding of health and illness and their varied outcomes (see also Kasl, 1977; Hinkle, 1977). Health psychologists can make a distinctive contribution by focusing on these important mediating variables, which other professionals tend to ignore.

The conceptual model can help to organize other bodies of research relating environmental factors to health, such as the effects of weather and other climatic variables on morbidity and mortality, of organizational variables like size and span of control on accident and absenteeism rates, of air and noise pollution on functional effectiveness, and so forth. Each of the sets of variables used earlier (see Figure 1) is important in understanding previous work and in formulating future work. For example, inconsistent or conflicting results on the relationship between physical-environmental and health indexes may be due to the influence of mediating social-environmental and/or person-related factors.

One of the major priorities is the development of systematic assessment and evaluation procedures for describing environments. Our recent work in constructing a Multiphasic Environmental Assessment Procedure (MEAP) to characterize sheltered-care settings for the elderly indicates that it is feasible to develop techniques that can assess the basic sets of environ-

mental variables reviewed earlier (Moos, 1977b). Identifying basic dimensions of human environments is a first step toward creating dependable
knowledge regarding the differential impacts of these environments and their
interaction with relevant mediating appraisal and coping variables.

Health psychologists need to be sensitized to the role of environmental and contextual variables, whereas ecologically oriented professionals
need to be sensitized to the role of social-environmental and person-related
variables. In my view, future attempts to understand health status and
health-related behavior must focus on environmental, personal background,
cognitive appraisal, and coping factors, and their interrelationships, insofar
as this is practically feasible. The model also suggests a number of possibilities for intervention, short of massive changes in the physical environment,
some of which will now be discussed.

Some Promising Practical Applications

Two major sets of suggestions for practical intervention have been developed from the foregoing literature; one focuses primarily on the individual, the other on the environment. Several investigators have emphasized
the importance of providing information to enhance people's sense of control over the environment and their reactions to it. Cohen, Glass, and Phillips
(1977) have suggested that feelings of helplessness and an inability to control
environmental stimuli may be more important than the actual characteristics
of the environment itself. They conclude that health can be improved by
helping people develop increased control over their environment through
more effective community organization. Langer and Saegert (1977) found
that the consequences of crowded environments could be ameliorated
through cognitive means. Providing information that explained and validated
the experience of arousal resulted in reducing the emotional and behavioral
consequences of crowding. This information even had a beneficial influence
in an uncrowded setting, suggesting that it would be useful to teach skills for
coping with different kinds of environments (see also Langer and Rodin,
1976; Pennebaker and others, 1977; Schulz, 1976).

Since the social environment has an important mediating influence on
the effects of other environmental variables, several investigators have suggested the desirability of changing the social climate, particularly by developing cohesion and support. Hinkle and Loring (1977) point to the relevance
of interventions to encourage acquaintance building and other primary rela-
tion-forming activities among "high risk" populations. McCarthy and Saegert
(1978) indicate that designers must try to create environmental units with
which residents can identify (see also Becker, 1977; Sommer, 1972; Steele,
1973). My own work has led me to identify several related areas in which a
social-ecological focus may be useful for evaluating and changing individuals
and community settings, and thus potentially for enhancing health and well-
being (Moos, 1976b).

Facilitating Environmental Change

Feedback and utilization of findings regarding social and physical environments can facilitate environmental change. The methods we use involve four simple steps: (1) a systematic assessment of the environment; (2) feedback to participating groups with particular stress on real-ideal setting differences; (3) planning and instituting specific changes in the setting; and (4) reassessment. Since there is no specific "end point" to this process, continual change and continual monitoring and reassessment may occur. Relevant demonstration studies using this method have been carried out in various settings. For example, the Community-Oriented Programs Environment Scale, which assesses the social environments of community-based psychiatric treatment programs, has been used to facilitate change in an adolescent residential center (Moos, 1974a, chap. 11), to monitor change in alcohol treatment programs (Bliss, Moos, and Bromet, 1976), and to evaluate program stability and change in a residential treatment program for acute schizophrenic patients (Mosher, Menn, and Matthews, 1975).

Information about environments can be used to identify settings in which preventive intervention might be particularly useful. Settings low in involvement, autonomy, and/or student influence, and high in competition, strictness, and control, tend to be characterized by high rates of "dysfunctional" behavior, such as complaints of physical symptoms, sick-call, dropout, and absenteeism rates, and the like. Since high-risk settings of various sorts appear to be characterized similarly by their inhabitants, health psychologists could focus their consultation and preventive intervention attempts on these environments. As the work environments of health care staff (such as intensive care units and terminal cancer wards) can be highly stressful (Moos, 1977a), health psychologists might also consider attempts to evaluate and change these settings for the benefit of both workers and patients.

Formulating Ecologically Relevant Clinical Case Descriptions

Systematic information about patients' environments, such as their work and family settings, should be used in clinical case descriptions and in overall treatment planning. Such information would help health care professionals to understand a patient's life situation better and to plan his or her treatment more rationally. Consider the enormous gain in information if we could describe the "ecological niche" in which an individual patient functions. For example, family cohesion and support are related to positive treatment outcome for alcoholism (Bromet and Moos, 1977), and some evidence indicates that the degree of expressiveness in a family is related to the outcome of treatment for schizophrenia (Brown, Birley, and Wing, 1972). These results suggest that it might be useful to assess the family environment of patients before their release from the hospital to identify those families in which preventive intervention and after-care services might be most beneficial. Similar considerations apply to the treatment and rehabilitation of major physical illnesses such as severe burns, heart attacks, strokes, and organ transplants.

Maximizing Environmental Information

The rapid growth of new social settings has increased the need for descriptions of these settings. Health care professionals know more about the characteristics of entering patients than those patients know about the health care facilities they plan to enter. Currently available descriptions of environments (usually compiled by people who wish to present "their" environment in a positive light) do not seem to give an adequate picture. This results in overly positive and inaccurate expectations, which, in turn, may result in disappointment, low morale, poor functioning, and increased absenteeism, dropout, and turnover rates.

Major ways of conceptualizing environments can provide useful guidelines for writing more accurate and complete descriptions of settings which can then help people select environments (Moos, 1974a, chap. 11). For example, the presentation of information about social environments to their prospective members can reduce discrepant perceptions and expectations and enhance successful adaptation (Leiberman, 1974). One example would involve providing prospective residents a "consumer's guide" to health care facilities, which would include descriptions of their physical and social environments.

Transcending Environmental Pressure

One better way in which to evaluate health care and community settings is to focus on how people cope with environmental stress and transcend environmental pressure. Many people conform to their environments, but some people do not. Studies of these "environmental resistors" and of the coping methods they use would be particularly informative. For example, we identified the personal characteristics that distinguished university students whose level of physical symptoms conformed to the symptom level of their living unit from those whose symptom level did not. Low-symptom females living in high-symptom living groups who did not themselves increase in symptoms ("environmental resistors") were higher in dominance and religious concern and lower in social participation than those who increased in symptoms (Nielsen and Moos, 1977). Further specification of the personal variables that relate to the degree of conformity or resistance to environmental influence is central to understanding the impact of health care and community settings.

Enhancing Environmental Competence

It is necessary to develop health care professionals who understand environments, the kinds of reactions people have in them, and the environmental dimensions and mediating mechanisms involved. When this information is combined with knowledge about how people generally cope with and adapt to different types of environments, then a new role of environmental educator can be implemented. At present, there are some examples of the use of information about social environments as an aid in teaching people who may become environmental educators. For example, the Ward Atmosphere Scale has been used to teach residents and interns about the functioning of psychiatric wards (Moos, 1974a), and the Family Environment Scale has been used as a teaching aid in a course on marriage and family living (Waters, 1976). However, the general utility of this approach remains largely unexplored.

The social climate perspective can sensitize us about what to look for in analyzing social settings. The three types of dimensions (relationship, personal growth or development, and system maintenance and system change) provide a useful way of understanding the confusing complexity of social settings. Understanding these dimensions may help individuals select a wide range of environments in which to participate in their everyday lives. In addition, those responsible for selecting the environments of others (such as for children or the elderly) can do so with a better awareness of the personal traits alternative environments may foster.

Although these areas are promising, I do not wish to minimize the inherent problems and contradictions involved. Willems (1977) has pointed out that seemingly promising interventions may have unintended consequences. For example, in one study, retirement home residents who had initially benefited from a short-term intervention that increased the control and predictability of the environment exhibited precipitous declines in health and psychological status once the study was terminated. In fact, the group of residents who gained most as a result of the interventions also declined most later on. Further work indicated that an intervention to effect a permanent increase in the predictability of the environment (through establishing an individualized orientation program that included detailed information about facility procedures, available services, directions on how to get to different areas of the facility, and the like) had a positive impact that persisted over time (Schulz and Hanusa, 1978).

The best we can do is to try to understand when unintended effects occur, to monitor their emergence, and to attempt to use the resulting information to develop more effective interventions. One general problem is that increased control for one person may lead to decreased control for another and thus to decreased cohesion and support. In addition, too strong a need to control the environment appears to be related to sustained elevation of catecholamines, cholesterol, and blood pressure, and thus to a greater probability of coronary heart disease (Glass, Snyder, and Hollis, 1974). These considerations underscore the necessity for caution and moderation.

Cassel (1976) points out that disease, with rare exceptions, has not been prevented by finding and treating sick individuals but rather by modifying environmental factors facilitating its occurrence. He suggests that we must focus directly on identifying and modifying social-environmental factors that affect disease rather than on screening and early detection. For example, it may be more immediately feasible to improve and strengthen social support than to reduce exposure to environmental stressors. Preventive health services might identify families and groups at high risk by virtue of lack of fit with their environment, and determine the nature and form of social supports that can and should be strengthened if such people are to be protected from disease outcomes. Cassel (1976, pp. 121-122) notes that this is not only economically feasible but also might do more to prevent a wide variety of diseases "than all the efforts currently being made through multiphasic screening and multi-risk cardiovascular intervention attempts." Although this view may be somewhat optimistic, a social-ecological approach to the concerns of health psychologists does hold considerable promise.

21 ∝∾

The Brain as a
Health Care System

Gary Schwartz

∾ This chapter considers some of the implications of theory and research in psychobiology for the emerging field of health psychology. The concept of the "brain as a health care system" is derived from general systems theory (von Bertalanffy, 1968) and cybernetic theory (Wiener, 1948). Recent chapters by the author (Schwartz, 1977b, 1977c, 1978, 1979) have illustrated some of the implications of this approach for biofeedback, psychotherapy, and behavioral medicine. The present chapter considers these ideas in the context of health psychology. We will argue that modern biological theory, rather than disparaging the importance of behavioral factors in health and illness, provides a strong justification and foundation for evaluating the importance of (and determining the mechanisms underlying) behavioral factors in the etiology, pathogenesis, diagnosis, treatment, and rehabilitation of disease processes.

General systems theory provides the basic framework underlying the present analysis; it utilizes systems concepts of feedback, self-regulation, and disregulation. We will focus especially on the general process of *disregulation*, a term used to describe the conditions under which normally integrated, self-regulatory systems (be they atomic, chemical, biological, or

Note: This chapter is adapted from Schwartz (1979).

social) may become imbalanced with regard to their underlying positive and negative feedback loops. Briefly stated, the attenuation or *disconnection* of regulatory, negative feedback loops among parts of a system can result in the process of disregulation. The effects of such disregulation are observable in the behavior of the system, which may become less stable, less rhythmic, and more disordered. Such disordered behavior of a physiological system is often labeled medically as "disease."

One psychological procedure for producing a disconnection within the human organism involves *disattention*. Hence, we can posit that disattention is one condition that can lead to a neuropsychological disconnection (between brain and body), resulting in disregulation. Disregulation is observed as a disordered relationship between brain and body which can contribute to disease. Therefore, Disattention → Disconnection → Disregulation → Disorder → Disease.

It follows that the converse reflects one condition in which the brain may act as an adaptive, health care system. When the brain attends to peripheral organs (thereby connecting itself neuropsychologically to the body) we should initiate self-regulatory processes. This self-regulation should lead to a more stable, balanced, ordered relationship between brain and body that may promote psychobiological health. Therefore, Attention → Connection → Self-Regulation → Order → "Ease" (or Health).

This chapter is both an introduction to and a progress report on this theoretical position. Systems and cybernetic theory in general, and the disregulation principle in particular, can help integrate diverse theories and findings in relevant health psychology areas such as biofeedback, suggest new experiments and procedures for analyzing and interpreting psychophysiological data, and provide the beginnings of a biobehavioral model of health and illness. Since the present framework grew out of the biofeedback literature, and since this literature is of special relevance to health psychology, the biofeedback approach will be used as a model system for presenting the framework. However, this chapter is not intended to be a comprehensive review of the basic or clinical literature on biofeedback (or other relevant areas in psychobiology) but rather is organized to illustrate some of the many directions and applications implicit in a psychobiological approach to health psychology.

General Systems Theory, Biofeedback, and Physiological Patterning

General systems theory, so termed by von Bertalanffy almost forty years ago, and well described in his book of that title (1968), is not really a theory per se but a metatheory. It should be thought of as a general approach or strategy, a way of thinking about defining and solving problems. An excellent book describing the systems approach is Weinberg's (1975) appropriately titled *Introduction to General Systems Thinking*. The reader interested in the systems approach should study these volumes for an introduction to the philosophy, mathematics, and applications of systems theory applied to all disciplines of science. The edited volume by Laszlo (1972) is also useful in this regard. More advanced presentations can be found in the set of volumes, *General Systems Yearbooks*, published annually since 1956 by the Society for General Systems Research. Journal articles reflecting the systems approach applied to all fields of science can be found in *Behavioral Science*, the official journal of the Society for General Systems Research.

As described by von Bertalanffy (1968), general systems theory is no stranger to engineering, biology, or behavior. On the contrary, systems theory evolved from the technology of engineering, in which mathematics for describing the *behavior* of machines were developed and applied to biological control systems. The concepts and mathematics were sufficiently general that they could be adapted to the study of larger systems such as economics. Within the behavioral sciences, systems theory was embraced by a group of psychiatrists concerned with multidisciplinary, biopsychosocial approaches to health and illness. According to Grinker (1967, p. ix): "If there be a third revolution (that is, after the psychoanalytic and behavioristic), it is in the development of a general (systems) theory."

It is impossible to present general systems theory briefly and do it justice. However, we should point out that at the most rudimentary level, general systems theory is concerned with the *behavior* of *any system* (atomic, chemical, cellular, organ, organism, social); hence, the selection of the title *Behavioral Science* for the journal of the Society for General Systems Research. The deep principle underlying systems theory, the one often missed or erroneously viewed as being trivial, is that the *behavior of a system emerges from dynamic interaction of its parts*. To understand how the system (any system) works as a *whole*, it becomes necessary to study its properties (its behavior) as a whole. This requires that the investigator appreciate the fact that complex and often unique *interactions* can occur between parts in a system. The parts, in interaction, are ultimately responsible for the unique properties or behaviors that occur when the system behaves as a whole. The concept of the "whole being greater than the sum of its parts but dependent upon the organization of the parts for its emergent properties as a whole" is at the heart of this realization.

This seemingly simple concept has important implications for scientific research in general, and health psychology research in particular. It implies that we must begin to develop conceptual (albeit tentative) models that consider the *set* of underlying components hypothesized to be relevant to the process of self-regulation (based on current knowledge). Then we must conduct research that examines the interactions of such components as they contribute to learned self-regulation. The study of the whole requires that we systematically examine combinations, and therefore patterns, of the parts.

Although this writer was not aware of it then (for example, Schwartz, 1975, 1976), the biofeedback research suggesting that self-regulation of patterns of responses could have different effects from those observed when controlling individual functions alone followed directly from systems theory.

Similarly, the concept that physiological patterning involves unique *interactions of components* that contribute to the *emergent experience* of consciousness and emotion (Schwartz, 1975, 1977a) also reflects a basic tenet of systems theory. The study of patterns (or combinations, or interactions of component parts) requires more complex experimental designs and more complex procedures for psychophysiological data analysis and interpretation than those currently in use.

These general points are well stated by von Bertalanffy (1968, p. 38):

> It looks, at first, as if the definition of systems as "sets of elements standing in interaction" is so general and vague that not much can be learned from it. This, however, is not true. For example, systems can be defined by certain families of differential equations and if, in the usual way of mathematical reasoning, more specified conditions are introduced, many important properties can be found of systems in general and more special cases.
>
> The mathematical approach followed in general systems theory is not the only possible or most general one. There are a number of related modern approaches, such as information theory, cybernetics, game, decision, and net theories, stochastic models, operations research, to mention only the most important ones. However, the fact that differential equations cover extensive fields in the physical, biological, economical, and probably also the behavioral sciences, makes them a suitable access to the study of generalized systems.

One frustrating aspect of general systems theory is that it not only teaches us how much we do not know but it also points out how many things we should know in order to do justice to the specific problems under investigation. Most behavioral scientists (this author included) have had no formal training in general systems theory. Specific training in the mathematics and biology relevant to systems theory is usually not a required part of the educational system of a psychologist. Fortunately, some of the principles of systems theory are sufficiently fundamental and intuitive that they can have an immediate impact on one's theory and research. At the same time, general systems theory stimulates the need for continued education required of investigators working on interdisciplinary problems.

At first glance, it may appear surprising to discover how little impact up to now general systems theory has had on the specific area of biofeedback. Given that the term *biofeedback* implies biological feedback—which implies cybernetics and techniques of mathematical descriptions of self-regulatory processes, which in turn implies general systems theory—one may wonder why the recognition of the relevance of systems thinking to biofeedback research has not been widely appreciated. As implied above, one likely explanation is that biofeedback grew primarily out of the behavioral sciences (particularly psychology). Until very recently, psychology based its science and training on the early models of physics as opposed to the more recent models of biology. Whereas classic physics emphasized simple, closed systems (for example, systems that are considered to be isolated from their environment), modern biology and modern physics have tended to emphasize open systems interacting with closed systems.

To paraphrase von Bertalanffy (1968), every living organism is essentially an open system, maintaining itself in a continuous inflow and outflow, a building up and breaking down of components. Open systems are never, so long as they are alive, in a state of chemical and thermodynamic equilibrium, but are maintained in a so-called steady state (which is distinct from the former). It should be noted that biofeedback brings closed-loop and open-loop system concepts together, adding complexity to the analysis but also potential richness to our understanding. In fact, as Mulholland (1977a, 1977b) has illustrated, the biofeedback experiment can be seen as a general model of the scientific method. This point is important for psychobiological research in health psychology and will be returned to in the next section.

The main point to be emphasized here is that the orientation of general systems theory should not be alien to researchers in health psychology. We propose that the general systems approach provides a useful framework for conceptualizing and investigating the interactions of parts of systems, which in the biofeedback literature has been referred to as *patterning* of responses or mechanisms of *multiple* processes. To understand specific mechanisms in health and illness, it becomes necessary to understand general mechanisms of feedback processes and interactions of component parts in systems. The concept of self-regulation in cybernetics—and its opposite, disregulation—can be a fruitful place to begin.

Cybernetic Theory, Biofeedback, and Self-Regulation

The concept of a self-regulating system is fundamental to the field of cybernetics (Wiener, 1948). Although general systems theory is sometimes equated with cybernetic theory, this is an error. Cybernetic theory is a *subset* of general systems theory, a part or component of the general systems perspective. Cybernetics is specifically concerned with how a system becomes self-regulatory, be the system mechanical, biological, or social.

Cybernetic theory, like general systems theory, evolved from a number of sources. Of particular relevance to research in biofeedback are these comments by von Bertalanffy (1968, p. 16): "It is true that cybernetics was not without precursors. Cannon's concept of homeostasis became a cornerstone in these considerations. Less well-known, detailed feedback models of physiological phenomena had been elaborated by the German physiologist Richard Wagner (1954) in the 1920s, the Swiss Nobel Prize winner W. R. Hess (1941, 1942) and in Eric von Holst's *Reafferenzprinzip*. The enormous popularity of cybernetics in science, technology, and general publicity is, of course, due to Wiener and his proclamation of the Second Industrial Revolution."

Cybernetics is concerned with a difficult, philosophically significant problem. How can a biological or mechanical system demonstrate intentionality, purpose, will? Must we view such discussions as being teleological and therefore beyond the scope of scientific study? Apparently not. Cybernetic theory proposes specific models or mechanisms for processes that, at first glance, may appear teleological. According to Frank and others (1948, p. 191): "The concept of teleological mechanisms, however it may be expressed in different terms, may be viewed as an attempt to escape from these older mechanistic formulations that now appear inadequate, and to provide new and more fruitful conceptions, and more effective methodologies for studying self-regulating processes, self-orientating systems and organisms, and self-directing personalities. Thus the terms *feedback, servomechanisms, circular processes* may be viewed as different but equivalent expressions of much the same basic conception."

The reader interested in cybernetic theory can find a useful introduction in von Bertalanffy's (1968) book, as well as in the elementary book written by Parsegian (1972). The classic volume by Wiener (1948) should be read for a more detailed presentation of the theory. A representative sample of advanced books on the properties and mathematics of control theory in biological systems includes volumes by Bayliss (1966), Grodins (1963), and Milsum (1966).

It is impossible to present cybernetic theory briefly and do it justice. However, we should point out that the basis of cybernetic self-regulation theory involves the operation of a negative feedback loop. A negative feedback loop serves the important function of stabilizing the behavior (output of the system) by correcting the input. Simply stated, the input to the system is modulated by feedback from the output. Undesired disruptions to the output are subtracted from the input (in the case of negative feedback) to correct or stabilize the system. Negative feedback, so to speak, removes the "error" at the output by altering the input accordingly. The concept of feedback, like the concept of system, is elegantly simple, but deceptively so.

If the concept of negative feedback is so simple, we can wonder why the theory and mathematics of cybernetics has had so little impact up to now on research in biofeedback. Part of the reason is likely due to the fact that cybernetic theory has not been a standard component of the training of behavioral scientists. However, there is another equally important reason. We propose that part of the reason has to do with our failure to grasp fully the fundamental significance of the general concept of negative feedback for self-regulation.

For example, one of the deep implications of negative feedback is that a self-regulatory system (when such a system is intact) acts in an *automatic* fashion. The system behaves in a self-regulatory (that is, purposeful) manner by the very nature of its own construction. In other words, the very connection of a negative feedback loop has automatic, self-regulatory consequences for the behavior (output) of the system. Once the loop is connected (if it is a negative loop, meaning attenuation of the input to the system is a function of the output), self-regulation occurs on its own.

When we apply this concept to a biofeedback situation, it follows that once the person is connected to a new *negative* biofeedback loop, *automatic* self-regulatory changes among brain, body, and the biofeedback should occur. Note that the person need not "try" to change the feedback to obtain these self-regulatory effects. In fact, the person need not be aware of the complex self-regulatory processes that will take place. Theoretically, all the person need do is attend to the feedback (which is how the loop is connected, so to speak, to the person's nervous system). Once the connection is made, the self-regulatory effects of the negative feedback should be automatic. Parenthetically, automatic effects should also occur if the feedback is of a positive nature, though the behavior of a person's physiology in a positive feedback loop will differ accordingly. Here too, the person need not "try" to control the feedback—the effects of a positive feedback loop should occur automatically, without conscious awareness, so long as the person processes the stimuli (attends to the feedback and thereby connects the loop).

This is the basis for the research program conducted by Mulholland (1977a, 1977b). In a series of elegant studies, Mulholland has connected the EEG alpha from various sites (left versus right, posterior versus anterior) to environmental stimuli (typically lights or slides) to create a negative feedback loop situation. For example, the slide might be turned ON whenever alpha in the left occipital region appeared, and the slide would remain ON so long as the alpha was present. Since light (visual stimuli), particularly when attended to by the subject, leads to attenuation of alpha in the occipital region (alpha blocking), then connecting the slide in a negative feedback pathway should result in the autonomic, self-regulatory process of cortical stabilizing as the "new" system begins a behavioral sequence of alpha ON/alpha OFF in synchrony with the slide OFF/slide ON loop connected. Note that *mean* alpha abundance need not be changed (if instructions to change alpha abundance are not given to the subjects) when compared to yoked feedback. Nonetheless, the *temporal pattern* of alpha ON/alpha OFF can still be changed by the connection of this new loop.

These self-regulatory, stabilizing effects of biofeedback occur *automatically* in the sense that the subject need not be told that he or she is connected to a feedback loop. Furthermore, the subject need not be instructed to try to regulate the slides, turning them ON and OFF in any particular fashion. The subject need only be instructed to attend to the feedback. These effects occur without the subject consciously attempting to control his or her EEG.

Mulholland proposes that such self-regulatory effects should be highly selective in the sense that only those parts of the nervous system relevant to the nature of the feedback loop (in the instance given, left occipital processes) should be self-regulated. Hence, Mulholland would predict that the stabilizing effects of the particular negative feedback loop just described should be greater for occipital EEG than parietal EEG, and greater for left hemisphere activity than right. One implication of such a finding is that it should be possible to use biofeedback as a research tool for understanding how the nervous system normally works. By discovering which components are spontaneously brought into self-regulation by establishing experimentally particular feedback loops, it should be possible to map the *pattern* of processes involved in the processing, registration, and interpretation of stimuli.

We must emphasize that these self-regulatory effects can only be detected if appropriate statistics for assessing temporal patterns of responses are employed. The use of simple means must be supplemented by measures of variability, such as standard deviation (and, ideally, more complex time series statistics) if the nature of these self-regulatory effects is to be observed and understood.

To summarize thus far, biofeedback can have automatic regulatory effects on the stabilization (or destabilization) of psychophysiological self-regulation as a function of the specific properties of the feedback loops connected. We should mention that these properties will be influenced not only by the nature of the *feedback* and the way it is connected to the output (for example, factors such as modality, complexity, intensity of stimuli, and the nature of the contingency or connection created—continuous, discrete, yoked) but also will be influenced by the nature of the *organism* and how he or she processes the stimuli (for example, factors such as the instructions used, state of the person—aroused, deprived of particular stimuli—personality and cognitive style, and so forth).

It seems unlikely that a complete understanding of biofeedback effects will emerge without our considering the concept of self-regulation more broadly. The basic concept of negative feedback and its effects on stabilizing a system has important implications for the kinds of research that are conducted, the ways in which the data are analyzed, and the depth of the conclusions that are drawn. In the same way that there is more to the self-regulation of patterns of processes than simply the control of individual functions alone (as described in the previous section), there is more to the regulation of parts in a system than changes in simple mean rates of the parts per unit period of time.

Even when subjects are subsequently instructed (or self-instruct themselves) to change the mean frequency of their behavior, we can hypothesize that they will do so by altering internal feedback loops, both within the brain and between the brain and body. Cybernetic theory would lead us to predict that both the mean and variability of the behavior will change as a result of (1) the new external feedback and (2) the new instruction or set of internal feedback connections. It should be noted, however, that simply quantifying response measures such as standard deviation and cross-correlations is of little value if we do not have a theoretical context in which to interpret such numbers. Cybernetics and systems theory provides such a framework.

Before we discuss the application of cybernetic theory to understanding some of the inherent health care properties of the nervous system and the conditions under which the nervous system can become disregulated and disordered, we should briefly consider some of the broader implications of cybernetic theory for developing a general systems model of scientific research. As Mulholland (1977a, 1977b) has illustrated, the terms (1) input, system, and output (in cybernetics) can be replaced by the terms (2) stimulus, organism, and response (in psychology) and can also be replaced by the terms (3) independent variable, system, and dependent variable (in science in general). Mulholland suggests that once this translation of terms is made, it becomes self-evident that we can have: (1) open- and/or closed-loop cybernetic systems (in the latter, negative feedback is connected from output to input); (2) open- and/or closed-loop conditions in psychology (in the latter, a case in point is the development of operant conditioning—for negative feedback, punishment—involving the establishment of a contingency or connection between the response and the stimulus; a more recent case is the development of biofeedback, where the "response" is now "physiological" and is connected via a contingency to produce an environmental stimulus); and therefore (3) open- and/or closed-loop paradigms (Kuhn, 1962) in science (in the latter, there is a systematic use of negative feedback, stabilizing loops placed between the dependent and independent variables with the goal of improving one's ability to uncover processes linking the independent and dependent variables).

The important point to recognize here is that the concept of feedback can be broadened in such a way as potentially to improve the basic process of scientific discovery itself. The challenge here is to develop research paradigms that make creative use of the unique properties of negative feedback loops in health psychology. Parenthetically, we might note that our very capacity to recognize the fundamental *commonality* underlying cybernetic theory, health psychology, and the nature of scientific discovery in general is an illustration of general systems thinking at work.

The Brain as a Health Care System

By drawing on systems theory in general, and cybernetic theory in particular, it is possible to develop a biobehavioral model of the brain and nervous system in its role as a health care system. Figure 1 shows a highly simplified block diagram for expressing the main subsystems linking a person (numbers 2, 3, and 4) to his or her external environment (numbers 1 and 5). In systems terms: Stage 1 in the external environment reflects input stimulation to the system. Stage 2 reflects the information-processing subsystem (the brain) of the system (note that, for convenience, the sensory receptors for registering the environmental inputs are not drawn in this diagram). Stage 3 depicts the output from the system.

It is important to recognize that the output (Stage 3) can be skeletal (as in a behavioral response, as defined by a psychologist) or it can be autonomic or glandular (as in a physiological or endocrine response, as defined by a biologist). The diagram was drawn deliberately so as not to separate behavioral responses from physiological responses. This is because from a

Figure 1. Simplified block diagram depicting (Stage 1) environmental demands
influencing—via exteroceptors, not shown—(Stage 2) the brain's regulation of its
(Stage 3) peripheral organ, and (Stage 4) negative feedback from the periphery back to
the brain. Disregulation can be initiated at each of these stages. Biofeedback (Stage 5)
is a parallel feedback loop to Stage 4, detecting the activity of the peripheral organs
(Stage 3) and converting it into environmental input (Stage 1) that can be used
by the brain (Stage 2) to increase self-regulation.

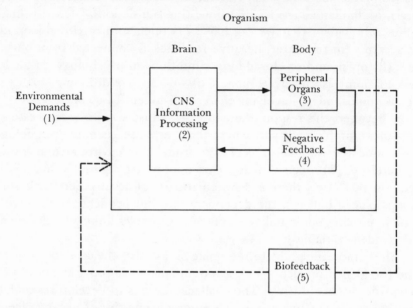

Note: CNS = central nervous system.

Source: Schwartz (1977c).

systems point of view, "behavior" to a psychologist is actually a patterned
combination of "physiological" parts (behavior *is* physiology); conversely,
what a physiologist studies is the "behavior" of the "physiological" parts!
Ultimately, psychologists and physiologists are dealing with the same system,
even though they may label it differently and may look at different parts or
combinations of the parts. From this perspective, "behavior" can play a
direct role in "physiological" health and illness.

It is also important to recognize that different parts can serve different
functions in the complete system. Obviously, a more complete diagram
would begin to subdivide. For example: Stage 3 outputs into different subsystems based on both anatomical and functional grounds. Stage 1 factors
would be subdivided into visual, auditory, or tactile stimulation (some of
these stimuli would be classified as psychosocial), whereas other Stage 1 factors would be subdivided into chemical, cellular, and other groupings (stimuli typically studied by biologists or biomedically trained persons). Of
course, the latter may (or may not) have a direct (immediate) effect on the
central nervous system or CNS (Stage 2). However, our goal at this point is
not to get lost, so to speak, in classifying the huge variety of trees making up
the forest (environment, brain, and body) without first appreciating the
basic components that define the forest (Stages 1 to 4).

If an organism consisted only of Stage 1, 2, and 3 processes, such an organism would be a simple, open-loop system consisting of input, processing, and output components. Such a system would be prone toward instability, since in response to Stage 1 inputs, the Stage 2 system would activate Stage 3 outputs without any 'knowledge or feedback of the ultimate Stage 3 effects. However, human organisms (and animals in general) are equipped with numerous Stage 4 input devices (biological transducers) that detect the status of the Stage 3 behavior and feed this information back to the brain (Stage 2) in a closed-loop fashion. For the most part, these feedback mechanisms operate as negative feedback loops. They act to stabilize, dampen, or buffer the behavior occurring at the output.

The connections linking Stages 2, 3, and 4 are fundamental to Cannon's (1932) concept of homeostasis. It is generally recognized that the self-regulatory properties of visceral and glandular homeostasis operate automatically in the sense that they occur quite reliably when the entire system is *functional and intact*. The capacity of the brain/body system (Stages 2 and 3) to maintain stability in light of insults from the external environment (Stage 1) requires the self-regulatory properties of an intact negative feedback, homeostatic system (Stage 4).

However, it is often not recognized that this same basic, automatic process is fundamental to the self-regulation of sensory and motor behavior as well. In fact, as reviewed in the important book by Powers (1973), the voluntary production of smooth, deliberate motor behaviors requires the automatic functioning of intact negative feedback mechanisms at various levels, from receptors in the skeletal muscles to neural circuits in the spinal cord, through loops in the cerebellum all the way to higher cortical centers.

The concept of the brain and body as a complex feedback system is not new. For example, Ashby (1960) has presented a useful introduction to this concept in his book *Design for a Brain*, and Arbib (1972) has extended this approach in his book *The Metaphorical Brain*. Unfortunately, despite the fact that most students of physiological psychology and medicine recognize these concepts, few seem to have taken them seriously in furthering the development of biobehavioral models of health and illness.

The concept of the human organism as being composed of essential self-regulatory feedback systems is emphasized in the work of A. R. Luria, a Russian neuropsychologist. Luria's work is based on the general concept of functional systems as proposed by Anokhin (1935). As Luria writes in *The Working Brain* (1973, p. 27):

> When we speak of the "function of digestion" or "function of respiration," it is abundantly clear that this cannot be understood as a function of a particular tissue. The act of digestion requires transportation of food to the stomach, processing of the food under the influence of gastric juice, the participation of the secretions of the liver and pancreas in this processing, the act of contraction of the walls of the stomach and intestines, the propulsion of the material to be assimilated along the

digestive tract, and finally, absorption of the processed components of the food by the walls of the small intestine.

It is exactly the same with the function of respiration.
The ultimate object of respiration is the supply of oxygen to
the alveoli into the blood. However, for this ultimate purpose to
be achieved, a complex muscular apparatus incorporating the
diaphragm and the intercostal muscles, capable of expanding
and contracting the chest and controlled by a complex of nervous structures in the brain stem and higher centers, is necessary.

It is obvious that the whole of this process is carried out,
not as a simple "function," but as a *complete functional system*
embodying many components belonging to different levels of
the secretory, motor, and nervous apparatus. [Italics in original.]

Luria argues that the basic concept of functional systems should be
applied equally to the structure of the brain itself. In the same way that
respiration cannot be localized solely in the lungs, or digestion solely in the
stomach, neither can the neural regulation of breathing be localized solely in
a single respiratory "center" in the brain. According to Luria, the brain coor-
dinates *multiple* areas (patterns) of neural tissues to meet specific functional
goals.

Luria (1973, p. 21) goes one step further by providing a foundation
for understanding the relationship between cognitive processes and multiple
systems in the brain: "Mental functions, as complex functional systems, cannot be localized in narrow zones of the cortex or in isolated cell groups, but
must be *organized in systems of concertedly working zones, each of which
performs its role in complex functional systems*, and which may be located
in completely different and often far distant areas of the brain" (italics in
original). However, how do these patterns of processes become organized?
Are they all interconnected at birth, or are additional neural functional
systems created in the individual brain through experience and feedback
from the external environment? Luria is very explicit on this point, emphasizing the special nature of the human brain to modify itself with external
feedback.

It is a short step for us to propose that *the brain engages continually
in self-regulatory behavior, most of which occurs at an unconscious level, for
the purpose of maintaining the health and well-being of itself and its body.*
The brain continually makes adjustments in its regulation of all the major
systems in the body (including respiratory, cardiovascular, and endocrine
systems) as a function of the feedback it receives from the periphery. This
feedback (Stage 4) must be intact and it must be appropriately registered and
processed by the brain (Stage 2) if the appropriate self-regulation of a
peripheral organ (Stage 3) is to be made. If an attenuation (or in extreme
forms, disconnection) occurs anywhere in this system, the system can become disregulated, go out of control, and its health care functions will
become disordered (Schwartz, 1977c, 1978, 1979).

It follows from this perspective that human beings are always acting as a complex health care system, even though, for the most part, they are not conscious of this fact. However, human beings may become aware of this self-regulatory process when the feedback is registered in consciousness. The everyday example of a normal, self-regulated person eating when "hungry" and stopping when "full" involves the operation of complex negative feedback systems between brain and body.

Similarly, if a part of the body becomes injured, for whatever reason (for example, by a germ or a physical assault from the external environment), the normal person may experience pain. The pain can act to *force* the person to *change* behavior for the sake of the injured organ. Consider the common example of breaking a limb. If localized pain is experienced by the brain, appropriate health-related behaviors may be instigated by the brain. In fact, a normal, adaptive person will learn *not* to use the limb for a period of time so that it may heal. The adaptive brain not only will *localize* where the limb is injured but will also learn to *anticipate* that particular commands to the limb may lead to pain and therefore should not be engaged in. Note that the potential for this self-correcting learning process to occur is built into the normal organism. It follows that if disruptions occur anywhere within Stages 2, 3, 4, the system can become disregulated and go out of control (Schwartz, 1977c).

When people "feel sick" (a negative feedback process), they typically do not randomly change their behavior but do so in a manner that ultimately reduces the experience of the negative feedback (Stage 4) and, in the process, we hope, eliminates the causes of the feedback (Stage 3). Note that whether people (1) use their eyes and ears to examine their bodies, (2) palpate sore parts of their bodies and feel their foreheads with their hands, or (3) take their temperature with a thermometer, they are engaged in a Stage 5 feedback process as diagrammed in Figure 1. Of course, there are great differences in complexity between taking one's pulse by hand and doing so with an EKG, especially if a health care professional is added to the loop as part of the Stage 5 process. Certainly, more information can be obtained in the latter case. Also, a greater selection of Stage 1 inputs (therapies) may be placed back into the system as a result. However, Figure 1 is deliberately drawn to focus our attention on the underlying commonality of (1) taking one's pulse by hand, (2) having a nurse take one's pulse by hand and tell one the value, or (3) having a cardiologist take an EKG and tell one the rate. Each of these three situations involves the implementation of a Stage 5 biofeedback process. What varies are (1) the information gathered, (2) the degree to which that information is fed back (directly or indirectly via the health care professional), and (3) the modifications in the environment (Stage 1) that are proposed to alter the behavior of the disordered system.

The general concept of the brain as a health care system has a number of important implications for specific research in biofeedback and, more broadly, health psychology. One implication is that from a biobehavioral, systems point of view, *all health behavior involves self-regulation and hence self-responsibility*. If the brain evolved with one of its primary functions being to preserve itself and its body, then it follows that we should be taught to recognize the fact that we are ultimately responsible for our own health. This need not imply that the person is always responsible for becoming sick or injured, even though the more that we learn about the role of the central nervous system in nutrition, immune functions, stress reactions, and the like, the more we can understand the contributing role that human behavior plays in susceptibility to disease. Rather, what we are suggesting is that, in the final analysis, the person is ultimately responsible for detecting feedback indicating that something is wrong and for seeking appropriate procedures to correct the problem. In fact, a systems analysis of the design of the brain and body provides us with one of the best arguments for placing health care in the hands (or more appropriately, the brains—Stage 2) of the individual.

A second implication of the concept of the brain as a health care system is that *all* treatments involve (at least indirectly) *all* five stages to varying degrees. Consider the role of the brain (Stage 2) in each of the following: Whether the treatment involves changing one's environment (Stage 1, such as reducing pollutants in the air or leaving the polluted environment), changing one's attitudes and behavior (Stage 2, such as developing better habits of eating or exercising or relaxing), changing one's body directly (Stage 3, undertaking surgery or taking drugs that reduce excitation of the peripheral organ in question), or changing the feedback (Stage 4, undergoing surgery for baroreceptor stimulation therapy)—all these techniques involve cooperation, if not active involvement, of the brain and nervous system. Note that it is the brain (Stage 2) that attempts to change the environment or leave it, engages in exercise or changes diet, decides to undergo surgery, or engages in the process of taking pills. All therapies involve patient compliance or, more appropriately stated, they all involve patient self-regulation. There is not a single intervention that does not in one way or another involve self-regulation on the part of the person. It follows that even surgery (a Stage 1 intervention directed often at Stage 3 without regard to Stage 2) should not be performed without considering the state of the person's cognitions and emotions (Stage 2). To summarize, *all* therapies can be seen as being ultimately *biobehavioral* in the sense that they all involve an interaction of Stage 2 processes with all other parts of the system comprising the organism in his or her environment.

The concept of the brain as a health care system provides a useful foundation for applying the paradigm of general systems theory to clinical research. For example, the concept of "holistic" medicine becomes more meaningful, and can conceivably become more systematic, when approached from an integrative biobehavioral systems point of view.

It follows from the preceding analysis that biofeedback (Stage 5) is ultimately a component in *all* therapies (Schwartz, 1978). This conclusion is not widely recognized. Typically, biofeedback is thought to apply only to the specific situation where the person is encouraged (via Stage 1 instructions) to use the feedback (Stage 5) to regulate his or her physiology (Stage 3) and therefore reduce symptoms (detected by Stage 4) by thought processes per se (Stage 2).

However, we propose that this is a very limited view of biofeedback. *From a systems point of view, biological feedback* (Stage 5), *to use a broader term, is actually employed in various ways in all therapies.* Patients learning new relaxation, exercise, or diet habits must obtain intermittent biological feedback (Stage 5) to determine whether the self-regulation regime is effective in controlling the response in question. In the case of high blood pressure, for example, one monitors blood pressure (Stage 5) to determine whether the particular diet, exercise, relaxation, psychotherapy, or other intervention is actually producing the desired end state. Even when a physician prescribes drugs based on whatever biological tests (Stage 5) were used, the physician must continually monitor the Stage 5 feedback to ensure that the prescribed drug treatment is having its desired effects.

When we propose that Stage 5 feedback processes are common to all therapies, we do not mean to imply that therefore all therapies are the same, or that all therapies work by the same mechanism. Such a conclusion would not only be ridiculous but would also reveal a failure to understand fully the general systems framework. Rather, the point we wish to emphasize here is that biological feedback plays an important common *role* in all therapies. Different therapies can share certain common goals using certain common processes (for example, feedback) even though they may employ different biobehavioral mechanisms to arrive at a similar end point (Stage 3, in the case of peripheral disease). Note that from this general perspective, it makes little sense for us to ask whether biofeedback per se is an "effective" therapy (since biofeedback is present in various degrees in *all* therapies). The question we should be asking instead is, *How* is biological feedback being used in particular instances? Are we using feedback optimally with our various intervention procedures?

The concept of the brain as a health care system has many other implications. It can help us delineate the various conditions that lead to breakdowns in self-regulatory processes, causing disregulation, disorder, and disease. Furthermore, as will be described, the general concept can stimulate specific hypotheses regarding the conditions under which different therapies (both biomedical and psychological) may have certain unexpected "side effects" that may inadvertently contribute to further disregulation and disorder.

Disregulation, Disordered Homeostasis, and Disease

It follows directly from cybernetic and systems theory that a normally self-regulatory system can become disordered when communication of essential information between specific parts of the system is, for whatever reasons, disrupted. We use the term *disregulation* to refer to the process whereby imbalances between positive and negative feedback loops occur (by whatever mechanisms) that cause the system in question to become disordered and go out of control. The simplest way of producing disregulation is to attenuate (or in the extreme form, disconnect) a necessary negative feedback loop within a stabilized, closed-loop system. We use the phrase "disconnection leading to disregulation leading to disorder" to highlight an extreme form of the process.

Stated in this fashion, the concept of disregulation may seem on first reading to be so obvious as to be trivial. However, in the same way that the general concepts of system, negative feedback, and self-regulation have each proved to be deceptively simple, so too is the general concept of disregulation. Interestingly, books on general systems theory, cybernetic theory, and control theory have tended to assume *implicitly* that disregulation must occur. However, these books do not *explicitly* and systematically describe the specific conditions whereby disconnections can lead to disregulation and disorder. The current difficulty in recognizing the general significance of the concept of disregulation is not unlike the previous difficulty in recognizing the general concept of stress (Selye, 1976). According to Selye, since it was common knowledge that patients who were ill shared an obvious characteristic in that they felt "sick," the general process of being sick was typically considered to be trivial. It was taken for granted and hence ignored. However, it is now recognized that the general characteristic of being sick has important implications for our understanding of health and illness. Within the framework of the present chapter, Selye's concept of the stress response can be viewed as being basic to the brain's ability to behave as a health care system. It is interesting to ponder how the most difficult concepts to appreciate are often those that appear to be the most obvious.

We believe that the general concept of disregulation is useful because it leads us to consider a range of different mechanisms whereby disconnections between people and the environment, as well as between various systems within people themselves, can contribute to disorder and disease. As described in detail in Schwartz (1977b, 1977c, 1978, 1979), the highly simplified diagram in Figure 1 can help integrate diverse theories of psychosomatic disease in terms of their contribution to disrupting the brain's role as a health care system.

For example, we can hypothesize that various environmental stressors —be they physical (electric shocks), chemical (poisons), or psychosocial ("crowding")—may lead to psychophysiological disease by producing a Stage 1 initiated disregulation. In the typical experiment, an organism is placed in a stressful environment (Stage 1) which, via Stages 2 and 3, results in Stage 4 stimulation back to the brain (Stage 2) that can be interpreted as fear, anger, distress, and/or pain. Under normal conditions, the adaptive response (behavior) to this negative feedback would be for the organism either to change the environment or leave it (thereby changing Stages 2 and 3 and reducing the Stage 4 feedback, and hence the distress). This self-regulatory biobehavioral process, however, is short-circuited if the organism (be it a lower animal or man) is forced by the experimental situation to remain in the stressful environment, being free neither to change it nor flee it. Under these conditions, the Stage 1 environment may promote the creation of a functional disconnection process in which the negative feedback (Stage 4) must, in one way or another, be ignored (since it cannot be heeded in the normal, adaptive fight or flight manner).

We propose that such a functional disconnection between visceral feedback and normal brain self-regulation underlies many research and real-life conditions whereby unavoidable, uncontrollable environmental stress contributes to physical illness. For example, the student who stays up late at night studying for an exam, fighting fatigue and trying to ignore a stomachache caused, in part, by eating an unbalanced diet under conditions of fatigue and fear (when the autonomic nervous system to the stomach is often inhibited), may be engaged in a disregulatory process whereby important negative feedback is ignored in order to meet the demands imposed by the environment. A similar suggestion is made by von Bertalanffy (1968, p. 193): "It does not look particularly 'homeostatic' when a businessman follows his restless activities in spite of the ulcers he is developing."

Another example, this one emphasizing Stage 2 processes, involves conditions where through experience (education, social training, and so on) and genetics—or more appropriately, an interaction of the two—the person ignores (neurophysiologically attenuates or disconnects) feedback (Stage 4) coming from the body (Stage 3). The classic descriptions of the repressive personality style (where the person denies anxiety and illness) may be re-translated into the language of cybernetic theory as involving a neuropsychological process whereby negative feedback signals are attenuated or ignored (and hence disconnected). As reviewed in Schwartz (1977c), the observations linking the repression of anger to hypertension can be examined from this framework. The fascinating question arises, What possible neuropsychological mechanisms exist that could cause normally self-regulatory, homeostatic processes to become disregulated?

One plausible theory applies research linking patterns of lateralization of brain function to patterns of cognitive and affective processes. Galin (1974) has proposed that the cognitive, affective, and personality characteristics of Freud's concepts of repression and hysteria can be understood as reflecting the productions of a functional disconnection syndrome in the brain. He proposes that mental events generated in the right hemisphere can, under certain conditions, become disconnected functionally from those of the left hemisphere. By the inhibition of neural transmission across the cerebral commissures, which connect the two hemispheres, each half can become disregulated by the other and thereby continue with a life of its own. To the extent that normal, verbal consciousness is localized primarily in the left hemisphere (for right-handed individuals), a functional disconnection of this sort would cause the left hemisphere to become unconscious of emotional processes occurring in the right hemisphere.

In accord with this theory, Schwartz, Davidson, and Maer (1975) have found that in response to emotional questions (primarily negative emotions), the average right-handed person tends to move his or her eyes to the left (suggesting relative activation of the right hemisphere). Extending this observation to denial and repression in psychosomatic disorders, Gur and Gur (1975) have reported that people who persistently move their eyes to the left (regardless of the type of question) tend to score higher on scales of denial and to report higher incidence of psychosomatic complaints. Taken together, such data suggest the intriguing hypothesis that the brain can, under certain conditions, learn to cope with negative affective physiological states by functionally severing communications across the two hemispheres. Under these conditions, the conscious brain would *perceive* a reduction in the affective processes. Unfortunately, if this process were to occur, the right hemisphere/affective processes might become accentuated and unstable since the inhibitory control of these processes by the left hemisphere was no longer being provided. Hence, a state of disregulation could exist.

It is not possible to present here a more detailed discussion of the concept of disregulation as it may be applied to health psychology. However, the specific examples described should illustrate the general concept of how disconnections can lead to the process of disregulation and the existence of disorder in biobehavioral systems. According to Greengard (1978, p. 146): "It seems probable that derangements of homeostatic processes are responsible for many disease states. Conversely, it seems likely that the effects of many therapeutic and toxic agents are exerted on such homeostatic systems." By such statements, biologists such as Greengard *imply* that breakdowns in self-regulatory processes occur in disease. When we propose that disattention (as is often required in uncontrollable, stressful environments—Stage 1; or as is inherently a part of the repressive personality style—Stage 2) may result in the production of a neurophysiological disconnection within a biobehavioral health care system (leading to disregulation between the brain and body, and between humans and their environment, producing disorder and thereby contributing to disease), we do so with the intent of illustrating how new hypotheses and research designs can be stimulated that integrate behavioral and biomedical approaches to disordered behavior (that is, disease).

Disregulation, like self-regulation, is a general concept. Disregulation can occur for various reasons in various parts of a system. In fact, it is possible for disregulation in one part of the system to lead to disregulation in other parts of the system. *Interactions* of disregulations can result from *patterns* of causes. For example, an individual exposed to a particular environmental stressor (Stage 1), who also happens to be a repressive individual (Stage 2), who also happens to have a genetically mediated hyperreactive vascular system (Stage 3), may in combination show more of a total disregulatory effect on the *entire* system than any of the components alone. In the area of hypertension, for example, it is possible that (1) excessive salt in the diet can disregulate part of the sympathetic control of blood pressure, *and* (2) organisms can be genetically predisposed to become disregulated by salt, *and* (3) exposure to intense, unavoidable environmental stress may functionally disregulate the system (for example, via excessive pressure on the baroreceptors). More importantly, these factors can *interact* with one another, leading to the greatest disregulation in the control of blood pressure, and hence increase the likelihood of developing hypertension.

Patterns, combinations, systems of disregulation—in the abstract, the general concept seems simple. However, in the concrete, the general concept forces us to appreciate the tremendous complexity inherent in the structure of living systems composed of millions of components with feedback loops interconnecting them. One goal for future research is to examine different theories (behavioral and biological) concerned with different combinations or levels within an organism, and to evolve a common, systems framework that can help us uncover redundancies, reduce irrelevant discrepancies, and promote integration of theories in health psychology.

There are numerous problems inherent in reaching such a lofty goal. One problem is conceptual in origin and deals with our ability to learn more about the cybernetics of self-regulation and about the specific conditions under which disregulation can occur. As von Bertalanffy (1968, p. 23) notes: "Concepts and models of equilibrium, homeostasis, adjustment, etc., are suitable for the maintenance of systems, but inadequate for phenomena of change, differentiation, evolution, negentropy, production of improbable states, creativity, building up of tensions, self-realization, emergence, etc.; as indeed Cannon realized when he acknowledged, beside homeostasis, a 'heterostasis' including phenomena of the latter nature." The concept of disregulation is a rephrasing of Cannon's "heterostasis." As suggested earlier, it would be a mistake for us to equate the concept of disregulation *solely* with disease. The *general* concept of disregulation may contribute not only to disease in specific instances but also to basic processes of disorder in numerous other systems.

A second problem is methodological in origin and involves the need to learn more about the mathematics of self-regulation and disregulation in order to develop appropriate research designs and data analysis procedures. For example, as mentioned previously, the complete measurement of a self-regulating system requires more than just an assessment of central tendency per se. It requires assessment of variability and, more importantly, regularity occurring over time (that is, temporal patterns). Mulholland (1977a, 1977b) illustrates how dividing the mean by the standard deviation provides a simple measure of stability in a self-regulating system.

As recently reviewed by Stoyva (1977), a major property of stress-related disorders is not reflected solely in the magnitude of the response to an environmental stressor per se but is reflected in recovery time following the response to the stressor. Measurement of this recovery effect is usually ignored because we lack the conceptual models for understanding how systems recover. Stoyva's proposal that the lengthened recovery times may indicate that a breakdown in homeostasis has occurred is an important first step. The next step is to consider systematically the role of specific subcomponents composing a self-regulating system that modulates response/recovery interactions to specific inputs.

The concept of disregulation implies that if a negative feedback loop has been attenuated or disconnected, one consequence of removing this regulatory constraint may be seen as a moderate increase in response amplitude (all other things being equal). However, a more dramatic effect of disregulation would be seen as a deficit in recovery time. Systematically assessing the relationship between response amplitude (including time to peak) and recovery time can be a mathematical procedure for examining whether disregulation (caused by an alteration of negative feedback) has occurred. The need for a more sophisticated, systems approach to the measurement of input/output relationships becomes apparent as we come to appreciate more fully the basic concepts of self-regulation and disregulation.

Self-Regulation, Disregulation, and Treatment

As previously mentioned, biofeedback can be conceptualized as being a central component in all treatments. However, this conceptualization need not imply that the specific treatment procedure is always used in a self-regulatory fashion. For example, if Stage 1 and Stage 2 processes are contributing in specific individuals to the etiology of stomachaches and ulcers, then the primary use of those treatments aimed *primarily* at changing Stage 3 processes (for example, certain drugs or surgery) can be viewed as being potentially disregulatory. As noted in Schwartz (1977c), drugs are sometimes inadvertently advertised to promote biobehavioral disregulation. For example, certain antacid commercials in the early 1970s showed a person overeating in a pie-eating contest, or shopping under stress, and developing a stomachache. However, the message of these commercials was not "The feedback is a signal telling you that you should change your environment (Stage 1) or behavior (Stage 2) for the sake of your stomach's health (Stage 3)," but rather "Eat, eat (or shop, shop) and if you get a stomachache, don't change your environment or behavior, take a drug instead."

From a systems point of view, using treatments that remove Stages 3 and 4 processes directly may remove the "symptoms" in the short run but leave intact Stages 1 and 2, the "causes." In fact, the more success we have in removing negative feedback per se (using peripheral drugs or nerve stimulators in biomedicine, or hypnosis and other cognitive self-control procedures in psychology), the greater should be the disregulation between the environment (Stage 1) and the organism (Stages 2, 3, 4). We can hypothesize that some of the biopsychosocial "side effects" found for certain drugs and behavioral procedures may reflect inadvertent disregulatory effects produced by the treatments themselves.

Whether or not specific psychophysiological self-regulation procedures such as meditation or biofeedback lead to generalized biobehavioral self-regulation should depend on exactly how these procedures are used. For example, if meditation is used to help individuals become more aware of their physiology and the stresses in their environment, with the goal of having patients *change their environment in relation to their behavior to maintain a healthy environment/person interaction*, then meditation can be viewed as promoting self-regulation (for example, establishing environmental/organism feedback loops). However, if meditation is used to help individuals short-circuit their physiological responses and simply cope with (for example, ignore) stresses in their environment, with the goal of helping patients remain in an unhealthy environment in relation to their behavior, then meditation can be viewed as promoting environment/person disregulation (especially in the long run). It follows that the study of biobehavioral approaches to treatment should not simply evaluate mechanisms and effectiveness in the abstract but should evaluate the concrete conditions under which such treatments promote self-regulation *and* disregulation within the individual and between the individual and his or her environment. A comprehensive theory of intervention should include the conditions under which the treatments can cause disorder as well as eliminate it.

On the Need for General Models in Biofeedback and Health Psychology

There is clearly a need to develop broader models that will not only stimulate new data and applications but also will help integrate disparate theoretical and empirical approaches in the area. Biofeedback (like health psychology in general) is an area of study that is inherently interdisciplinary. It places the investigator face to face with complex issues of mind/brain/body/environment relationships. It requires that the investigator (1) consider cognitive processes of attention, perception, learning, memory, and imagery, (2) link these processes to emotional processes (including motivation), and (3) relate these processes to the underlying biological substrates (neural, endocrine, and physiological) that are involved. As reviewed in Schwartz (1979), diverse concepts such as operant conditioning, biological constraints, cognitive self-control, feedback, instructions, and consciousness are currently used in the literature with little order or cohesion. It should be clear that the need for basic empirical research is not being questioned here. Rather, what is being questioned is the extent to which progress in basic empirical research is being hampered by our lack of organizing concepts that can provide direction, integration, and clarity to the research.

The need for a unifying approach to help direct research and application is not unique to biofeedback. It is present in modern psychology at large and is particularly apparent in the emerging area of health psychology. The need to develop syntheses of biochemical, physiological, neurological, behavioral, and social levels of analysis becomes self-evident when all these levels are found to be relevant to the solution of a particular problem (for example, disease). The task of translating one theoretical language to another within psychology (for example, operant conditioning to feedback terminology, or cognitive processes to information-processing terms) is complex enough. The development of collaborative research efforts in health psychology that cut across neuroendocrine, physiological, neurological, and behavioral disciplines makes the task of translation between theories even more complex (for example, homeostasis to operant conditioning, or the biochemistry of immune reactions to cognitive processes).

The task of making meaningful translations between theories is neither esoteric nor unimportant. On the contrary, this issue mediates the kinds of research that are conducted and the nature of the interpretation of results that are obtained. As described in Schwartz (1978), there are numerous instances of unrecognized confusions between behavioral and biomedical scientists that are caused by a failure to recognize the problems of translation. For example, in pharmacology, the term *direct* has a precise meaning, describing the condition where a drug makes contact with particular sites of "action." Any consequence of the drug that is not due to the "direct action" of the drug is called an "indirect effect." Using this terminology, drugs do not have a direct action on blood pressure per se but may have direct actions on organs or systems controlling the organs. Certain drugs can have a direct action on the vascular beds and thereby have an indirect effect on blood pressure. Other drugs can have a direct action on the central nervous system, thereby having an indirect effect on the vascular beds and eventually an indirect effect on the blood pressure. Note that in using this terminology, the words *direct* and *effect* should never be used together. When a pharmacologist reads the behavioral literature in which statements are made about biofeedback having "direct effects" on blood pressure, this can cause confusion. In fact, from a pharmacologic perspective, environmental contingencies *never* have a direct effect (or even a direct action) on "behavior." Rather, environmental contingencies have a direct action on the sensory receptors (the eyes). Only then can they have an indirect effect on the central nervous system (thalamus to occipital cortex and relevant association areas), followed by a chain of indirect effects from motor cortex to skeletal muscle (behavior). Numerous other unrecognized sources of problems in translation are described in detail in Schwartz (1978). General systems theory (von Bertalanffy, 1968) can provide a framework for recognizing and minimizing such difficulties.

Summary and Conclusions

This chapter has introduced general systems theory as it relates to biofeedback and health psychology. We have further illustrated how specific concepts from cybernetic theory can be useful in conceptualizing mechanisms by which self-regulation may develop. We have considered the role of the brain as a health care system and have suggested that biofeedback plays a fundamental role in both behavioral and biomedical approaches to treatment. The concept of disregulation was introduced as a means of conceptualizing how normally self-regulatory systems can break down, leading to disorder and disease. We have considered how various behavioral and biomedical procedures may either promote self-regulation or inadvertently promote disregulation, depending upon the conditions under which the treatments are employed.

We have not discussed here how distinctions between mind, brain, and body contribute to the split between behavioral and biological approaches to biofeedback and health psychology (see Schwartz, 1978), nor have we presented in detail the application of systems concepts to specific content areas such as hypertension (see Schwartz and others, forthcoming). The purpose of this chapter was to provide for the reader an introduction and progress report regarding a general systems framework that is clearly in its early stages of evolution and evaluation.

We believe that the general systems framework proposed by von Bertalanffy (1968) implies a shift in scientific paradigm (Kuhn, 1962) that can have profound implications for theory and research in biofeedback and health psychology. The reader may wish to reflect upon some of the implications of a systems approach to health psychology, using the general concept of the brain as a natural health care system, for developing broader bio-behavioral models of (1) health and illness behavior, (2) the roles that practitioners and educators play in aiding the brain in its functioning as a health care system, and (3) the extent to which the prevailing models of health care and illness (including their effects on the nature of training, hospital design and functioning, and health insurance) undermine and possibly disregulate the brain's role as a health care system. Whether these implications prove to be valid and useful is clearly for future research to decide. If this chapter helps to stimulate interest in exploring the potential value of concepts of systems theory in general, and cybernetic and control theory in particular, in the conduct of future research linking psychobiology with health psychology, then it will have achieved its goal.

22

Themes and Professional Prospects in Health Psychology

Nancy E. Adler

Frances Cohen

George C. Stone

It is now time to face some questions about the prospects for the development of a new field in psychology that has to do with the application of psychological concepts and methods to the problems of the health system. We will begin by reflecting on some of the major themes that have emerged from the chapters of this book. We will then consider what health psychology is and how it relates to other psychological approaches to illness, to other social science disciplines, and to the rest of psychology. In doing so, we present our argument about the usefulness of health psychology as an area of specialization in psychology and go on to consider issues of training and prospects for employment of future health psychologists.

Psychologists did not discover, but they have listened and learned about, an apparent historical shift now taking place in the definition of the fundamental aims of the health care system. Chapter One describes a long-term historical shift, beginning 2,000 years ago, away from a holistic emphasis on balance and harmony in living as the source of health to a focus on specific diseases, their causes, and their cures. Now, as many of the authors in this volume have noted, we have learned how to deal effectively with most of the acute and specific diseases, and our attention is turning once more to the chronic, degenerative conditions. Whereas formerly the emphasis was almost totally on diagnosis and treatment, there is now a growing interest in prevention. It becomes increasingly apparent that this change of focus has major consequences for all aspects of the health system. This theme, although noted by many of the authors, is not specifically a psychological issue. However, it provides one aspect of the context within which more specifically psychological themes arise. Presented here are five specific themes discussed in this volume that psychologists have identified as significant issues in the health system.

General Themes in Health Psychology

Importance of Stress and Coping Perspectives

Many chapters in this volume have focused on the central role of stress and coping factors in influencing both the development of and recovery from illness and in affecting transactions in the health care environment. Both the types of threats or stresses involved in medical transactions and the nature of the coping efforts used to deal with these stresses have been discussed in Chapters Five, Nine, Ten, Sixteen, and Nineteen. Models, from the stress and coping perspective, such as the one outlined by Moos in Chapter Twenty, have been used to illustrate how psychological factors may be involved in the development of illness and how they affect the seeking of and response to medical treatment.

Regarding the *development of illness*, Cohen (Chapter Four) evaluates the evidence that links stress, modes of coping, and other psychological factors to the development of disease and provides an outline of various models that implicate biological and psychological mechanisms as mediating variables in these relationships. Regarding the *patient's response* to the intrusion of illness, Cohen and Lazarus (Chapter Nine), Haan (Chapter Five), and Mages and Mendelsohn (Chapter Ten) describe in detail the types of threat that illness can bring, the adaptive tasks necessary for effective adaptation, and the types of coping strategies used. From different perspectives, these authors and Janis and Rodin (Chapter Nineteen) have tried to answer the questions: What factors can reduce stress in medical transactions? What is adaptive coping in the face of stressful medical illnesses and procedures? Their respective answers to these questions differ.

For example, there is controversy about the adaptiveness of vigilance as compared with avoidance-denial strategies in health-relevant situations. Janis and Rodin argue that vigilant strategies are most adaptive in health situations where pain and other physical discomforts must be endured in the present for the expectation of future benefits. However, Cohen and Lazarus discuss evidence that avoidance strategies may be quite adaptive in particular health crisis situations, such as while awaiting general surgery or during the initial adjustment to polio or severe burns. Mages and Mendelsohn discuss how avoidance strategies can aid adjustment in particular stages of the cancer process. Similar disagreement exists regarding the adaptiveness of specific defense mechanisms such as denial. Further research is necessary to test out these seemingly contradictory hypotheses.

There is also controversy about the effects of interventions designed to encourage active involvement by the patient. This issue is relevant to efforts to gain the patient's active cooperation in treatment regimens, as discussed by Kirscht and Rosenstock (Chapter Eight). It is also important with respect to the emotional components of the patient's adaptation to the treatment situation. Haan suggests that involving the patient as a full, active partner in health decisions and treatment plans reduces stress and benefits the patient. Yet patients often express the sentiment that they do not want to know details of their diagnosis and treatment. Are there short-run harms (for example, confusion, increased anxiety, traumatic avoidance of risky but necessary medical procedures) and/or long-run benefits (increasing patients' sense of control and their ability to take greater responsibility for their health) of active involvement procedures? Cohen and Lazarus (Chapter Nine) and Mages and Mendelsohn (Chapter Ten) argue that individual differences and situational factors must be taken into account in evaluating adaptive outcomes and in planning psychological interventions. How difficult is it to aid the patient in taking on the role of a full and active partner in the health process? Janis and Rodin (Chapter Nineteen) discuss how attempts to aid patients in gaining personal control can boomerang, resulting in increased rather than decreased stress responses. Cohen and Lazarus suggest that there may be some medical situations in which it is difficult, if not impossible, to give patients any sense of real control, and Mages and Mendelsohn illustrate this difficulty in the case of cancer.

We have described briefly some issues about stress and coping that focus on stresses of the patient. Cartwright (Chapter Sixteen) and Haan (Chapter Five) both discuss stress and coping issues from the *viewpoint of the provider*, illustrating the stresses to which health care professionals are subject and how these stresses affect their health, well-being, capacities to maintain optimal cognitive functioning and human sensitivity, and their effectiveness in communicating with patients. They describe common coping strategies used by physicians—such as detachment, intellectualization, and avoidance—and suggest that these may be devices necessary to help physicians maintain their own equilibrium in response to stress. However, such strategies may exacerbate the patient's distress in the medical transaction.

Emphasis on Positive Human Adaptive Capacities

A second related theme reflects the recent call by Engel (1977) for an approach to health care that recognizes humans as biopsychosocial totalities and emphasizes the importance of their powerful adaptive capacities—biological, social, and moral—in their striving toward health. There are two aspects to this theme. One centers on the powerful effects that faith, the will to live, and the support of significant others can have on the healing process (as described by Frank, 1975, and Cousins, 1976). Although the topic of healing and the importance of placebo effects are not addressed fully in this volume, brief examples are provided where these processes were thought to have had important influences. Further, Cohen and Lazarus (Chapter Nine), Rosenstock and Kirscht (Chapter Seven), and Cohen (Chapter Four) discuss the role that social supports can play in aiding adaptation, affecting utilization of health services, and improving health status. Haan (Chapter Five) views these adaptive capacities as ever striving for expression; she describes people's insistent efforts to maintain their sense of agency or control in threatening health-relevant situations.

A second aspect of this theme concerns how the expression of human adaptive capacities can be encouraged in medical environments. Haan argues strongly that patients should be taken as full, responsible partners in the health care process, suggesting that this will mobilize these important psychological processes. Janis and Rodin (Chapter Nineteen) discuss similar issues concerning how personal control can play a vital role in improving coping efforts in medical situations. In addition, Schwartz (Chapter Twenty-One) considers the potential hazards to a person's adaptive capacity that arise when the natural feedback about the body's "dis-ease" is interrupted by medical interventions.

Problem of Rationality Versus Irrationality in Psychological Models

A third theme, also related to some issues discussed earlier, centers on the use of rational versus irrational assumptions and models about human behavior and health care processes. A major strand of human history has to do with the emergence of a self-aware, rational basis for selecting among alternative paths of action, and many psychological models assume that patients will be rational decision makers and assimilators of information. Yet when we look at people's behavior, we may be more struck by the lapses and failures of rationality than by its successes. Elstein and Bordage (Chapter Thirteen), Hunt and MacLeod (Chapter Twelve), and Janis and Rodin (Chapter Nineteen) describe how distortions and biases that occur in basic cognitive processes—biases of "availability" and "representativeness," for example—can influence the types of decisions made by patients and physicians. As these authors discuss, humans are subject to bounded rationality because of their inability to process all the information available to them at any given time; thus, their decisions are subsequently affected. This inability to process information may be exacerbated in situations in which fear is aroused or conflicts produced, as discussed in Chapter Nineteen, interfering even further with an individual's ability to comprehend and act on information and to make decisions that will have a beneficial effect on his or her health. Along these lines, Adler and Milstein (Chapter Fifteen) discuss the dilemma of using rational versus irrational models in health planning analyses. They describe how intrapsychic conflicts and defenses may distort the true expression of needs in health-planning situations.

We tend to be dismayed when we confront the evidence of irrationality in ourselves and others. The occurrence of self-destructive behavior and maladaptive failures to follow sound health practices for prevention and cure of illness provide the focus for several chapters and are addressed briefly in several others. Henderson, Hall, and Lipton (Chapter Six) cite extensively the evidence concerning the great difficulty in changing self-destructive behavior and its seeming inaccessibility to reasoned approaches. Kirscht and Rosenstock (Chapter Eight) survey the difficulties of finding one's way into the health care system and then in following the recommendations that are given there. A number of authors comment on the difficulty that people have in adopting preventive health behaviors, which may involve significant short-term costs in exchange for promises of later benefits. However, "irrational" behaviors may serve adaptive functions, as has been discussed by Cohen and Lazarus (Chapter Nine) regarding defenses such as denial. It is to be hoped that theoreticians will continue to struggle with these issues and will provide better guidelines as to when rational or irrational models are most applicable.

Importance of Good Communication Between Patient and Provider

Another key theme focuses on the important role that proper communication plays in influencing outcomes of health transactions and on the factors that aid such communication. We have previously mentioned the contributions of Haan and Cartwright in this area. In addition, Hunt and MacLeod emphasize how cognitive factors influence the nature of the communications of patient and provider. They offer suggestions for altering communications so as to obtain needed information, presenting important advice effectively, and dealing with patients whose cognitive abilities are diminished. From a counseling viewpoint, Kagan (Chapter Eighteen) describes a method for teaching interpersonal skills. He discusses various specific techniques that would encourage effective communication, such as ways of encouraging patients to elaborate their concerns. Janis and Rodin provide suggestions on how health care professionals can effectively use their power as significant reference persons to motivate patients to carry out recommended courses of action. They discuss different phases that patient decision makers must surmount and recommend communication strategies for the practitioner to follow.

Complexity of the Issues and Psychological Processes Hypothesized

A final theme, less substantive in nature, emphasizes the complexity of many of the psychological processes studied by health psychologists. For example, although many popular authors write facilely about stress as the major killer of this era, Cohen's discussion emphasizes that the relationship between stress and the development of illness is not at all simple or straight-forward, and that many other variables must be taken into account. As mentioned earlier, Janis and Rodin discuss how attempts to aid patients in gaining personal control can boomerang, resulting in increased rather than decreased stress responses. Schwartz discusses the tremendous complexity of the functioning of living systems.

As our understanding of communications in health transactions grows, we may find it harder to make recommendations. For example, those who, like Kagan, have taught communications skills to counselors stress the value of "exploratory questions" and other means that leave the structuring of the communication to the client while providing emotional support. Hunt and MacLeod, however, point to situations in which vigorous structuring of the transaction is necessary to support patients whose cognitive capacities may be overstressed. These two apparently contradictory approaches to the struc-turing of situations can be resolved only by the development of more com-plex rules regarding the degree to which the experts' framework should dominate or recede into the background.

These data suggest the importance of taking a multidimensional ap-proach to research, the evaluation of adaptive outcomes, and the structuring of health transactions. We must also consider the need for nonlinear models and for models that incorporate feedback loops, as Schwartz emphasizes in Chapter Twenty-One. As several authors have discussed, factors of situation (or environment, as described by Moos in Chapter Twenty), individual differ-ence, and culture all affect the psychological processes found in health care transactions. For example, Mages and Mendelsohn (Chapter Ten) point out how the nature of the cancer itself strongly influences the adaptive tasks re-quired and the types of coping strategies utilized. They also illustrate how the age, sex, and personal history of the person influence the degree to which the person is stressed and the nature of his or her response. From another perspective, Bibace and Walsh (Chapter Eleven) illustrate how a child's level of cognitive development influences his or her understanding of medical procedures and why health practitioners should take these differ-ences into account in their health communications with children. Schofield (Chapter Seventeen) describes methods for assessing many of the relevant individual difference factors and discusses their use in medical settings. Sechrest and Cohen (Chapter Fourteen) point out the difficulty and com-plexity involved in assessments of health outcomes.

Another important variable, alluded to only briefly by several authors, involves cultural belief systems and sociocultural practices and customs. The degree to which these variables have important health influences has been extensively discussed by medical anthropologists (see Chapter Two).

General Conclusions

The themes that have emerged from this book point the way to impor-tant areas of needed research. They also suggest some conclusions that can be useful to those engaged in health care. As health psychologists, we make several general points that we hope will be helpful to those involved in patient contact: (1) In order to mobilize the strengths of particular patients, it may be helpful to involve them as responsible participants in the health care process. This involvement will require some shifts in the role definitions that have prevailed during the past hundred years or more. It will also require that we learn to distinguish those patients and those circumstances where such a shift of responsibilities is or is not to the patient's benefit. (2) Health care providers need to understand the psychological processes that underlie the behavior of their patients, but they must be aware, as must psychologists, of the great complexity of these processes. For example, interactions among personal characteristics of patients, their sociocultural background, and situational factors are the rule. As another example, beliefs can influence emotional reactions and can change as a function of emotional states; fear may be mobilizing under some circumstances and immobilizing under others. (3) Understanding of psychological processes must be linked with interpersonal skills of communicating information and offering support in order to be effective. Knowledge is of little value until it can be implemented. (4) Health care providers need to recognize that their patients are often operating under conditions of overload with regard to information and at levels of emotional and physiological arousal in which the processing of information is impaired. Not only do providers need to make allowance for this state of affairs in their presentation of information but they also need to provide mechanisms whereby these burdens can be lightened. Because of the stigma associated with referral to mental health personnel and facilities, other, more intrinsic sources of psychological assistance need to be provided. (Psychological research personnel may be one source of such help, as Mages and Mendelsohn indicate.) (5) Finally, the greater understanding of psychological processes gained by health care personnel must be used with sensitivity to ethical problems that are raised whenever one person attempts to influence the beliefs or behaviors of others. For example, when we know how to be persuasive or to develop "referent power," we must use our knowledge with great care. Many of the authors in this volume have commented on this source of ethical concerns, as well as on the seeming dilemma posed by those situations in which deception or covert manipulation would appear to be a means of motivating fallible patients to act in their own best interest.

The Domain of Health Psychology

Having looked at the general themes that have emerged in this book, it is time to step back and consider the field of health psychology per se. As noted in Chapter Three, psychologists have been working in the health field for many years, but only recently has there been a self-conscious awareness that there might be a field or discipline called *health psychology*. In reflecting on the possible form and future of such a discipline, it may be helpful to consider how it relates to (1) other psychological approaches to questions of health and illness, (2) other social science disciplines that are also engaged in health-related research, and (3) other specialties of psychology.

Relationship to Other Psychological Approaches to Health

Three terms in addition to *health psychology* are used to describe the involvement of psychologists in the health system: medical psychology, psychosomatic medicine, and behavioral medicine. It is our belief that health psychology is broader than any of these more circumscribed fields and will provide a better framework on which to develop a discipline.

Medical psychology has several meanings. In England, it refers to psychiatry. In the United States, it has generally been applied to clinical psychologists who work in hospital settings or are otherwise involved in service delivery to ill patients. In any event, its meaning is tied to a clinical orientation and service delivery.

Psychosomatic medicine studies the impact of emotional states and responses to stress on the development of somatic symptoms and illness. Until about twenty years ago, attention was paid to a limited number of diseases. Subsequently, the focus was broadened with growing recognition of the pervasive effects of stress on physical states. Thus, psychosomatic medicine currently assumes that all diseases have psychological components and that all of medicine should be encompassed by psychosomatic medicine. It may well be that as the trend toward broadening the focus of psychosomatic medicine continues, there will be difficulty in differentiating it from an emerging field —behavioral medicine.

Behavioral medicine is a recent term and is being used more and more frequently by psychologists involved in research related to medical care. At a recent conference on behavioral medicine, a formal definition was adopted: "the field concerned with the development of behavioral science knowledge and techniques relevant to the understanding of physical health and illness and the application of this knowledge and these techniques to prevention, diagnosis, treatment, and rehabilitation" (Schwartz and Weiss, 1977, p. 379). Although most of the aspects of behavioral medicine incorporated in this definition would also hold true of health psychology, we believe that it differs in two important ways. First, the use of the term *psychology* does remove it from an interdisciplinary field to one that is more firmly grounded in psychological perspectives, theories, and research. Second, and more importantly, the use of the term *health* instead of *medicine* has significant implications for the scope of the field. Although medicine is being viewed in broader terms recently and there have been calls for a less restrictive view of the field (Engel, 1977), the use of the term still suggests the traditional medical model. Medicine is still seen primarily in terms of the application of the art and science of medical experts to problems of health (and, in fact, more usually to illness) of a target population. Within the framework of the health system presented in Chapter One of this book, medicine encompasses only a portion of the total health system. It looks primarily at activities of health care providers (and, in most cases, just a portion of actual care givers) in relation to targets and does not consider, to any great extent, the other aspects of health. The use of the term *health* also removes us from the orientation toward pathology associated with a medical approach and the stress on expert responsibility associated with medicine.

Other social science disciplines, such as anthropology and sociology, have designated their subspecialties with the term *medical*. But there is growing awareness of the limitations of this term and suggestions for change. Rosen (1972, p. 52), in his review of the history of medical sociology, concludes: "A review of the literature clearly shows that the term *medical sociology* is not satisfactory. . . . Perhaps, one should endeavor to introduce a new designation: *the sociology of health.*" Since we are not yet enmeshed in traditional or habitual use of a term, we would argue that psychology should also adopt the use of the term *health* rather than *medical* in describing that specialty that concerns problems of health as well as illness and treatment. In this regard, we note with pleasure the recent establishment by the American Psychological Association of a division of health psychology.

Relationship to Other Social Science Disciplines

In Chapter Two, we described other social science approaches to the health system and identified those aspects of the system that each examined. Health psychology will deal with many aspects of the health system and consequently will overlap these disciplines. However, the nature of the questions asked about any aspect of the system will be different. For example, both economists and psychologists may be interested in resources. As noted by Fuchs (1974), economics concerns itself with the means by which values might be maximized and would address itself to the optimum allocation of resources. Psychologists would be far more likely to be interested in how those values arose and might study values associated with health and their relationship to other values, beliefs, and attitudes. Thus, the two disciplines would be complementary in their approach to the same area of the health system.

Of the four social science disciplines studying the health system, psychology most resembles sociology. The fields are similar in the breadth of their interests, methods, and research. In neither field is there a single organizing framework or theory. Both can span the range from small scale to large scale, qualitative to quantitative, and laboratory to field (although more psychologists are likely to be engaged in laboratory work and relatively more sociologists in fieldwork). It is thus instructive to consider the implications for health psychology of the differentiation that is drawn between sociology *in* medicine and sociology *of* medicine (Straus, 1957).

As noted in Chapter Two, sociology in medicine is the application of sociological principles to the solution of medical problems. Research in this area tends to accept medical definitions of problems. In contrast, sociology of medicine takes an outsider's perspective and asks questions about the institution of medicine itself. Straus and others have noted a tension between the two since one requires adoption of the perspective of medical colleagues in order to obtain close collaboration, and the other necessitates some independence of judgment and perspective and may well antagonize those who are engaged in the practice of medicine. Much of the psychological research to date has been within the framework of medicine. It has focused on individuals as targets and has considered such questions as how to improve patient compliance with prescribed regimens (Chapter Eight) and how to change self-destructive habits (Chapter Six). Whereas psychology in medicine would be likely to deal with people as targets of health interventions, health psychology would be more likely to consider people as agents and examine the psychological dynamics involved in the processes of seeking, maintaining, and recovering health and of providing health services. Chapters Thirteen and Sixteen in this volume are examples of a psychological appraisal of medical behavior. Similarly, Chapter Fifteen investigates psychological dimensions of broader health behavior—health planning. There is also a great deal of research on the role of individuals as agents in their own health care; some of the research on stress, coping, and adaptation takes an independent look at individuals as they struggle with problems of health and illness. Although little research has been done to date, psychologists could also be involved in the examination of health hazards and how people as agents seek to reduce the risks associated with these hazards.

Relationship to Other Specialties of Psychology

Each of the social science disciplines has a different pattern of socialization and training for its members who are interested in questions of health. Medical sociology, the field with the longest history, trains researchers in the specific subdiscipline, as does medical anthropology. Economics, in contrast, does not provide special graduate programs in health economics; rather, students are trained in general economics and may later apply their general knowledge to problems of the health market. Few of the specialties have developed their own unique set of theories or methods. Instead, they apply the general principles of the parent discipline as they are appropriate to issues in the health field. An exception to this is "grounded theory" (Glaser and Strauss, 1967) in sociology, which is rooted in medical sociology.

What should be the relationship of health psychology to the rest of psychology? It is likely that it will have the same relationship to the larger discipline as specialties like medical sociology do to sociology. All theoretical fields of psychology—such as physiological, developmental, social, cognitive, and personality—as well as all methodological approaches—such as experimental, psychometric, and clinical—could make important contributions to the solution of health problems. Individuals working within any of the areas of psychology or with any psychological theory may, on occasion, want to test their hypotheses or apply the theory in regard to a health problem. Thus, there will likely be many psychologists who will not identify with health psychology per se but who will spend some of their professional lives investigating problems within the health field. In most cases, their interest will be in the testing of their hypotheses and not in the solution of any particular health problem. For example, a social psychologist interested in issues of attitude change might choose to test a hypothesis relating attitude change to degree of threat in a health setting. Such research could well provide useful information to those working within the health setting who are concerned with modifying patient attitudes toward taking medications on schedule, but that would not be the purpose of the research from the psychologist's point of view. There are dangers in such an approach, however, namely: (1) researchers not familiar with the health setting may find it difficult to obtain access to the appropriate population; (2) even when researchers have gained access to a setting, they may, because of lack of knowledge or insensitivity to the special characteristics of that setting, alienate the health professionals or actually harm the patients; and (3) the results may never be fed back into the setting to be applied. More effective research may be accomplished by those who are familiar with the health setting as well as with theoretical issues that could be tested in the setting.

In addition to the historical definition of fields in psychology that encompass theoretical areas, there has been a growing trend toward the development of substantive areas. In recent years, specialties such as population, environmental psychology, and psychology of religion have been established. Health psychology also constitutes a substantive specialty. As of this time, there are no theories or methods peculiar to the field, but it draws upon the range of theories and methods of psychology. What sets health psychologists apart from other psychologists is their primary commitment to problems of the health field and their knowledge of the people, settings, customs, problems, and issues of the health system. By formally recognizing a domain of specialization in this area as the other social and behavioral sciences have done or are doing, we can facilitate the entry of more psychologists into the health system. In the next sections, we will consider the training of specialists in health psychology and their prospects for employment.

Training of Health Psychologists

The work reported in this book reflects the great variety of ways in which individual psychologists relate to the domain of health psychology. Some are anchored firmly in one of the core fields of psychology, with primary identities as social psychologists, developmental psychologists, cognitive psychologists, and so on. Others have committed themselves to a particular problem or issue and pursue its resolution across boundaries of specialization and even of the discipline of psychology. Since, in the past, there have been no formal training programs in health psychology, all of those who currently function in the field have come from one of the existing specializations. Now, however, it is important to consider the kind of training that is appropriate for those who will be the next generation of health psychologists. As we view the field, it is broad and complex and many different kinds of psychologists will be necessary to meet its various needs. If every core field of psychology is relevant to health psychology, then we need training that will adapt the theories and methods of these core fields to the requirements of work in the health system. Postdoctoral training may be most appropriate as a means of preparing psychologists already educated in a specialization to utilize their skills in health-related areas. Regular graduate departments may facilitate the efforts of students who desire to undertake their dissertation research on a health problem in preparation for a career in the health system, and may offer courses and seminars focusing on health issues. Such a pattern of training is already being explored at a number of universities: the University of Michigan, Michigan State, the University of Minnesota, Yale, Florida State, the University of Houston, and the University of California at Riverside, among others. However, predoctoral course work specifically in health psychology areas may be of value in training researchers who can address some of the core problems of the health care system. It may be particularly useful to develop programs that teach students psychology within the context of a health setting: such programs could emphasize health care issues in many basic courses as well. The examples and problems that give substance to the development of conceptual frameworks could be drawn, in considerable part, from the day-to-day operations of the health system. Students of learning could investigate the mastery of anatomy and biochemistry by students of the health professions, rather than drawing their lists of words or sentences from haphazard sources and presenting them to beginning students in psychology courses. Survey methodology could be learned in interviews of health agents and health targets about their beliefs and values with regard to health issues. It is at least plausible that this kind of education could produce a *tacit knowledge* (Polyani, 1967) that would enable its graduates to extend psychological theories in ways that are maximally relevant to the health system. It is certain that it could bring significant human resources to the task of acquiring a body of factual knowledge about the psychological aspects of the health system.

Such programs in health psychology would train students to perform all of the principal activities in which psychologists engage: basic research and the development of theory; teaching knowledge and theory in introductory and practical courses in psychology (in this case, also teaching students preparing for careers as health agents); consultation and applied research with people and organizations at work in both academic and nonacademic settings; and the direct application of psychological skills to the problems of individual patients or clients.

Some psychologists doubt the desirability of conducting doctoral education of psychologists in medical environments. They express concern about the small number of psychology faculty and the limited availability of courses in departments such as mathematics, languages, philosophy, and the humanities if the medical center is remote from a general campus. These concerns about resources raise questions that need to be answered. Can a truly excellent doctoral program in psychology be provided in a setting where health psychologists are segregated from the main body of graduate education in psychology? As a corollary to that question, we may ask whether health psychology programs of this kind can avoid risking the separate and unequal status that for many years afflicted educational psychologists.

The answers to these questions depend on the degree to which psychologists working in medical settings retain their primary professional identity as psychologists. If this identity is not preserved by health psychologists through membership in a general department of psychology, then it will be especially important for them to maintain strong associations with the discipline through communication with colleagues, professional organizations, and the like. Faculty in programs of health psychology must be strongly encouraged to read and publish in core psychological journals and to see that their students do so as well.

With regard to the number of psychologists available to serve as faculty, there are enough psychologists now present in a number of medical schools to permit the development of programs in health psychology. A recent survey by Lubin, Nathan, and Matarazzo (1978) found twenty-seven medical schools with twenty or more full-time psychologists on their faculties. What of the absence of courses in the liberal arts? Most of the medical schools are actually close enough to a general campus to make it possible for students to take such additional courses elsewhere. In our own program at the University of California at San Francisco, students with special needs or interests can and do enroll in courses at the general campus in Berkeley, which is thirty-five minutes away. There are undeniable limitations. Offsetting them, however, are a wealth of special opportunities at the medical center—programs in medical anthropology, medical sociology, history of medicine, ethics, biomathematics and statistics, medical genetics (or molecular genetics), and so on—in which the knowledge of other fields and disciplines is organized in such a way as to make their relevance to the health system more readily apparent than would be true of more general courses offered in the same areas.

The problem that we find at our campus is not a limitation on breadth of learning opportunities but rather a limitation on the time of our students. To learn about psychology and about the health system adds up to a considerable load. Our health psychology program offers three quarters of orienting courses, as well as colloquia and research placements. These are in addition to what might be expected in a general graduate program in psychology. Much of the health-related learning is embedded in other more basic courses, essentially without cost of time. The health system sometimes functions as the context in which the psychological material is presented—but such material must always be presented in some context. Thus, strong specialization in health psychology may limit the range of contexts in which application of psychological principles is made but it limits hardly at all the range of principles and concepts from within or outside of psychology upon which the student can draw.

Employment Opportunities for Health Psychologists

Both prospective students and organizations that are asked to support new educational ventures inquire sharply, in these days of gloomy forecasts, about the employment prospects of graduates. The National Science Foundation (1975), using statistics drawn mostly from the period 1962 to 1972, projected an oversupply of doctorates of 7 to 10 percent in the life sciences and 42 to 49 percent in the social sciences by 1985. But this report does observe that forecasts may not be applicable to specific fields or disciplines. Even less so will they be applicable to a new specialty area within our discipline.

Will health psychologists be in demand? What kinds of occupational niches can they expect to find or create in the health system? These questions cannot be answered with assurance now, nor do we want to represent ourselves as expert in forecasting trends. We will set forth certain facts in such a way that they may give some sense of the possibilities that exist. In many cases, the realization of these possibilities will depend on the competence and imagination that health psychologists display in their work. We will consider first possibilities in replacement, and then new roles for psychologists.

Estimates of Replacement Needs

Recent surveys (Gottfredson and Dyer, 1978; Kleinknecht, Klepac, and Bernstein, 1976; Lubin, Nathan, and Matarazzo, 1978) provide some information on the number of psychologists now at work in the health system, which can be used to estimate replacement possibilities. By making some estimates and assumptions, one can conclude that there are approximately 1,000 psychologists whose principal employment is in a medical school and another 1,000 who work in schools of dentistry, general medical hospitals, and other more specialized health settings. Thus, we estimate that there are about 2,000 persons who might be considered as health psychologists at the present time.

A widely used attrition factor, cited in the forecast made by the National Science Foundation (1975), assumes that 1.5 percent of a labor pool will die or retire in any single year. Thus, without allowing for growth, we would expect to see 300 psychologists recruited over the next ten years into medical school facilities and other currently filled niches in the health system. How many of these will be trained as health psychologists depends on factors that we cannot predict. This estimate will be high to the degree that present health psychologists are younger than working people as a whole, or otherwise lower in attrition. The estimate will be low to the extent that there is growth. But that is our next topic.

Estimates of Growth in Demand for Health Psychologists

The four major activities in which we expect that health psychologists will engage are research, teaching, consultation, and provision of direct service to patients. The places where they will probably find employment are on faculties, in hospitals and clinics, health maintenance organizations, consulting firms, and private practice. How can we possibly predict what will happen with respect to all these activities and settings?

To begin, we might take a very global approach. Total expenditures on health in the United States in 1976 were $139 billion. Of this total, $120 billion was for personal health care of individuals. By how much could this amount be reduced through the effective application of psychological knowledge? Follette and Cummings (1967) studied patients with high utilization rates in a health maintenance organization. They found a reduction of up to 50 percent over a five-year period in the number of outpatient visits and the number of days of hospitalization among those who had made use of outpatient psychiatric services. Goldberg, Krantz, and Locke (1970) found a 30 percent reduction in a highly selected group of patients from another prepaid plan during a twelve-month period following a brief course of psychotherapy compared to the twelve months that preceded it. Some estimates of the proportion of all health services consumed by patients whose complaints physicians consider to be medically inconsequential run as high as 20 percent. A reduction of this component by half could save 10 percent of $120 billion, or $12 billion. This is not a prediction but an indication of the magnitude of potential savings. Another area of possible savings is in the shortening of hospital stays. For example, Egbert and others (1964, p. 826) found that a program aimed at reducing postoperative pain by instruction, suggestion, and encouragement also reduced the average duration of hospitalization by 2.7 days. In 1973, there were eighteen million hospitalizations for surgical operations in the United States. If only a single day, on the average, were cut from the average stay of these patients, a saving of about $2.7 billion would be realized.

These figures—and there are presumably others that could be developed in terms of increased efficiency in care through better communications, higher rates of adherence, reduced stress on health care professionals, reduced incidence of preventable illness, and the like—suggest that an effective application of health psychology to such problems could result in savings equal to the combined salaries of many thousands of health psychologists.

One general problem that can only be mentioned here is that most of the potential savings would arise from changes that would affect the working patterns, role performances, self-images, and incomes of many providers of health care services. To be effective, health psychologists must recognize this fact and include as part of their task the facilitation of the necessary changes. Some psychologists will no doubt be employed by organizations that function by bringing pressure to bear on the health care system. The large majority are likely to work in health care organizations and secondary organizations of the health care system such as health professional schools or to practice under circumstances that will often involve referral of clients from a health organization. To be effective, they will have to work in close and sympathetic cooperation with the physicians, dentists, nurses, dietitians, hospital administrators and staff, and so on, whose behavior must change along with that of the patients if savings are to be realized.

Where are the jobs to develop? Medical schools might employ psychologists both on their teaching faculties and in government-supported research positions. If all medical schools were to hire health psychologists to bring the number of their full-time paid faculty up to the median number (9) now employed in schools of medicine, about 260 new positions would be created. Other schools of the health professions and occupations might add psychologists to their faculties. We have not been able to find good figures on the numbers now in such schools, nor, for the most part, on the number of schools involved. However, we can estimate that there were about 800,000 students, exclusive of those in medicine, in all of the health educational programs listed by the Bureau of the Census in 1976. If psychologists were added even at the rate of 1 per 1,000 students, that would create 800 positions. Some positions may be created at the undergraduate level as well. Despite the shortage of academic positions in psychology, growing interest in health issues among undergraduates may create pressure for courses and provide opportunities for health psychologists in liberal arts settings.

Basic research positions are another possible source of employment. Such positions would probably be added mostly in conjunction with federally supported research. Even those who are responsible for distributing such funds find it hard to anticipate what will happen to support levels from year to year. We believe that as the contributions of health psychologists become visible, substantial increases in health psychological research will be supported. Part of this support will be in what is classified as biomedical research, and part in health services research. The National Research Council (1976) forecast a marked overproduction of researchers in the areas of biomedical research and behavioral sciences, relative to the number of replacement positions anticipated, so severe competition can be expected by health psychologists who want to work in fields that are categorized under these rubrics. However, the Council cited estimated needs for from 1,200 to 2,000 new persons in the field of health services research by 1980, with an anticipated production of "Ph.D.s in public health" at the rate of about 100 per year (National Research Council, 1976, p. 60). The report indicated that "most health services researchers practicing at this time entered from such academic disciplines as economics, sociology, statistics, epidemiology, and public health" (p. 59). Psychology, notably absent from this list, might be able to contribute at least a proportional share in the years ahead, and, if so, 200 to 300 positions would be created.

A job market that has great potential for expansion is that of the general hospital. If the research and consultation of a psychologist within such an organization can reduce costs of providing quality care by as little as 1 percent, every hospital of seventy-five beds or more should have at least one psychologist on its staff. If only a fourth of such hospitals realized this fact, there would still be 800 new jobs created.

Adding these optimistic, but not unjustifiable guesses together, we find a total of about 2,400 new jobs in the next ten years, without even considering the potential growth in the provision of direct psychological services to general medical patients. This is a remarkably rosy picture for a period of generally gloomy employment prospects. It is based in considerable part upon our belief that the effective application of psychology can increase the effectiveness and efficiency of the health system. In order to realize this agreeable future, health psychologists will have to demonstrate their value.

Will all of these new positions be filled by persons who emerge from doctoral or postdoctoral programs that are labeled as health psychology or one of its subdivisions? Even if we include pediatric psychology and rehabilitation psychology as specializations within health psychology, the answer to that question must be, assuredly not. Many persons will continue to move into a specialization in the health field from more general backgrounds in clinical psychology, social psychology, organizational psychology, and the like. If we envision a continuing need for about 200 health psychologists per year, it might be reasonable to train half of them in specialized predoctoral programs. Such programs will probably be relatively small, typically graduating perhaps five students a year, from each of about twenty programs. We do not add the faculty for these programs to our forecasts of new jobs, since we strongly suspect that the personnel required are already among the present cohort of health psychologists, actively planning the inauguration of such training. As the field grows, however, this may be a source of some new positions.

A Final Word

Psychology can do a great deal to improve the quality of health care. Psychologists can participate in the development of more rational approaches to the total deployment of resources to improve the health of populations. Psychologists can help increase the satisfactions and decrease the personal costs for those who follow careers as providers of health care and health services. Psychologists who specialize for such work—health psychologists—would amply justify their existence by providing such benefits to the society at large. But let us consider how health psychologists can also make significant contributions to the development of psychology as a scientific discipline.

We have earlier taken note of the view that psychology needs to strengthen its theories by testing them against the complexities of real and relevant problems (Deutsch, 1976; Glaser, 1973). The health system offers an opportunity for such tests but it also offers other special advantages as a real-world laboratory that are not shared by the educational, industrial, recreational, and political sectors of our society. We have already mentioned some of the special problems of doing research in health settings—problems that arise, in part, from the salience of ethical issues in health contexts and from the deep concern for the protection of the rights and sensibilities of patients and their families in times of great stress. But these very difficulties also provide opportunities that can be developed as we find ways to do research with fundamental respect and human concern for those from whom we garner data. There is no need to deceive people in order to have a chance to observe them under conditions of stress. The stress is present in every degree, ready to inform us when we have methods of sufficient delicacy. Similarly, normal taboos regarding privacy are greatly reduced in the contexts of health care, giving access to material that may normally be hidden. Here too we must work from a basis of respect and caring for those whom we observe, so that, in our desire to gain knowledge, we do not add to their burdens. This risk exists in all medical research, but there appear to be offsetting, direct values for some participants in psychological research. The chance to talk with a skilled listener about the emotional burdens of severe illness and its treatment without having to ask for counseling services is often much appreciated by those who are interviewed.

Another advantage of the health setting as a research site is the relative coherence of values that prevail. In education, there are great differences of opinion and philosophy as to what constitutes a valued outcome. In industry and politics, there are often overtly conflicting values among the different parties. In the health system, such differences are not entirely absent but they are substantially reduced. This greater agreement enhances possibilities for cooperation, not only among researchers and professionals in the health care system but also among researchers and potential research subjects. People who cooperate are more willing than those in conflict to talk about their motives, plans, and expectations and to subject their beliefs to empirical test. Their willingness provides a favorable situation for the study of the processes through which people reach decisions, plan for their implementation, and often fall short in their efforts to bring their plans to completion.

Thus, the health system offers us opportunities for learning about the behavior of humans who are engaged fully in poignant struggles to preserve and develop their human capacities in the face of challenge and adversity. Health psychology, as that part of the discipline of psychology that deals with the special qualities and problems presented by the health system as a setting for human behavior, can greatly enrich the range of phenomena that we as psychologists are able to observe and can extend our theories into regions inaccessible to laboratory study.

References

Aakster, C. W. "Psycho-Social Stress and Health Disturbances." *Social Science and Medicine*, 1974, *8*, 77-90.

Abelson, R. P., and Rosenberg, M. J. "Symbolic Psychologic: A Model of Attitudinal Cognition." *Behavioral Science*, 1958, *3*, 51-73.

Abram, H. S. (Ed.). "Psychological Aspects of Surgery." *International Psychiatry Clinics*, 1967, *4* (2).

Abram, H. S. "Survival by Machine: The Psychological Stress of Chronic Hemodialysis." *Psychiatry in Medicine*, 1970, *1*, 37-51.

Abram, H. S., and Gill, B. F. "Predictions of Postoperative Psychiatric Complications." *New England Journal of Medicine*, 1961, *265*, 1123-1128.

Abrams, H. L. *Angiography.* Vol. 1 (2nd ed.). Boston: Little, Brown, 1971.

Abrams, R. D. "The Patient with Cancer—His Changing Patterns of Communication." *New England Journal of Medicine*, 1966, *274*, 317-322.

Abrams, R. D., and Finesinger, J. "Guilt Reactions in Patients with Cancer." *Cancer*, 1953, *6*, 474-482.

Abse, D. W., Wilkins, M. M., Van de Castle, R. L., Buxton, W. D., Demars, J., Brown, R. S., and Kirschner, L. G. "Personality and Behavioral Characteristics of Lung Cancer Patients." *Journal of Psychosomatic Research*, 1974, *18*, 101-113.

Ackerknecht, E. A. *A Short History of Medicine.* New York: Ronald Press, 1968.

Adair, J., Deuschle, K., and McDermott, W. "Patterns of Health and Disease Among the Navaho." *Annals of the American Academy of Political and Social Science,* 1957, *311,* 80-94.

Aday, L. A., and Andersen, R. "A Framework for the Study of Access to Medical Care." *Health Services Research,* 1974, *9* (3), 208-220.

Aday, L. A., and Andersen, R. *Access to Medical Care.* Ann Arbor, Mich.: Health Administration Press, 1975.

Aday, L. A., and Eichhorn, R. L. *The Utilization of Health Services: Indices and Correlates—A Research Bibliography.* DHEW Publication No. (HSM) 73-3003. Washington, D.C.: U.S. Government Printing Office, 1972.

Ader, R. "Plasma Pepsinogen Level as a Predictor of Susceptibility to Gastric Erosions in the Rat." *Psychosomatic Medicine,* 1963, *25,* 221-232.

Ader, R. "The Role of Developmental Factors in Susceptibility to Disease." *International Journal of Psychiatry in Medicine,* 1974, *5,* 367-376.

Ader, R., and Grota, L. J. "Adrenocortical Mediation of the Effects of Early Life Experiences." *Progress in Brain Research,* 1973, *39,* 395-405.

Adesso, V. J. "Correlates Between Cigarette Smoking and Alcohol Use." Paper presented at annual meeting of the American Psychological Association, San Francisco, August 1977.

Adler, A. *The Science of Living.* New York: Greenberg, 1929.

Adriani, J., and Lief, V. F. "Psychological Aspects of Anesthesia." In H. I. Lief, V. F. Lief, and N. R. Lief (Eds.), *The Psychological Basis of Medical Practice.* New York: Harper & Row, 1963.

Adsett, C. A. "Emotional Reactions to Disfigurement from Cancer Therapy." *Canadian Medical Association Journal,* 1963, *89,* 385-391.

Aiken, L. H. "Systematic Relaxation to Reduce Preoperative Stress." *The Canadian Nurse,* 1972, *68,* 38-42.

Aiken, L. H., and Henrichs, T. F. "Systematic Relaxation as a Nursing Intervention Technique with Open-Heart Surgery Patients." *Nursing Research,* 1971, *20,* 212-217.

Alford, R. R. *Health Care Politics: Ideological and Interest Group Barriers to Reform.* Chicago: University of Chicago Press, 1975.

Allan, J., Townley, R., and Phelan, P. "Family Response to Cystic Fibrosis." *Australian Pediatric Journal,* 1974, *10,* 136-146.

Allen, T. W. "Physical Health: An Expanding Horizon for Counselors." *Personnel and Guidance Journal,* 1977, *57,* 40-43.

Almond, G. A. "Political Theory and Political Science." In I. Pool (Ed.), *Contemporary Political Science.* New York: McGraw-Hill, 1967.

Alpert, J., Kosa, J., Haggerty, R. J., Robertson, L. S., and Heagarty, M. C. "The Types of Families That Use an Emergency Service." *Medical Care,* 1969, *7,* 55-61.

Alpert, J., Kosa, J., Haggerty, R. J., Robertson, L. S., and Heagarty, M. C. "Attitudes and Satisfactions of Low-Income Families Receiving Comprehensive Pediatric Care." *American Journal of Public Health,* 1970, *60,* 499-506.

Altman, I. "Crowding: Historical and Contemporary Trends in Crowding Research." In A. Baum and Y. Epstein (Eds.), *Human Responses to Crowding.* Hillsdale, N.J.: Lawrence Erlbaum, 1977.

American Board of Professional Psychology. *Directory of Diplomates.* Rochester, N.Y.: American Board of Professional Psychology, 1974.

American Psychological Association, Task Force on Health Research. *Newsletter #2.* Washington, D.C.: American Psychological Association, 1974a.

American Psychological Association, Task Force on Health Research. *Newsletter #3.* Washington, D.C.: American Psychological Association, 1974b.

American Psychological Association, Task Force on Health Research. "Contributions of Psychology to Health Research: Patterns, Problems, and Potentials." *American Psychologist,* 1976, *31,* 263-274.

American Psychological Association. *Directory: 1978.* Washington, D.C.: American Psychological Association, 1978a.

American Psychological Association, Task Force on Continuing Evaluation in National Health Insurance. "Continuing Evaluation and Accountability Controls for a National Health Insurance System." *American Psychologist,* 1978b, *33,* 305-313.

Amkraut, A., and Solomon, G. F. "From the Symbolic Stimulus to the Pathophysiologic Response: Immune Mechanisms." *International Journal of Psychiatry in Medicine,* 1974, *5,* 541-563.

Anant, S. S. "A Note on the Treatment of Alcoholics by a Verbal Aversion Technique." *Canadian Psychologist,* 1967, *8,* 19-22.

Andersen, R. *A Behavioral Model of Families' Use of Health Services.* Research Series No. 25. Chicago: Center for Health Administration Studies, University of Chicago, 1968.

Andersen, R. A., Anderson, D. W., and Smedby, B. "Perception of and Response to Symptoms of Illness in Sweden and the United States." *Medical Care,* 1968, *6* (1), 18-30.

Anderson, J., and Bartkus, D. "Choice of Medical Care: A Behavioral Model of Health and Illness Behavior." *Journal of Health and Social Behavior,* 1973, *14,* 348-362.

Anderson, J. R., and Bower, G. H. *Human Associative Memory.* Washington, D.C.: Winston-Wiley, 1973.

Andreasen, N. J. C., and Norris, A. S. "Long-Term Adjustment and Adaptation Mechanisms in Severely Burned Adults." *Journal of Nervous and Mental Disease,* 1972, *154,* 352-362.

Andreasen, N. J. C., Noyes, R., Jr., and Hartford, C. E. "Factors Influencing Adjustment of Burn Patients During Hospitalization." *Psychosomatic Medicine,* 1972, *34,* 517-525.

Andrew, J. M. "Coping Styles, Stress-Relevant Learning, and Recovery from Surgery." Unpublished doctoral dissertation, University of California, Los Angeles, 1967.

Andrew, J. M. "Recovery from Surgery, With and Without Preparatory Instruction, for Three Coping Styles." *Journal of Personality and Social Psychology,* 1970, *15,* 223-226.

Andrew, J. M. "Delay of Surgery." *Psychosomatic Medicine,* 1972, *34,* 345-354.

Andrus, L. H., Hyde, D. F., and Fischer, E. "Smoking by High School Students—Failure of a Campaign to Persuade Adolescents Not to Smoke." *California Medicine,* 1964, *101,* 246-247.

Anliker, J. "Biofeedback from the Perspectives of Cybernetics and Systems Science." In J. Beatty and H. Legewie (Eds.), *Biofeedback and Behavior.* New York: Plenum Press, 1977.

Anokhin, P. K. *Problems of Center and Periphery in the Physiology of Nervous Activity.* Gorki: Gosizdat, 1935.

Antley, R. M., and Hartlage, L. C. "Psychological Response to Genetic Counseling for Down's Syndrome." *Clinical Genetics,* 1976, *9,* 257-265.

Antonovsky, A. "Conceptual and Methodological Problems in the Study of Resistance Resources and Stressful Life Events." In B. S. Dohrenwend and B. P. Dohrenwend (Eds.), *Stressful Life Events: Their Nature and Effects.* New York: Wiley, 1974.

Antonovsky, A., and Hartman, H. "Delay in the Detection of Cancer: A Review of the Literature." *Health Education Monographs,* 1974, *2* (2), 98-125.

Arbib, M. A. *The Metaphorical Brain.* New York: Wiley, 1972.

Archer, J., Jr., and Kagan, N. "Teaching Interpersonal Relationship Skills on Campus: A Pyramid Approach." *Journal of Counseling Psychology,* 1973, *20,* 534-541.

Argyris, C., and Schön, D. A. *Theory in Practice: Increasing Professional Effectiveness.* San Francisco: Jossey-Bass, 1974.

Armstrong, M., and others. "Double Blind Control Study of Hypertensive Agents." *Archives of Internal Medicine,* 1962, *110,* 222-239.

Arnold, M. "Use of Management Tools for Health Planning." *Public Health Reports,* 1968, *83,* 820-826.

Artiss, K. L., and Levine, A. S. "Doctor-Patient Relation in Severe Illness." *New England Journal of Medicine,* 1973, *288,* 1210-1214.

Ashby, W. R. *Design for a Brain.* New York: Wiley, 1960.

Asken, M. J. "Medical Psychology: Psychology's Neglected Child." *Professional Psychology,* 1975, *6,* 155-160.

Atkinson, R. C., and Shiffrin, R. M. "Human Memory: A Proposed System and Its Control Processes." In K. W. Spence and J. T. Spence (Eds.), *The Psychology of Learning and Motivation.* Vol. 2. New York: Academic Press, 1968.

Attkisson, C. C., and Hargreaves, W. A. "A Conceptual Model for Program Evaluation in Health Organizations." In H. C. Schulberg and F. Baker (Eds.), *Program Evaluation in the Health Fields.* Vol. 2. New York: Behavioral Publications, 1976.

Aubrey, R. F. "Historical Development of Guidance and Counseling and Implications for the Future." *Personnel and Guidance Journal,* 1977, *55,* 288-295.

Audy, J. R. "Measurement and Diagnosis of Health." In P. Shepard and D. McKinley (Eds.), *Environ/Mental.* Boston: Houghton Mifflin, 1971.

Auerbach, S. M., Kendall, P. C., Cuttler, H. F., and Levitt, N. R. "Anxiety, Locus of Control, Type of Preparatory Information, and Adjustment to Dental Surgery." *Journal of Consulting and Clinical Psychology,* 1976, *44,* 809-818.

Auerbach, S. M., and Kilmann, P. R. "Crisis Intervention: A Review of Outcome Research." *Psychological Bulletin,* 1977, *84,* 1189-1217.

Austin, S. H. "Coping and Psychological Stress in Pregnancy, Labor, and Delivery, with 'Natural Childbirth' and 'Medicated' Patients." Unpublished doctoral dissertation, University of California, Berkeley, 1974.

Averill, J. R. "Personal Control over Aversive Stimuli and Its Relationship to Stress." *Psychological Bulletin,* 1973, *80,* 286-303.

Averill, J. R. "A Selective Review of Cognitive and Behavioral Factors Involved in the Regulation of Stress." In R. A. Depue (Ed.), *The Psychobiology of Depressive Disorders: Implications for the Effects of Stress.* New York: Academic Press, in press.

Averill, J. R., and Opton, E. M., Jr. "Psychophysiological Assessment: Rationale and Problems." In P. McReynolds (Ed.), *Advances in Psychological Assessment.* Vol. 1. Palo Alto, Calif.: Science and Behavior Books, 1968.

Azrin, N. H. "A Strategy for Applied Research." *American Psychologist,* 1977, *32,* 140-149.

Backus, R., and Dudley, D. "Observations of Psychosocial Factors and Their Relationship to Organic Disease." *International Journal of Psychiatry in Medicine,* 1974, *5,* 499-515.

Bacon, C. L., Renneker, R., and Cutler, M. "A Psychosomatic Survey of Cancer of the Breast." *Psychosomatic Medicine,* 1952, *14,* 453-460.

Baddeley, A. D. *The Psychology of Memory.* New York: Academic Press, 1976.

Baddeley, A. D. "A Three-Minute Reasoning Test Based on Grammatical Transformations." *Psychonomic Science,* 1968b, *10,* 341-342.

Baddeley, A. D. "Information Processing and Alcohol: A Field Experiment." Paper presented at the first Scandinavian Symposium on Information Processing and Performance, Uppsala, Sweden, 1977.

Baekeland, F., and Lundwall, L. "Dropping Out of Treatment: A Critical Review." *Psychological Bulletin,* 1975, *82,* 738-783.

Baekeland, F., Lundwall, L., and Kissin, B. "Methods for the Treatment of Chronic Alcoholism: A Critical Appraisal." In Y. Israel (Ed.), *Research Advances in Alcohol and Drug Problems.* Vol. 2. New York: Wiley, 1975.

Baekeland, F., Lundwall, L., and Shanahan, T. "Correlates of Patient Attrition in the Outpatient Treatment of Alcoholism." *Journal of Nervous and Mental Disease,* 1973, *157,* 99-107.

Bahnson, C. B. "Psychophysiological Complementarity in Malignancies: Past

Work and Future Vistas." *Annals of the New York Academy of Sciences,* 1969, *164* (Art. 2), 319-333.

Bahnson, C. B., and Bahnson, M. B. "Role of the Ego Defenses: Denial and Repression in the Etiology of Malignant Neoplasm." *Annals of the New York Academy of Sciences,* 1966, *125* (Art. 3), 827-845.

Bahnson, M. B., and Bahnson, C. B. "Ego Defenses in Cancer Patients." *Annals of the New York Academy of Sciences,* 1969, *164* (Art. 2), 546-557.

Bailey, R. Personal Communication, 1978.

Baker, L. *Out on a Limb.* New York: McGraw-Hill, 1946.

Balance, W. D. G., Hirschfield, P. P., and Bringman, W. G. "Mental Illness: Myth, Metaphor, or Model." *Professional Psychology,* 1970, *1,* 133-137.

Ball, T. S., and Vogler, R. E. "Uncertain Pain and the Pain of Uncertainty." *Perceptual and Motor Skills,* 1971, *33,* 1195-1203.

Bandura, A. *Principles of Behavior Modification.* New York: Holt, Rinehart and Winston, 1969.

Bandura, A. *Social Learning Theory.* Englewood Cliffs, N.J.: Prentice-Hall, 1976.

Bandura, A., and Walters, R. H. *Social Learning and Personality Development.* New York: Holt, Rinehart and Winston, 1963.

Banks, F., and Keller, M. "Symptom Experience and Health Action." *Medical Care,* 1971, *9* (6), 498-502.

Barber, T. X. "Death by Suggestion: A Critical Note." *Psychosomatic Medicine,* 1961, *23,* 153-155.

Bard, M. "The Sequence of Emotional Reactions in Radical Mastectomy Patients." *Public Health Reports,* 1952, *67,* 1144-1148.

Bard, M. "The Price of Survival for Cancer Victims." In A. Strauss (Ed.), *Where Medicine Fails.* Chicago: Aldine, 1970.

Bard, M., and Sutherland, A. M. "Psychological Impact of Cancer and its Treatment: IV. Adaptation to Radical Mastectomy." *Cancer,* 1955, *8,* 656-672.

Baric, L. "Recognition of the 'At Risk' Role—A Means to Influence Health Behavior." *International Journal of Health Education,* 1969, *12,* 24-34.

Barker, R. G., and Associates. *Habitats, Environments, and Human Behavior: Studies in Ecological Psychology and Eco-Behavioral Science.* San Francisco, Calif.: Jossey-Bass, 1978.

Barker, R. G., and Schoggen, P. *Qualities of Community Life: Methods of Measuring Environment and Behavior Applied to an American and an English Town.* San Francisco, Calif.: Jossey-Bass, 1973.

Barnett, E. M. "Behavioral Therapy in the Effective Management of Periodontal Disease—An Introduction to Behavioral Dentistry." *Dental Digest,* 1970, *76,* 506-511.

Baron, R., and Rodin, J. "Perceived Control and Crowding Stress." In A. Baum, J. E. Singer, and S. Valins (Eds.), *Advances in Environmental Psychology.* Hillsdale, N.J.: Lawrence Erlbaum, 1978.

Barrows, H. S., and Bennett, K. "Experimental Studies on the Diagnostic

(Problem-Solving) Skill of the Neurologist: Their Implications for Neurological Training." *Archives of Neurology,* 1972, *26,* 273-277.

Barrows, H. S., Feightner, J. W., Neufeld, V. R., and Norman, G. R. "Analysis of the Clinical Methods of Medical Students and Physicians." Hamilton, Ontario: School of Medicine, McMaster University, 1978.

Barrows, H. S., Norman, G. R., Neufeld, V. R., and Feightner, J. W. "Studies of the Clinical Reasoning Process of Medical Students and Physicians." In *Proceedings of the Sixteenth Annual Conference on Research in Medical Education.* Washington, D.C.: Association of American Medical Colleges, 1977.

Bartlett, F. C. *Remembering.* Cambridge, England: Cambridge University Press, 1932.

Baum, A., and Davis, G. "Spatial and Social Aspects of Crowding Perception." *Environment and Behavior,* 1976, *8,* 527-544.

Baum, A., and Greenberg, C. "Waiting for a Crowd: The Behavioral and Perceptual Effects of Anticipated Crowding." *Journal of Personality and Social Psychology,* 1975, *32,* 671-679.

Baum, A., Harpin, R., and Valins, S. "The Role of Group Phenomena in the Experience of Crowding." *Environment and Behavior,* 1975, *7,* 185-198.

Baum, A., and Koman, S. "Differential Response to Anticipated Crowding: Psychological Effects of Social and Spatial Density." *Journal of Personality and Social Psychology,* 1976, *34,* 526-536.

Baum, A., and Valins, S. (Eds.). *Advances in Environmental Research.* Hillsdale, N.J.: Lawrence Erlbaum, 1977.

Baumann, B. "Diversities in Conceptions of Health and Physical Fitness." *Journal of Health and Human Behavior,* 1961, *2,* 39-46.

Bayliss, L. E. *Living Control Systems.* San Francisco: W. H. Freeman, 1966.

Beach, B. H. "Expert Judgment About Uncertainty: Bayesian Decision Making in Realistic Settings." *Organizational Behavior and Human Performance,* 1975, *14,* 10-59.

Bearman, J. E., Loewenson, R. B., and Gullen, W. H. "Muench's Postulates, Laws, and Corollaries." In *Biometrics Note 4.* Bethesda, Md.: National Eye Institute, 1974.

Beatty, J., and Legewie, H. (Eds.). *Biofeedback and Behavior.* New York: Plenum Press, 1977.

Beck, E., Blaichman, S., Scriver, C. R., and Clow, C. L. "Advocacy and Compliance in Genetic Screening." *New England Journal of Medicine,* 1974, *291,* 1166-1172.

Becker, F. "User Participation, Personalization, and Environmental Meaning: Three Field Studies." *Program in Urban and Regional Studies.* Ithaca, N.Y.: Cornell University Press, 1977.

Becker, H. S., and Geer, B. "The Fate of Idealism in Medical School." *American Sociological Review,* 1958, *23,* 50-60.

Becker, H. S., Geer, B., Hughes, E. C., and Strauss, A. L. *Boys in White: Student Culture in Medical School.* Chicago: University of Chicago Press, 1961.

Becker, M. H. (Ed.). "The Health Belief Model and Personal Health Behavior." *Health Education Monographs,* 1974a, *2* (Whole no. 4).

Becker, M. H. "The Health Belief Model and Sick Role Behavior." *Health Education Monographs,* 1974b, *2* (4), 409-419.

Becker, M. H. "Sociobehavioral Determinants of Compliance." In D. L. Sackett and R. B. Haynes (Eds.), *Compliance with Therapeutic Regimens.* Baltimore: Johns Hopkins University Press, 1976.

Becker, M. H., Drachman, R. H., and Kirscht, J. P. "Motivations as Predictors of Health Behavior." *Health Services Reports,* 1972a, *87,* 852-862.

Becker, M. H., Drachman, R. H., and Kirscht, J. P. "Predicting Mothers' Compliance with Pediatric Medical Regimens." *Journal of Pediatrics,* 1972b, *81* (4), 843-854.

Becker, M. H., Drachman, R. H., and Kirscht, J. P. "A Field Experiment to Evaluate Various Outcomes of Continuity of Physician Care." *American Journal of Public Health,* 1974, *64* (11), 1062-1070.

Becker, M. H., Haefner, D. P., Kasl, S. V., Kirscht, J. P., Maiman, L. A., and Rosenstock, I. M. "Selected Psychosocial Models and Correlates of Individual Health-Related Behaviors." *Medical Care,* 1977a, *15* (suppl.), 27-48.

Becker, M. H., Kaback, M., Rosenstock, I. M., and Ruth, M. "Some Influences on Public Participation in a Genetic Screening Program." *Journal of Community Health,* 1975, *1,* 3-14.

Becker, M. H., and Maiman, L. A. "Sociobehavioral Determinants of Compliance with Health and Medical Care Recommendations." *Medical Care,* 1975, *13* (1), 10-24.

Becker, M. H., Maiman, L. A., Kirscht, J. P., Haefner, D. P., and Drachman, R. H. "The Health Belief Model and Dietary Compliance: A Field Experiment." *Journal of Health and Social Behavior,* 1977b, *18,* 348-366.

Beecher, H. K. *Measurement of Subjective Responses.* New York: Oxford University Press, 1959.

Beeson, D. Personal Communication, August 19, 1977.

"Behavioral Sciences and Medical Education." DHEW Publication No. (NIH) 72-41. Washington, D.C.: U.S. Government Printing Office, 1972.

Beiser, M., Feldman, J., and Engelhoff, C. "Assets and Affects." *Archives of General Psychiatry,* 1972, *27,* 545-549.

Bell, C. R. "Additional Data on Animistic Thinking." *Scientific Monthly,* 1954, *79,* 67-69.

Bell, R. A. "The Use of the Convergent Assessment Model in the Determination of Health Status and Assessment of Need." In R. A. Bell, M. Sundel, J. F. Aponte, and S. A. Murrel (Eds.), *Need Assessment in Health and Human Services: Proceedings of the Louisville National Conference,* University of Louisville, Louisville, Ky., March 9-12, 1976. (Expanded version to be published by Human Sciences Press, 1979.)

Bellack, A. S. "Behavior Therapy for Weight Reduction: An Evaluative Review." *Addictive Behaviors: An International Journal,* 1975, *1,* 73-82.

Bennette, G. "Psychic and Cellular Aspects of Isolation and Identity Impair-

References 599

ment in Cancer: A Dialectic of Alienation." *Annals of the New York Academy of Sciences,* 1969, *164* (Art. 2), 352-363.

Benney, M., Riesman, D., and Star, S. "Age and Sex in the Interview." *American Journal of Sociology,* 1956, *62,* 143-152.

Benor, D., and Ditman, K. S. "Tranquilizers in the Management of Alcoholics: A Review of the Literature to 1964, Part I." *Journal of New Drugs,* 1964, *6,* 319-337.

Berecz, J. "Smoking, Stuttering, Sex, and Pizza. Is there a Commonality?" Paper presented at annual meeting of the American Association for Behavior Therapy, New York, 1974.

Berg, R. L. *Health Status Indexes.* Chicago: Hospital Research and Educational Trust, 1973.

Bergler, E. "Psychopathology of Compulsive Smoking." *Psychiatric Quarterly,* 1946, *20,* 297-321.

Bergler, E. "Smoking and Its Infantile Precursors." *International Journal of Sexology,* 1953, *6,* 214-220.

Bergner, L., and Yerley, A. S. "Low Income Barriers to Use of Health Services." *New England Journal of Medicine,* 1968, *278,* 541-546.

Bergner, M., Bobbitt, R. A., Pollard, W. E., Martin, M. A., and Gilson, B. S. "The Sickness Impact Profile: Validation of a Health Status Measure." *Medical Care,* 1976, *14,* 57-67.

Berkanovic, E. "Lay Conceptions of the Sick Role." *Social Forces,* 1972, *51,* 53-64.

Berkman, L. F. "Social Networks, Host Resistance, and Mortality: A Follow-Up Study of Alameda County Residents." Unpublished doctoral dissertation, University of California, Berkeley, 1977.

Berle, B. B., Pinsky, R. H., Wolf, S., and Wolff, H. G. "A Clinical Guide to Prognosis in Stress Diseases." *Journal of the American Medical Association,* 1952, *149,* 1624-1628.

Berne, E. *Games People Play.* New York: Grove, 1964.

Bernstein, A. C., and Cowan, P. A. "Children's Concepts of How People Get Babies." *Child Development,* 1975, *46,* 77-91.

Bernstein, I. L. "Taste Aversions in Children Receiving Chemotherapy." *Science,* 1978, *200,* 1302-1303.

Berscheid, E., and Walster, E. H. *Interpersonal Attraction.* Reading, Mass.: Addison-Wesley, 1969.

Betaque, N. E., and Gorry, G. A. "Automating Judgmental Decision Making for a Serious Medical Problem." *Management Science,* 1971, *17,* B421-B434.

Bibace, R., and Walsh, M. E. "Children's Conceptions of Health and Illness." Paper presented at annual meeting of the American Psychological Association, San Francisco, August 1977.

Bickman, L., Teger, A., Gabriele, T., McLaughlin, C., Berger, M., and Sunaday, E. "Dormitory Density and Helping Behavior." *Environment and Behavior,* 1973, *5,* 465-490.

Binger, C. M., Arlin, A. R., Feuerstein, R. C., Kushner, J. H., Zoger, S., and

Mikkelsen, C. "Childhood Leukemia." *New England Journal of Medicine*, 1969, *280*, 414-418.

Bion, W. R. *Experiences in Groups*. London: Tavistock Publications, 1961.

Bissell, L. "The Alcoholic Physician: A Survey." *American Journal of Psychiatry*, 1976, *133*, 1142-1146.

Blachly, P. H., Disher, W., and Roduner, G. "Suicide by Physicians." *Bulletin of Suicidology*, December 1968, pp. 1-18.

Blachly, P. H., Osterud, H. T., and Josslin, R. "Suicide in Professional Groups." *New England Journal of Medicine*, 1963, *268*, 1278-1282.

Blackburn, H. "Prediction and Prognostication in Coronary Heart Disease." *New England Journal of Medicine*, 1974, *290*, 1315-1316.

Blacker, R. S. "Losses of Internal Organs." In B. Schoenberg, A. C. Carr, D. Peretz, and A. H. Kutscher (Eds.), *Loss and Grief: Psychological Management in Medical Practice*. New York: Columbia University Press, 1970.

Blackwell, B. "Drug Therapy: Patient Compliance." *New England Journal of Medicine*, 1973, *289*, 249-253.

Blake, B. G. "The Application of Behavior Therapy to the Treatment of Alcoholism." *Behavior Research and Therapy*, 1965, *3*, 75-85.

Blake, B. G. "A Follow-Up of Alcoholics Treated by Behavior Therapy." *Behavior Research and Therapy*, 1967, *5*, 89-94.

Blane, H. T., and Meyers, W. R. "Behavioral Dependence and Length of Stay in Psychotherapy Among Alcoholics." *Quarterly Journal of Studies on Alcohol*, 1963, *24*, 503-510.

Blank, L. "Clinical Psychology Training, 1945-1962: Conferences and Issues." In L. Blank and H. P. David (Eds.), *Sourcebook for Training in Clinical Psychology*. New York: Springer, 1964.

Blaug, S. M., Gold, B., Sonnedecker, G., Suarstad, B., Knapp, D. E., Morris, L. A., Knapp, D. A., and Palumbo, F. B. "Interdisciplinary Panel Discussion: A Realistic Appraisal of the Potential Contribution of the Social and Behavioral Sciences to Professional Education in Pharmacy." *American Journal of Pharmaceutical Education*, 1975, *39*, 593-595.

Blischke, W. R., Bush, J. W., and Kaplan, R. M. "A Successive Analysis of Social Preference Measures for a Health Status Index." *Health Services Research*, 1975, *10*, 181-198.

Bliss, R., Moos, R. H., and Bromet, E. "Monitoring Change in Community-Oriented Treatment Programs." *Journal of Community Psychology*, 1976, *4*, 315-326.

Block, J. "Some Reasons for the Apparent Inconsistency of Personality." *Psychological Bulletin*, 1968, *70*, 210-212.

Bloom, B. "The Use of Social Indicators in the Estimation of Health Needs." In R. A. Bell, M. Sundel, J. F. Aponte, and S. A. Murrel (Eds.), *Need Assessment in Health and Human Services: Proceedings of the Louisville National Conference*, University of Louisville, Louisville, Ky., March 9-12, 1976. (Expanded version to be published by Human Sciences Press, 1979.)

Bloom, S. W. "From Learned Profession to Policy Science: A Trend Analysis of Sociology in the Medical Education of the United States." In M. Sokolowska, J. Holowka, and A. Ostrowska (Eds.), *Health, Medicine, and Society*. Boston: D. Reidel, 1976.

Blum, H. L. *Planning for Health*. New York: Human Services Press, 1974a.

Blum, H. L. "Evaluating Health Care." *Medical Care*, 1974b, *121*, 999-1011.

Blumberg, B. D., and Golbus, M. S. "Psychological Sequelae of Elective Abortion." *Western Journal of Medicine*, 1975, *3* (123), 188-193.

Blumberg, E. M., West, P. M., and Ellis, F. W. "A Possible Relationship Between Psychological Factors and Human Cancer." *Psychosomatic Medicine*, 1954, *16*, 277-286.

Blumenthal, J. A., Kong, Y., Rosenman, R. H., and others. "Type A Behavior Pattern and Angiographically Documented Coronary Disease." Paper presented at the meeting of the American Psychosomatic Society, New Orleans, March 1975. (Referenced in Jenkins, 1976).

Bobbitt, J. M. "Opening Remarks." In *Conference on Graduate Education in Psychology*. Washington, D.C.: American Psychological Association, 1959.

Boffey, P. M. "Smallpox: Outbreak in Somalia Slows Rapid Progress Toward Eradication." *Science*, 1977, *196*, 1298-1299.

Boltuch, B. S. "The Effects of a Pre-Practicum Skill Training Program, *Influencing Human Interaction*, on Developing Counselor Effectiveness in a Master's Level Practicum." Unpublished doctoral dissertation, New York University, 1975.

Booth, A., and Edwards, J. "Crowding and Family Relations." *American Sociological Review*, 1976, *41*, 308-321.

Bordage, G., Elstein, A. S., Vinsonhaler, J., and Wagner, C. "Computer-Aided and Computer-Simulated Medical Diagnosis." In *Proceedings of the First IEEE Symposium on Computer Application in Medical Care*. Washington, D.C.: 1977.

Bornstein, P. H., Carmody, R. P., Relinger, H., Zohn, J. C., Devine, D. A., and Bugge, I. D. "Reduction of Smoking Behavior Through Token Reinforcement Procedures." Unpublished manuscript, University of Montana, 1975.

Borsky, P., and Sagen, O. "Motivations Toward Health Examinations." *American Journal of Public Health*, 1959, *49*, 514-527.

Bortz, W. M. "Metabolic Consequences of Obesity." *Annals of Internal Medicine*, 1969, *71*, 833-843.

Bott, E. A. "Teaching of Psychology in the Medical Course." *Bulletin of the Association of American Medical Colleges*, 1928, *3*, 289-304.

Boulding, K. "The Concept of Need for Health Services." *Milbank Memorial Fund Quarterly*, 1960, *44*, 202-223.

Bourne, P. G., Rose, R. M., and Mason, J. W. "Urinary 17-OHCS Levels." *Archives of General Psychiatry*, 1967, *17*, 104-110.

Bowden, C. H., and Burstein, A. G. *Doctor-Patient Interaction in the Practice of Medicine*. Baltimore: Johns Hopkins University Press, 1974.

Bowen, H. R., and Jeffers, J. R. "The Economics of Health Services in the

United States." In M. M. Hauser (Ed.), *The Economics of Medical Care.* London: Allen & Unwin, 1972.

Bowen, W. T., and Adroes, L. "A Follow-Up Study of 79 Alcoholic Patients: 1963-1965." *Bulletin of the Menninger Clinic,* 1968, *32,* 26-34.

Bower, G. H. "Cognitive Psychology: An Introduction." In W. K. Estes (Ed.), *Handbook of Learning and Cognitive Processes.* Hillsdale, N.J.: Lawrence Erlbaum, 1975.

Bowers, K. G. "Pain, Anxiety, and Perceived Control." *Journal of Consulting and Clinical Psychology,* 1968, *32,* 596-602.

Boyar, J. I., and Gramlich, E. P. "Unusual Postsurgical Pain." *Surgical Clinics of North America,* 1970, *50* (2), 309-318.

Boyd, I., Yeager, M., and McMillan, M. "Personality Styles in the Postoperative Course." *Psychosomatic Medicine,* 1973, *35,* 23-40.

Boyle, B. P., and Coombs, R. H. "Personality Profiles Related to Emotional Stress in the Initial Year of Medical School." *Journal of Medical Education,* 1974, *46,* 882-887.

Brammer, L. *The Helping Relationship: Process and Skills.* Englewood Cliffs, N.J.: Prentice-Hall, 1973.

Bransford, J. D., and Franks, J. J. "The Abstraction of Linguistic Ideas." *Cognitive Psychology,* 1971, *2,* 331-350.

Bray, G. A. "Management of Subcutaneous Fat Cells from Obese Patients." *Annals of Internal Medicine,* 1970, *73,* 565-569.

Breen, D. *The Birth of a First Child: Towards an Understanding of Femininity.* London: Tavistock, 1975.

Brehm, J. W. *A Theory of Psychological Reactance.* New York: Academic Press, 1966.

Brehm, S. *The Application of Social Psychology to Clinical Practice.* Washington, D.C.: Hemisphere, 1976.

Brener, J. "Sensory and Perceptual Determinants of Voluntary Visceral Control." In G. E. Schwartz and J. Beatty (Eds.), *Biofeedback: Theory and Research.* New York: Academic Press, 1977a.

Brener, J. "Visceral Perception." In J. Beatty and H. Legewie (Eds.), *Biofeedback and Behavior.* New York: Plenum Press, 1977b.

Breslow, L. "An Historical Review of Multiphasic Screening." *Preventive Medicine,* 1973, *2,* 177-196.

Bressler, B. "Suicide and Drug Abuse in the Medical Community." *Suicide and Life Threatening Behavior,* 1976, *6,* 169-178.

Breuer, S. R. "Feeling of Physical Well Being and Mood Level in Chronically Ill Patients." Unpublished master's thesis, Northwestern University, 1974.

Brew, J. O. (Ed.). *One Hundred Years of Anthropology.* Cambridge: Harvard University Press, 1968.

Brightwell, D. R. "One Year Follow-Up of Obese Subjects Treated with Behavior Therapy." *Diseases of the Nervous System,* 1976, *37,* 593-594.

Brightwell, D. R., and Sloan, C. L. "Long-Term Results of Behavior Therapy for Obesity." *Behavior Therapy,* 1977, *8* (5), 898-905.

Brodie, B. "Views of Healthy Children Toward Illness." *American Journal of Public Health,* 1974, *64,* 1156-1159.

Brodman, K., Erdmann, A. J., Lorge, I., Gershenson, C. P., and Wolff, H. G. "The Cornell Medical Index-Health Questionnaire: III. The Evaluation of Emotional Disturbances." *Journal of Clinical Psychology,* 1952a, *8,* 119-124.

Brodman, K., Erdmann, A. J., Lorge, I., Gershenson, C. P., and Wolff, H. G. "The Cornell Medical Index-Health Questionnaire: IV. The Recognition of Emotional Disorders in a General Hospital." *Journal of Clinical Psychology,* 1952b, *8,* 289-293.

Bromet, E., and Moos, R. H. "Environmental Resources and the Posttreatment Functioning of Alcoholic Patients." *Journal of Health and Social Behavior,* 1977, *18,* 326-338.

Bronfenbrenner, U. "Toward an Experimental Ecology of Human Development." *American Psychologist,* 1977, *32,* 513-531.

Brook, R. H. "Quality of Care Assessment: A Comparison of Five Methods of Peer Review." DHEW Publication No. (HRA) 74-3100. Washington, D.C.: U.S. Government Printing Office, 1973.

Brook, R. H., and Davies-Avery, A. *Mechanisms for Assuring Quality of U.S. Medical Care Services: Past, Present, and Future.* Rand Paper Series, R-1939. Santa Monica, Calif.: Rand Corporation, 1977.

Brown, B. *New Mind, New Body.* New York: Harper & Row, 1975.

Brown, E. D. "The Role of Expectancy in Ratings of Consumer Satisfaction with Mental Health Services." Prospectus for doctoral dissertation, Florida State University, 1978.

Brown, E. L. "Meeting Patients' Psychosocial Needs in the General Hospital." In J. K. Skipper, Jr., and R. C. Leonard (Eds.), *Social Interaction and Patient Care.* Philadelphia: Lippincott, 1965.

Brown, E. R., and Margo, G. E. "Health Education: Can the Reformers Be Reformed?" *International Journal of Health Services,* 1978, *8,* 3-26.

Brown, G. W. "Meaning, Measurement, and Stress of Life Events." In B. S. Dohrenwend and B. P. Dohrenwend (Eds.), *Stressful Life Events: Their Nature and Effects.* New York: Wiley, 1974.

Brown, G. W., Birley, J. L. T., and Wing, J. "Influence of Family Life in the Course of Schizophrenic Disorders: A Replication." *British Journal of Psychiatry,* 1972, *121,* 241-258.

Brownell, K. D., Heckerman, C. L., Westlake, R. J., Hayes, S. C., and Monte, P. M. "The Effect of Couples' Training and Partner Cooperativeness in the Behavioral Treatment of Obesity." Paper presented at annual meeting of the Association for the Advancement of Behavior Therapy, Atlanta, 1977.

Bruce-Briggs, B. "Child Care: The Fiscal Time Bomb." *The Public Interest,* 1977, *49,* 87-102.

Bruch, H. *Eating Disorders.* New York: Basic Books, 1973.

Bruegel, M. A. "Relationship of Preoperative Anxiety to Perception of Postoperative Pain." *Nursing Research,* 1971, *20,* 26-31.

Bruhn, J. G., Chandler, B., and Wolf, S. "A Psychological Study of Survivors and Nonsurvivors of Myocardial Infarction." *Psychosomatic Medicine,* 1969, *31,* 8-19.

Bruhn, J. G., and Parsons, O. A. "Medical Student Attitudes Toward Four Medical Specialties." *Journal of Medical Education,* 1964, *39,* 40-49.

Bruhn, J. G., and Parsons, O. A. "Attitudes Toward Medical Specialties: Two Follow-Up Studies." *Journal of Medical Education,* 1965, *40,* 40-49.

Bruner, J., and Goodman, C. G. "Value and Need as Organizing Factors in Perception." *Journal of Abnormal and Social Psychology,* 1947, *42,* 33-44.

Brunswik, E. "Representative Design and Probabilistic Theory in a Functional Psychology." *Psychological Review,* 1955, *62,* 193-217.

Brzezinski, Z. J. "Comparison of Physical Health Assessments Using Questionnaires and Medical Records." Unpublished manuscript, Human Population Laboratory, California Department of Public Health, Berkeley, 1965.

Buchanan, J. R. "Five Year Psychoanalytic Study of Obesity." *American Journal of Psychoanalysis,* 1973, *33,* 30-38.

Buck, R. L. "Behavioral Scientists in Schools of Medicine." *Journal of Health and Human Behavior,* 1961, *2,* 59-64.

Bullough, B. "Poverty, Ethnic Identity, and Preventive Health Care." *Journal of Health and Social Behavior,* 1972, *13,* 347-359.

Bulman, R. J., and Wortman, C. B. "Attribution of Blame and Coping in the 'Real World': Severe Accident Victims React to Their Lot." *Journal of Personality and Social Psychology,* 1977, *35,* 351-363.

Bultz, B. D. "The Use of Psychometrics in Predicting Surgical Recovery." *Dissertation Abstracts International,* 1975, *35* (7B), 3571.

Bunker, J. P., Barnes, B. A., and Mosteller, F. (Eds.). *Costs, Risks, and Benefits of Surgery.* New York: Oxford University Press, 1977.

Burke, J. B., and Kagan, N. "Influencing Human Interaction in Urban Schools." Final report NIMH grant MH13526-02. Unpublished paper, Department of Counseling Psychology, Michigan State University, East Lansing, Mich., 1976.

Burnum, J. F. "Outlook for Treatment of Patients with Self-Destructive Habits." *Annals of Internal Medicine,* 1974, *81,* 387-393.

Bursten, B., and Russ, J. J. "Preoperative Psychological State and Corticosteroid Levels of Surgical Patients." *Psychosomatic Medicine,* 1965, *27,* 309-316.

Burton, I. "Culture and Personality Variables in the Perception of Natural Hazards." In J. F. Wohlwill and D. H. Carson (Eds.), *Environment and the Social Sciences.* Washington, D.C.: American Psychological Association, 1972.

Busse, E. W., and Pfeiffer, E. (Eds.). *Behavior and Adaptation in Late Life.* Boston: Little, Brown, 1969.

Butler, R. N. "The Life Review: An Interpretation of Reminiscence in the Aged." *Psychiatry,* 1963, *26,* 65-76.

Butler, R. N. "Psychiatry and Psychology of the Middle Aged." In A. Freedman, H. Kaplan, and B. Sadock (Eds.), *Comprehensive Handbook of Psychiatry II*. Vol. 2 (2nd ed.). Baltimore: Williams and Wilkins, 1975a.

Butler, R. N. *Why Survive? Being Old in America*. New York: Harper & Row, 1975b.

Bykov, K. M. "The Effect of the Cerebral Cortex on Visceral and Tissue Activity." *Izbrannye Proizvedeniia*, 1937, *1*, 141-156.

Byrne, D. "The Repression-Sensitization Scale: Rationale, Reliability, and Validity." *Journal of Personality*, 1961, *29*, 334-349.

Byrne, D. "Repression-Sensitization as a Dimension of Personality." In B. A. Maher (Ed.), *Progress in Experimental Personality Research*. Vol. 1. New York: Academic Press, 1964.

Byrne, D. *The Attraction Paradigm*. New York: Academic Press, 1971.

Caffrey, B. "Factors Involving Interpersonal and Psychological Characteristics: A Review of Empirical Findings." In S. L. Syme and L. G. Reeder (Eds.), "Social Stress and Cardiovascular Disease." *Milbank Memorial Fund Quarterly*, 1967, *45* (2), 119-139.

Calden, G., Dupertuis, C. W., Hokanson, J. E., and Lewis, W. C. "Psychosomatic Factors in the Rate of Recovery from Tuberculosis." *Psychosomatic Medicine*, 1960, *22*, 345-355.

Caldwell, J., Cobb, S., Dowling, M. D., and Jongh, D. D. "The Dropout Problem in Antihypertensive Therapy." *Journal of Chronic Diseases*, 1970, *22*, 579-592.

Cameron, A., and Hinton, J. "Delay in Seeking Treatment for Mammary Tumors." *Cancer*, 1968, *21*, 1121-1126.

Campbell, J. D. "Illness Is a Point of View: The Development of Children's Concepts of Illness." *Child Development*, 1975, *46*, 92-100.

Campbell, J. P., Dunnette, M. D., Lawler, E. E., III, and Weick, K. E., Jr. *Managerial Behavior Performance and Organizational Effectiveness*. New York: McGraw-Hill, 1970.

Campbell, R. J., Kagan, N., and Krathwohl, D. R. "The Development and Validation of a Scale to Measure Affective Sensitivity (Empathy)." *Journal of Counseling Psychology*, 1971, *18*, 407-412.

Canfield, R. C., Powell, G. L., and Weinstein, P. "Facilitating the Transition to Dental School." *Journal of Dental Education*, 1976, *40*, 269-271.

"Can Hypertension Be Induced by Stress?" *Journal of Human Stress*, 1977, *3* (1), 4-11.

Cannell, C. F., and MacDonald, J. C. "The Impact of Health News on Attitudes and Behavior." *Journalism Quarterly*, 1956, *33*, 315-323.

Cannon, W. B. *Wisdom of the Body*. New York: Norton, 1932.

Cannon, W. B. "Voodoo Death." *American Anthropologist*, 1942, *44*, 169-181.

Canter, A., Imboden, J. B., and Cluff, L. E. "The Frequency of Physical Illness as a Function of Prior Psychological Vulnerability and Contemporary Stress." *Psychosomatic Medicine*, 1966, *28*, 344-350.

Caplan, G. *Principles of Preventive Psychiatry*. New York: Basic Books, 1974.

Caplan, G., and Killilea, M. (Eds.). *Support Systems and Mutual Help.* New York: Grune & Stratton, 1976.

Caplan, R., Robinson, E. A. R., French, J. R. P., Jr., Caldwell, J. R., and Shinn, M. *Adhering to Medical Regimens.* Ann Arbor: Institute for Social Research, University of Michigan, 1976.

Carkhuff, R. R. *Helping and Human Relations.* Vols. 1 and 2. New York: Holt, Rinehart and Winston, 1969.

Carlson, H. S. "The AASPB Story." *American Psychologist,* 1978, *33,* 486-495.

Carlson, L. A., and Bollinger, L. E. "Ischaemic Heart Disease in Relation to Fasting Values of Plasma Triglyceride and Cholesterol: Stockholm Prospective Study." *Lancet,* 1972, *1,* 865-868.

Carnahan, J., and Nugent, C. "The Effects of Self-Monitoring by Patients on the Control of Hypertension." *American Journal of Medical Science,* 1975, *269,* 69-73.

Caron, H., and Roth, H. "Objective Assessment of Cooperation with an Ulcer Diet: Relation to Antacid Intake and to Assigned Physician." *American Journal of Medical Science,* 1971, *261,* 61-66.

Carroll, J. G., and Monroe, J. "Teaching the Interpersonal Skills of Medical Interviewing: A Review of the Literature." Paper presented at the Conference on Research in Medical Education, Association of American Medical Colleges, New Orleans, 1978.

Carter, C., Fraser-Roberts, J., Evans, K., and Buck, A. "Genetic Clinic: A Follow-Up." *Lancet,* 1971, *2,* 281-285.

Cartwright, A. *Patients and Their Doctors: A Study of General Practice.* London: Routledge and Kegan Paul, 1967.

Cartwright, D. (Ed.). *Field Theory in Social Science: Selected Theoretical Papers by Kurt Lewin.* New York: Harper & Row, 1951.

Cartwright, D., and Zander, A. (Eds.). *Group Dynamics: Research and Theory.* (3rd ed.) New York: Harper & Row, 1968.

Cartwright, L. K. "Personality Differences in Male and Female Medical Students." *Psychiatry in Medicine,* 1972, *3,* 213-218.

Cartwright, L. K. "Personality Changes in a Sample of Young Women Physicians." *Journal of Medical Education,* 1977, *52,* 467-474.

Cartwright, L. K. "Attitudes of a Sample of California Physicians Towards Criteria of High Quality Care." *Journal of Medical Education,* 1978a, *53,* 321-329.

Cartwright, L. K. "Career Satisfaction and Role Harmony in a Sample of Young Women Physicians." *Journal of Vocational Behavior,* 1978b, *12,* 184-196.

Cartwright, L. K. "Career Satisfaction in the Male Physician." Unpublished research report, Institute of Personality Assessment and Research, University of California, Berkeley, 1978c.

Cartwright, L. K. "The Kinds of Patients Doctors Don't Like to See." Unpublished research report, Institute of Personality Assessment and Research, University of California, Berkeley, 1978d.

Cassel, J. "Factors Involving Sociocultural Incongruity and Change: Appraisal and Implications for Theoretical Development." In S. L. Syme and L. G. Reeder (Eds.), "Social Stress and Cardiovascular Disease." *Milbank Memorial Fund Quarterly,* 1967, *45* (2), 41-45.

Cassel, J. "The Contribution of the Social Environment to Host Resistance." *American Journal of Epidemiology,* 1976, *104,* 107-123.

Cassel, J. "The Relation of the Urban Environment to Health: Toward a Conceptual Frame and a Research Strategy." In L. Hinkle and W. Loring (Eds.), *The Effects of the Man-Made Environment on Health and Behavior.* Washington, D.C.: U.S. Government Printing Office, 1977.

Catalano, R., and Dooley, D. "Economic Predictors of Depressed Mood and Stressful Life Events." *Journal of Health and Social Behavior,* 1977, *18,* 292-307.

Cater, D. "An Overview." In D. Cater and P. R. Lee (Eds.), *The Politics of Health.* New York: MedCom Press, 1972.

Cater, D., and Lee, P. R. *The Politics of Health.* New York: MedCom Press, 1972.

Caudhill, W. "Applied Anthropology in Medicine." In A. L. Kroeber (Ed.), *Anthropology Today.* Chicago: University of Chicago Press, 1953.

Cauffman, J. G., Lloyd, J. S., Lyons, M. L., Cortese, P. A., Beckwith, R. L., Petit, D. W., Wehrle, P. F., McBroom, E., and McIntire, J. R. "A Study of Health Referral Patterns." *American Journal of Public Health,* 1974, *64,* 331-356.

Chamberlain, T. C. "The Method of Multiple Working Hypotheses." *Science,* 1965, *148,* 754-759. (Originally published 1890.)

Chambers, L. W., Spitzer, W. O., Hill, G. B., and Helliwell, B. E. "Underreporting of Cancer in Medical Surveys: A Source of Systematic Error in Cancer Research." *American Journal of Epidemiology,* 1976, *104,* 141-145.

Chapman, C. R., and Cox, G. B. "Anxiety, Pain, and Depression Surrounding Elective Surgery: A Multivariate Comparison of Abdominal Surgery Patients with Kidney Donors and Recipients." *Journal of Psychosomatic Research,* 1977, *21,* 7-15.

Charney, E., Bynum, R., Eldredge, D., MacWhinney, J. B., McNabb, N., Scheiner, A., Sumpter, E. A., and Iker, H. "How Well Do Patients Take Oral Penicillin? A Collaborative Study in Private Practice." *Pediatrics,* 1967, *40,* 188-195.

Chen, M., Bush, J. W., and Patrick, D. L. "Social Indicators for Health Planning and Policy Analysis." *Policy Science,* 1975, *6,* 71-105.

Chodoff, P., Friedman, S. B., and Hamburg, D. A. "Stress, Defenses, and Coping Behavior: Observations in Parents of Children with Malignant Disease." *American Journal of Psychiatry,* 1964, *120,* 743-749.

Cipolla, C. M. *Public Health and the Medical Profession in the Renaissance.* New York: Cambridge University Press, 1976.

Clayton, P. J. "Mortality and Morbidity in the First Year of Widowhood." *Archives of General Psychiatry,* 1974, *30,* 747-750.

Cleary, P. J. "Life Events and Disease: A Review of Methodology and Findings." *Reports from the Laboratory for Clinical Stress Research* (No. 37),

Departments of Medicine and Psychiatry, Karolinska Sjukhuset, Stockholm, November 1974.

Clements, J., and Wakefield, J. "Symptoms and Uncertainty." *International Journal of Health Education,* 1972, *15,* 113-122.

Clow, C., Fraser, F., Laberge, C., and Scriver, C. "On the Application of Knowledge to the Patient with Genetic Disease." *Progress in Medical Genetics,* 1973, *9,* 159-213.

Cobb, A. B. *Medical and Psychological Aspects of Disability.* Springfield, Ill.: Thomas, 1973.

Cobb, S. "A Model for Life Events and their Consequences." In B. S. Dohrenwend and B. P. Dohrenwend (Eds.), *Stressful Life Events: Their Nature and Effects.* New York: Wiley, 1974.

Cobb, S. "Social Support as a Moderator of Life Stress." *Psychosomatic Medicine,* 1976, *38,* 300-314.

Coelho, G. V., Hamburg, D. A., and Adams, J. E. (Eds.). *Coping and Adaptation.* New York: Basic Books, 1974.

Cohen, F. "Psychological Preparation, Coping, and Recovery from Surgery." Unpublished doctoral dissertation, University of California, Berkeley, 1975.

Cohen, F., and Lazarus, R. S. "Active Coping Processes, Coping Dispositions, and Recovery from Surgery." *Psychosomatic Medicine,* 1973, *35,* 375-389.

Cohen, L. "Graduate Degree Training in Medical Schools: 1976-1977." Paper presented at annual meeting of the American Psychological Association, San Francisco, August 1977.

Cohen, O. H. Personal Communication, 1978.

Cohen, R. Y. "The Role of Psychologists in the Management of Diabetes Mellitus." Unpublished manuscript, Florida State University, 1976.

Cohen, R. Y. "The Development of a Group Education and Management Program for Low-Income Diabetic and Hypertensive Patients." Unpublished doctoral dissertation, Florida State University, 1977.

Cohen, S. "Environmental Load and the Allocation of Attention." In A. Baum and S. Valins (Eds.), *Advances in Environmental Research.* Hillsdale, N.J.: Lawrence Erlbaum, 1978.

Cohen, S., Glass, D., and Phillips, S. "Environment and Health." In H. Freeman, S. Levine, and L. Reeder (Eds.), *Handbook of Medical Sociology.* Englewood Cliffs, N.J.: Prentice-Hall, 1977.

Cohen, S., Glass, D., and Singer, J. "Apartment Noise, Auditory Discrimination, and Reading Ability in Children." *Journal of Experimental Social Psychology,* 1973, *9,* 407-422.

Coker, R. E., Back, R. W., Donnelly, T. G., and Miller, N. "Patterns of Influence: Medical School Faculty Members and the Values and Specialty Interest of Medical Students." *Journal of Medical Education,* 1960, *35,* 518-527.

Collen, M. F. "Guidelines for Multiphasic Health Checkups." *Archives of Internal Medicine,* 1971, *127,* 99-100.

Colleti, G., and Kopel, S. "The Relative Efficacy of Participant Modeling,

Participant-Observer, and Self-Modeling Procedures as Maintenance Strategies Following a Positive Behaviorally Based Treatment for Smoking Reduction." Unpublished doctoral dissertation, Rutgers University, 1977.

Collins, J., Kasap, H., and Holland, W. "Environmental Factors in Child Mortality in England and Wales." *American Journal of Epidemiology*, 1971, *93*, 10-22.

Colson, A. C. "A Model for a Comprehensive Low-Cost Health Program in Rural Malaysia." *Medical Anthropology Newsletter*, 1976, 7 (4), 13-18.

Colson, A. C., and Selby, K. E. "Medical Anthropology." In B. J. Siegel (Ed.), *Annual Review of Anthropology*. Palo Alto, Calif.: Annual Reviews, 1974.

Colten, M. E., and Janis, I. L. "Effects of Self-Disclosure and the Decisional Balance-Sheet Procedure in a Weight Reduction Clinic." In I. Janis (Ed.), *Counseling on Personal Decisions: Theory and Field Research on Helping Relationships*. New Haven, Conn.: Yale University Press, in press.

Cook, R. L., and Stewart, T. R. "A Comparison of Seven Methods of Obtaining Subjective Descriptions of Judgmental Policy." *Organizational Behavior and Human Performance*, 1975, *13*, 31-45.

Cooley, A. "Psychiatric Considerations in Surgery." *Journal of the International College of Surgeons*, 1961, *35*, 745-751.

Coombs, R. H. "Sex Education for Physicians: Is it Adequate?" *Family Life Coordinator*, 1968, *17*, 271-277.

Coombs, R. H. "The Medical Marriage." In R. H. Coombs and C. E. Vincent (Eds.), *Psychosocial Aspects of Medical Training*. Springfield, Ill.: Thomas, 1971.

Coombs, R. H., and Vincent, C. E. *Psychosocial Aspects of Medical Training*. Springfield, Ill.: Thomas, 1971.

Corman, H. H., Hornick, E. J., Kritchman, M., and Terestman, N. "Emotional Reactions of Surgical Patients to Hospitalization." *American Journal of Surgery*, 1958, *96*, 646-653.

Council on Mental Health. "The Sick Physician: Impairment by Psychiatric Disorders including Alcoholism and Drug Dependence." *Journal of the American Medical Association*, 1973, *223*, 684-687.

Cousins, N. "Anatomy of an Illness (as Perceived by the Patient)." *New England Journal of Medicine*, 1976, *295*, 1458-1463.

Cowie, B. "The Cardiac Patient's Perception of His Heart Attack." *Social Science and Medicine*, 1976, *10*, 87-96.

Cozby, P. "Effects of Density, Activity, and Personality on Environmental Preferences." *Journal of Research in Personality*, 1973, 7, 45-60.

Craig, A. G., and Pitts, F. N. "Suicide by Physicians." *Diseases of the Nervous System*, 1968, *29*, 763-772.

Craig, T. J., Comstock, G. W., and Geiser, P. B. "The Quality of Survival in Breast Cancer: A Case-Control Comparison." *Cancer*, 1974, *33*, 1451-1457.

Craik, F. I. M., and Lockhart, R. S. "Levels of Processing: A Framework for Memory Research." *Journal of Verbal Learning and Verbal Behavior*, 1972, *11*, 671-684.

Crannel, C. W. "The Responses of College Students to a Questionnaire of Animistic Thinking." *Scientific Monthly,* 1954, *78,* 54-56.

Crary, W. G., and Steger, H. G. "Prescriptive and Consultative Approaches to Psychological Evaluation." *Professional Psychology,* 1972, *3,* 105-109.

Cravioto, J., and Delicardie, E. "Mental Performance in School Age Children: Findings Offer Recovery from Early Severe Malnutrition." *American Journal of Diseases of Children,* 1970, *120,* 404-410.

Crew, F. A. E. *Health, Its Nature and Conservation.* New York: Pergamon Press, 1965.

Criddle, R. *Love Is Not Blind.* New York: Norton, 1953.

Crisp, A. H. "Some Psychosomatic Aspects of Neoplasia." *British Journal of Medical Psychology,* 1970, *43,* 313-331.

Crites, J. O. "A Comprehensive Model of Career Development in Early Adulthood." *Journal of Vocational Behavior,* 1976, *9,* 105-118.

Croog, S. H., Shapiro, D. S., and Levine, S. "Denial Among Male Heart Patients: An Empirical Study." *Psychosomatic Medicine,* 1971, *33,* 385-397.

Crowell, D. H. "Personality and Physical Disease: A Test of the Dunbar Hypothesis Applied to Rheumatic Fever and Diabetes Mellitus." *Genetic Psychology Monographs,* 1953, *48,* 117-153.

Cuadra, C. A. "A Psychometric Investigation of Control Factors in Psychological Adjustment." Unpublished doctoral dissertation, University of California, Berkeley, 1953.

Cumming, E., and Henry, W. H. *Growing Old: The Process of Disengagement.* New York: Basic Books, 1961.

Cummings, K., Jette, A., Brock, B., and Haefner, D. "Psycho-Social Determinants of Immunization Behavior in a Swine Influenza Campaign." *Medical Care,* in press.

Cummings, N. A. "The Health Model as Entree to the Human Service Model in Psychotherapy." *Clinical Psychologist,* 1975, *29,* 19-21.

Dabbs, J., and Kirscht, J. P. "Internal Control and the Taking of Influenza Shots." *Psychological Reports,* 1971, *28,* 959-962.

Damrell, J., Lewin, E., and Peguillan, V. "Doing Nursing: The Life, Work, and Career of the Post-Baccalaureate Nurse." Grant NU004-94-02. Division of Nursing Resources, U.S. Public Health Service, 1977.

Danaher, B. G. "Rapid Smoking and Self-Control in the Modification of Smoking Behavior." *Journal of Consulting and Clinical Psychology,* 1977, *45* (6), 1068-1075.

Daniel, R. W., and Louttit, C. M. *Professional Problems in Psychology.* New York: Prentice-Hall, 1953.

Danish, S. J., and Brodsky, S. L. "Training Policemen in Emotional Control and Awareness." *American Psychologist,* 1970, *25,* 368-369.

Danish, S. J., and Hauer, A. L. *Helping Skills: A Basic Training Program.* New York: Human Sciences Press, 1973.

Danish, S. J., and Kagan, N. "Measurement of Affective Sensitivity: Toward a Valid Measure of Interpersonal Perception." *Journal of Counseling Psychology,* 1971, *18,* 51-54.

D'Atri, E. "Psychophysiological Responses to Crowding." *Environment and Behavior,* 1975, *7,* 237-252.

Davidson, R. J., and Schwartz, G. E. "Brain Mechanisms Subserving Self-Generated Imagery: Electrophysiological Specificity and Patterning." *Psychophysiology,* 1977, *14,* 598-602.

Davies, R. K., Quinlan, D. M., McKegney, F. P., and Kimball, C. P. "Organic Factors and Psychological Adjustment in Advanced Cancer Patients." *Psychosomatic Medicine,* 1973, *35,* 464-471.

Davis, F. *Passage Through Crisis.* Indianapolis: Bobbs-Merrill, 1963.

Davis, F., and Olesen, V. "Initiation into a Woman's Profession." *Sociometry,* 1963, *26,* 89-101.

Davis, K. *National Health Insurance: Benefits, Costs, and Consequences.* Washington, D.C.: The Brookings Institution, 1975.

Davis, M. S. "Variations in Patients' Compliance with Doctors' Orders: Analysis of Congruence Between Survey Responses and Results of Empirical Investigations." *Journal of Medical Education,* 1966, *41,* 1037-1048.

Davis, M. S. "Variations in Patients' Compliance with Doctors' Advice: An Empirical Analysis of Patterns of Communication." *American Journal of Public Health,* 1968, *58,* 274-288.

Davis, M. S., and Eichhorn, R. "Compliance with Medical Regimens: A Panel Study." *Journal of Health and Human Behavior,* 1963, *4,* 240-249.

Davis, M. S., and Von der Lippe, R. P. "Discharge from Hospital Against Medical Advice: A Study of Reciprocity in the Doctor-Patient Relationship." *Social Science and Medicine,* 1967, *1,* 336-344.

Davis, R., Buchanan, B., and Shortliffe, E. "Production Rules as a Representation for a Knowledge-Based Consultation Program." *Artificial Intelligence,* 1977, *8,* 15-42.

Davis, R. B. "Stress and Hemostatic Mechanisms." In R. S. Eliot (Ed.), "Stress and the Heart." *Contemporary Problems in Cardiology,* 1974, *1,* 97-122.

Davison, G. C., and Valins, S. "Maintenance of Self-Attributed and Drug-Attributed Behavior Change." *Journal of Personality and Social Psychology,* 1969, *11,* 25-33.

Dawes, R. M. "A Case Study of Graduate Admissions: Application of Three Principles of Human Decision Making." *American Psychologist,* 1971, *26,* 180-188.

Dawes, R. M. "Case-by-Case Versus Rule-Generated Procedures for the Allocation of Scarce Resources." In M. F. Kaplan and S. Schwartz (Eds.), *Human Judgment and Decision Processes in Applied Settings.* New York: Academic Press, 1977.

Dawes, R. M., and Corrigan, B. "Linear Models in Decision Making." *Psychological Bulletin,* 1974, *81,* 95-106.

Dean, L., Pugh, W., and Gunderson, E. "Spatial and Perceptual Components of Crowding Effects on Health and Satisfaction." *Environment and Behavior,* 1975, *7,* 225-236.

de Araujo, G., van Arsdel, P. P., Holmes, T. H., and Dudley, D. L. "Life

Change, Coping Ability and Chronic Intrinsic Asthma." *Journal of Psychosomatic Research,* 1973, *17,* 359-363.

Decker, B., and Bonner, P. *Criteria in Peer Review.* Cambridge, Mass.: A. D. Little, n.d.

de Groot, A. D. *Thought and Choice in Chess.* The Hague, Netherlands: Mouton, 1965.

de Groot, A. D. "Perception and Memory Versus Thought: Some Old Ideas and Recent Findings." In B. Kleinmuntz (Ed.), *Problem Solving: Research, Method, and Theory.* New York: Wiley, 1966.

Delbecq, A. L. "The Use of the Nominal Group Method in the Assessment of Community Needs." In R. A. Bell, M. Sundel, J. F. Aponte, and S. A. Murrel (Eds.), *Need Assessment in Health and Human Services: Proceedings of the Louisville National Conference,* University of Louisville, Louisville, Ky., March 9-12, 1976. (Expanded version to be published by Human Sciences Press, 1979.)

DeLong, D. R. "Individual Differences in Patterns of Anxiety Arousal, Stress-Relevant Information, and Recovery from Surgery." Unpublished doctoral dissertation, University of California, Los Angeles, 1970.

Demone, H. W. "Translating Need Assessment and Resource Identification Data into Human Service Goals." In R. A. Bell, M. Sundel, J. F. Aponte, and S. A. Murrel (Eds.), *Need Assessment in Health and Human Services: Proceedings of the Louisville National Conference,* University of Louisville, Louisville, Ky., March 9-12, 1976. (Expanded version to be published by Human Sciences Press, 1979.)

Denenberg, V. H. "Discussion." *Physiology, Emotion, and Psychosomatic Illness.* Ciba Foundation Symposium, new series 8. Amsterdam: Associated Scientific Publishers, 1972, p. 78.

Dennerll, R. D., Broeder, J., and Sokolov, S. I. "WISE and WAIS Factors in Children and Adults with Epilepsy." *Journal of Clinical Psychology,* 1964, *20,* 236-240.

Dennis, W. *Current Trends in the Relation of Psychology to Medicine.* Pittsburgh: University of Pittsburgh Press, 1950.

Dennis, W. "Animistic Thinking Among College and University Students." *Scientific Monthly,* 1953, *76,* 247-249.

Dennis, W. "Animistic Thinking Among College and High School Students in the Near East." *Journal of Educational Psychology,* 1957, *48,* 193-198.

Derogatis, L. R., and Abeloff, M. D. "Psychological Coping Mechanisms and Survival Time in Metastatic Breast Cancer." Abstract presented at meeting of the American Society of Clinical Oncology, Washington, D.C., April 1978.

Detmer, D. E., Fryback, D. G., and Gassner, K. "Heuristics and Biases in Medical Decision Making." *Journal of Medical Education,* 1978, *53,* 682-683.

Deutsch, H. "Some Psychoanalytic Observations in Surgery." *Psychosomatic Medicine,* 1942, *4,* 105-115.

Deutsch, M. "On Making Social Psychology More Useful." *Social Science Research Council: Items,* 1976, *30* (1), 1-6.

Deutsch, M., and Gerard, H. "A Study of Normative and Informational Social Influences on Individual Judgment." *Journal of Abnormal and Social Psychology,* 1955, *51,* 629-636.

DeWolfe, A. S., Barrell, R. P., and Cummings, J. W. "Patient Variables in Emotional Response to Hospitalization for Physical Illness." *Journal of Consulting Psychology,* 1966, *30,* 68-72.

DiCicco, L., and Apple, D. "Health Needs and Opinions of Older Adults." In D. Apple (Ed.), *Sociological Studies of Health and Sickness.* New York: McGraw-Hill, 1960.

Dickinson, F. G., and Martin, L. W. "Physician Mortality, 1949-1951." *Journal of the American Medical Association,* 1956, *162* (16), 1462-1468.

Dimsdale, J. E., Eckenrode, J., Haggerty, R. J., Kaplan, B. H., Cohen, F., and Dornbusch, S. "The Impact of Social Supports on Medical Care and Health." Paper adapted from a report prepared for the Task Panel on Community Support Systems for the President's Commission on Mental Health, 1978.

Dirks, J. F., Jones, N. F., and Kinsman, R. A. "Panic-Fear: A Personality Dimension Related to Intractability in Asthma." *Psychosomatic Medicine,* 1977, *39,* 120-126.

Dirks, J. F., Kinsman, R. A., Horton, D. J., Fross, K. H., and Jones, N. F. "Panic-Fear in Asthma: Rehospitalization Following Intensive Long-Term Treatment." *Psychosomatic Medicine,* 1978, *40,* 5-13.

Dirks, J. F., Kinsman, R. A., Jones, N. F., Spector, S. L., Davidson, P. T., and Evans, N. W. "Panic-Fear: A Personality Dimension Related to Length of Hospitalization in Respiratory Illness." *Journal of Asthma Research,* 1977, *14,* 61-71.

Djerassi, E. "Some Problems of Occupational Diseases of Dentists." *International Dental Journal,* 1971, *21,* 252-269.

Doberneck, R. C., Griffen, W. O., Papermaster, A. A., Bonello, F. J., and Wangensteen, O. H. "Hypnosis as an Adjunct to Surgical Therapy." *Surgery,* 1959, *46,* 299-304.

Doberneck, R. C., McFee, A. S., Bonello, F. J., Papermaster, A. A., and Wangensteen, O. H. "The Prevention of Postoperative Urinary Retention by Hypnosis." *American Journal of Clinical Hypnosis,* 1961, *3,* 235-237.

Dohrenwend, B. S. "Stressful Life Events and Illness: Implications for Needs Assessment." In R. A. Bell, M. Sundel, J. F. Aponte, and S. A. Murrel (Eds.), *Need Assessment in Health and Human Services: Proceedings of the Louisville National Conference,* University of Louisville, Louisville, Ky., March 9-12, 1976. (Expanded version to be published by Human Sciences Press, 1979.)

Dohrenwend, B. S., and Dohrenwend, B. P. "Overview and Prospects for Research on Stressful Life Events." In B. S. Dohrenwend and B. P. Dohrenwend (Eds.), *Stressful Life Events: Their Nature and Effects.* New York: Wiley, 1974a.

Dohrenwend, B. S., and Dohrenwend, B. P. (Eds.). *Stressful Life Events: Their Nature and Effects.* New York: Wiley, 1974b.

Donabedian, A. "Evaluating the Quality of Medical Care." *Milbank Memorial Fund Quarterly,* 1966, *44* (2), 166-206.

Donabedian, A. *Medical Care Appraisal—Quality and Utilization. A Guide to Medical Care Administration.* Vol. 2. New York: American Public Health Association, 1969.

Donabedian, A., and Rosenfeld, L. "Follow-Up Study of Chronically Ill Patients Discharged from Hospital." *Journal of Chronic Diseases,* 1964, *17,* 847-862.

Dörken, H. "The Practicing Psychologist: A Growing Force in Private Sector Health Care Delivery." *Professional Psychology,* 1977, *8,* 269-274.

Dörken, H., and Whiting, F. "Psychologists as Health-Service Providers." *Professional Psychology,* 1974, *5,* 309-319.

Doyle, B. J., and Ware, J. E. "Physician Conduct and Other Factors that Affect Consumer Satisfaction with Medical Care." *Journal of Medical Education,* 1977, *52,* 793-801.

Drew, F. L., Moriarty, R. W., and Shapiro, A. P. "An Approach to the Measurement of the Pain and Anxiety Responses of Surgical Patients." *Psychosomatic Medicine,* 1968, *30,* 826-836.

Drolet, G., and Porter, D. *Why Patients in Tuberculosis Hospitals Leave Against Medical Advice.* New York: New York Tuberculosis and Health Association, 1949.

Drotar, D. "Clinical Psychological Practice in a Pediatric Hospital." *Professional Psychology,* 1977, *8,* 72-80.

Druss, R. G., O'Connor, J. F., and Stern, L. C. "Psychologic Response to Colectomy: II. Adjustment to a Permanent Colostomy." *Archives of General Psychiatry,* 1969, *20,* 419-427.

Dubos, R. J. *Man Adapting.* New Haven, Conn.: Yale University Press, 1965.

Dubourg, G. O. "After-Care for Alcoholics—A Follow-Up Study." *British Journal of the Addictions,* 1969, *64,* 155-163.

Duché, D. J., Rausch de Traubenberg, N., and Bouras, A. "Value of Psychological Techniques in the Examination for Detection of Visual Disturbances in the Three- to Six-Year-Old Child." *Revue de Neuropsychiatrie Infantile et d'Hygiène Mentale de l'Enfance,* 1971, *19,* 49-56.

Dudley, D. L., Verhey, J. W., Masuda, M., Martin, C. J., and Holmes, T. H. "Long-Term Adjustment, Prognosis, and Death in Irreversible Diffuse Obstructive Pulmonary Syndromes." *Psychosomatic Medicine,* 1969, *31,* 310-325.

Dumas, R. G., Anderson, B. J., and Leonard, R. C. "The Importance of the Expressive Function in Preoperative Preparation." In J. K. Skipper and R. C. Leonard (Eds.), *Social Interaction and Patient Care.* Philadelphia: Lippincott, 1965.

Dumas, R. G., and Leonard, R. C. "The Effect of Nursing on the Incidence of Postoperative Vomiting." *Nursing Research*, 1963, *12*, 12-15.

Duncker, K. "On Problem Solving." *Psychological Monographs*, 1945, *58* (Whole no. 270).

Dunnel, K., and Cartwright, A. *Medicine Takers, Prescribers, and Hoarders.* London: Routledge and Kegan Paul, 1972.

Durkheim, E. *Suicide.* New York: Free Press, 1951.

Easson, W. M. "Care of the Young Patient Who Is Dying." *Journal of the American Medical Association*, 1968, *205*, 203-207.

Easton, D. *The Political System: An Inquiry into the State of Political Science.* New York: Knopf, 1953.

Easton, D. *A Systems Analysis of Political Life.* New York: Wiley, 1965.

Easton, D. "The New Revolution in Political Science." *American Political Science Review*, 1969, *63*, 1051-1061.

Eastwood, M. R., and Trevelyan, M. H. "Stress and Coronary Heart Disease." *Journal of Psychosomatic Research*, 1971, *15*, 289-292.

Eastwood, M. R., and Trevelyan, M. H. "Relationship Between Physical and Psychiatric Disorder." *Psychological Medicine*, 1972, *2*, 363-372.

Edlin, J. V., Johnson, R. H., Hletko, P., and Heilbrunn, G. "The Conditioned Aversion Treatment of Chronic Alcoholism (Preliminary Report)." *Archives of Neurology and Psychiatry*, 1945, *53*, 85-87.

Edwards, J., and Booth, A. "Crowding and Human Sexual Behavior." *Social Forces*, 1977, *55*, 791-808.

Edwards, M. T., and Zimet, C. N. "Problems and Concerns Among Medical Students." *Journal of Medical Education*, 1976, *51*, 619-625.

Edwards, W. "The Theory of Decision Making." *Psychological Bulletin*, 1954, *51*, 380-417.

Edwards, W. "Behavioral Decision Theory." *Annual Review of Psychology*, 1961, *12*, 473-498.

Edwards, W. "Conservatism in Human Information Processing." In B. Kleinmuntz (Ed.), *Formal Representation of Human Judgment.* New York: Wiley, 1968.

Edwards, W., Guttentag, M., and Snapper, K. "A Decision Theoretic Approach to Evaluation Research." In E. L. Struening and M. Guttentag (Eds.), *Handbook of Evaluation Research.* Vol. 1. Beverly Hills, Calif.: Sage, 1975.

Edwards, W., Lindman, H., and Phillips, L. D. "Emerging Technologies for Making Decisions." In F. Barron (Ed.), *New Directions in Psychology.* Vol. 2. New York: Holt, Rinehart and Winston, 1965.

Edwards, W., and Tversky, A. (Eds.). *Decision Making.* Baltimore: Penguin, 1967.

Egbert, L. D., Battit, G. E., Welch, C. E., and Bartlett, M. K. "Reduction of Postoperative Pain by Encouragement and Instruction of Patients." *New England Journal of Medicine*, 1964, *270*, 825-827.

Eggan, F. "One Hundred Years of Ethnology and Social Anthropology." In

J. O. Brew (Ed.), *One Hundred Years of Anthropology.* Cambridge: Harvard University Press, 1968.

Ehrenreich, B., and Ehrenreich, J. *The American Health Empire: Power, Profits, and Politics.* New York: Random House, 1971.

Ehrenreich, B., and English, D. *For Her Own Good.* New York: Doubleday, 1978.

Ehrlich, J., and Riesman, D. "Age and Authority in the Interview." *Public Opinion Quarterly,* 1961, *25,* 39-56.

Eich, J. E., Weingartner, H., Stillman, R. C., and Gillin, J. C. "State-Dependent Accessibility of Retrieval Cues in the Retention of a Categorized List." *Journal of Verbal Learning and Verbal Behavior,* 1975, *14,* 408-417.

Einhorn, H. J. "The Use of Nonlinear, Noncompensatory Models in Decision Making." *Psychological Bulletin,* 1970, *73,* 221-230.

Einhorn, H. J. "Expert Measurement and Mechanical Combination." *Organizational Behavior and Human Performance,* 1972, *7,* 86-106.

Einhorn, H. J. "Expert Judgment: Some Necessary Conditions and an Example." *Journal of Applied Psychology,* 1974a, *59,* 562-571.

Einhorn, H. J. "Cue Definition and Residual Judgment." *Organizational Behavior and Human Performance,* 1974b, *12,* 30-49.

Einhorn, H. J., and Schacht, S. "Decisions Based on Fallible Clinical Judgment." In M. F. Kaplan and S. Schwartz (Eds.), *Human Judgment and Decision Processes in Applied Settings.* New York: Academic Press, 1977.

Eisenberg, L. "The Social Imperative of Medical Research." *Science,* 1977, *198,* 1105-1110.

Eisendrath, R. M. "The Role of Grief and Fear in the Death of Kidney Transplant Patients." *American Journal of Psychiatry,* 1969, *126,* 381-387.

Ekblom, B. "Significance of Socio-Psychological Factors with Regard to Risk of Death Among Elderly Persons." *Acta Psychiatrica Scandinavica,* 1963, *39,* 627-633.

Ekman, P. "Universals and Cultural Differences in Facial Expressions of Emotion." In *Nebraska Symposium on Motivation.* Omaha: University of Nebraska Press, 1972.

Elinson, J., Henshaw, S., and Cohen, S. "Responses by a Low-Income Population to a Multiphasic Screening Program: A Sociological Analysis." *Preventive Medicine,* 1976, *5,* 414-424.

Elling, R., Whittemore, R., and Green, M. "Patient Participation in a Pediatric Program." *Journal of Health and Human Behavior,* 1960, *1,* 183-191.

Elmore, A. M., and Tursky, B. "A Model and Improved Methodology to Enhance Biofeedback's Therapeutic Success." *Psychophysiology,* 1977, *14,* 118 (abstract).

Elms, A. C. *Personality and Politics.* New York: Harcourt Brace Jovanovich, 1976.

Elstein, A. S. "Clinical Judgment: Psychological Research and Medical Practice." *Science,* 1976, *194,* 696-700.

Elstein, A. S., Kagan, N., Shulman, L., Jason, H., and Loupe, M. J. "Methods and Theory in the Study of Medical Inquiry." *Journal of Medical Education,* 1972, *47,* 85-92.

Elstein, A. S., Shulman, L. S., and Sprafka, S. A. *Medical Problem Solving: An Analysis of Clinical Reasoning.* Cambridge: Harvard University Press, 1978.

Emery, A. "Genetic Counseling or What Can We Tell Parents?" *The Practitioner,* 1974, *213,* 641-646.

Emery, A., Watt, M. S., and Clark, E. R. "The Effects of Genetic Counseling on Duchenne Muscular Dystrophy." *Clinical Genetics,* 1972, *3,* 147-150.

Emrick, C. D. "A Review of Psychologically Oriented Treatment of Alcoholism: II. The Relative Effectiveness of Different Treatment Approaches and the Effectiveness of Treatment Versus No Treatment." *Journal of Studies on Alcohol,* 1975, *36,* 88-108.

Ends, E. J., and Page, C. W. "A Study of Three Types of Group Psychotherapy with Hospitalized Male Inebriates." *Quarterly Journal of Studies on Alcohol,* 1957, *18,* 263-277.

Ends, E. J., and Page, C. W. "Group Psychotherapy and Concomitant Psychological Change." *Psychological Monographs,* 1959, *73* (Whole no. 480).

Engel, G. L. *Psychological Development in Health and Disease.* Philadelphia: Saunders, 1962.

Engel, G. L. "A Life Setting Conducive to Illness: The Giving Up-Given Up Complex." *Bulletin of the Menninger Clinic,* 1968, *32,* 355-365.

Engel, G. L. "Sudden and Rapid Death During Psychological Stress: Folklore or Folk Wisdom?" *Annals of Internal Medicine,* 1971, *74,* 771-782.

Engel, G. L. "Enduring Attributes of Medicine Relevant for the Education of the Physician." *Annals of Internal Medicine,* 1973, *78,* 587-593.

Engel, G. L. "The Need for a New Medical Model: A Challenge for Biomedicine." *Science,* 1977, *196,* 129-136.

Engel, G. L., and Schmale, A. H. "Psychoanalytic Theory of Somatic Disorder." *Journal of the American Psychoanalytic Association,* 1967, *15,* 344-363.

Epstein, C. F. "Encountering the Male Establishment: Sex-Status Limits on Women's Careers in the Profession." *American Journal of Sociology,* 1974, *120,* 95-100.

Epstein, M. N., and Kaplan, E. B. "Criteria for Clinical Decision Making." In W. Schneider and A. L. Sagvall-Hein (Eds.), *Computational Linguistics in Medicine.* New York: North Holland, 1977.

Epstein, S., and Clarke, S. "Heart Rate and Skin Conductance During Experimentally Induced Anxiety: Effects of Anticipated Intensity of Noxious Stimulation and Experience." *Journal of Experimental Psychology,* 1970, *84,* 105-112.

Epstein, S., and Fenz, W. D. "The Detection of Areas of Emotional Stress Through Variations in Perceptual Threshold and Physiological Arousal." *Journal of Experimental Research in Personality,* 1967, *2,* 191-199.

Erickson, N. T. "The Influence of Health Factors on Psychological Variables Predicting Complications of Pregnancy, Labor, and Delivery." *Journal of Psychosomatic Research,* 1976, *20,* 21-24.

Erikson, E. H. *Childhood and Society.* New York: Norton, 1950.

Erikson, E. H. "The Problem of Ego Identity." *Journal of the American Psychoanalytic Association,* 1956, *4,* 58-121.

Erikson, E. H. "Identity and the Life Cycle." *Psychological Issues,* 1959, *1,* 18-164.

Erikson, E. H. "Reflections on Dr. Borg's Life Cycle." *Daedalus,* 1976, *105,* 1-28.

Eron, L. D. "Effect of Medical Education on Medical Students' Attitudes." *Journal of Medical Education,* 1955, *30,* 559-566.

Espmark, S. "Stroke Before 50: A Follow-Up Study of Vocational and Psychological Adjustment." *Scandinavian Journal of Rehabilitation Medicine,* 1973, *5* (Whole suppl. no. 2).

Eulau, H. "Introduction: Drift of a Discipline." *American Behavioral Scientist,* 1977, *21,* 5-10.

Evans, R. I. "Discussion Facilitation Statement for Session 'A'—Life Style Development and Modification Session." In S. M. Weiss (Ed.), *Proceedings of the National Heart and Lung Institute Working Conference on Health Behavior.* DHEW Publication No. (NIH) 76-868. Washington, D.C.: U.S. Government Printing Office, 1975.

Evans, R. I., Rozell, R. M., Lasater, T. M., Dembroski, T. M., and Allen, B. P. "Fear Arousal, Persuasion, and Actual Versus Implied Behavioral Change: New Perspective Utilizing a Real-Life Dental Hygiene Program." *Journal of Personality and Social Psychology,* 1970, *16,* 220-227.

Everson, R. B., and Fraumeni, J. F. "Mortality Among Medical Students and Young Physicians." *Journal of Medical Education,* 1975, *50,* 809-811.

Eysenck, H. J. *Smoking, Health, and Personality.* New York: Basic Books, 1965.

Fabrega, H., Jr. "Medical Anthropology." In B. J. Siegel (Ed.), *Biennial Review of Anthropology, 1971.* Stanford, Calif.: Stanford University Press, 1972.

Fabrega, H., Jr. *Disease and Social Behavior.* Cambridge: M.I.T. Press, 1974.

Fanning, D. "Families in Flats." *British Medical Journal,* 1967, *18,* 382-386.

Fanshel, S., and Bush, J. W. "A Health-Status Index and Its Application to Health Services Outcomes." *Operations Research,* 1970, *18,* 1021-1066.

Farrar, C. H., Powell, B. J., and Martin, L. K. "Punishment of Alcohol Consumption by Apneic Paralysis." *Behavior Research and Therapy,* 1968, *6,* 13-16.

Federal Register. March 26, 1976, *41* (60), 12812-12834.

Feigenbaum, E. A. "The Art of Artificial Intelligence: Themes and Case Studies of Knowledge Engineering." In *Proceedings of the Fifth Joint Conference on Artificial Intelligence,* 1977, pp. 1014-1029.

Fein, R. "Health Manpower: Some Economic Considerations." *Journal of Dental Education,* 1976, *40,* 655-661.

Feinstein, A. R. "Clinical Biostatistics, XXVII: The Derangements of the 'Range of Normal.' " *Clinical Pharmacology and Therapeutics,* 1974, *15,* 528-540.

Feinstein, A., Wood, H. F., Epstein, J. A., Taranta, A., Simpson, R., and Tursky, E. "A Controlled Study of Three Methods of Prophylaxis Against Streptococcal Infection in a Population of Rheumatic Children: II. Results of the First Three Years of the Study, Including Methods for Evaluating the Maintenance of Oral Prophylaxis." *New England Journal of Medicine,* 1959, *260,* 697-702.

Feldman, J. *The Dissemination of Health Information.* Chicago: Aldine, 1966.

Ferrare, N. A. "Institutionalization and Attitude Change in an Aged Population." Unpublished doctoral dissertation, Western Reserve University, 1962.

Ferster, C. B., Nurnberger, J. I., and Levitt, E. B. "The Control of Eating." *Journal of Mathetics,* 1962, *1,* 87-109.

Festinger, L. *A Theory of Cognitive Dissonance.* Stanford, Calif.: Stanford University Press, 1957.

Fiedler, F. *Leadership.* New York: General Learning Press, 1971.

Fink, D., Malloy, M. J., Cohen, M., Greycloud, M. A., and Martin, F. "Effective Patient Care in the Pediatric Ambulatory Setting: A Study of the Acute Care Clinic." *Pediatrics,* 1969, *43,* 927-935.

Fink, R., Shapiro, S., and Roeser, R. "Impact of Efforts to Increase Participation in Repetitive Screenings for Early Breast Cancer Detection." *American Journal of Public Health,* 1972, *62,* 328-336.

Finnerty, F. A., Jr., Mattie, E., and Finnerty, F. A., III. "Hypertension in the Inner City: I. Analysis of Clinic Dropouts." *Circulation,* 1973a, *47,* 73-75.

Finnerty, F. A., Jr., Shaw, L., and Himmelsbach, C. "Hypertension in the Inner City: II. Detection and Follow-Up." *Circulation,* 1973b, *47,* 76-78.

Fisch, R., Conley, J., Eysenbach, S., and Chang, P. "Contact with Phenylketonurics and Their Families Beyond Pediatric Age: Conclusions from a Survey and Conference." *Mental Retardation,* 1977, *15,* 10-12.

Fischhoff, B. "Decision Analysis: Clinical Art or Clinical Science?" Paper presented at Sixth Research Conference on Subjective Probability, Utility, and Decision Making, Warsaw, Poland, 1977.

Fischhoff, B., Slovic, P., and Lichtenstein, S. "Knowing with Certainty: The Appropriateness of Extreme Confidence." *Journal of Experimental Psychology: Human Perception and Performance,* 1977, *3,* 552-564.

Fishbein, M. "An Investigation of the Relationship Between Beliefs About an Object and Attitude Toward that Object." *Human Relations,* 1963, *16,* 233-239.

Fishbein, M., and Ajzen, I. *Belief, Attitude, Intention, and Behavior.* Reading, Mass.: Addison-Wesley, 1975.

Fisher, J. "Situation Specific Variables as Determinants of Perceived Environmental Esthetic Quality and Perceived Crowdedness." *Journal of Research in Personality,* 1974, *8,* 177-188.

Fisher, S. "Motivation for Patient Delay." *Archives of General Psychiatry,* 1967, *16,* 676-678.

Fletcher, C. R. "Study of Behavioral Science Teaching in Schools of Medicine." *Journal of Medical Education,* 1974, *49,* 188-189.

Fletcher, S., Appel, F., and Bourgois, M. "Improving Emergency-Room Patient Follow-Up in a Metropolitan Teaching Hospital." *New England Journal of Medicine,* 1974, *291,* 385-388.

Flook, E. E., and Sanazaro, P. J. *Health Services Research and R and D in Perspective.* Ann Arbor, Mich.: Health Administration Press, 1973.

Folkard, S. "Diurnal Variation in Logical Reasoning." *British Journal of Psychology,* 1976, *66,* 1-8.

Folkins, C. "Temporal Factors and the Cognitive Mediators of Stress Reactions." *Journal of Personality and Social Psychology,* 1970, *14,* 173-184.

Folkman, S., Schaefer, C., and Lazarus, R. S. "Cognitive Processes as Mediators of Stress and Coping." In V. Hamilton and D. M. Warburton (Eds.), *Human Stress and Cognition: An Information-Processing Approach.* London: Wiley, in press.

Follette, W., and Cummings, N. A. "Psychiatric Services and Medical Utilization in a Prepaid Health Plan Setting." *Medical Care,* 1967, *5,* 25-35.

Foote, A., and Erfurt, J. "Controlling Hypertension: A Cost-Effective Model." *Preventive Medicine,* 1977, *6,* 319-343.

Fordyce, W. E. *Behavioral Methods for Chronic Pain and Illness.* St. Louis, Mo.: Mosby, 1976.

Foreyt, J. P., and Kennedy, W. A. "Treatment of Overweight by Aversion Therapy." *Behaviour Research and Therapy,* 1971, *9,* 29-34.

Forsham, P. H. "Some Endocrine Anomalies in Obesity." In L. D. Rubin (Ed.), *Understanding and Successfully Managing Obesity.* A Postgraduate Medicine Symposium. Cincinnati: Merrell-National Laboratories, 1974.

Foster, G. M. "Medical Anthropology: Some Contrasts with Medical Sociology." *Social Science and Medicine,* 1975, *9,* 427-432.

Foster, G. M. "Medical Anthropology and International Health Planning." *Medical Anthropology Newsletter,* 1976, *7* (1), 12-18.

Fowler, R. D. "The Current Status of Computer Interpretation of Psychological Tests." *American Journal of Psychiatry,* 1969, *125* (suppl.), 21-27.

Fox, B. H. "Premorbid Psychological Factors as Related to Cancer Incidence." *Journal of Behavioral Medicine,* 1978, *1,* 45-133.

Fox, V., and Smith, M. A. "Evaluation of a Chemopsychotherapeutic Program for the Rehabilitation of Alcoholics: Observation Over a Two-Year Period." *Quarterly Journal of Studies on Alcohol,* 1959, *20,* 767-780.

Francis, V., Korsch, B., and Morris, M. "Gaps in Doctor-Patient Communication: Patients' Response to Medical Advice." *New England Journal of Medicine,* 1969, *280,* 535-540.

Frank, J. D. "The Faith that Heals." *Johns Hopkins Medical Journal,* 1975, *137,* 127-131.

Frank, L. K., Hutchinson, G. E., Livingstone, W. K., McCulloch, W. S., and

Wiener, N. "Teleological Mechanisms." *Annals of the New York Academy of Sciences*, 1948, *50* (Art. 4), 187-278.

Frankenhaeuser, M. "Behavior and Circulating Catecholamines." *Brain Research*, 1971, *31*, 241-262.

Frankenhaeuser, M. "Sympathetic-Adrenomedullary Activity, Behaviour, and the Psychosocial Environment." In P. H. Venables and M. J. Christie (Eds.), *Research in Psychophysiology*. New York: Wiley, 1975.

Frankenhaeuser, M. "The Role of Peripheral Catecholamines in Adaptation to Understimulation and Overstimulation." In G. Serban (Ed.), *Psychopathology of Human Adaptation*. New York: Plenum Press, 1976.

Frankenhaeuser, M., and Gardell, B. "Underload and Overload in Working Life: Outline of a Multidisciplinary Approach." *Journal of Human Stress*, 1976, *2* (3), 35-46.

Frankenhaeuser, M., and Johansson, G. "Task Demand as Reflected in Catecholamine Excretion and Heart Rate." *Journal of Human Stress*, 1976, *2* (1), 15-23.

Frankl, V. *The Doctor and the Soul*. New York: Knopf, 1955.

Frankl, V. *Man's Search for Meaning*. New York: Washington Square Press, 1963.

Franklin, B., and McLemore, S. "Factors Affecting the Choice of Medical Care Among University Students." *Journal of Health and Social Behavior*, 1970, *11*, 311-326.

Franz, S. I. "The Present Status of Psychology in Medical Education and Practice." *Journal of the American Medical Association*, 1912, *53*, 909-911.

Franz, S. I. "On Psychology and Medical Education." *Science*, 1913, *37*, 555-566.

Fras, I., Litin, E. M., and Pearson, J. S. "Comparison of Psychiatric Symptoms in Carcinoma of the Pancreas with Those in Some Other Intra-Abdominal Neoplasms." *American Journal of Psychiatry*, 1967, *123*, 1553-1562.

Freeborn, D. K., Pope, C. R., Davis, M. A., and Mullooly, J. P. "Health Status, Socioeconomic Status, and Utilization of Outpatient Services for Members of a Prepaid Group Practice." *Medical Care*, 1977, *15* (2), 115-128.

Freeman, G. "Gaps in Doctor-Patient Communication: Doctor-Patient Interaction Analysis." *Pediatric Research*, 1971, *5*, 298-311.

Freeman, H. E., Levine, S., and Reeder, L. G. "Present Status of Medical Sociology." In H. E. Freeman, S. Levine, and L. G. Reeder (Eds.), *Handbook of Medical Sociology*. (2nd ed.) Englewood Cliffs, N.J.: Prentice-Hall, 1972.

Freidson, E. *Patients' Views of Medical Practice*. New York: Russell Sage Foundation, 1961.

Freidson, E. *Professional Dominance: The Social Structure of Medical Care*. Chicago: Aldine, 1970a.

Freidson, E. *Profession of Medicine*. New York: Harper & Row, 1970b.

French, J. R., and Raven, B. "The Bases of Social Power." In D. Cartwright (Ed.), *Studies in Social Power*. Ann Arbor: University of Michigan Press, 1959.

Fretz, B. R. (Ed.). "Professional Identity." *Counseling Psychologist*, 1977, *7* (2), 1-110.

Freudenberger, H. J. "Staff Burn-Out." *Journal of Social Issues*, 1974, *30*, 159-165.

Friedman, G. D., Ury, H. K., Klatsky, A. L., and Siegelaub, A. M. "A Psychological Questionnaire Predictive of Myocardial Infarction: Results from the Kaiser-Permanente Epidemiologic Study of Myocardial Infarction." *Psychosomatic Medicine*, 1974, *36*, 327-343.

Friedman, M. "Stress, Type A Behavior, and Your Heart." Paper presented at conference on the Nature and Management of Stress, University of California Extension, Santa Cruz, April 1978.

Friedman, M., and Rosenman, R. H. *Type A Behavior and Your Heart*. New York: Knopf, 1974.

Friedman, M., Rosenman, R. H., and Carroll, V. "Changes in the Serum Cholesterol and Blood Clotting Time in Men Subjected to Cyclic Variation of Occupational Stress." *Circulation*, 1958, *17*, 852-861.

Friedman, S. B., and Glasgow, L. A. "Psychologic Factors and Resistance to Infectious Disease." *Pediatric Clinics of North America*, 1966, *13* (2), 315-335.

Friedman, S. B., Glasgow, L. A., and Ader, R. "Psychosocial Factors Modifying Host Resistance to Experimental Infections." *Annals of the New York Academy of Sciences*, 1969, *164* (Art. 2), 381-392.

Friedman, S. B., Mason, J. W., and Hamburg, D. A. "Urinary 17-Hydroxy-corticosteroid Levels in Parents of Children with Neoplastic Disease: A Study of Chronic Psychological Stress." *Psychosomatic Medicine*, 1963, *25*, 364-376.

Froelich, R. E., and Bishop, F. M. *Medical Interviewing: A Programmed Manual*. St. Louis, Mo.: Mosby, 1972.

Fryback, D. G. "Use of Radiologists' Subjective Probability Estimates in a Medical Decision Making Problem." Ann Arbor: Mathematical Psychology Program, Department of Psychology, University of Michigan, 1974.

Fryback, D. G., and Thornbury, J. R. "Evaluation of a Computerized Bayesian Model for Diagnosis of Renal Cyst Versus Tumor Versus Normal Variant from Excretory Urogram Information." *Investigative Radiology*, 1976, *11*, 102-111.

Fuchs, V. R. *Who Shall Live?* New York: Basic Books, 1974.

Fuller, G. D. "Current Status of Biofeedback in Clinical Practice." *American Psychologist*, 1978, *33*, 39-48.

Funkenstein, D. H. "Medical Students, Medical Schools, and Society During Three Eras." In R. H. Coombs and C. E. Vincent (Eds.), *Psychosocial Aspects of Medical Training*. Springfield, Ill.: Thomas, 1971.

Furst, S. S. "Psychic Trauma: A Survey." In S. S. Furst (Ed.), *Psychic Trauma*. New York: Basic Books, 1967.

Futterman, E. H., and Hoffman, I. "Crisis and Adaptation in the Families of

Fatally Ill Children." In E. J. Anthony and C. Koupernik (Eds.), *The Child in His Family: The Impact of Disease and Death*. New York: Wiley, 1973.

Gabrielson, I., Levin, L., and Ellison, M. "Factors Affecting School Health Follow-Up." *American Journal of Public Health*, 1967, *57*, 48-54.

Gal, R., and Lazarus, R. S. "The Role of Activity in Anticipating and Confronting Stressful Situations." *Journal of Human Stress*, 1975, *1* (4), 4-20.

Galdston, I. "The Natural History of Specialism in Medicine." *Journal of the American Medical Association*, 1959, *170* (3), 294-297.

Galdston, I. "The Third Revolution: Prelude and Polemic." In E. F. Torrey (Ed.), *Ethical Issues in Medicine*. Boston: Little, Brown, 1968.

Galin, D. "Implications of Left-Right Cerebral Lateralization for Psychiatry: A Neurophysiological Context for Unconscious Processes." *Archives of General Psychiatry*, 1974, *9*, 412-418.

Galle, O., Gove, W., and McPherson, J. "Population Density and Pathology: What Are the Relations for Man?" *Science*, 1972, *176*, 23-30.

Gambrill, E. D. *Behavior Modification: Handbook of Assessment, Intervention, and Evaluation*. San Francisco: Jossey-Bass, 1977.

Garcia, J., Hankins, W. G., and Rusiniak, K. W. "Behavioral Regulation of the Milieu Interne in Man and Rat." *Science*, 1974, *185*, 824-832.

Garcia, J., and Rusiniak, K. W. "Visceral Feedback and the Taste Signal." In J. Beatty and H. Legewie (Eds.), *Biofeedback and Behavior*. New York: Plenum Press, 1977.

Gardner, G. G. (Ed.). *Society of Pediatric Psychology Newsletter 1*. New York: Cornell University Medical College, 1969.

Gardner, R. W., Holzman, P. S., Klein, G. S., Linton, H. B., and Spence, D. P. "Cognitive Control: A Study of Individual Consistencies in Cognitive Behavior." *Psychological Issues*, 1959, *1* (4).

Garfield, S. R. "The Delivery of Medical Care." *Scientific American*, 1970, *222*, 15-23.

Garrity, T. F., Somes, G. W., and Marx, M. B. "Personality Factors in Resistance to Illness After Recent Life Changes." *Journal of Psychosomatic Research*, 1977, *21*, 23-32.

Gates, S., and Colburn, D. "Lowering Appointment Failures in a Neighborhood Health Center." *Medical Care*, 1976, *14*, 263-267.

Gath, A. "The Impact of an Abnormal Child upon the Parents." *British Journal of Psychiatry*, 1977, *130*, 405-410.

Geertsma, R. H., and Grinols, D. R. "Specialty Choice in Medicine." *Journal of Medical Education*, 1972, *47*, 509-517.

Gellert, E. "Children's Conceptions of the Content and Functions of the Human Body." *Genetic Psychology Monographs*, 1962, *65*, 293-405.

Georgopoulos, B. S. *Hospital Organization Research: Review and Source Book*. Philadelphia: Saunders, 1975.

Gerard, D. L., and Saenger, G. *Out-Patient Treatment of Alcoholism: A Study of Outcome and Its Determinants*. Toronto, Ontario: University of Toronto Press, 1966.

Gerard, H. B., and Rabbie, J. M. "Fear and Social Comparison." *Journal of Abnormal and Social Psychology*, 1961, *62*, 586-592.

Gerbert, B. "Wives of Podiatric Medical Students: Their Attitudes, Life Styles, and Values." *Journal of Podiatric Medicine,* 1977, *8,* 26-31.

Gersten, J. C., Langner, T. S., Eisenberg, J. G., and Orzeck, L. "Child Behavior and Life Events: Undesirable Change or Change Per Se?" In B. S. Dohrenwend and B. P. Dohrenwend (Eds.), *Stressful Life Events: Their Nature and Effects.* New York: Wiley, 1974.

Giancalone, J. J., and Hudson, J. I. "A Health Status Assessment System for a Rural Navajo Population." *Medical Care,* 1975, *13,* 722-735.

Gibson, G. "Emergency Medical Services: The Research Gaps." *Health Services Research,* 1974, *9,* 6-21.

Gilberstadt, H., and Sako, Y. "Intellectual and Personality Changes Following Open-Heart Surgery." *Archives of General Psychiatry,* 1967, *16,* 210-214.

Gilbert, J. P., McPeek, B., and Mosteller, F. "Statistics and Ethics in Surgery and Anesthesia." *Science,* 1977, *198,* 684-689.

Gill, P. W., Leaper, D. J., Guillou, P. J., Staniland, J. R., Horrocks, J. C., and de Dombal, F. T. "Observer Variation in Clinical Diagnosis—A Computer-Aided Assessment of Its Magnitude and Importance in 552 Patients with Abdominal Pain." *Methods of Information in Medicine,* 1973, *12,* 108-113.

Giller, D. W. "Some Psychological Correlates of Recovery from Surgery." *Texas Reports on Biology and Medicine,* 1962, *20* (3), 366-373.

Gillis, A. "High-Rise Housing and Psychological Strain." *Journal of Health and Social Behavior,* 1977, *18,* 418-431.

Gillis, L. S., and Keet, M. "Prognostic Factors and Treatment Results in Hospitalized Alcoholics." *Quarterly Journal of Studies on Alcohol,* 1969, *30,* 426-437.

Gilson, B. S., Gilson, J. S., Bergner, M., Bobbitt, R. A., Kressel, S., Pollard, W. E., and Vesselago, M. "The Sickness Impact Profile: Development of an Outcome Measure of Health Care." *American Journal of Public Health,* 1975, *65,* 1304-1325.

Ginsberg, A. S., and Offensend, F. L. "An Application of Decision Theory to a Medical Diagnosis-Treatment Problem." *IEEE Transactions on Systems Science and Cybernetics,* 1968, *SSC-4,* 355-362.

Girodo, M. "Self-Talk: Mechanisms in Anxiety and Stress Management." In C. Spielberger and I. G. Sarason (Eds.), *Stress and Anxiety.* Vol. 4. Washington, D.C.: Hemisphere, 1977.

Girodo, M., and Roehl, J. "Preparatory Information and Self-Talk in Coping with the Stress of Flying." Unpublished manuscript, University of Ottawa, Ontario, 1976.

Glaser, B. G., and Strauss, A. L. *Awareness of Dying.* Chicago: Aldine, 1965.

Glaser, B. G., and Strauss, A. L. *The Discovery of Grounded Theory.* Chicago: Aldine, 1967.

Glaser, R. "Educational Psychology and Education." *American Psychologist,* 1973, *28,* 557-566.

Glass, D. *Behavior Patterns, Stress and Coronary Disease.* Hillsdale, N.J.: Lawrence Erlbaum, 1977.

Glass, D., Singer, J., and Pennebaker, J. "Behavioral and Physiological Effects of Uncontrollable Environmental Events." In D. Stokols (Ed.), *Perspectives on Environment and Behavior.* New York: Plenum Press, 1977.

Glass, D., Snyder, M., and Hollis, J. "Time Urgency and Type A Coronary Prone Behavior Pattern." *Journal of Applied Social Psychology,* 1974, *4,* 125-140.

Glazer, N. "Paradoxes of Health Care." *The Public Interest,* 1971, *22,* 62-77.

Glover, E. "Medical Psychology or Academic (Normal) Psychology: A Problem in Orientation." *British Journal of Medical Psychology,* 1934, *14,* 31-49.

Gochman, D. S. "Some Steps Toward a Psychological Matrix for Health Behavior." *Canadian Journal of Behavioral Science,* 1971, *3,* 88-101.

Goffman, E. *Stigma.* Englewood Cliffs, N.J.: Prentice-Hall, 1963.

Gold, M. "A Crisis of Identity: The Case of Medical Sociology." *Journal of Health and Social Behavior,* 1977, *18,* 160-168.

Goldberg, I. D., Krantz, G., and Locke, B. Z. "Effects of a Short-Term Outpatient Psychiatric Therapy Benefit on Utilization of Medical Services in a Prepaid Group Practice Medical Program." *Medical Care,* 1970, *8,* 419-427.

Goldberg, L. R. "Diagnosticians Versus Diagnostic Signs: The Diagnosis of Psychosis Versus Neurosis from the MMPI." *Psychological Monographs,* 1965, *79* (9, Whole no. 602).

Goldberg, L. R. "Simple Models or Simple Processes? Some Research on Clinical Judgments." *American Psychologist,* 1968, *23,* 483-496.

Goldberg, L. R. "The Search for Configural Relationships in Personality Assessment: The Diagnosis of Psychosis Versus Neurosis from the MMPI." *Multivariate Behavioral Research,* 1969, *4,* 523-536.

Goldberg, L. R. "Man Versus Model of Man: A Rationale, Plus Some Evidence for a Method of Improving on Clinical Inferences." *Psychological Bulletin,* 1970, *73,* 422-432.

Goldberg, L. R. "Five Models of Clinical Judgment: An Empirical Comparison Between Linear and Non-Linear Representations of the Human Inference Process." *Organizational Behavior and Human Performance,* 1971, *6,* 458-479.

Goldberg, L. R. "Admission to the Ph.D. Program in the Department of Psychology at the University of Oregon." *American Psychologist,* 1977, *32,* 663-668.

Golden, J. S., and Johnston, G. D. "Problems of Distortion in Doctor-Patient Communications." *Psychiatry in Medicine,* 1970, *1,* 127-149.

Goldfried, M. R. M. "Prediction of Improvement in an Alcoholism Outpatient Clinic." *Quarterly Journal of Studies on Alcohol,* 1969, *30,* 129-139.

Goldschmidt, W. "Ethology, Ecology, and Ethnological Realities." In G. V.

Coelho, D. A. Hamburg, and J. E. Adams (Eds.), *Coping and Adaptation.* New York: Basic Books, 1974.

Goldsmith, C. "The Effect of Differing Compliance Distributions on the Planning and Statistical Analysis of Therapeutic Trials." In D. Sackett and R. Haynes (Eds.), *Compliance with Therapeutic Regimens.* Baltimore: Johns Hopkins University Press, 1976.

Goldstein, A. M. "Denial and External Locus of Control as Mechanisms of Adjustment in Chronic Medical Illness." *Essence,* 1976, *1,* 5-22.

Goldstein, M. J. "The Relationship Between Coping and Avoiding Behavior and Response to Fear-Arousing Propaganda." *Journal of Abnormal and Social Psychology,* 1959, *58,* 247-252.

Goldstein, M. J., Jones, R. B., Clemens, T. L., Flagg, G., and Alexander, F. "Coping Style as a Factor in Psychophysiological Response to a Tension-Arousing Film." *Journal of Personality and Social Psychology,* 1965, *1,* 290-302.

Gordis, L. "Methodologic Issues in the Measurement of Patient Compliance." In D. L. Sackett and R. B. Haynes (Eds.), *Compliance with Therapeutic Regimens.* Baltimore: Johns Hopkins University Press, 1976.

Gordis, L., and Markowitz, M. "Evaluation of the Effectiveness of Comprehensive and Continuous Pediatric Care." *Pediatrics,* 1971, *48,* 766-776.

Gordis, L., Markowitz, M., and Lilienfeld, A. "The Inaccuracy of Using Interviews to Estimate Patient Reliability in Taking Medications at Home." *Medical Care,* 1969a, *7,* 49-54.

Gordis, L., Markowitz, M., and Lilienfeld, A. "Why Patients Don't Follow Medical Advice: A Study of Children on Long-Term Antistreptococcal Prophylaxis." *Journal of Pediatrics,* 1969b, *75,* 957-968.

Gordon, D. W. "Ambulatory Patient Care in the General Medical Clinic." *Medical Care,* 1974, *12,* 648-658.

Gordon, G. *Role Theory and Illness: A Sociological Perspective.* New Haven, Conn.: College and University Press, 1966.

Gordon, R. E. "Psychiatric Screening Through Multiphasic Health Testing." *American Journal of Psychiatry,* 1971, *128,* 559-563.

Gordon, T. L. "DATAGRAM: Applicants for the 1976-77 First-Year Medical School Class." *Journal of Medical Education,* 1977, *52,* 780-782.

Gordon, T. L., and Dubé, W. F. "Medical School Enrollment, 1971-72 Through 1975-76." *Journal of Medical Education,* 1976, *51,* 144-146.

Gore, S. "The Influence of Social Support and Related Variables in Ameliorating the Consequences of Job Loss." Unpublished doctoral dissertation, University of Michigan, 1973.

Gottfredson, G. D., and Dyer, S. E. "Health Service Providers in Psychology." *American Psychologist,* 1978, *33,* 314-338.

Gough, H. G. *The Adjective Check List.* Palo Alto, Calif.: Consulting Psychologists Press, 1952.

Gough, H. G. *California Psychological Inventory.* Palo Alto, Calif.: Consulting Psychologists Press, 1956.

Gough, H. G. *Manual for the California Psychological Inventory.* Palo Alto, Calif.: Consulting Psychologists Press, 1957.

Gough, H. G. "Clinical Versus Statistical Prediction in Psychology." In L. Postman (Ed.), *Psychology in the Making.* New York: Knopf, 1962.

Gough, H. G. "The Recruitment and Selection of Medical Students." In R. H. Coombs and C. E. Vincent (Eds.), *Psychological Aspects of Medical Training.* Springfield, Ill.: Thomas, 1971.

Gough, H. G. "A Factorial Study of Medical Specialty Preference." *British Journal of Medical Education,* 1975, *9,* 78-85.

Gough, H. G. "What Happens to Creative Medical Students?" *Journal of Medical Education,* 1976, *51,* 461-467.

Gough, H. G. "Doctors' Estimates of the Percentage of Patients Whose Problems Do Not Require Medical Attention." *Medical Education,* 1977, *11,* 380-384.

Gough, H. G., and Ducker, D. G. "Social Class in Relation to Medical School Performance and Choice of Specialty." *Journal of Psychology,* 1977, *96,* 31-43.

Gough, H. G., and Hall, W. B. "A Prospective Study of Personality Changes in Students of Medicine, Dentistry, and Nursing." *Research in Higher Education,* 1973, *1,* 127-140.

Gough, H. G., and Hall, W. B. "A Comparison of Medical Students from Medical and Nonmedical Families." *Journal of Medical Education,* 1977a, *52,* 541-547.

Gough, H. G., and Hall, W. B. "Physicians' Retrospective Evaluations of Their Medical Education." *Research in Higher Education,* 1977b, *7,* 29-42.

Gough, H. G., and Heilbrun, A. B. *The Adjective Check List Manual.* Palo Alto, Calif.: Consulting Psychologists Press, 1965.

Graduate Education in Psychology. Report of a conference held in Miami Beach, Fla., 1958. Washington, D.C.: American Psychological Association, 1959.

Graham, S. "The Sociological Approach to Epidemiology." *American Journal of Public Health,* 1974, *64,* 1046-1049.

Gray, R. M., Newman, W. R. E., and Reinhardt, A. M. "The Effect of Medical Specialization on Physicians' Attitudes." *Journal of Health and Human Behavior,* 1966, *7,* 128-132.

Green, G. H. "Some Notes on Smoking." *International Journal of Psychoanalysis,* 1923, *4,* 323-324.

Green, L. *Status Identity and Preventive Health Behavior.* Pacific Health Education Report No. 1. Berkeley: University of California, 1970.

Green, L., Werlin, S. H., Schauffler, H. H., and Avery, C. H. "Research and Demonstration Issues in Self-Care: Measuring the Decline of Medicocentrism." *Health Education Monographs,* 1977, *5,* 161-189.

Greenberg, I. M., Weltz, S., Spitz, C., and Bizzozero, O. J. "Factors of Adjustment in Chronic Hemodialysis Patients." *Psychosomatics,* 1975, *16,* 178-184.

Greene, W. A. "Psychological Factors and Reticuloendothelial Disease: I. Preliminary Observations on a Group of Males with Lymphomas and Leukemias." *Psychosomatic Medicine,* 1954, *16,* 220-230.

Greene, W. A. "The Psychosocial Setting of the Development of Leukemia and Lymphoma." *Annals of the New York Academy of Sciences,* 1966, *125* (Art. 3), 794-801.

Greene, W. A., Young, L. E., and Swisher, S. N. "Psychological Factors and Reticuloendothelial Disease: II. Observations on a Group of Women with Lymphomas and Leukemias." *Psychosomatic Medicine,* 1956, *18,* 284-303.

Greenfield, N. S., Roessler, R., and Crosley, A. P. "Ego Strength and Length of Recovery from Infectious Mononucleosis." *Journal of Nervous and Mental Disease,* 1959, *128,* 125-128.

Greengard, P. "Phosphorylated Proteins and Physiological Effectors." *Science,* 1978, *199,* 146-152.

Greer, S., and Morris, T. "Psychological Attributes of Women Who Develop Breast Cancer: A Controlled Study." *Journal of Psychosomatic Research,* 1975, *19,* 147-153.

Grinker, R. R. (Ed.). *Toward a Unified Theory of Human Behavior.* (2nd ed.) New York: Basic Books, 1967.

Grinker, R. R., Albee, G. W., Shachter, J., Garmezy, N., Thrasher, R. H., and Mensh, I. N. "Emergency Conceptions of Mental Illness and Models of Treatment." *Professional Psychology,* 1971, *2,* 129-144.

Grodins, F. S. *Control Theory and Biological Systems.* New York: Columbia University Press, 1963.

Gruen, W. "Effects of Brief Psychotherapy During the Hospitalization Period on the Recovery Process in Heart Attacks." *Journal of Consulting and Clinical Psychology,* 1975, *43,* 223-232.

"Guidelines. Clinical Services Manpower Training Programs in Psychology." Division of Manpower and Training Programs, National Institute of Mental Health. Bethesda, Md.: Alcohol, Drug Abuse, and Mental Health Administration, July 1977.

Gunderson, E. K. E., and Rahe, R. H. (Eds.). *Life Stress and Illness.* Springfield, Ill.: Thomas, 1974.

Gur, R., and Gur, R. "Defense Mechanisms, Psychosomatic Symptomatology, and Conjugate Lateral Eye Movements." *Journal of Consulting and Clinical Psychology,* 1975, *43,* 416-420.

Gustafson, D. H., and Huber, G. P. "Behavioral Decision Theory and the Health Delivery System." In M. F. Kaplan and S. Schwartz (Eds.), *Human Judgment and Decision Processes in Applied Settings.* New York: Academic Press, 1977.

Gustafson, D. H., Kestly, J. J., Greist, J. H., and Jansen, N. M. "Initial Evaluation of a Subjective Bayesian Diagnostic System." *Health Service Research,* 1971, *6,* 204-213.

Guthrie, G. M. "A Study of the Personality Characteristics Associated with the Disorders Encountered by an Internist." Unpublished doctoral dissertation, University of Minnesota, Minneapolis, 1949.

Guttmacher, S., and Elinson, J. "Ethno-Religious Variation in Perceptions of Illness." *Social Science and Medicine,* 1971, *5,* 117-125.

Haan, N. "Proposed Model of Ego Functioning: Coping and Defense Mechanisms in Relationship to IQ Change." *Psychological Monographs,* 1963, *77* (8, Whole no. 571).

Haan, N. "A Tripartite Model of Ego Functioning: Values and Clinical Research Applications." *Journal of Nervous and Mental Disease,* 1969, *148,* 14-30.

Haan, N. *Coping and Defending: Processes of Self-Environment Organization.* New York: Academic Press, 1977.

Haan, N. "Two Moralities in Action Contexts: Relationships to Thought, Ego Regulation, and Development." *Journal of Personality and Social Psychology,* 1978, *36,* 286-305.

Haas, J. D., and Harrison, G. G. "Nutritional Anthropology and Biological Adaptation." *Annual Review of Anthropology,* 1977, *6,* 69-101.

Hackett, T. P., and Cassem, N. H. "Psychological Management of the Myocardial Infarction Patient." *Journal of Human Stress,* 1975, *1* (3), 25-38.

Hackett, T. P., Cassem, N. H., and Raker, J. W. "Patient Delay in Cancer." *New England Journal of Medicine,* 1973, *289,* 14-20.

Hackett, T. P., Cassem, N. H., and Wishnie, H. A. "The Coronary-Care Unit: An Appraisal of Its Psychologic Hazards." *New England Journal of Medicine,* 1968, *279,* 1365-1370.

Hackett, T. P., and Weisman, A. D. "Reactions to the Imminence of Death." In G. H. Grosser, H. Wechsler, and M. Greenblatt (Eds.), *The Threat of Impending Disaster.* Cambridge, Mass.: M.I.T. Press, 1964.

Haefner, D., Kegeles, S. S., Kirscht, J. P., and Rosenstock, I. M. "Preventive Actions Concerning Dental Disease, Tuberculosis, and Cancer." *Public Health Reports,* 1967, *82,* 451-459.

Haefner, D., and Kirscht, J. P. "Motivational and Behavioral Effects of Modifying Health Beliefs." *Public Health Reports,* 1970, *85,* 478-484.

Hagen, R. L. "Group Therapy Versus Bibliotherapy in Weight Reduction." *Behavior Therapy,* 1974, *5,* 222-234.

Haggerty, R., and Roghmann, K. "Noncompliance and Self-Medication: Two Neglected Aspects of Pediatric Pharmacology." *Pediatric Clinics of North America,* 1972, *19,* 101-115.

Hagnell, L. "The Premorbid Personality of Persons Who Develop Cancer in a Total Population Investigated in 1947 and 1957." *Annals of the New York Academy of Sciences,* 1966, *125* (Art. 3), 846-855.

Hall, R. G., Sachs, D. L., and Hall, S. M. "Medical Risk and Therapeutic Effectiveness of Rapid Smoking." *Behavior Therapy,* in press.

Hall, S. M., Bass, A., and Monroe, J. "Confirmed Contact and Monitoring as Follow-Up Strategies: A Long-Term Study of Obesity Treatment." *Addictive Behavior,* 1978, *3,* 139-147.

Hall, S. M., and Hall, R. G. "Outcome and Methodological Considerations in Behavioral Treatment of Obesity." *Behavior Therapy,* 1974, *5,* 59-68.

Hall, S. M., and Hall, R. G. "Maintaining Change." In J. Fergusen and C. B. Taylor (Eds.), *Comprehensive Handbook of Behavioral Medicine.* New York: Spectrum, in press.

Hall, S. M., Hall, R. G., Borden, B. L., and Hanson, R. W. "Follow-Up Strategies in the Behavioral Treatment of Overweight." *Behavior Research and Therapy,* 1975, *13,* 167-172.

Hall, S. M., Hall, R. G., DeBoes, G., and Okalitch, P. "Self and External Management Compared with Psychotherapy in the Control of Obesity." *Behavior Research and Therapy,* 1977, *15,* 89-95.

Hall, S. M., Hall, R. G., Hansen, R. W., and Borden, B. L. "Performance of Two Self-Managed Treatments of Overweight in University and Community Populations." *Journal of Consulting and Clinical Psychology,* 1974, *42,* 781-786.

Hall, Y. F., Stamler, J., Mojonnier, L., Shekelle, R. B., Berkson, D. M., and Stamler, A. "Long-Term Effect of A.H.A.-Type Diet on Hypertriglyceridemia and Hypercholesterolemia." *Circulation,* 1971, *44* (suppl. no. 2), 87.

Hallauer, D. "Illness Behavior—An Experimental Investigation." *Journal of Chronic Diseases,* 1972, *25,* 599-610.

Halstead, W. C. *Brain and Intelligence.* Chicago: University of Chicago Press, 1947.

Hamburg, D. A., and Adams, J. E. "A Perspective on Coping Behavior: Seeking and Utilizing Information in Major Transitions." *Archives of General Psychiatry,* 1967, *17,* 277-284.

Hamburg, D. A., Coelho, G. V., and Adams, J. E. "Coping and Adaptation: Steps Toward a Synthesis of Biological and Social Perspectives." In G. V. Coelho, D. A. Hamburg, and J. E. Adams (Eds.), *Coping and Adaptation.* New York: Basic Books, 1974.

Hamburg, D. A., Hamburg, B., and deGoza, S. "Adaptive Problems and Mechanisms in Severely Burned Patients." *Psychiatry,* 1953, *16,* 1-20.

Hammerschlag, C. A., Fisher, S., DeCosse, J., and Kaplan, E. "Breast Symptoms and Patient Delay: Psychological Variables Involved." *Cancer,* 1964, *17,* 1480-1485.

Hammond, E. "Some Preliminary Findings on Physical Complaints from a Prospective Study of 1,064,000 Men and Women." *American Journal of Public Health,* 1964, *54,* 11-23.

Hammond, K. R. "Probabilistic Functioning and the Clinical Method." *Psychological Review,* 1955, *62,* 255-262.

Hammond, K. R. "Social Judgment Theory: Its Use in the Study of Psychoactive Drugs." In K. R. Hammond and C. R. B. Joyce (Eds.), *Psychoactive Drugs and Social Judgment: Theory and Research.* New York: Wiley, 1975.

Hammond, K. R. "Social Judgment Theory: Application in Policy Formation." In M. F. Kaplan and S. Schwartz (Eds.), *Human Judgment and Decision Processes in Applied Settings.* New York: Academic Press, 1977.

Hammond, K. R., and Adelman, L. "Science, Values, and Human Judgment." *Science,* 1976, *194,* 389-396.

Hammond, K. R., and Joyce, C. R. B. *Psychoactive Drugs and Social Judgment: Theory and Research.* New York: Wiley, 1975.

Hammond, K. R., Stewart, T. R., Brehmer, B., and Steinmann, D. D. "Social Judgment Theory." In M. F. Kaplan and S. Schwartz (Eds.), *Human Judgment and Decision Processes.* New York: Academic Press, 1975.

Hammond, K. R., and Summers, D. A. "Cognitive Control." *Psychological Review,* 1972, *79,* 58-67.

Hanft, R. Address given at Workshop on Rural Health Care Evaluations, National Center for Health Services Research, Annapolis, Md., January 1978.

Hanson, R. W., Borden, B. L., Hall, S. M., and Hall, R. G. "Use of Programmed Instruction in Teaching Self-Management Skills to Overweight Adults." *Behavior Therapy,* 1976, *7,* 366-373.

Hare, A. P. "A Study of Interaction and Consensus in Different Sized Groups." *American Sociological Review,* 1952, *17,* 261-267.

Hare, A. P. *Handbook of Small Group Research.* (2nd ed.) New York: Free Press, 1976.

Harmatz, M. G., and Lapuc, P. "Behavior Modification of Overeating in a Psychiatric Population." *Journal of Consulting and Clinical Psychology,* 1968, *32,* 583-589.

Harper, D. A. "Take My Word—Patient Follow-Up of Medical Advice, a Literature Review." *Journal of the Kansas Medical Society,* 1971, *72* (5), 265-274.

Harrington, R. L. "Mental Health Component of Multiphasic Health Testing Services." In M. F. Collen (Ed.), *Multiphasic Health Testing Services.* New York: Wiley, 1978.

Harris, M. "History and Significance of the Emic/Etic Distinction." *Annual Review of Anthropology,* 1976, *5,* 329-350.

Harris, M. B. "Self-Directed Program for Weight Control: A Pilot Study." *Journal of Abnormal Psychology,* 1969, *74,* 263-270.

Harris, M. B., and Bruner, C. G. "A Comparison of a Self-Control and a Contract Procedure for Weight Control." *Behaviour Research and Therapy,* 1971, *9,* 347-354.

Harris, R. J. "The Comprehension of Pragmatic Implications in Advertising." *Journal of Applied Psychology,* in press.

Harris, S. E. *The Economics of Health Care.* Berkeley, Calif.: McCutchan, 1975.

Harvey, W. *Exercitatio Anatomica de Motu Cordis et Sanguinis in Animalibus* [Essay on the Movement of the Heart and Blood in Animals]. Frankfurt, Germany: 1628. (F. A. Willius and T. E. Keys, Trans., in *Cardiac Classics.* St. Louis: Mosby, 1941.)

Hathaway, K. B. *The Little Locksmith.* New York: Coward-McCann, 1943.

Hathaway, S. R. "A Study of Human Behavior: The Clinical Psychologist." *American Psychologist,* 1958, *13,* 257-265.

Hauser, M. M. "Summary of Main Points Raised in Discussion." In M. M. Hauser (Ed.), *The Economics of Medical Care.* London: Allen & Unwin, 1972.

Havinghurst, R. J., Neugarten, B., and Tobin, S. S. "Disengagement and Patterns of Aging." In B. L. Neugarten (Ed.), *Middle Age and Aging.* Chicago: University of Chicago Press, 1968.

Hay, D., and Oken, D. "The Psychological Stresses of Intensive Care Unit Nursing." *Psychosomatic Medicine,* 1972, *34,* 109-118.

Hayman, M. "Current Attitudes to Alcoholism of Psychiatrists in Southern California." *American Journal of Psychiatry,* 1956, *112,* 485-493.

Haynes, R. B. "A Critical Review of the 'Determinants' of Patient Compliance with Therapeutic Regimens." In D. L. Sackett and R. B. Haynes (Eds.), *Compliance with Therapeutic Regimens.* Baltimore: Johns Hopkins University Press, 1976.

Haynes, R. B., Sackett, D. L., Gibson, E. S., Taylor, D. W., Hackett, B. C., Roberts, R. S., and Johnson, A. L. "Improvement of Medication Compliance in Uncontrolled Hypertension." *Lancet,* 1976, *1,* 1265-1268.

Healy, K. "Does Preoperative Instruction Make a Difference?" *American Journal of Nursing,* 1968, *68,* 62-67.

Heinzelmann, F. "Determinants of Prophylaxis Behavior With Respect to Rheumatic Fever." *Journal of Health and Human Behavior,* 1962, *3,* 73-81.

Heller, J., Groff, B., and Solomon, S. "Toward an Understanding of Crowding: The Role of Physical Interaction." *Journal of Personality and Social Psychology,* 1977, *35,* 183-190.

Heller, S. S., Frank, K. A., Malm, J. R., Bowman, F. O., Jr., Harris, P. D., Charlton, M. H., and Kornfeld, D. S. "Psychiatric Complications of Open-Heart Surgery: A Reexamination." *New England Journal of Medicine,* 1970, *283,* 1015-1020.

Henderson, J. B., and Enelow, A. J. "The Coronary Risk Factor Problem: A Behavioral Perspective." *Preventive Medicine,* 1976, *5,* 128-148.

Henrichs, T. F., MacKenzie, J. W., and Almond, C. H. "Psychological Adjustment and Acute Response to Open-Heart Surgery." *Journal of Nervous and Mental Disease,* 1969, *148,* 158-164.

Herman, M. "The Poor: Their Medical Needs and the Health Services Available to Them." *Annals of the American Academy of Political and Social Science,* 1972, *399,* 12-21.

Herrera, L. F., and Kiser, C. V. "Social and Psychological Factors Affecting Fertility: XIII. Fertility in Relation to Fertility Planning and Health of Wife, Husband, and Children." *Milbank Memorial Fund Quarterly,* 1951, *29,* 375-420.

Herzlich, C. *Health and Illness: A Social-Psychological Analysis.* New York: Academic Press, 1973.

Hess, W. R. "Die Motorik als Organisations Problem." *Biologisches Zentralblatt,* 1941, *61,* 545-572.

Hess, W. R. "Biomotorik als Organisations Problem, I, II." *Naturwissenschaften,* 1942, *30,* 441-448 and 537-541.

Hetherington, R., and Hopkins, C. "Symptom Sensitivity: Its Social and Cultural Correlates." *Health Services Research,* 1969, *4,* 63-70.

Hiatt, R. B. "Preparation of the Patient for Surgery." In H. I. Lief, V. F. Lief, and N. R. Lief (Eds.), *The Psychological Basis of Medical Practice.* New York: Harper & Row, 1963.

Higbee, K. L. *Your Memory: How It Works and How to Improve It.* Englewood Cliffs, N.J.: Prentice-Hall, 1977.

Hill, M. I., and Blane, H. T. "Evaluation of Psychotherapy with Alcoholics: A Critical Review." *Quarterly Journal of Studies on Alcohol,* 1967, *28,* 76-104.

Hill, O. W. (Ed.). *Modern Trends in Psychosomatic Medicine.* Vol. 2. New York: Appleton-Century-Crofts, 1970.

Hill, O. W. (Ed.). *Modern Trends in Psychosomatic Medicine 3.* London: Butterworths, 1976.

Hinde, R. A. "Discussion." *Physiology, Emotion, and Psychosomatic Illness.* Ciba Foundation Symposium, new series 8. Amsterdam: Associated Scientific Publishers, 1972, p. 78.

Hinkle, L. E., Jr. "The Effect of Exposure to Culture Change, Social Change, and Changes in Interpersonal Relationships on Health." In B. S. Dohrenwend and B. P. Dohrenwend (Eds.), *Stressful Life Events: Their Nature and Effects.* New York: Wiley, 1974.

Hinkle, L. E., Jr. "Measurement of the Effects of the Environment upon the Health and Behavior of People." In L. E. Hinkle, Jr., and W. C. Loring (Eds.), *The Effect of the Man-Made Environment on Health and Behavior.* DHEW Publication No. (CDC) 77-8318. Washington, D.C.: U.S. Government Printing Office, 1977.

Hinkle, L. E., Jr., Christenson, W. N., Benjamin, B., Kane, F. D., Plummer, N., and Wolff, H. G., with the collaboration of Schaefer, M., and Widelock, D. "The Occurrence of Illness Among 24 'Normal' Women: Evidences of Differences in Susceptibility to Acute Respiratory and Gastrointestinal Syndromes." Paper presented at annual scientific meeting of American College of Physicians, Miami Beach, Fla., May 10, 1961. [Referenced in Hinkle, 1974.]

Hinkle, L. E., Jr., Christenson, W. N., Kane, F. D., Ostfeld, A. M., Thetford, W. N., and Wolff, H. G. "An Investigation of the Relation Between Life Experience, Personality Characteristics, and General Susceptibility to Illness." *Psychosomatic Medicine,* 1958, *20,* 278-295.

Hinkle, L. E., Jr., Kane, F. D., Christenson, W. N., and Wolff, H. G. "Hungarian Refugees: Life Experiences and Features Influencing Participation in the Revolution and Subsequent Flight." *American Journal of Psychiatry,* 1959, *116,* 16-19.

Hinkle, L. E., Jr., and Loring, W. C. (Eds.). *The Effects of the Man-Made Environment on Health and Behavior.* DHEW Publication No. (CDC) 77-8318. Washington, D.C.: U.S. Government Printing Office, 1977.

Hinkle, L. E., Jr., Pinsky, R. H., Bross, I., and Plummer, N. "The Distribution of Sickness Disability in a Homogeneous Group of 'Healthy Adult Men.'" *American Journal of Hygiene, 1956, 64,* 220-242.

Hinkle, L. E., Jr., Plummer, N., Metraux, R., Richter, P., Gittinger, J. W., Thetford, W. N., Ostfeld, A. M., Kane, F. D., Goldberger, L., Mitchell, W. E., Leichter, H., Pinsky, R., Goebel, D., Bross, I., and Wolff, H. G. "Factors Relevant to the Occurrence of Bodily Illness and Disturbances in Mood, Thought, and Behavior in Three Homogeneous Population Groups." *American Journal of Psychiatry, 1957, 114,* 212-220.

Hinkle, L. E., Jr., and Wolff, H. G. "The Nature of Man's Adaptation to His Total Environment and the Relation of This to Illness." *Archives of Internal Medicine, 1957, 99,* 442-460.

Hinton, J. *Dying.* Baltimore: Penguin Books, 1967.

Hinton, J. "Bearing Cancer." *British Journal of Medical Psychology, 1973, 46,* 105-113.

Hochbaum, G. *Public Participation in Medical Screening Programs: A Sociopsychological Study.* Public Health Service Publication No. 572. Washington, D.C.: Superintendent of Public Documents, 1958.

Hodges, A. *Psychosocial Counseling in General Medical Practice.* Lexington, Mass.: Heath, 1977.

Hodgkin, J. E., Balchum, O. J., Kass, I., Glaser, E. M., Miller, W. F., Haas, A., Shaw, D. B., Kimbel, P., and Petty, T. L. "Chronic Obstructive Airway Diseases: Current Concepts in Diagnosis and Comprehensive Care." *Journal of the American Medical Association, 1975, 232,* 1243-1260.

Hofer, M. A., Wolff, C. T., Friedman, S. B., and Mason, J. W. "A Psychoendocrine Study of Bereavement: Part I. 17-Hydroxy-Corticosteroid Excretion Rates of Parents Following Death of Their Children from Leukemia." *Psychosomatic Medicine, 1972a, 34,* 481-491.

Hofer, M. A., Wolff, C. T., Friedman, S. B., and Mason, J. W. "A Psychoendocrine Study of Bereavement: Part II. Observations on the Process of Mourning in Relation to Adrenocortical Function." *Psychosomatic Medicine, 1972b, 34,* 492-504.

Hoffman, H. E. "Use of Avoidance and Vigilance by Repressors and Sensitizers." *Journal of Consulting and Clinical Psychology, 1970, 34,* 91-96.

Hoffman, P. J. "The Paramorphic Representation of Clinical Judgment." *Psychological Bulletin, 1960, 57,* 116-131.

Hoffman, P. J. "Cue-Consistency and Configurality in Human Judgment." In B. Kleinmuntz (Ed.), *Formal Representation of Human Judgment.* New York: Wiley, 1968.

Hoffman, P. J., Slovic, P., and Rorer, I. G. "An Analysis-of-Variance Model for the Assessment of Configural Cue Utilization in Clinical Judgment." *Psychological Bulletin, 1968, 69,* 338-349.

Holahan, C. *Environment and Behavior: A Synthesis.* New York: Plenum Press, 1978.

Holland, J. "Psychological Aspects of Cancer." In J. F. Holland and E. Frei, III (Eds.), *Cancer Medicine.* Philadelphia: Lea and Febiger, 1973.

Hollander, J., and Yeostros, S. "The Effect of Simultaneous Variations of Humidity and Barometric Pressure on Arthritis." *Bulletin of the American Meterological Society,* 1963, *44,* 489-494.

Hollingshead, A. B. "Medical Sociology: A Brief Review." *Milbank Memorial Fund Quarterly,* 1973, *51,* 531-542.

Holmes, T. H., and Masuda, M. "Life Change and Illness Susceptibility." In B. S. Dohrenwend and B. P. Dohrenwend (Eds.), *Stressful Life Events: Their Nature and Effects.* New York: Wiley, 1974.

Holmes, T. H., and Rahe, R. H. *Schedule of Recent Experiences.* Seattle: School of Medicine, University of Washington, 1967a.

Holmes, T. H., and Rahe, R. H. "The Social Readjustment Rating Scale." *Journal of Psychosomatic Research,* 1967b, *11,* 213-218.

Holmes, T. H., and Rahe, R. H. "Life Crisis and Disease Onset: II. Qualitative and Quantitative Definition of the Life Crisis and Its Association with Health Change." Unpublished manuscript, School of Medicine, University of Washington, n.d.

Holt, H., and Winick, C. "Group Psychotherapy with Obese Women." *Archives of General Psychiatry,* 1961, *5,* 156-158.

Holt, R. R. "Clinical and Statistical Prediction: A Reformulation and Some New Data." *Journal of Abnormal and Social Psychology,* 1958, *56,* 1-12.

Hoppock, R. R. *Occupational Information.* New York: McGraw-Hill, 1957.

Horan, J. J., Hackett, G., Nicholov, W. C., Linberg, S. E., Stone, C. I., and Lukaski, H. C. "Rapid Smoking: A Cautionary Note." *Journal of Consulting and Clinical Psychology,* 1977, *45,* 341-343.

Horan, J. J., and Johnson, R. G. "Covert Conditioning Through a Self-Management Application of the Premack Principle: Its Effect on Weight Reduction." *Journal of Behavior Therapy and Experimental Psychiatry,* 1971, *2,* 243-249.

Hornblow, A. R., Kidson, M. A., and Jones, K. V. "Measuring Medical Students' Empathy: A Validation Study." *Medical Education,* 1977, *11,* 7-12.

Horowitz, M. J. *Educating Tomorrow's Doctors.* New York: Appleton-Century-Crofts, 1964.

Horowitz, M. J. *Stress Response Syndromes.* New York: Aronson, 1976.

Horowitz, M. J., Schaefer, C., Hiroto, D., Wilner, N., and Levin, B. "Life Event Questionnaires for Measuring Presumptive Stress." *Psychosomatic Medicine,* 1977, *39,* 413-431.

Horton, E., Danforth, E., Sims, E., and Salans, L. "Endocrine and Metabolic Alterations in Spontaneous and Experimental Obesity." In G. A. Bray (Ed.), *Obesity in Perspective.* Washington, D.C.: U.S. Government Printing Office, 1975.

Horwitz, N. "Post-Op Patients Forget, Fabricate, Even Deny Having Consent Talks." *Hospital Tribune,* March 22, 1976, pp. 1, 17.

Hosack, A. "A Comparison of Crises: Mothers' Early Experiences with Normal and Abnormal Firstborn Infants." Unpublished doctoral dissertation, School of Public Health, Harvard University, 1968.

Houston, B. K. "Control Over Stress, Locus of Control, and Response to Stress." *Journal of Personality and Social Psychology,* 1972, *21,* 249-255.

Howard, J. H., Cunningham, D. A., and Rechnitzer, P. A. "Health Patterns Associated with Type A Behavior: A Managerial Population." *Journal of Human Stress,* 1976, *2,* 24-31.

Howard, J. H., Cunningham, D. A., Rechnitzer, P. A., and Goode, R. C. "Stress in the Job and Career of a Dentist." *Journal of the American Dental Association,* 1976, *93,* 630-636.

Howe, H. F. "Application of Automated Multiphasic Health Testing in Clinical Medicine: The Current State of the Art." *Journal of the American Medical Association,* 1972, *219,* 885-889.

Hoyt, M. F., and Janis, I. L. "Increasing Adherence to a Stressful Decision via a Motivational Balance-Sheet Procedure: A Field Experiment." *Journal of Personality and Social Psychology,* 1975, *31,* 833-839.

Hsia, Y. E. "Parental Reaction to Genetics Counseling." *Contemporary Obstetrics/Gynecology,* 1974, *4,* 99-106.

Hsu, J. J. "Electroconditioning Therapy of Alcoholics: A Preliminary Report." *Quarterly Journal of Studies on Alcohol,* 1965, *26,* 449-459.

Hudgens, R. W. "Personal Catastrophe and Depression." In B. S. Dohrenwend and B. P. Dohrenwend (Eds.), *Stressful Life Events: Their Nature and Effects.* New York: Wiley, 1974.

Huesmann, L. (Ed.). "Learned Helplessness as a Model of Depression." *Journal of Abnormal Psychology,* 1978, *87,* 1-198.

Huggan, R. E. "Neuroticism, Distortion, and Objective Manifestations of Anxiety in Males with Malignant Disease." *British Journal of Social and Clinical Psychology,* 1968, *7,* 280-285.

Hulka, B. S. "Correlates of Satisfaction and Dissatisfaction with Medical Care: A Community Perspective." *Medical Care,* 1975, *13,* 648-658.

Hulka, B. S., Cassel, J. C., and Kupper, L. "Disparities Between Medications Prescribed and Consumed Among Chronic Disease Patients." In L. Lasagna (Ed.), *Patient Compliance.* Mt. Kisco, N.Y.: Futura, 1976.

Hulka, B. S., Zyzanski, S. J., Cassell, J. C., and Thompson, S. J. "Scale for the Measurement of Attitudes Toward Physicians and Primary Medical Care." *Medical Care,* 1970, *8,* 429-436.

Hunt, E. B. "What Kind of Computer Is Man?" *Cognitive Psychology,* 1971, *2,* 57-98.

Hunt, E. B. "The Memory We Must Have." In R. Schank and K. Colby (Eds.), *Computer Models of Thought and Language.* San Francisco: W. H. Freeman, 1973.

Hunt, E. B. "The Mechanics of Verbal Ability." *Psychological Review,* 1978, *85,* 109-130.

Hunt, G. M., and Azrin, N. H. "Community Reinforcement Approach to Alcoholism." *Behavior Research and Therapy,* 1973, *11,* 99-104.

Hunt, W. A., Barnett, L. W., and Branch, L. G. "Relapse Rates in Addiction Programs." *Journal of Clinical Psychology,* 1971, *27,* 455-456.

Hunt, W. A., and Matarazzo, J. D. "Three Years Later: Recent Developments in the Experimental Modification of Smoking Behavior." *Journal of Abnormal Psychology*, 1973, *81*, 107-114.

Hunter, R. C. A., Prince, R. H., and Schwartzman, A. E. "Comments on Emotional Disturbances in a Medical Undergraduate Population." *Canadian Medical Association Journal*, 1961, *85*, 989-992.

Hurtado, A., Greenlick, M., and Columbo, T. "Determinants of Medical Care Utilization: Failure to Keep Appointments." *Medical Care*, 1973, *11*, 189-198.

Hutchins, E. B., and Morris, W. W. "A Follow-Up Study of Nonentrants and High Ability Rejected Applicants to the 1958-59 Entering Class of U.S. Medical Schools." *Journal of Medical Education*, 1963, *38*, 1023-1028.

Hutchinson, J. W., and Lockhead, G. R. "Similarity as Distance: A Structural Principle for Semantic Memory." *Journal of Experimental Psychology: Human Learning and Memory*, 1977, *3*, 660-678.

Hyman, H. H., Cobb, W. H., Feldman, J. J., Hart, C. W., and Stember, C. H. *Interviewing in Social Research*. Chicago: University of Chicago Press, 1954.

Hyman, M. "Some Links Between Economic Status and Untreated Illness." *Social Science and Medicine*, 1970, *4*, 387-399.

Imboden, J. B. "Psychosocial Determinants of Recovery." *Advances in Psychosomatic Medicine*, 1972, *8*, 142-155.

Imboden, J. B., Canter, A., and Cluff, L. E. "Convalescence from Influenza." *Archives of Internal Medicine*, 1961, *108*, 393-399.

Imboden, J. B., Canter, A., and Cluff, L. E. "Separation Experiences and Health Records in a Group of Normal Adults." *Psychosomatic Medicine*, 1963, *25*, 433-440.

Imboden, J. B., Canter, A., Cluff, L. E., and Trever, R. W. "Brucellosis: III. Psychologic Aspects of Delayed Convalescence." *Archives of Internal Medicine*, 1959, *103*, 406-414.

Indian Health Service EMCRO. *Fourth Quarterly and Annual Report*. Tucson, Ariz., 1975.

Insko, C. A., Arkoff, A., and Insko, V. M. "Effects of High and Low Fear Arousing Communications upon Opinions Toward Smoking." *Journal of Experimental Social Psychology*, 1965, *1*, 256-266.

Inter-Society Commission for Heart Disease Resources. "Primary Prevention of the Artherosclerotic Diseases." *Circulation*, 1970, *42*, A55-A95.

Inui, T., Yourtee, E., and Williamson, J. "Improved Outcomes in Hypertension After Physician Tutorials." *Annals of Internal Medicine*, 1976, *84*, 646-651.

Ireton, H., and Thwing, E. "Appraising the Development of a Preschool Child by Means of a Standardized Report Prepared by the Mother." *Clinical Pediatrics*, 1976, *15*, 875-882.

Ivey, A., and Authier, J. *Microcounseling: Innovations in Interviewing, Counseling, Psychotherapy, and Psychoeducation*. Springfield, Ill.: Thomas, 1978.

Izsak, F. C., Engel, J., and Medalie, J. H. "Comprehensive Rehabilitation of the Patient with Cancer—Five Years Home Care." *Journal of Chronic Diseases,* 1973, *26,* 363-374.

Izsak, F. C., and Medalie, J. H. "Comprehensive Follow-Up of Carcinoma Patients." *Journal of Chronic Diseases,* 1971, *24,* 179-191.

Jacobs, M. A., Spilken, A. Z., and Norman, M. "Relationship of Life Change, Maladaptive Aggression, and Upper Respiratory Infection in Male College Students." *Psychosomatic Medicine,* 1969, *31,* 31-44.

Jacobs, S., and Ostfeld, A. M. "An Epidemiological Review of the Mortality of Bereavement." *Psychosomatic Medicine,* 1977, *39,* 344-357.

Jaggard, R. S., Zager, L. L., and Wilkins, D. S. "Clinical Evaluation of Analgesic Drugs." *Archives of Surgery,* 1950, *61,* 1073-1082.

Janis, I. L. *Psychological Stress: Psychoanalytic and Behavioral Studies of Surgical Patients.* New York: Wiley, 1958.

Janis, I. L. "Psychological Effects of Warnings." In G. W. Baker and D. W. Chapman (Eds.), *Man and Society in Disaster.* New York: Basic Books, 1962.

Janis, I. L. "Effect of Fear Arousal on Attitude Change: Recent Developments in Theory and Research." In L. Berkowitz (Ed.), *Advances in Experimental Social Psychology.* Vol. 3. New York: Academic Press, 1967.

Janis, I. L. *Stress and Frustration.* New York: Harcourt Brace Jovanovich, 1971.

Janis, I. L. *Victims of Groupthink.* Boston: Houghton Mifflin, 1972.

Janis, I. L. "Effectiveness of Social Support for Stressful Decisions." In M. Deutsch and H. Hornstein (Eds.), *Applying Social Psychology: Implications for Research, Practice, and Training.* Hillsdale, N.J.: Lawrence Erlbaum, 1975a.

Janis, I. L. "Reaction" to section titled "Public Opinion, Attitude Research and Health Problems." In A. J. Enelow and J. B. Henderson (Eds.), *Applying Behavioral Science to Cardiovascular Risk.* New York: American Heart Association, 1975b.

Janis, I. L. (Ed.). *Counseling on Personal Decisions: Theory and Research on Helping Relationships.* New Haven, Conn.: Yale University Press, in press.

Janis, I. L., and Feshbach, S. "Effects of Fear-Arousing Communications." *Journal of Abnormal and Social Psychology,* 1953, *48,* 78-92.

Janis, I. L., and Leventhal, H. "Psychological Aspects of Physical Illness and Hospital Care." In B. B. Wolman (Ed.), *Handbook of Clinical Psychology.* New York: McGraw-Hill, 1965.

Janis, I. L., and Mann, L. "Effectiveness of Emotional Role-Playing in Modifying Smoking Habits and Attitudes." *Journal of Experimental Research in Personality,* 1965, *1,* 84-90.

Janis, I. L., and Mann, L. *Decision Making: A Psychological Analysis of Conflict, Choice, and Commitment.* New York: Free Press, 1977.

Janis, I. L., and Terwilliger, R. "An Experimental Study of Psychological Resistance to Fear-Arousing Communications." *Journal of Abnormal and Social Psychology,* 1962, *65,* 403-410.

Jarvik, M. E., Cullen, J. W., Gritz, E. R., Vogt, T. M., and West, J. L. *Re-*

search on Smoking Behavior. Rockville, Md.: National Institute on Drug Abuse, 1977.

Jeffrey, D. B. "Additional Methodological Considerations in the Behavioral Treatment of Obesity: A Reply to the Hall and Hall Review of Obesity." *Behavior Therapy,* 1975, *6,* 96-97.

Jeffrey, D. B., and Christensen, E. R. "The Relative Efficacy of Behavior Therapy, Will Power, and No-Treatment Control Procedures in the Modification of Obesity." In a symposium on "Behavior Modification Approaches to the Treatment of Obesity: Recent Trends and Developments" presented at the Association for the Advancement of Behavior Therapy, Miami Beach, Fla., 1972.

Jenkins, C. D. "Factors Involving Interpersonal and Psychological Characteristics: Appraisal and Implications for Theoretical Development." In S. L. Syme and L. G. Reeder (Eds.), "Social Stress and Cardiovascular Disease." *Milbank Memorial Fund Quarterly,* 1967, *45* (2), 141-149.

Jenkins, C. D. "Psychologic and Social Precursors of Coronary Disease." *New England Journal of Medicine,* 1971, *284,* 244-255 and 307-317.

Jenkins, C. D. "Psychology in Epidemiology: The Growing Edge." In G. T. Steward (Ed.), *Trends in Epidemiology.* Springfield, Ill.: Thomas, 1972.

Jenkins, C. D. "Recent Evidence Supporting Psychologic and Social Risk Factors for Coronary Disease." *New England Journal of Medicine,* 1976, *294,* 987-994 and 1033-1038.

Jenkins, C. D., Hames, C. G., Zyzanski, S. J., Rosenman, R. H., and Friedman, M. "Psychological Traits and Serum Lipids." *Psychosomatic Medicine,* 1969, *31,* 115-128.

Jenkins, C. D., Rosenman, R. H., and Friedman, M. "Development of an Objective Psychological Test for the Determination of the Coronary-Prone Behavior Pattern in Employed Men." *Journal of Chronic Diseases,* 1967, *20,* 371-379.

Jenkins, C. D., Rosenman, R. H., and Zyzanski, S. J. Letter to the Editor. *Journal of the American Medical Association,* 1974a, *229,* 1284.

Jenkins, C. D., Rosenman, R. H., and Zyzanski, S. J. "Prediction of Clinical Coronary Heart Disease by a Test for the Coronary-Prone Behavior Pattern." *New England Journal of Medicine,* 1974b, *290,* 1271-1275.

Jenkins, C. D., Zyzanski, S. J., and Rosenman, R. H. "Coronary-Prone Behavior: One Pattern or Several?" *Psychosomatic Medicine,* 1978, *40,* 25-43.

Jenkins, C. D., Zyzanski, S. J., Ryan, T. J., Flessas, A., and Tannenbaum, S. I. "Social Insecurity and Coronary-Prone Type A Responses as Identifiers of Severe Atherosclerosis." *Journal of Consulting and Clinical Psychology,* 1977, *45,* 1060-1067.

Johannsen, W., Hellmuth, G., and Sorauf, T. "On Accepting Medical Recommendations." *Archives of Environmental Health,* 1966, *12,* 63-69.

Johns, M. W., Dudley, H. A. F., and Masterton, J. P. "Psychosocial Problems in Surgery." *Journal of the Royal College of Surgeons of Edinburgh,* 1973, *18,* 91-102.

Johnson, C. A., Hammel, R. J., and Heinen, J. S. "Levels of Satisfaction Among Hospital Pharmacists." *American Journal of Hospital Pharmacy,* 1977, *34,* 241-247.

Johnson, D. G., and Hutchins, E. B. "Doctor or Dropout? A Study of Medical Student Attrition." *Journal of Medical Education,* 1966, *41,* 1099-1269.

Johnson, H. J., and Schwartz, G. E. "Suppression of GSR Activity Through Operant Reinforcement." *Journal of Experimental Psychology,* 1967, *73,* 307-312.

Johnson, J. E. "The Influence of Purposeful Nurse-Patient Interaction on the Patient's Postoperative Course." *A.N.A. Monograph Series No. 2: Exploring Medical-Surgical Nursing Practice.* New York: American Nurses' Association, 1966.

Johnson, J. E. "Stress Reduction Through Sensation Information." In I. G. Sarason and C. D. Spielberger (Eds.), *Stress and Anxiety.* Vol. 2. New York: Wiley, 1975.

Johnson, J. E., and Leventhal, H. "Effects of Accurate Expectations and Behavioral Instructions on Reactions During a Noxious Medical Examination." *Journal of Personality and Social Psychology,* 1974, *29,* 710-718.

Johnson, J. E., Leventhal, H., and Dabbs, J. "Contribution of Emotional and Instrumental Response Processes in Adaptation to Surgery." *Journal of Personality and Social Psychology,* 1971, *20,* 55-64.

Johnson, J. E., Rice, V. H., Fuller, S. S., and Endress, M. P. "Sensory Information, Behavioral Instruction, and Recovery from Surgery." Paper presented at annual meeting of the American Psychological Association, San Francisco, August 1977.

Jonas, S. "Appointment-Breaking in a General Medical Clinic." *Medical Care,* 1971, *9,* 82-88.

Jones, E. E. *Ingratiation: A Social Psychological Analysis.* New York: Appleton-Century-Crofts, 1964.

Jones, E. E., and Nisbett, R. E. *The Actor and the Observer: Divergent Perceptions of the Causes of Behavior.* Morristown, N.J.: General Learning Press, 1971.

Juan, I. R., and Haley, H. B. "High and Low Levels of Dogmatism in Relation to Personality, Intellectual, and Environmental Characteristics of Medical Students." *Psychological Reports,* 1970, *26,* 535-544.

Juan, I. R., Paiva, R. E. A., Haley, H. B., and O'Keefe, R. D. "High and Low Levels of Dogmatism in Relation to Personality Characteristics of Medical Students: A Follow-Up Study." *Psychological Reports,* 1974, *34,* 313-315.

Kagan, A. R., and Levi, L. "Health and Environment—Psychosocial Stimuli: A Review." *Social Science and Medicine,* 1974, *8,* 225-241.

Kagan, N. "Can Technology Help Us Toward Reliability in Influencing Human Interaction?" *Educational Technology,* 1973, *13,* 44-51.

Kagan, N. "Influencing Human Interaction—Eleven Years with IPR." *Canadian Counsellor,* 1975, *9,* 74-97.

Kagan, N. *Elements of Facilitating Communication* (film and manual). Mason, Mich.: Mason Media, 1976a.

Kagan, N. *Influencing Human Interaction.* Mason, Mich.: Mason Media, 1976b.

Kagan, N., and Krathwohl, D. R. *Studies in Human Interaction: Interpersonal Process Recall Stimulated by Videotape.* East Lansing: Educational Publication Services, Michigan State University, 1967. (Currently available on microfiche through the ERIC System.)

Kagan, N., Krathwohl, D. R., and Miller, R. "Stimulated Recall in Therapy Using Videotape: A Case Study." *Journal of Counseling Psychology,* 1963, *10,* 237-243.

Kagan, N., and Schauble, P. G. "Affect Simulation in Interpersonal Process Recall." *Journal of Counseling Psychology,* 1969, *16,* 309-313.

Kahana, R. J. "Studies in Medical Psychology: A Brief Survey." *Psychiatry in Medicine,* 1972, *3,* 1-22.

Kahana, R. J., and Bibring, G. L. "Personality Types in Medical Management." In N. E. Zinberg (Ed.), *Psychiatry and Medical Practice in a General Hospital.* New York: International Universities Press, 1964.

Kahn, A. *Theory and Practice of Social Planning.* New York: Russell Sage Foundation, 1969.

Kahn, L., Anderson, M., and Perkoff, G. "Patients' Perceptions and Uses of a Pediatric Emergency Room." *Social Science and Medicine,* 1973, *7,* 155-160.

Kahn, R. L., and Cannell, C. F. *The Dynamics of Interviewing: Theory, Technique, and Cases.* New York: Wiley, 1957.

Kahn, R. L., Zarit, S., Hilbert, N., and Niederehe, G. "Memory Complaint and Impairment in the Aged." *Archives of General Psychiatry,* 1975, *32,* 1569-1573.

Kahneman, D. *Attention and Effort.* Englewood Cliffs, N.J.: Prentice-Hall, 1973.

Kahneman, D., and Tversky, A. "Subjective Probability: A Judgment of Representativeness." *Cognitive Psychology,* 1972, *3,* 430-454.

Kahneman, D., and Tversky, A. "On the Psychology of Prediction." *Psychological Review,* 1973, *80,* 237-251.

Kalmer, H. (Ed.). "Reviews of Research and Studies Related to Delay in Seeking Diagnosis of Cancer." *Health Education Monographs,* 1974, *2* (Whole no. 2).

Kamiya, J. "Operant Control of the EEG Alpha Rhythm and Some of Its Reported Effects on Consciousness." In C. T. Tart (Ed.), *Altered States of Consciousness.* New York: Wiley, 1969.

Kanfer, F., and Seider, M. L. "Self-Control: Factors Enhancing Tolerance of Noxious Stimulation." *Journal of Personality and Social Psychology,* 1973, *25,* 381-389.

Kant, F. "The Use of Conditioned Reflexes in the Treatment of Alcohol Addicts." *Wisconsin Medical Journal,* 1945, *44,* 217-221.

Kaplan, B. H., Cassel, J. C., and Gore, S. "Social Support and Health." *Medical Care,* 1977, *15* (5, suppl.), 47-58.

Kaplan, M. F., and Schwartz, S. (Eds.). *Human Judgment and Decision Processes*. New York: Academic Press, 1975.

Kaplan, M. F., and Schwartz, S. (Eds.). *Human Judgment and Decision Processes in Applied Settings*. New York: Academic Press, 1977.

Kaplan, R. M., Bush, J. W., and Berry, C. C. "Health Status: Types of Validity for an Index of Well-Being." *Health Services Research*, 1976, *11*, 478-507.

Kaplan-de Nour, A., and Czaczkes, J. W. "Personality Factors in Chronic Hemodialysis Patients Causing Noncompliance with Medical Regimen." *Psychosomatic Medicine*, 1972, *34*, 334-344.

Kasl, S. V. "The Health Belief Model and Behavior Related to Chronic Illness." *Health Education Monographs*, 1974, *2*, 433-454.

Kasl, S. V. "Issues in Patient Adherence to Health Care Regimens." *Journal of Human Stress*, 1975a, *1* (3), 5-17.

Kasl, S. V. "Social-Psychological Characteristics Associated with Behaviors Which Reduce Cardiovascular Risk." In A. J. Enelow and J. B. Henderson (Eds.), *Applying Behavioral Science to Cardiovascular Risk*. New York: American Heart Association, 1975b.

Kasl, S. V. "The Effects of the Residential Environment on Health and Behavior: A Review." In L. E. Hinkle, Jr., and W. C. Loring (Eds.), *The Effects of the Man-Made Environment on Health and Behavior*. Washington, D.C.: U.S. Government Printing Office, 1977.

Kasl, S. V., and Cobb, S. "Health Behavior, Illness Behavior, and Sick Role Behavior." *Archives of Environmental Health*, 1966, *12*, 246-266 and 531-541.

Kasl, S. V., and Cobb, S. "Blood Pressure Changes in Men Undergoing Job Loss: A Preliminary Report." *Psychosomatic Medicine*, 1970, *32*, 19-38.

Kassebaum, G., and Baumann, B. "Dimensions of the Sick Role in Chronic Illness." *Journal of Health and Human Behavior*, 1965, *6*, 16-27.

Katz, D., Sarnoff, I., and McClintock, C. G. "Ego-Defense and Attitude Change." *Human Relations*, 1956, *9*, 27-46.

Katz, J. L., Weiner, H., Gallagher, T. G., and Hellman, L. "Stress, Distress, and Ego Defenses." *Archives of General Psychiatry*, 1970, *23*, 131-142.

Katz, R., and Zlutnick, S. (Eds.). *Behavior Therapy and Health Care*. Elmsford, N.Y.: Pergamon Press, 1975.

Katz, S., Akpom, C. A., Papsidero, J. A., and Weiss, S. T. "Measuring the Health Status of Populations." In R. L. Berg (Ed.), *Health Status Indexes*. Chicago: Hospital Research and Educational Trust, 1973.

Katz, S., Ford, A. B., Moskowitz, R. W., Jackson, B. A., and Jaffe, M. W. "Studies of Illness of the Aged: The Index of ADL, a Standardized Measure of Biological and Psychological Function." *Journal of American Medical Association*, 1963, *185*, 914-919.

Kaufman, G. M., and Thomas, H. *Modern Decision Analysis*. New York: Penguin Books, 1977.

Kaufman, H. "The Politics of Health Planning." *American Journal of Public Health*, 1969, *59*, 795-797.

Kaufman, I. C. "Mother-Infant Separation in Monkeys: An Experimental Model." In J. P. Scott and E. C. Senay (Eds.), *Separation and Depression.* Washington, D.C.: American Association for the Advancement of Science, 1973.

Kaufman, I. C., and Rosenblum, L. A. "The Reaction to Separation in Infant Monkeys: Anaclitic Depression and Conservation-Withdrawal." *Psychosomatic Medicine,* 1967, *29,* 648-675.

Kegeles, S., Kirscht, J. P., Haefner, D., and Rosenstock, I. M. "Survey of Beliefs About Cancer Detection and Taking Papanicolaou Tests." *Public Health Reports,* 1965 (September), *80,* 815-824.

Kegeles, S., Lotzkar, S., and Andrews, L. "Dental Care for the Chronically Ill and Aged: II. Some Factors Relevant for Predicting the Acceptance of Dental Care by Nursing Home Residents." Unpublished manuscript, Public Health Service, U.S. Department of Health, Education, and Welfare, 1959.

Kehrer, B. "Professional and Practice Characteristics of Men and Women Physicians." In *Profile of Medical Practice.* Chicago: Center for Health Services Research and Development, American Medical Association, 1974.

Keith, R. A. "Personality and Coronary Heart Disease: A Review." *Journal of Chronic Diseases,* 1966, *19,* 1231-1243.

Kelley, H. H. *Attribution in Social Interaction.* Morristown, N.J.: General Learning Press, 1971.

Kelman, H., and Lane, D. "Use of Hospital Emergency Room in Relation to Use of Private Physicians." *American Journal of Public Health,* 1976, *66* (9), 891-894.

Kendall, P. L. "Medical Specialization: Trends and Contributing Factors." In R. Coombs and C. E. Vincent (Eds.), *Psychosocial Aspects of Medical Training.* Springfield, Ill.: Thomas, 1971.

Kendall, P. L., and Merton, R. K. "Medical Education as a Social Process." In E. G. Jaco (Ed.), *Patients, Physicians, and Illness.* New York: Free Press, 1958.

Kenton, C. "Health Indices in the United States." Literature Search Number 73-7. National Library of Medicine, U.S. Department of Health, Education, and Welfare, 1973.

Kerr, T. A., Schapira, K., and Roth, M. "The Relationship Between Premature Death and Affective Disorders." *British Journal of Psychiatry,* 1969, *115,* 1277-1282.

Kessner, D. M., Kalk, C. E., and Singer, J. "Assessing Health Quality—The Case for Tracers." *New England Journal of Medicine,* 1973, *288,* 189-194.

Kiesler, C. A. (Ed.). *The Psychology of Commitment.* New York: Academic Press, 1971.

Kilpatrick, D. G., Miller, W. C., Allain, A. N., Huggins, M. B., and Lee, W. H., Jr. "The Use of Psychological Test Data to Predict Open-Heart Surgery Outcome: A Prospective Study." *Psychosomatic Medicine,* 1975, *37,* 62-73.

Kimball, C. P. "Psychological Responses to the Experience of Open-Heart Surgery: I." *American Journal of Psychiatry,* 1969, *126,* 348-359.

Kimmel, K. "Stress Situation in Dental Practice." *Quintessence International,* 1973, *11,* 77-82.

King, D. L., and Pontious, R. H. "Time Relations in the Recall of the Events of the Day." *Psychonomic Science,* 1969, *17,* 330-340.

King, H. "Health in the Medical and Other Learned Professions." *Journal of Chronic Diseases,* 1970, *23,* 257-281.

King, H., and Bailar, J. C. "Mortality Among Lutheran Clergymen." *Milbank Memorial Fund Quarterly,* 1968, *46,* 527-548.

King, H., Zafros, G., and Hass, R. "Further Inquiry into Protestant Mortality Patterns." *Journal of Biosocial Science,* 1975, *7,* 243-254.

King, S. *Perceptions of Illness and Medical Practice.* New York: Russell Sage Foundation, 1962.

Kingdon, M. A. "A Cost/Benefit Analysis of the Interpersonal Process Recall Technique." *Journal of Counseling Psychology,* 1975, *22,* 353-357.

Kingsley, R. G., and Wilson, G. T. "Behavior Therapy for Obesity: A Comparative Investigation of Long-Term Efficacy." *Journal of Consulting and Clinical Psychology,* 1977, *45,* 288-298.

Kinsman, R. A., Dahlem, N. W., Spector, S., and Staudenmayer, H. "Observations on Subjective Symptomatology, Coping Behavior, and Medical Decisions in Asthma." *Psychosomatic Medicine,* 1977, *39,* 102-119.

Kiresuk, T. J., and Sherman, R. E. "Goal Attainment Scaling: A General Method for Evaluating Comprehensive Community Health Programs." *Community Mental Health Journal,* 1968, *4,* 443-453.

Kirscht, J. P. "The Health Belief Model and Illness Behavior." *Health Education Monographs,* 1974, *2* (4), 387-408.

Kirscht, J. P., Becker, M., and Eveland, J. "Psychological and Social Factors as Predictors of Medical Behavior." *Medical Care,* 1976, *14* (5), 422-431.

Kirscht, J. P., Haefner, D., and Eveland, J. "Public Response to Various Written Appeals to Participate in Health Screening." *Public Health Reports,* 1975, *90,* 539-543.

Kirscht, J. P., Haefner, D., Kegeles, S., and Rosenstock, I. M. "A National Study of Health Beliefs." *Journal of Health and Human Behavior,* 1966, *7,* 248-254.

Kirscht, J. P., and Rosenstock, I. M. "Patient Adherence to Antihypertensive Medical Regimens." *Journal of Community Health,* 1977, *3,* 115-124.

Kish, G. B., and Hermann, H. T. "The Fort Meade Alcoholism Treatment Program: A Follow-Up Study." *Quarterly Journal of Studies on Alcohol,* 1971, *32,* 628-635.

Kissen, D. M. "Personality Characteristics in Males Conducive to Lung Cancer." *British Journal of Medical Psychology,* 1963, *36,* 27-36.

Kissen, D. M. "The Significance of Personality in Lung Cancer in Men." *Annals of the New York Academy of Sciences,* 1966, *125* (Art. 3), 820-826.

Kissen, D. M., Brown, R. I. F., and Kissen, M. "A Further Report on Personality and Psychosocial Factors in Lung Cancer." *Annals of the New York Academy of Sciences,* 1969, *164* (Art. 2), 535-544.

Kissin, B., Platz, A., and Su, W. H. "Selective Factors in Treatment Choice and Outcome in Alcoholics." In N. K. Mello and H. H. Mendelson (Eds.), *Recent Advances in Studies of Alcoholism.* DHEW Publication No. (HSM) 71-9045. Washington, D.C.: U.S. Government Printing Office, 1971.

Klarman, H. E. "Trends and Tendencies in Health Economics." In H. E. Klarman (Ed.), *Empirical Studies in Health Economics.* Baltimore: Johns Hopkins University Press, 1968.

Klebba, A. J., Maurer, J. D., and Glass, E. J. *Mortality Trends: Age, Color, and Sex: United States, 1950-1969.* DHEW Publication No. (HRA) 74-1852. Washington, D.C.: U.S. Government Printing Office, 1973.

Klebba, A. J., Maurer, J. D., and Glass, E. J. *Mortality Trends for Leading Causes of Death: United States, 1950-1969.* DHEW Publication No. (HRA) 74-1853. Washington, D.C.: U.S. Government Printing Office, 1974.

Klein, D. C., and Lindemann, E. "Preventive Intervention in Individual and Family Crisis Situations." In G. Caplan (Ed.), *Prevention of Mental Disorders in Children.* New York: Basic Books, 1961.

Kleinknecht, R. A., Klepac, R. K., and Bernstein, D. A. "Psychology and Dentistry: Potential Benefits from a Health Care Liaison." *Professional Psychology,* 1976, *6,* 585-592.

Kleinman, A. M. "Explanatory Model Transactions in Health Care Relationships." In *Health of the Family: 1974 International Health Conference.* Washington, D.C.: National Council for International Health, 1975.

Kleinman, A. M. "Lessons from a Clinical Approach to Medical Anthropological Research." *Medical Anthropology Newsletter,* 1977, *8* (4), 11-15.

Kleinman, J. C., and Wilson, R. W. "Are 'Medically Underserved Areas' Medically Underserved?" *Health Services Research,* 1977, *12,* 147-162.

Kleinmuntz, B. "MMPI Decision Rules for the Identification of College Maladjustment: A Digital Computer Approach." *Psychological Monographs,* 1963, *77* (14, Whole no. 577).

Kleinmuntz, B. "The Processing of Clinical Information by Man and Machine." In B. Kleinmuntz (Ed.), *Formal Representation of Human Judgment.* New York: Wiley, 1968.

Kleinmuntz, B. *Clinical Information Processing by Computer.* New York: Holt, Rinehart and Winston, 1969.

Klemp, G. O., and Rodin, J. "Effects of Uncertainty, Delay, and Focus of Attention on Reactions to an Aversive Situation." *Journal of Experimental Social Psychology,* 1976, *12,* 416-421.

Klopfer, B. "Psychological Variables in Human Cancer." *Journal of Projective Techniques,* 1957, *21,* 331-340.

Kluckhohn, C., and Murray, H. A. "Personality Formation: The Determinants." In C. Kluckhohn, H. A. Murray, and D. M. Schneider (Eds.), *Personality in Nature, Society, and Culture.* (2nd ed.) New York: Knopf, 1953.

Knapp, D. A. "Pharmacist as a Health Professional." *Wisconsin Pharmacist,* 1974, pp. 270-273.

Knapp, D. E., and Knapp, D. A. "Disillusionment in Pharmacy Students." *Social Science and Medicine,* 1968, *1,* 445-447.

Knapp, D. E., Knapp, D. A., and Edwards, J. D. "The Pharmacist as Perceived by Physicians, Patrons, and Other Pharmacists." *Journal of the American Pharmaceutical Association,* 1969, *NS9,* 80-84.

Kneppreth, N. P., Gustafson, D. H., Leifer, R. P., and Johnson, E. M. "Techniques for the Assessment of Worth." Technical paper 254. Arlington, Va.: U.S. Army Research Institute for the Behavioral and Social Sciences, 1974.

Kohut, H. *The Analysis of the Self.* New York: International Universities Press, 1971.

Kolouch, F. T. "Hypnosis and Surgical Convalescence: A Study of Subjective Factors in Postoperative Recovery." *American Journal of Clinical Hypnosis,* 1964, *7,* 120-129.

Koos, E. *The Health of Regionville.* New York: Columbia University Press, 1954.

Kopel, S. A. "Effects of Self-Control, Booster Sessions, and Cognitive Factors in the Maintenance of Smoking Reduction." Unpublished doctoral dissertation, University of Oregon, 1974.

Koran, L. M. "The Reliability of Clinical Methods, Data, and Judgments." *New England Journal of Medicine,* 1975, *293,* 642-646 and 695-701.

Kornfeld, D. S. "The Hospital Environment: Its Impact on the Patient." *Advances in Psychosomatic Medicine,* 1972, *8,* 252-270.

Kornfeld, D. S., Heller, S. S., Frank, K. A., and Moskowitz, R. "Personality and Psychological Factors in Postcardiotomy Delirium." *Archives of General Psychiatry,* 1974, *31,* 249-253.

Korsch, B. M., Gozzi, E. K., and Francis, V. "Gaps in Doctor-Patient Communication: I. Doctor-Patient Interaction and Patient Satisfaction." *Pediatrics,* 1968, *42,* 855-871.

Korte, C., Ypma, I., and Toppen, A. "Helpfulness in Dutch Society as a Function of Urbanization and Environmental Input Level." *Journal of Personality and Social Psychology,* 1975, *32,* 996-1003.

Kosa, J., and Coker, R. E. "The Female Physician in Public Health: Conflict of the Sex and Professional Roles." *Sociology and Social Research,* 1965, *49,* 294-305.

Kosa, J., and Robertson, L. "The Social Aspects of Health and Illness." In J. Kosa and I. Zola (Eds.), *Poverty and Health: A Sociological Analysis.* (rev. ed.) Cambridge, Mass.: Harvard University Press, 1975.

Kramer, M. *Reality Shock: Why Nurses Leave Nursing.* St. Louis: Mosby, 1974.

Krant, M. *Dying and Dignity.* Springfield, Ill.: Thomas, 1974.

Krant, M. Personal Communication, 1976.

Krasnoff, A. "Psychological Variables and Human Cancer: A Cross-Validational Study." *Psychosomatic Medicine,* 1959, *21,* 291-295.

Kreitler, H., and Kreitler, S. "Children's Concepts of Sex and Birth." *Child Development,* 1966, *37,* 363-378.

Kristt, D. A., and Engel, B. T. "Learned Control of Blood Pressure in Patients with High Blood Pressure." *Circulation*, 1975, *51*, 370-378.

Kritzer, H., and Zimet, C. N. "A Retrospective View of Medical Specialty Choice." *Journal of Medical Education*, 1967, *42*, 47-53.

Kroeber, T. C. "The Coping Functions of the Ego Mechanism." In R. W. White (Ed.), *The Study of Lives*. Englewood Cliffs, N.J.: Prentice-Hall, 1963.

Krumboltz, J. D. (Ed.). *Revolution in Counseling*. Boston: Houghton Mifflin, 1966.

Kübler-Ross, E. *On Death and Dying*. New York: Macmillan, 1969.

Kuhn, T. S. *The Structure of Scientific Revolutions*. Chicago: University of Chicago Press, 1962.

Kulcar, Z., Seso, M., and Majnaric, V. "Group Therapy of Chronic Patients in General Medicine." *Medical Journal*, 1966, *88* (7), 14-24.

Kushner, R. *Breast Cancer: A Personal History and an Investigative Report*. New York: Harcourt Brace Jovanovich, 1975.

Kutner, B. "Surgeons and Their Patients: A Study in Social Perception." In E. G. Jaco (Ed.), *Patients, Physicians, and Illness*. New York: Free Press, 1958.

Kutner, D. "Overcrowding: Human Responses to Density and Visual Exposure." *Human Relations*, 1973, *26*, 31-50.

Kutner, N. G. "Medical Students' Orientation Toward the Chronically Ill." *Journal of Medical Education*, 1978, *53*, 111-118.

Kvis, F. J. "Need and Use of Health Services in Underserved Areas." Research Grant Proposal No. HS 02778. Washington, D.C.: U.S. Public Health Service, Department of Health, Education, and Welfare, 1976.

La Barba, R. C. "Experiential and Environmental Factors in Cancer: A Review of Research with Animals." *Psychosomatic Medicine*, 1970, *32*, 259-276.

Laframboise, H. L. "Health Policy: Breaking the Problem Down into More Manageable Segments." *Canadian Medical Association Journal*, 1973, *108*, 388-393.

Lalonde, M. *A New Perspective on the Health of Canadians*. Ottawa, Ontario: Ministry of National Health and Welfare, 1974.

Lane, M. F., Barbarite, R. V., Bergner, L., and Harris, D. "Child-Resistant Medicine Containers: Experience in the Home." *American Journal of Public Health*, 1971, *61*, 1861-1868.

Langer, E. J., Janis, I. L., and Wolfer, J. A. "Reduction of Psychological Stress in Surgical Patients." *Journal of Experimental Social Psychology*, 1975, *11*, 155-165.

Langer, E. J., and Rodin, J. "The Effects of Choice and Enhanced Personal Responsibility for the Aged: A Field Experiment in an Institutional Setting." *Journal of Personality and Social Psychology*, 1976, *34*, 191-198.

Langer, E. J., and Saegert, S. "Crowding and Cognitive Control." *Journal of Personality and Social Psychology*, 1977, *35*, 175-182.

Langlie, J. "Social Networks, Health Beliefs, and Preventive Health Behavior." *Journal of Health and Social Behavior,* 1977, *18,* 244-260.

La Patra, J. W. *Health Care Delivery Systems.* Springfield, Ill.: Thomas, 1975.

Larson, T. A. "Datagram: Ethnic Group Members on U.S. Medical School Faculties." *Journal of Medical Education,* 1976, *51,* 69-70.

Lasswell, H. D. *The Future of Political Science.* New York: Prentice-Hall, 1963.

Laszlo, E. (Ed.). *The Relevance of General Systems Theory.* New York: Braziller, 1972.

Latiolais, C., and Berry, C. "Misuse of Prescription Medications by Outpatients." *Drug Intelligence and Clinical Pharmacy,* 1969, *3,* 270-277.

Laurendeau, M., and Pinard, A. *Causal Thinking in the Child.* New York: International Universities Press, 1962.

Lave, L. "Incentives Affecting Use of Emergency and Other Acute Medical Services." In S. J. Mushkin (Ed.), *Consumer Incentives for Health Care.* New York: Prodist, 1974.

Laverty, S. G. "Aversion Therapies in the Treatment of Alcoholism." *Psychosomatic Medicine,* 1966, *28,* 651-666.

Lawson, D. M., and May, R. B. "Three Procedures for the Extinction of Smoking Behavior." *Psychological Record,* 1970, *20,* 151-157.

Lawton, M. P., and Nahemow, L. "Ecology and the Aging Process." In C. Eisdorfer and P. Lawton (Eds.), *The Psychology of Adult Development and Aging.* Washington, D.C.: American Psychological Association, 1973.

Layne, O. L., Jr., and Yudofsky, S. C. "Postoperative Psychosis in Cardiotomy Patients." *New England Journal of Medicine,* 1971, *284,* 518-520.

Lazarus, H. R., and Hagens, J. H. "Prevention of Psychosis Following Open-Heart Surgery." *American Journal of Psychiatry,* 1968, *124,* 1190-1195.

Lazarus, R. S. *Psychological Stress and the Coping Process.* New York: McGraw-Hill, 1966.

Lazarus, R. S. "Psychological Stress and Coping in Adaptation and Illness." *International Journal of Psychiatry in Medicine,* 1974, *5,* 321-333.

Lazarus, R. S. "The Self-Regulation of Emotion." In L. Levi (Ed.), *Emotions —Their Parameters and Measurement.* New York: Raven Press, 1975.

Lazarus, R. S. "The Stress and Coping Paradigm." Paper presented at conference organized by C. Eisdorfer, A. Kleinman, and D. Cohen, Department of Psychiatry and Behavioral Sciences, University of Washington, on "The Critical Evaluation of Behavioral Paradigms for Psychiatric Science," Gleneden Beach, Ore., November 3-6, 1978.

Lazarus, R. S., and Alfert, E. "The Short-Circuiting of Threat by Experimentally Altering Cognitive Appraisal." *Journal of Abnormal and Social Psychology,* 1964, *69,* 195-205.

Lazarus, R. S., Averill, J. R., and Opton, E. M., Jr. "Towards a Cognitive Theory of Emotion." In M. B. Arnold (Ed.), *Feelings and Emotions.* New York: Academic Press, 1970.

Lazarus, R. S., Averill, J. R., and Opton, E. M., Jr. "The Psychology of Coping: Issues of Research and Assessment." In G. V. Coelho, D. A. Hamburg, and J. E. Adams (Eds.), *Coping and Adaptation*. New York: Basic Books, 1974.

Lazarus, R. S., and Cohen, J. B. "Environmental Stress." In I. Altman and J. F. Wohlwill (Eds.), *Human Behavior and the Environment: Current Theory and Research*. New York: Plenum Press, 1977.

Lazarus, R. S., Cohen, J. B., Folkman, S., Kanner, A., and Schaefer, C. "Psychological Stress and Adaptation: Some Unresolved Issues." In H. Selye (Ed.), *Guide to Stress Research*. New York: Van Nostrand Reinhold, in press.

Lazarus, R. S., and Launier, R. "Stress-Related Transactions Between Person and Environment." In L. A. Pervin and M. Lewis (Eds.), *Perspectives in Interactional Psychology*. New York: Plenum Press, 1978.

Leaper, D. J., Horrocks, J. C., Staniland, J. R., and de Dombal, F. T. "Computer-Assisted Diagnosis of Abdominal Pain Using 'Estimates' Provided by Clinicians." *British Medical Journal*, 1972, *2*, 350-354.

Leavell, H. R. "Contributions of the Social Sciences to the Solution of Health Problems." *New England Journal of Medicine*, 1952, *247*, 885-897.

LeBow, M. D. "Operant Conditioning-Based Behavior Modification: One Approach to Treating Somatic Disorders." *International Journal of Psychiatry in Medicine*, 1975, *6* (1/2), 241-254.

Lee, P. R. "Do We Need a Federal Department of Health?" In D. Cater and P. R. Lee (Eds.), *The Politics of Health*. New York: MedCom Press, 1972.

Lefcourt, H. "The Functions of Illusions of Control and Freedom." *American Psychologist*, 1973, *28* (3), 417-425.

Leiberman, M. "Relocation Research and Social Policy." *Gerontologist*, 1974, *14*, 494-501.

Leon, G. R. "Current Directions in the Treatment of Obesity." *Psychological Bulletin*, 1976, *83*, 557-578.

Leon, G. R., and Roth, L. "Obesity: Psychological Causes, Correlations, and Speculations." *Psychological Bulletin*, 1977, *84*, 117-139.

Leonard, C. O., Chase, G., and Childs, B. "Genetic Counseling: A Consumer's View." *New England Journal of Medicine*, 1972, *287* (9), 433-439.

Lepawsky, A. "Medical Science and Political Science." *Journal of Medical Education*, 1967, *42*, 1-13.

Lerner, M. J. "Evaluation of Performance as a Function of Performer's Reward and Attractiveness." *Journal of Personality and Social Psychology*, 1965, *1*, 355-360.

Lerner, M. "Conceptualization of Health and Social Well Being." In R. L. Berg (Ed.), *Health Status Indexes*. Chicago: Hospital Research and Educational Trust, 1973.

Lerner, M. "Social Differences in Physical Health." In J. Kosa and I. Zola (Eds.), *Poverty and Health: A Sociological Analysis*. (rev. ed.) Cambridge, Mass.: Harvard University Press, 1975.

Lerner, M., and Anderson, O. *Health Progress in the United States, 1900-1960: A Report of the Health Information Foundation*. Chicago: University of Chicago Press, 1963.

Lerner, M. J. *Deserving Versus Justice: A Contemporary Dilemma*. Report No. 24. Waterloo, Ontario: University of Waterloo, 1971.

Lerner, M. J., and Matthews, G. "Reactions to Suffering of Others Under Conditions of Indirect Responsibility." *Journal of Personality and Social Psychology*, 1967, *5*, 319-325.

Lerner, M. J., and Simmons, C. "Observer's Reaction to the 'Innocent Victim': Compassion or Rejection?" *Journal of Personality and Social Psychology*, 1966, *4*, 203-210.

LeShan, L. L. "Psychological States as Factors in the Development of Malignant Disease: A Critical Review." *Journal of the National Cancer Institute*, 1959, *22*, 1-18.

LeShan, L. L., and Worthington, R. E. "Personality as a Factor in Pathogenesis of Cancer: A Review of the Literature." *British Journal of Medical Psychology*, 1956, *29*, 49-56.

Leventhal, H. "Findings and Theory in the Study of Fear Communications." *Advances in Experimental Social Psychology*, 1970, *5*, 119-186.

Leventhal, H. "Changing Attitudes and Habits to Reduce Risk Factors in Chronic Disease." *American Journal of Cardiology*, 1973, *31*, 571-580.

Leventhal, H. "The Consequences of Depersonalization During Illness and Treatment." In J. Howard and A. Strauss (Eds.), *Humanizing Health Care*. New York: Wiley, 1975.

Leventhal, H., Hochbaum, G., and Rosenstock, I. "Epidemic Impact on the General Population in Two Cities." In *The Impact of Asian Influenza on Community Life: A Study in Five Cities*. DHEW, PHS, Publication No. 766. Washington, D.C.: U.S. Government Printing Office, 1960.

Leventhal, H., Singer, R. P., and Jones, S. "Effects of Fear and Specificity of Recommendation upon Attitudes and Behavior." *Journal of Personality and Social Psychology*, 1965, *2*, 20-29.

Levi, L. "The Urinary Output of Adrenalin and Noradrenalin During Pleasant and Unpleasant Emotional States." *Psychosomatic Medicine*, 1965, *27*, 80-85.

Levi, L. "Psychosocial Stress and Disease: A Conceptual Model." In E. K. E. Gunderson and R. H. Rahe (Eds.), *Life Stress and Illness*. Springfield, Ill.: Thomas, 1974.

Levin, L. "Focus and Issues in the Revival of Interest in Self-Care." *Health Education Monographs*, 1977, *5*, 115-120.

Levine, M., and Spivack, G. *The Rorschach Index of Repressive Style*. Springfield, Ill.: Thomas, 1964.

Levine, S., Scotch, N. A., and Vlasak, G. J. "Unraveling Technology and Culture in Public Health." *American Journal of Public Health*, 1969, *59*, 237-244.

Levinger, G., and Breedlove, J. "Interpersonal Attraction and Agreement: A

Study of Marriage Partners." *Journal of Personality and Social Psychology*, 1966, *3*, 367-372.

Levinson, T., and Sereny, G. "An Experimental Evaluation of 'Insight Therapy' for the Chronic Alcoholic." *Canadian Psychiatric Association Journal*, 1969, *14*, 143-145.

Levit, E. J., Sabshin, M., and Mueller, C. B. "Trends in Graduate Medical Education and Specialty Certification." *New England Journal of Medicine*, 1974, *290*, 545-549.

Levitz, L., and Stunkard, A. J. "A Therapeutic Coalition for Obesity: Behavior Modification and Patient Self-Help." *American Journal of Psychiatry*, 1974, *131*, 423-427.

Levy, J. M., and McGee, R. K. "Childbirth as Crises: A Test of Janis' Theory of Communication and Stress Resolution." *Journal of Personality and Social Psychology*, 1975, *31*, 171-179.

Levy, L., and Herzog, A. "Effects of Population Density and Crowding on Health and Social Adaptation in the Netherlands." *Journal of Health and Social Behavior*, 1974, *15*, 228-240.

Ley, P. "Comprehension, Memory, and the Success of Communications with the Patient." *Journal of Institutional Health Education*, 1972a, *10*, 23-29.

Ley, P. "Primacy, Rated Importance, and the Recall of Medical Statements." *Journal of Health and Social Behavior*, 1972b, *13*, 311-317.

Ley, P. "Toward Better Doctor-Patient Communications." In A. E. Bennett (Ed.), *Communication Between Doctors and Patients*. New York: Oxford University Press, 1976.

Ley, P., and Spelman, M. S. "Communications in an Outpatient Setting." *British Journal of Social and Clinical Psychology*, 1965, *4*, 115-125.

Ley, P., and Spelman, M. S. *Communicating with the Patient*. St. Louis, Mo.: Green, 1967.

Li, F. P. "Suicide Among Chemists." *Archives of Environmental Health*, 1969, *19*, 518-520.

Lichtenstein, E., and Danaher, B. G. "Modification of Smoking Behavior: A Critical Analysis of Theory, Research, and Practice." In M. Hersen, R. M. Eisler, and P. M. Miller (Eds.), *Progress in Behavior Modification*. Vol. 3. New York: Academic Press, 1976.

Lichtenstein, E., and Rodrigues, M. P. "Long-Term Effects of Rapid-Smoking Treatment for Dependent Cigarette Smokers." *Addictive Behaviors*, 1977, *2*, 109-112.

Lidz, T. *The Person: His Development Throughout the Life Cycle*. New York: Basic Books, 1968.

Lieban, R. W. "Medical Anthropology." In J. H. Honigman (Ed.), *Handbook of Social and Cultural Anthropology*. Chicago: Rand McNally, 1973.

Lieberman, M., and Straetz, R. "Health Policy Studies by Political Scientists." *Policy Studies Journal*, 1974, *3*, 195-200.

Lieberson, S. "Ethnic Groups and the Practice of Medicine." *American Sociological Review*, 1958, *23*, 542-549.

Lief, H. I. "Sexual Attitudes and Behavior of Medical Students: Implications from Medical Practice." In E. M. Nash (Ed.), *Marriage Counseling in Medical Practice.* Chapel Hill: University of North Carolina Press, 1964.

Lief, H. I. "Personality Characteristics of Medical Students." In R. H. Coombs and C. E. Vincent (Eds.), *Psychosocial Aspects of Medical Training.* Springfield, Ill.: Thomas, 1971.

Lief, H. I., and Fox, R. C. "Training for 'Detached Concern' in Medical Students." In H. I. Lief, V. F. Lief, and N. R. Lief (Eds.), *The Psychological Basis of Medical Practice.* New York: Harper & Row, 1963.

Liem, J. H., and Liem, R. "Life Events, Social Supports, and Physical and Psychological Well-being." Paper presented at annual meeting of the American Psychological Association, Washington, D.C., 1976.

"Life's Good Times Can Be Dangerous." *San Francisco Chronicle,* October 19, 1978, p. 24.

Lima, J., Nazarian, L., Charney, E., and Lahti, C. "Compliance with Short-Term Antimicrobial Therapy: Some Techniques that Help." *Pediatrics,* 1976, *57,* 383-386.

Lindeman, C. A., and Stetzer, S. L. "Effect of Preoperative Visits by Operating Room Nurses." *Nursing Research,* 1973, *22,* 4-16.

Lindeman, C. A., and Van Aernam, B. "Nursing Intervention with the Presurgical Patient—The Effects of Structured and Unstructured Preoperative Teaching." *Nursing Research,* 1971, *20,* 319-332.

Lindemann, E. "Symptomatology and Management of Acute Grief." *American Journal of Psychiatry,* 1944, *101,* 414-447.

Linduska, N. *My Polio Past.* Chicago: Pellegrini and Cudahy, 1947.

Linkewich, J. A., Catalano, R. B., and Flack, H. L. "The Effect of Packaging and Instruction on Outpatient Compliance with Medication Regimens." *Drug Intelligence and Clinical Pharmacy,* 1974, *8,* 10-15.

Linksy, A. S. "The Changing Public Views on Alcoholism." *Quarterly Journal of Studies on Alcohol,* 1970, *31,* 692-704.

Linn, E. L. "Women Dentists: Career and Family." *Social Problems,* 1971, *18,* 393-404.

Linn, L. "State Hospital Environment and Rates of Patient Discharge." *Archives of General Psychiatry,* 1970, *23,* 346-351.

Linn, L. S. "Primex Trainees Under Stress." *Journal of Nursing Education,* 1975, *14,* 10-19.

Linn, M. W., and Linn, B. S. "Narrowing the Gap Between Medical and Mental Health Evaluation." *Medical Care,* 1975, *13,* 607-614.

Lipowski, Z. J. "Psychosocial Aspects of Disease." *Annals of Internal Medicine,* 1969, *71,* 1197-1206.

Lipowski, Z. J. "Physical Illness, the Individual, and the Coping Process." *Psychiatry in Medicine,* 1970, *1,* 91-102.

Lipowski, Z. J. "Affluence, Information Inputs, and Health." *Social Science and Medicine,* 1973a, *7,* 517-529.

Lipowski, Z. J. "Psychosomatic Medicine in a Changing Society: Some Current Trends in Theory and Research." *Comprehensive Psychiatry*, 1973b, *14*, 203-215.

Lipowski, Z. J. "Physical Illness, the Patient, and His Environment: Psychosocial Foundations of Medicine." In S. Arieti (Ed.), *American Handbook of Psychiatry*. Vol. 4 (2nd ed.). New York: Basic Books, 1975.

Lipowski, Z. J. "Psychosomatic Medicine: An Overview." In O. W. Hill (Ed.), *Modern Trends in Psychosomatic Medicine 3*. London: Butterworths, 1976.

Lipowski, Z. J. "Psychosomatic Medicine in the Seventies: An Overview." *American Journal of Psychiatry*, 1977, *134*, 233-244.

Litman, T. "The Family as a Basic Unit in Health and Medical Care." *Social Science and Medicine*, 1974, *8*, 495-519.

Little, S. W., and Cohen, L. D. "Goal Setting and Behavior of Asthmatic Children and Their Mothers." *Journal of Personality*, 1951, *19*, 376-389.

Livingston, P. B., and Zimet, C. N. "Death Anxiety, Authoritarianism, and Choice of Specialty in Medical Students." *Journal of Nervous and Mental Disease*, 1965, *140*, 222-230.

Lloyd, G. G., and Deakin, H. G. "Phobias Complicating Treatment of Uterine Cancer." *British Medical Journal*, 1975, *4*, 440.

Lloyd, R. W., and Salzberg, H. C. "Controlled Social Drinking." *Psychological Bulletin*, 1975, *82*, 815-842.

Loftus, E. F. "Leading Questions and the Eyewitness Report." *Cognitive Psychology*, 1975, *7*, 560-572.

Lohr, W. "Effects of Medicaid." *Evaluation Research Methodology*, 1974, *13*, 299-303.

Lopate, C. *Women in Medicine*. Baltimore: Johns Hopkins University Press, 1968.

Loring, W. C. "Public Health and the Residential Environment." In L. E. Hinkle, Jr., and W. C. Loring (Eds.), *The Effects of the Man-Made Environment on Health and Behavior*. Washington, D.C.: U.S. Government Printing Office, 1977.

Lothrop, W. W. "Relationship Between Bender-Gestalt Test Scores and Medical Success with Duodenal Ulcer Patients." *Psychosomatic Medicine*, 1958, *20*, 30-32.

Lounsbury, F. G. "One Hundred Years of Anthropological Linguistics." In J. O. Brew (Ed.), *One Hundred Years of Anthropology*. Cambridge, Mass.: Harvard University Press, 1968.

Lovibond, S. H., and Caddy, G. "Discriminated Aversive Control in the Moderation of Alcoholics' Drinking Behavior." *Behavior Therapy*, 1970, *1*, 437-444.

Lowe, J. C., and Moryadas, S. *Special Interaction: The Geography of Movement*. New York: Houghton Mifflin, 1975.

Lowenthal, M. F., Thurnher, M., and Chiriboga, D. *Four Stages of Life: A Comparative Study of Women and Men Facing Transitions*. San Francisco: Jossey-Bass, 1975.

Lowi, T. "Distribution, Regulation, Redistribution: The Function of Government." In R. Ripley (Ed.), *Public Policies and Their Politics.* New York: Martin, 1969.

Lowrie, D. G. "Additional Data on Animistic Thinking." *Scientifici Monthly,* 1954, *79,* 69-70.

Lubin, B., Nathan, R. G., and Matarazzo, J. D. "Psychologists in Medical Education: 1976." *American Psychologist,* 1978, *33,* 339-343.

Luborsky, L., Docherty, J. P., and Penick, S. "Onset Conditions for Psychosomatic Symptoms: A Comparative Review of Immediate Observation with Retrospective Research." *Psychosomatic Medicine,* 1973, *35,* 187-204.

Luborsky, L., Todd, T. C., and Katcher, A. H. "A Self-Administered Social Assets Scale for Predicting Physical and Psychological Illness and Health." *Journal of Psychosomatic Research,* 1973, *17,* 109-120.

Lucente, F. E., and Fleck, S. "A Study of Hospitalization Anxiety in 408 Medical and Surgical Patients." *Psychosomatic Medicine,* 1972, *34,* 302-312.

Ludwig, E., and Adams, S. "Patient Cooperation in a Rehabilitation Center: Assumption of the Client Role." *Journal of Health and Social Behavior,* 1968, *9,* 328-336.

Ludwig, E., and Gibson, G. "Self-Perception of Sickness and Seeking of Medical Care." *Journal of Health and Social Behavior,* 1969, *10,* 125-133.

Lundberg, U. "Urban Commuting: Crowdedness and Catechol Amine Excretion." *Journal of Human Stress,* 1976, *2,* 26-32.

Lundberg, U., Theorell, T., and Lind, E. "Life Changes and Myocardial Infarction: Individual Differences in Life Change Scaling." *Journal of Psychosomatic Research,* 1975, *19,* 27-32.

Luria, A. R. *The Working Brain.* New York: Basic Books, 1973.

Lusted, L. B. *Introduction to Medical Decision Making.* Springfield, Ill.: Thomas, 1968.

Lynn, R. *Personality and National Character.* Oxford, England: Pergamon Press, 1971.

McAlister, A. L., Farquhar, J. W., Thoresen, C. E., and Maccoby, N. "Behavioral Science Applied to Cardiovascular Health: Progress and Research Needs in the Modification of Risk-Taking Habits in Adult Populations." *Health Education Monographs,* 1976, *4,* 45-74.

McAllister, T. A., and Philip, A. E. "The Clinical Psychologist in a Health Centre: One Year's Work." *British Medical Journal,* 1975, *4,* 513-514.

McCain, G., Cox, V., and Paulus, P. "The Relationship Between Illness Complaints and Degree of Crowding in Prison Environments." *Environment and Behavior,* 1976, *8,* 283-290.

McCarthy, D., and Saegert, S. "Residential Density, Social Overload, and Withdrawal." *Human Ecology,* 1978, *6,* 253-272.

McCartney, J. L. "On Being Scientific: Changing Styles of Presentation of Sociological Research." *American Sociologist,* 1970, *5,* 30-35.

Maccoby, E. E., and Jacklin, C. N. *The Psychology of Sex Differences.* Stanford, Calif.: Stanford University Press, 1974.

Maccoby, N., and Farquhar, J. "Communication for Health: Unselling Heart Disease." *Journal of Communication,* 1975, *25,* 114-126.

McCoy, J. W. "Psychological Variables and Onset of Cancer." Unpublished doctoral dissertation, Oklahoma State University, 1976.

McCrae, W. M., Cull, M., Burton, L., and Dodge, J. "Cystic Fibrosis: Parents' Responses to the Genetic Basis of the Disease." *Lancet,* 1973, *7,* 141-143.

McDaniel, J. V. *Physical Disability and Human Behavior.* Elmsford, N.Y.: Pergamon Press, 1969.

MacDonald, A. P. "Internal-External Locus of Control and the Practice of Birth Control." *Psychological Reports,* 1970, *27,* 206.

McFall, R. M., and Hammen, L. "Motivation, Structure, and Self-Monitoring: Role of Nonspecific Factors in Smoking Reduction." *Journal of Consulting and Clinical Psychology,* 1971, *37,* 80-86.

McGuire, W. J. "Selective Exposure: A Summing Up." In R. P. Abelson, E. Aronson, W. J. McGuire, T. M. Newcomb, M. J. Rosenberg, and P. H. Tannenbaum (Eds.), *Theories of Cognitive Consistency: A Sourcebook.* Chicago: Rand McNally, 1968.

Macht, D. I. "Psychosomatic Allusions in the Book of Proverbs." *Bulletin of the History of Medicine,* 1945, *18,* 301-327.

McIntire, C. "The Importance of the Study of Medical Sociology." *Bulletin of the American Academy of Medicine,* 1894, *1,* 425-434.

McIntosh, J. "Processes of Communication, Information Seeking, and Control Associated with Cancer: A Selective Review of the Literature." *Social Science and Medicine,* 1974, *8,* 167-187.

McKay, A. "View on Genetic Counseling and Family Planning." In *First International Conference on the Mental Health Aspects of Sickle Cell Anemia.* DHEW Publication No. (HSM) 73-9141. Washington, D.C.: U.S. Government Printing Office, 1974.

McKenney, J., Slining, J. M., Henderson, H. R., Devins, D., Barr, M., Stern, M. P., Farquhar, J. W., Maccoby, N., and Russell, S. H. "The Effect of Clinical Pharmacy Services on Patients with Essential Hypertension." *Circulation,* 1973, *48,* 1104-1111.

McKinlay, J. "Some Approaches and Problems in the Study of the Use of Services—An Overview." *Journal of Health and Social Behavior,* 1972, *13,* 115-152.

McKinlay, J. "Who Is Really Ignorant—Physician or Patient?" *Journal of Health and Social Behavior,* 1975, *16,* 3-11.

McKinley, J. B., and Dutton, D. B. "Social-Psychological Aspects of Consumer Use." In S. J. Mushkin (Ed.), *Consumer Incentives for Health Care.* New York: Watson, 1974.

MacKintosh, E., West, S., and Saegert, S. "Two Studies of Crowding in Urban Public Places." *Environment and Behavior,* 1975, *7,* 159-184.

McLean, E., and Tarnopolsky, A. "Noise, Discomfort, and Mental Health: A

Review of the Socio-Medical Implications of Disturbance by Noise." *Psychological Medicine,* 1977, *7,* 19-62.

MacLeod, C. M., Dekaban, A. S., and Hunt, E. B. "Memory Impairment in Epileptic Patients: Selective Effects of Phenobarbital Level." Technical Report, University of Washington, 1978.

McMillan, J. J. "Agenda for the 70s in Professional Affairs." *Professional Psychology,* 1970, *1,* 181-183.

McReynolds, W. T., Lutz, R. N., Paulsen, B. K., and Kohrs, M. B. "Weight Loss Resulting from Two Behavior Modification Procedures with Nutritionists as Therapists." *Behavior Therapy,* 1976, *7,* 283-291.

Maddison, D., and Viola, A. "The Health of Widows in the Year Following Bereavement." *Journal of Psychosomatic Research,* 1968, *12,* 297-306.

Maguire, P. "The Psychological and Social Sequellae of Mastectomy." In J. G. Howells (Ed.), *Modern Perspectives in the Psychiatric Aspects of Surgery.* New York: Brunner/Mazel, 1976.

Mahoney, M. J. *Cognition and Behavior Modification.* Cambridge, Mass.: Ballinger, 1974a.

Mahoney, M. J. "Self-Reward and Self-Monitoring Techniques for Weight Control." *Behavior Therapy,* 1974b, *45,* 48-57.

Mahoney, M. J. "The Behavioral Treatment of Obesity." In A. J. Enelow and J. B. Henderson (Eds.), *Applying Behavioral Science to Cardiovascular Risk.* New York: American Heart Association, 1975.

Mahoney, M. J., and Mahoney, K. *Permanent Weight Control.* New York: Norton, 1976.

Maier, N. R. F. "Reasoning in Humans: II. The Solution of a Problem and Its Appearance in Consciousness." *Journal of Experimental Psychology,* 1931, *12,* 181-194.

Malahy, B. "The Effect of Instruction and Labeling on the Number of Medication Errors Made by Patients at Home." *American Journal of Hospital Pharmacy,* 1966, *23,* 283-292.

Mann, L., and Janis, I. L. "A Follow-Up Study on the Long-Term Effects of Emotional Role Playing." *Journal of Personality and Social Psychology,* 1968, *8,* 339-342.

Margolis, J. R., Kannel, W. B., Feinleib, M., Dawber, T. R., and McNamara, P. M. "Clinical Features of Unrecognized Myocardial Infarction—Silent and Symptomatic. Eighteen Year Follow-Up: The Framingham Study." *American Journal of Cardiology,* 1973, *32,* 1-7.

Marks, R. U. "Factors Involving Social and Demographic Characteristics: A Review of Empirical Findings." In S. L. Syme and L. G. Reeder (Eds.), "Social Stress and Cardiovascular Disease." *Milbank Memorial Fund Quarterly,* 1967, *45* (2), 51-108.

Markush, R. E., and Favero, R. V. "Epidemiologic Assessment of Stressful Life Events, Depressed Mood, and Psychophysiological Symptoms—A Preliminary Report." In B. S. Dohrenwend and B. P. Dohrenwend (Eds.), *Stressful Life Events: Their Nature and Effects.* New York: Wiley, 1974.

Marmer, M. J. "Hypnoanalgesia and Hypnoanesthesia for Cardiac Surgery." *Journal of the American Medical Association*, 1959, *171*, 512-517.

Marmor, J. "The Feeling of Superiority: An Occupational Hazard in the Practice of Psychotherapy." *American Journal of Psychiatry*, 1953, *110*, 370-376.

Marsella, A., Escudero, M., and Gordon, P. "Effects of Dwelling Density on Mental Disorders in Filipino Men." *Journal of Health and Social Behavior*, 1970, *11*, 288-294.

Marston, M. V. "Compliance with Medical Regimens. A Review of the Literature." *Nursing Research*, 1970, *19*, 312-323.

Martin, D. P., Gilson, B. S., Bergner, M., Bobbitt, R. A., Pollard, W. E., Conn, J. R., and Cole, N. A. "The Sickness Impact Profile: Potential Use of a Health Status Instrument for Physician Training." *Journal of Medical Education*, 1976, *51*, 942-944.

Marx, M. H., and Hillix, W. A. *Systems and Theories in Psychology.* (2nd ed.) New York: McGraw-Hill, 1973.

Maslach, C. "Burned-Out." *Human Behavior*, 1976, *5* (9), 16-22.

Maslach, C. "The Burn-Out Syndrome and Patient Care." In C. Garfield (Ed.), *Psychosocial Care of the Dying.* New York: McGraw-Hill, 1978.

Maslow, A. H. *Motivation and Personality.* New York: Harper & Row, 1954.

Mason, J. W. "Over-All Hormonal Balance as a Key to Endocrine Organization." *Psychosomatic Medicine*, 1968a, *30*, 791-808.

Mason, J. W. "A Review of Psychoendocrine Research on the Pituitary-Adrenal Cortical System." *Psychosomatic Medicine*, 1968b, *30*, 576-607.

Mason, J. W. "A Re-Evaluation of the Concept of 'Non-Specificity' in Stress Theory." *Journal of Psychiatric Research*, 1971, *8*, 323-333.

Mason, J. W. "Specificity in the Organization of Neuroendocrine Response Profiles." In P. Seeman and G. M. Brown (Eds.), *Frontiers in Neurology and Neuroscience Research.* First International Symposium of the Neuroscience Institute. Toronto, Ontario: University of Toronto, 1974.

Mason, J. W. "A Historical View of the Stress Field: Part I." *Journal of Human Stress*, 1975a, *1* (1), 6-12.

Mason, J. W. "A Historical View of the Stress Field: Part II." *Journal of Human Stress*, 1975b, *1* (2), 22-36.

Mason, R. C., Clark, G., Reeves, R. B., and Wagner, B. "Acceptance and Healing." *Journal of Religion and Health*, 1969, *8*, 123-142.

Masuda, M., and Holmes, T. H. "Life Events: Perceptions and Frequencies." *Psychosomatic Medicine*, 1978, *40*, 236-261.

Matarazzo, J. D. "The Role of the Psychologist in Medical Education and Practice." *Human Organization*, 1955, *14* (2), 9-14.

Matarazzo, J. D., and Daniel, R. S. "The Teaching of Psychology by Psychologists in Medical Schools." *Journal of Medical Education*, 1957, *32*, 410-415.

Matarazzo, J. D., Lubin, B., and Nathan, R. G. "Psychologists' Membership on the Medical Staff of University Teaching Hospitals." *American Psychologist*, 1978, *33*, 23-29.

Mattsson, A. "Long-Term Physical Illness in Childhood: A Challenge to Psychosocial Adaptation." *Pediatrics,* 1972, *50,* 801-811.

Mausner, B., and Platt, E. S. *Smoking: A Behavioral Analysis.* Elmsford, N.Y.: Pergamon Press, 1971.

Mausner, J. S., and Steppacher, R. C. "Suicide in Professionals: A Study of Male and Female Psychologists." *American Journal of Epidemiology,* 1973, *98,* 436-445.

Mayer, J., and Myerson, D. J. "Outpatient Treatment of Alcoholics: Effects of Status, Stability, and Nature of Treatment." *Quarterly Journal of Studies on Alcohol,* 1971, *32,* 620-627.

Mayer, R. E. *Thinking and Problem Solving: An Introduction to Human Cognition and Learning.* Glenview, Ill.: Scott, Foresman, 1977.

Mayou, R. "Chest Pain, Angina Pectoris, and Disability." *Journal of Psychosomatic Research,* 1973, *17,* 287-291.

Mazzullo, J. "Methods of Improving Patient Compliance." In L. Lasagna (Ed.), *Patient Compliance.* Mt. Kisco, N.Y.: Futura, 1976.

Mechanic, D. *Students Under Stress.* New York: Free Press, 1962a.

Mechanic, D. "The Concept of Illness Behavior." *Journal of Chronic Diseases,* 1962b, *15,* 189-194.

Mechanic, D. "The Influence of Mothers on Their Children's Health Attitudes and Behaviors." *Pediatrics,* 1964, *33,* 444-453.

Mechanic, D. *Medical Sociology.* New York: Free Press, 1968.

Mechanic, D. *Public Expectations and Health Care.* New York: Wiley, 1972a.

Mechanic, D. "Social Psychologic Factors Affecting the Presentation of Bodily Complaints." *New England Journal of Medicine,* 1972b, *286,* 1132-1139.

Mechanic, D. "Discussion of Research Programs on Relations Between Stressful Life Events and Episodes of Physical Illness." In B. S. Dohrenwend and B. P. Dohrenwend (Eds.), *Stressful Life Events: Their Nature and Effects.* New York: Wiley, 1974a.

Mechanic, D. "Social Structure and Personal Adaptation: Some Neglected Dimensions." In G. V. Coelho, D. A. Hamburg, and J. E. Adams (Eds.), *Coping and Adaptation.* New York: Basic Books, 1974b.

Mechanic, D. "Some Problems in the Measurement of Stress and Social Readjustment." *Journal of Human Stress,* 1975, *1* (3), 43-48.

Mechanic, D. *Medical Sociology.* (2nd ed.) New York: Free Press, 1978.

Mechanic, D., and Newton, M. "Some Problems in the Analysis of Morbidity Data." *Journal of Chronic Diseases,* 1965, *18,* 569-580.

Mechanic, D., and Volkart, E. H. "Stress, Illness Behavior, and the Sick Role." *American Sociological Review,* 1961, *26,* 51-58.

Medalie, J. H., Snyder, M., Groen, J. J., Neufeld, H. N., Goldbourt, U., and Riss, E. "Angina Pectoris Among 10,000 Men: 5-Year Incidence and Univariate Analysis." *American Journal of Medicine,* 1973, *55,* 583-594.

Meehl, P. E. *Clinical Versus Statistical Prediction.* Minneapolis: University of Minnesota Press, 1954.

Meichenbaum, D. *Cognitive-Behavior Modification: An Integrative Approach.* New York: Plenum Press, 1977.

Meichenbaum, D., and Cameron, R. "An Examination of Cognitive and Contingency Variables in Anxiety Relief Procedures." Unpublished manuscript, University of Waterloo, Ontario, 1973.

Meichenbaum, D., Turk, D., and Burstein, S. "The Nature of Coping with Stress." In I. Sarason and C. Spielberger (Eds.), *Stress and Anxiety.* Vol. 2. New York: Wiley, 1975.

Meier, P. "The Biggest Public Health Experiment Ever: The 1954 Trial of the Salk Poliomyelitis Vaccine." In J. M. Tanur and others (Eds.), *Statistics: A Guide to the Unknown.* San Francisco: Holden-Day, 1972.

Melton, A. W. "The Situation with Respect to the Spacing of Repetitions and Memory." *Journal of Verbal Learning and Verbal Behavior,* 1970, *9,* 596-606.

Meltzer, J. W., and Hochstim, J. R. "Reliability and Validity of Survey Data on Physical Health." *Public Health Reports,* 1970, *83,* 1075-1086.

Mensh, I. N. "Psychology in Medical Education." *American Psychologist,* 1953, *8,* 83-85.

Merton, R. J., Reader, R., and Kendall, P. L. (Eds.). *The Student-Physician: Studies in the Sociology of Medical Education.* Cambridge, Mass.: Harvard University Press, 1957.

Meyer, A. "The Value of Psychology in Psychiatry." *Journal of the American Medical Association,* 1912, *53,* 911-914.

Meyer, A. J., and Henderson, J. B. "Multiple Risk Factor Reduction in the Prevention of Cardiovascular Disease." *Preventive Medicine,* 1972, *3,* 225-236.

Meyer, B. C. "Some Psychiatric Aspects of Surgical Practice." *Psychosomatic Medicine,* 1958, *20,* 203-214.

Meyer, B. C. "Some Considerations of the Doctor-Patient Relationship in the Practice of Surgery." In H. S. Abram (Ed.), "Psychological Aspects of Surgery." *International Psychiatry Clinics,* 1967, *4* (2), 17-35.

Meyer, R. J., and Haggerty, R. J. "Streptococcal Infections in Families: Factors Altering Individual Susceptibility." *Pediatrics,* 1962, *29,* 539-549.

Mezei, A., and Németh, G. "Regression as an Intervening Mechanism: A System-Theoretical Approach." *Annals of the New York Academy of Sciences,* 1969, *164* (Art. 2), 560-567.

Michelson, W. "From Congruence to Antecedent Conditions: A Search for the Basis of Environmental Improvement." In D. Stokols (Ed.), *Perspectives on Environment and Behavior.* New York: Plenum Press, 1977.

Miller, M. M. "Treatment of Chronic Alcoholism by Hypnotic Aversion." *Journal of the American Medical Association,* 1959, *171,* 1492-1495.

Miller, N. E. "Learning of Visceral and Glandular Responses." *Science,* 1969, *163,* 434-445.

Miller, N. E. "Behavioral Medicine as a New Frontier: Opportunities and Danger." In S. M. Weiss (Ed.), *Proceedings of the National Heart and Lung*

Institute Working Conference on Health Behavior, Bayse, Va., May 12-15, 1975. DHEW Publication No. (NIH) 76-868. Washington, D.C.: U.S. Government Printing Office, 1975.

Miller, R. G., Rubin, R. T., Clark, B. R., Crawford, W. R., and Arthur, R. J. "The Stress of Aircraft Carrier Landings: I. Corticosteroid Responses in Naval Aviators." *Psychosomatic Medicine, 1970, 32,* 581-588.

Miller, W. R. "Behavioral Self-Control: Training in the Treatment of Problem Drinkers." In R. B. Stuart (Ed.), *Behavioral Self-Management: Strategies, Techniques, and Outcomes.* New York: Brunner/Mazel, 1977.

Mills, J., Meltzer, R., and Clark, M. "Effect of Number of Options on Recall of Information Supporting Different Decision Strategies." *Personality and Social Psychology Bulletin, 1977, 3* (2), 213-218.

Milner, B. "Amnesia Following Operation on the Temporal Lobes." In O. L. Zangwill and C. M. W. Whitty (Eds.), *Amnesia.* London: Butterworths, 1967.

Milsum, J. H. *Biological Control Systems Analysis.* New York: McGraw-Hill, 1966.

Minckley, B. B. "Physiologic and Psychologic Responses of Elective Surgical Patients." *Nursing Research, 1974, 23,* 392-401.

Mindlin, D. F. "Characteristics of Alcoholics as Related to Prediction of Therapeutic Outcome." *Quarterly Journal of Studies on Alcohol, 1959, 20,* 604-619.

Mindlin, D. F., and Belden, E. "Attitude Changes with Alcoholics in Group Therapy." *California Mental Health Research Digest, 1965, 3,* 102-103.

Minsky, M. "A Framework for Representing Knowledge." In P. Winston (Ed.), *The Psychology of Computer Vision.* New York: McGraw-Hill, 1975.

Mitchell, R. "Some Social Implications of High-Density Housing." *American Sociological Review, 1971, 36,* 18-29.

Mitchell, W. D. "Medical Student Career Choice: A Conceptualization." *Social Science and Medicine, 1975, 9,* 641-653.

Mitchell, W. E. "Changing Others: The Anthropological Study of Therapeutic Systems." *Medical Anthropology Newsletter, 1977, 8* (3), 15-20.

Modlin, H. C., and Montes, A. "Narcotics Addiction in Physicians." *American Journal of Psychiatry, 1964, 121,* 358-369.

Molidor, J. B. "The Use of Objective and Subjective Weights to Model a Medical School Admissions Task." Unpublished doctoral dissertation, Michigan State University, 1978.

Money, J., and Granoff, D. "IQ and the Somatic Stigmata of Turner's Syndrome." *American Journal of Mental Deficiency, 1965, 70,* 69-77.

Monk, M., Tayback, M., and Gordon, J. "Evaluation of an Antismoking Program Among High School Students." *American Journal of Public Health and the Nation's Health, 1965, 55,* 994-1004.

Monk, M. A., and Terris, M. "Factors in Student Choice of General or Specialty Practice." *New England Journal of Medicine, 1956, 255,* 1135-1140.

Monk, M. A., and Thomas, C. B. "Personal and Social Factors Related to Medical Specialty Practice." *Johns Hopkins Medical Journal,* 1973, *133,* 19-29.

Monteiro, L. "Expense Is No Object . . . : Income and Physician Visits Reconsidered." *Journal of Health and Social Behavior,* 1973, *14,* 99-115.

Monto, A., and Johnson, K. "A Community Study of Respiratory Infections in the Tropics: III. Introduction and Transmissions of Infections Within Families." *American Journal of Epidemiology,* 1968, *88,* 69-79.

Moore, D. C., Holton, C. P., and Marten, G. W. "Psychological Problems in the Management of Adolescents with Malignancy." *Clinical Pediatrics,* 1969, *8,* 464-473.

Moore, J. R. "Accuracy of a Health Interview Survey in Measuring Chronic Illness Prevalence." *Health Services Research,* 1975, *10,* 162-167.

Moore, M. F., Aitchison, J., Parker, L. S., and Taylor, T. R. "Use of Information in Thyrotoxicosis Treatment Allocation." *Methods of Information in Medicine,* 1974, *13,* 88-92.

Moore, R. A., and Ramseur, F. "Effects of Psychotherapy in an Open-Ward Hospital in Patients with Alcoholism." *Quarterly Journal of Studies on Alcohol,* 1960, *21,* 233-252.

Moos, R. H. *Evaluating Treatment Environments: A Social Ecological Approach.* New York: Wiley-Interscience, 1974a.

Moos, R. H. "Psychological Techniques in the Assessment of Adaptive Behavior." In G. V. Coelho, D. A. Hamburg, and J. E. Adams (Eds.), *Coping and Adaptation.* New York: Basic Books, 1974b.

Moos, R. H. *Evaluating Correctional and Community Settings.* New York: Wiley-Interscience, 1975.

Moos, R. H. *The Human Context: Environmental Determinants of Behavior.* New York: Wiley-Interscience, 1976a.

Moos, R. H. "Evaluating and Changing Community Settings." *American Journal of Community Psychology,* 1976b, *4,* 313-326.

Moos, R. H. (Ed.). *Coping with Physical Illness.* New York: Plenum Press, 1977a.

Moos, R. H. "Evaluating Sheltered Care Settings for the Elderly." Paper presented at VA/NASA conference on Habitability in Extended Care Environments, Minneapolis, September 1977b.

Moos, R. H. *Evaluating Educational Environments: Procedures, Measures, Findings, and Policy Implications.* San Francisco: Jossey-Bass, 1979.

Moos, R. H., and Moos, B. "Classroom Social Climate and Student Absences and Grades." *Journal of Educational Psychology,* 1978, *70,* 263-269.

Moos, R. H., and Tsu, V. "The Crisis of Physical Illness: An Overview." In R. H. Moos (Ed.), *Coping with Physical Illness.* New York: Plenum Press, 1977.

Moos, R. H., and Van Dort, B. "Student Physical Symptoms and the Social Climate of College Living Groups." *American Journal of Community Psychology,* in press.

Moos, W. "The Effects of 'Foehn' Weather on Accident Rates in the City of Zurich (Switzerland)." *Aerospace Medicine,* 1964, *35,* 643-645.

Moran, P. A. "An Experimental Study of Pediatric Admission." Unpublished master's thesis, School of Nursing, Yale University, 1963.

Morris, J., and Laurence, K. "The Effectiveness of Genetic Counseling for Neural-Tube Malformations." *Developmental Medicine and Child Neurology,* 1976, *18* (suppl. no. 37), 157-163.

Morrison, R. F. "Career Adaptivity: The Effective Adaptation of Managers to Changing Role Demands." *Journal of Applied Psychology,* 1977, *62,* 549-558.

Morse, R. M., and Litin, E. M. "Postoperative Delirium: A Study of Etiologic Factors." *American Journal of Psychiatry,* 1969, *126,* 388-395.

Mosher, L. R., Menn, A., and Matthews, S. "Soteria: Evaluation of a Home-Based Treatment for Schizophrenia." *American Journal of Orthopsychiatry,* 1975, *45,* 455-467.

Moss, G. E. *Illness, Immunity, and Social Interaction.* New York: Wiley, 1973.

Mulholland, T. B. "Biofeedback as Scientific Method." In G. E. Schwartz and J. Beatty (Eds.), *Biofeedback: Theory and Research.* New York: Academic Press, 1977a.

Mulholland, T. B. "Biofeedback Method for Locating the Most Controlled Responses of EEG Alpha to Visual Stimulation." In J. Beatty and H. Legewie (Eds.), *Biofeedback and Behavior.* New York: Plenum Press, 1977b.

Muller, C. "Income and Receipt of Medical Care." *American Journal of Public Health,* 1965, *55,* 256-268.

Mumford, E. *From Students to Physicians.* Cambridge, Mass.: Harvard University Press, 1970.

Murphy, L. B. "Coping, Vulnerability, and Resilience in Childhood." In G. V. Coelho, D. A. Hamburg, and J. E. Adams (Eds.), *Coping and Adaptation.* New York: Basic Books, 1974.

Musante, G. J. "The Dietary Rehabilitation Clinic: Evaluation Report of a Behavioral and Dietary Treatment of Obesity." *Behavior Therapy,* 1976, *7,* 198-204.

Mutter, A. Z., and Schleifer, M. J. "The Role of Psychological and Social Factors in the Onset of Somatic Illness in Children." *Psychosomatic Medicine,* 1966, *28,* 333-343.

Myers, E. D., and Calvert, E. J. "The Effect of Forewarning on the Occurrence of Side-Effects and Discontinuance of Medication in Patients on Dothiepin." *Journal of International Medical Research,* 1976, *4,* 237-240.

Myers, I. B., and Davis, J. A. "Relation of Medical Students' Psychological Type to Their Specialties Twelve Years Later." Research Memorandum RM 64-15. Princeton, N.J.: Educational Testing Service, 1964.

Myers, J. D., and Pople, H. E. "Internist: A Consultative Diagnostic Program in Internal Medicine." In *Proceedings of the First IEEE Symposium on Computer Application in Medical Care,* Washington, D.C., 1977.

Myers, J. K., and Schaeffer, L. "Social Stratification and Psychiatric Practice: A Study of an Out-Patient Clinic." *American Sociological Review,* 1954, *19,* 307-310.

Nadelson, T. "The Psychiatrist in the Surgical Intensive Care Unit: I. Postoperative Delirium." *Archives of Surgery,* 1976, *111,* 113-117.

Nagy, M. "Children's Birth Theories." *Journal of Genetic Psychology,* 1953a, *83,* 217-226.

Nagy, M. "Children's Conceptions of Some Bodily Functions." *Journal of Genetic Psychology,* 1953b, *83,* 199-216.

Nagy, M. "The Meaning of Death." In H. Feifel (Ed.), *The Meaning of Death.* New York: McGraw-Hill, 1959.

Nall, F., and Speilberg, J. "Social and Cultural Factors in Responses of Mexican-Americans to Medical Treatment." *Journal of Health and Social Behavior,* 1967, *8,* 299-308.

Nash, J. "Curbing Drop-Out from Treatment for Obesity." Paper presented at the Association for the Advancement of Behavior Therapy, San Francisco, 1976.

Nathanson, C. "Sex, Illness, and Medical Care." *Social Science and Medicine,* 1977, *11,* 13-25.

National Analysts. *A Study of Health Practices and Opinions.* PHS Publication No. PB-210-978. Washington, D.C.: U.S. Government Printing Office, 1972.

National Institute of Alcohol Abuse and Alcoholism (NIAAA). "Alcohol and Health." 2nd Report. Rockville, Md.: Alcoholism Treatment Center Monitoring System, Department of Health, Education, and Welfare, 1974.

National Register of Health Service Providers in Psychology. Washington, D.C.: Council for the National Register of Health Service Providers, 1976.

National Research Council. *Personnel Needs and Training for Biomedical and Behavioral Research.* Washington, D.C.: National Academy of Sciences, 1976.

National Science Foundation. *Projections of Science and Engineering Doctorate Supply and Utilization: 1980 and 1985.* Publication No. NSF 75-301. Washington, D.C.: Superintendent of Documents, 1975.

Navarro, V. "Social Class, Political Power, and the State and Their Implications in Medicine." *Social Science and Medicine,* 1976, *10,* 437-457.

Neely, E., and Patrick, M. "Problems of Aged Persons Taking Medications at Home." *Nursing Research,* 1968, *17,* 52-55.

Neufeld, V. R., and Barrows, H. S. The McMaster Philosophy: An Approach to Medical Education. *Journal of Medical Education,* 1974, *49,* 1040-1050.

Neugarten, B. L. (Ed.). *Middle Age and Aging.* Chicago: University of Chicago Press, 1968a.

Neugarten, B. L. "Adult Personality: Toward a Psychology of the Life Cycle." In B. L. Neugarten (Ed.), *Middle Age and Aging.* Chicago: University of Chicago Press, 1968b.

Neugarten, B. L. "The Awareness of Middle Age." In B. L. Neugarten (Ed.), *Middle Age and Aging.* Chicago: University of Chicago Press, 1968c.

Neuhauser, C., Amsterdam, B., Hines, P., and Steward, M. "Children's Concepts of Healing: Cognitive Development and Locus of Control Factors." *American Journal of Orthopsychiatry*, 1978, *48*, 335-341.

Neuhauser, D. "Cost-Effective Clinical Decision Making: Implications for the Delivery of Health Services." In J. P. Bunker, B. A. Barnes, and F. Mosteller (Eds.), *Costs, Risks, and Benefits of Surgery*. New York: Oxford University Press, 1977.

Neuhauser, D., and Lewicki, A. M. "What Do We Gain from the Sixth Stool Guaiac?" *New England Journal of Medicine*, 1975, *293*, 226-228.

Neutra, R. "Indications for the Surgical Treatment of Suspected Acute Appendicitis: A Cost-Effectiveness Approach." In J. P. Bunker, B. A. Barnes, and F. Mosteller (Eds.), *Costs, Risks, and Benefits of Surgery*. New York: Oxford University Press, 1977.

Neutra, R., and Neff, R. "Fetal Death in Eclampsia: II. The Effect of Non-Therapeutic Factors." *British Journal of Obstetrics and Gynecology*, 1975, *82*, 390-396.

Newell, A., and Simon, H. A. *Human Problem Solving*. Englewood Cliffs, N.J.: Prentice-Hall, 1972.

Newhouse, J. P. "A Design for a Health Insurance Experiment." *Inquiry*, 1974, *5*, 5-27.

Newmark, C. S., and Raft, D. "Using an Abbreviated MMPI as a Screening Device for Medical Patients." *Psychosomatics*, 1976, *17*, 45-48.

Nguyen, T. D., Attkisson, C. C., and Bottino, M. J. "Definition and Identification of Human Service Need in a Community Context." In R. A. Bell, M. Sundel, J. F. Aponte, and S. A. Murrel, *Need Assessment in Health and Human Services: Proceedings of the Louisville National Conference*. University of Louisville, Ky., March 9-12, 1976. (Expanded version to be published by Human Sciences Press, 1979.)

Nielsen, D., and Moos, R. H. "Student-Environment Interaction in the Development of Physical Symptoms." *Research in Higher Education*, 1977, *6*, 139-156.

Nisbett, R. E., and Schachter, S. "Cognitive Manipulations of Pain." *Journal of Experimental Social Psychology*, 1966, *2*, 227-236.

Nisbett, R. E., and Valins, S. *Perceiving the Causes of One's Own Behavior*. Morristown, N.J.: General Learning Press, 1971.

Nisbett, R. E., and Wilson, T. "Telling More Than We Can Know—Verbal Reports on Mental Processes." *Psychological Review*, 1977, *84*, 231-259.

Norton, J. E. "Treatment of a Dying Patient." *Psychoanalytic Study of the Child*, 1963, *18*, 541-560.

Novik, B. R. "The Effects of Teaching Interview Skills and Affective Sensitivity to Family Medicine Residents: A Pilot Study." Unpublished doctoral dissertation, Michigan State University, 1978.

Nuckolls, K. B., Cassel, J., and Kaplan, B. H. "Psychosocial Assets, Life Crisis, and the Prognosis of Pregnancy." *American Journal of Epidemiology*, 1972, *95*, 431-441.

Olbrisch, M. E. "Psychotherapeutic Interventions in Physical Health: Effectiveness and Economic Efficiency." *American Psychologist*, 1977, *32*,

761-777.

Olesen, V. L. "Convergences and Divergences: Anthropology and Sociology in Health Care." *Social Science and Medicine,* 1975, *9,* 421-425.

Olesen, V. L., and Davis, F. "Baccalaureate Students' Images of Nursing: A Follow-Up Report." *Nursing Research,* 1966, *15* (2), 182.

Olesen, V. L., and Whittaker, E. W. *The Silent Dialogue: A Study in the Social Psychology of Professional Socialization.* San Francisco: Jossey-Bass, 1968.

Olin, H. S., and Hackett, T. P. "The Denial of Chest Pain in 32 Patients with Acute Myocardial Infarction." *Journal of the American Medical Association,* 1964, *190,* 977-981.

Olmstead, A. G., and Paget, M. A. "Theoretical Issues in Professional Socialization." *Journal of Medical Education,* 1969, *4,* 663-669.

Olsen, D. M. "A Controlled Trial of Multiphasic Screening." *New England Journal of Medicine,* 1976, *294,* 925-930.

O'Neill, D. *Modern Trends in Psychosomatic Medicine.* London: Butterworths, 1955.

Opton, E. M., Jr. "Psychological Stress and Coping Methods in Surgical Patients: A Preliminary Report." Unpublished manuscript, University of California, Berkeley, n.d.

Osgood, C. E., and Tannenbaum, P. H. *The Measurement of Meaning.* Urbana: University of Illinois Press, 1958.

Oskamp, S. "Overconfidence in Case-Study Judgments." *Journal of Consulting Psychology,* 1965, *29,* 261-265.

Ostfeld, A. M., Lebovits, B. Z., Shekelle, R. B., and Paul, P. "A Prospective Study of the Relationship Between Personality and Coronary Heart Disease." *Journal of Chronic Diseases,* 1964, *17,* 265-276.

Ota, W., and Bang, F. "A Continuous Study of Viruses in the Respiratory Tract in Families of Calcutta Bustee: II. Family Patterns of the Infection and Illness in a Crowded Environment." *American Journal of Epidemiology,* 1972, *95,* 384-391.

Otis, G., Quenk, N., Weiss, J., Albert, M. Offir, J., and Richardson, C. *Medical Specialty Selection: A Review.* DHEW Publication No. (HRA) 75-8. Washington, D.C.: U.S. Government Printing Office, 1975.

Paiva, R. E. A., and Haley, H. B. "Intellectual, Personality, and Environmental Factors in Career Specialty Preferences." *Journal of Medical Education,* 1971, *46,* 281-289.

Paivio, A. *Imagery and Verbal Processes.* New York: Holt, Rinehart and Winston, 1971.

Palmer, B. B., and Lewis, C. E. "Development of Health Attitudes and Behaviors." Paper presented at annual meeting of the American School Health Association, Denver, Colo., October 1975.

Palmer, R. D. "Patterns of Defensive Response to Threatening Stimuli." *Journal of Abnormal Psychology,* 1968, *73,* 30-36.

Pancheri, P., Bellaterra, M., Matteoli, S., Cristofari, M., Polizzi, C., and Puletti, N. "Infarct as a Stress Agent: Life History and Personality Characteristics in Improved Versus Non-Improved Patients After Severe Heart

Attack." *Journal of Human Stress,* 1978, *4* (1), 16-22 and 41-42.

Papper, E. M., Brodie, B. B., and Rovenstine, E. A. "Postoperative Pain: Its Use in the Comparative Evaluation of Analgesics." *Surgery,* 1952, *32,* 107-109.

Parad, H. J. (Ed.). *Crisis Intervention: Selected Readings.* New York: Family Service Association of America, 1965.

Parbrook, G. D., Dalrymple, D. G., and Steel, D. F. "Personality Assessment and Postoperative Pain and Complications." *Journal of Psychosomatic Research,* 1973, *17,* 277-285.

Parens, H., McConville, B. J., and Kaplan, S. M. "The Prediction of Frequency of Illness from the Response to Separation." *Psychosomatic Medicine,* 1966, *28,* 162-176.

Parker, A. W., Walsh, J. W., and Coon, M. A. "Normative Approach to the Definition of Primary Health Care." *Milbank Memorial Fund Quarterly,* 1976, *54,* 415-438.

Parker, B. R., and Srinivasan, V. "A Consumer Preference Approach to the Planning of Rural Primary Health-Care Facilities." *Operations Research,* 1976, *24,* 991-1025.

Parker, E. S., Birnbaum, I. M., and Noble, E. P. "Alcohol and Memory: Storage and State Dependency." *Journal of Verbal Learning and Verbal Behavior,* 1976, *15,* 691-702.

Parkes, C. M. "Psychosocial Transitions: A Field for Study." *Social Science and Medicine,* 1971, *5,* 101-115.

Parkes, C. M. *Bereavement: Studies of Grief in Adult Life.* New York: International Universities Press, 1972.

Parkes, C. M. "The Emotional Impact of Cancer on Patients and Families." *Journal of Laryngology and Otology,* 1975, *89,* 1271-1279.

Parkes, C. M., Benjamin, B., and Fitzgerald, R. G. "Broken Heart: A Statistical Study of Increased Mortality Among Widowers." *British Medical Journal,* 1969, *1,* 740-743.

Parkes, C. M., and Brown, R. J. "Health After Bereavement: A Controlled Study of Young Boston Widows and Widowers." *Psychosomatic Medicine,* 1972, *34,* 449-461.

Parsegian, V. L. *This Cybernetic World of Men and Machines and Earth Systems.* New York: Anchor Books, 1972.

Parsons, T. "Illness and the Role of the Physician: A Sociological Perspective." *American Journal of Orthopsychiatry,* 1951a, *21,* 452-460.

Parsons, T. *The Social System.* New York: Free Press, 1951b.

Parsons, T. "Definitions of Health and Illness in the Light of American Values and Social Structure." In E. G. Jaco (Ed.), *Patients, Physicians, and Illness.* (2nd ed.) New York: Free Press, 1972.

Parsons, T., and Fox, R. "Illness, Therapy, and the Modern Urban American Family." *Journal of Social Issues,* 1952, *8* (4), 31-44.

Pascal, G. R., and Thoroughman, J. C. "Relation Between Bender-Gestalt Test Scores and the Response of Patients with Intractable Duodenal Ulcer to Surgery." *Psychosomatic Medicine,* 1964, *26,* 625-627.

Patrick, D. L., Bush, J. W., and Chen, M. "Toward an Operational Definition of Health." *Journal of Health and Social Behavior,* 1973, *14,* 6-23.

Pauker, S. G. "Coronary Artery Surgery: The Use of Decision Analysis." *Annals of Internal Medicine,* 1976, *82,* 8-18.

Paulus, P., Cox, V., McCain, G., and Chandler, J. "Some Effects of Crowding in a Prison Environment." *Journal of Applied Social Psychology,* 1975, *5,* 86-91.

Paulus, P., Annis, A. B., Seta, J. J., Schkade, J. K., and Matthews, R. W. "Density Does Affect Task Performance." *Journal of Personality and Social Psychology,* 1976, *34,* 248-253.

Pearlin, L., and Schooler, C. "The Structure of Coping." *Journal of Health and Social Behavior,* 1978, *19,* 2-21.

Pearson, J. S., and Steinhilber, R. M. "Psychological Assessment of Therapy in Coronary Artery Disease." *Journal of the American Medical Association,* 1971, *217,* 72-74.

Penick, S. F., Filion, R., Fox, S., and Stunkard, A. J. "Behavior Modification in the Treatment of Obesity." *Psychosomatic Medicine,* 1971, *33,* 49-55.

Pennebacker, J. W., Burnam, M. A., Schaeffer, M. A., and Harper, D. C. "Lack of Control as a Determinant of Perceived Physical Symptoms." *Journal of Personality and Social Psychology,* 1977, *35,* 167-174.

Perkins, F. *My Fight with Arthritis.* New York: Random House, 1964.

Perlman, D. "Heart Doctors Clash over Coronary Risk Factors." *San Francisco Chronicle,* January 22, 1975, p. 4.

Perlman, M. "Economic History and Health Care in Industrialized Nations." In M. Perlman (Ed.), *The Economics of Health and Medical Care.* New York: Wiley, 1974.

Perricone, P. J. "Social Concern in Medical Students: A Reconsideration of the Eron Assumption." *Journal of Medical Education,* 1974, *49,* 541-553.

Perrin, G. M., and Pierce, I. R. "Psychosomatic Aspects of Cancer." *Psychosomatic Medicine,* 1959, *21,* 397-421.

Perrin, G. M., and Pierce, I. R. "Letter to the Editor." *Psychosomatic Medicine,* 1961, *23,* 262-264.

Pervin, L. A. "The Need to Predict and Control Under Conditions of Threat." *Journal of Personality,* 1963, *34,* 570-587.

Peterson, O. L., Andrews, L. T., Spain, R. S., and Greenberg, B. G. "An Analytical Study of North Carolina General Practice, 1953-1954." *Journal of Medical Education,* 1956, *31,* (12, Part 2), 1-165.

Petrie, A. *Individuality in Pain and Suffering.* Chicago: University of Chicago Press, 1967.

Phillips, L. D. *Bayesian Statistics for Social Scientists.* New York: Crowell, 1973.

Piaget, J. *The Child's Conception of the World.* New York: Harcourt Brace Jovanovich, 1929.

Piaget, J. *The Origins of Intelligence in Children.* New York: International Universities Press, 1952.

Pickett, R. M., and Triggs, T. J. (Eds.), *Human Factors in Health Care.* Lexington, Mass.: Heath, 1975.

Pinneau, S. R., Jr. "Effects of Social Support on Psychological and Physiological Strains." Unpublished doctoral dissertation, University of Michigan, 1975.

Pinneau, S. R., Jr. "Effects of Social Support on Occupational Stresses and Strains." Paper presented at annual meeting of the American Psychological Association, Washington, D.C., 1976.

Platt, J. R. "Strong Inference." *Science,* 1964, *146,* 347-352.

Pliskin, J. S., and Beck, C. H. "Decision Analysis in Individual Clinical Decision Making: A Real-World Application in Treatment of Renal Disease." *Methods of Information in Medicine,* 1976, *15,* 43-46.

Podell, R. *Physician's Guide to Compliance in Hypertension.* Summit, N.J.: Merck, 1975.

Pokorny, A. D., Miller, B. A., and Cleveland, S. E. "Response to Treatment of Alcoholism: A Follow-Up Study." *Quarterly Journal of Studies on Alcohol,* 1968, *29,* 364-381.

Polgar, S. "Health and Human Behavior: Areas of Interest Common to the Social and Medical Sciences." *Current Anthropology,* 1962, *2,* 159-205.

Polivy, J. "Psychological Effects of Mastectomy on a Woman's Feminine Self-Concept." *Journal of Nervous and Mental Disease,* 1977, *164,* 77-87.

Pollard, W. E., Bobbitt, R. A., Bergner, M., Martin, D. P., and Gilson, B. S. "The Sickness Impact Profile: Reliability of a Health Status Measure." *Medical Care,* 1976, *14,* 146-155.

Polyani, M. *The Tacit Dimension.* New York: Doubleday, 1967.

Pool, I. deS. *Contemporary Political Science.* New York: McGraw-Hill, 1967.

Pope, B., and Lisansky, E. T. "The Psychologist as a Colleague of the Practicing Physician." *Modern Treatment,* 1969, *6,* 866-884.

Pople, H. "The Formation of Composite Hypotheses in Diagnostic Problem Solving: An Exercise in Synthetic Reasoning." In *Proceedings of the Fifth International Conference on Artificial Intelligence.* Cambridge, Mass.: MIT Press, 1977.

Porter, A. "Drug Defaulting in a General Practice." *British Medical Journal,* 1969, *1,* 218-222.

Porter, L., and Lawler, R. "Properties of Organization Structure in Relation to Job Attitudes and Job Behavior." *Psychological Bulletin,* 1965, *64,* 23-51.

Porter, L., and Steers, R. "Organizational, Work, and Personal Factors in Employee Turnover and Absenteeism." *Psychological Bulletin,* 1973, *80,* 151-176.

Powell, M. "Occupational Problems of Professional Men: Dentists and Pharmacists." *Occupational Psychology,* 1972, *45,* 52-66.

Powers, W. T. *Behavior: The Control of Perception.* Chicago: Aldine, 1973.

Pranulis, M., Dabbs, J., and Johnson, J. "General Anesthesia and the Patient's Attempts at Control." *Social Behavior and Personality,* 1975, *3,* 49-54.

Pratt, J. H. "The Influence of the Emotions in the Causations and Cure of Psychoneuroses." *International Clinics,* 1934, *4* (Series 44), 1-16.

Pratt, L. "The Relationship of Socioeconomic Status to Health." *American Journal of Public Health,* 1971, *61,* 281-291.

Pratt, L., Seligmann, A., and Reader, G. "Physicians' Views on the Level of Medical Information Among Patients." *American Journal of Public Health,* 1957, *47,* 1277-1283.

Price, D. B., Thaler, M., and Mason, J. W. "Preoperative Emotional States and Adrenal Cortical Activity." *AMA Archives of Neurology and Psychiatry,* 1957, *77,* 646-656.

Price, K. P. "The Application of Behavior Therapy to the Treatment of Psychosomatic Disorders: Retrospect and Prospect." *Psychotherapy: Theory, Research, and Practice,* 1974, *11,* 138-155.

Price, P. B., Taylor, C. W., Nelson, D. E., Lewis, E. G., Loughmiller, G. C., Mathiesen, R., Murray, S. L., and Maxwell, J. G. *Measurement and Predictors of Physician Performance.* Salt Lake City, Utah: LLR Press, 1971.

Prince, M. "The New Psychology and Therapeutics." *Journal of the American Medical Association,* 1912, *53,* 918-921.

Pritchard, M. "Further Studies of Illness Behaviour in Long-Term Haemodialysis." *Journal of Psychosomatic Research,* 1977, *21,* 41-48.

Proshansky, H., and O'Hanlon, T. "Environmental Psychology: Origins and Development." In D. Stokols (Ed.), *Perspectives on Environment and Behavior.* New York: Plenum Press, 1977.

Psathas, G. "The Fate of Idealism in Nursing School." *Journal of Health and Social Behavior,* 1968, *9,* 52-64.

"Psychology and National Health Care." *American Psychologist,* 1971, *26,* 1025-1026.

"Psychophysiological Aspects of Cancer." *Annals of the New York Academy of Sciences,* 1966, *125* (Art. 3).

Querido, A. "Forecast and Follow-Up: An Investigation into the Clinical, Social, and Mental Factors Determining the Results of Hospital Treatment." *British Journal of Preventive and Social Medicine,* 1959, *13,* 33-49.

Rabinowitz, D. "Some Endocrine and Metabolic Aspects of Obesity." *Annual Review of Medicine,* 1970, *21,* 241-258.

Rabkin, J. G., and Struening, E. L. "Life Events, Stress, and Illness." *Science,* 1976, *194,* 1013-1020.

Rahe, R. H. "Subjects' Recent Life Changes and Their Near-Future Illness Susceptibility." *Advances in Psychosomatic Medicine,* 1972, *8,* 2-19.

Rahe, R. H. "The Pathway Between Subjects' Recent Life Changes and Their Near-Future Illness Reports: Representative Results and Methodological Issues." In B. S. Dohrenwend and B. P. Dohrenwend (Eds.), *Stressful Life Events: Their Nature and Effects.* New York: Wiley, 1974.

Rahe, R. H., and Arthur, R. H. "Life Change and Illness Studies." *Journal of Human Stress,* 1978, *4* (1), 3-15.

Rahe, R. H., Gunderson, E., Pugh, W. M., Rubin, R. T., and Arthur, R. J. "Illness Prediction Studies: Use of Psychosocial and Occupational Characteristics as Predictors." *Archives of Environmental Health,* 1972, *25,* 192-197.

Rahe, R. H., McKean, J. D., and Arthur, R. J. "A Longitudinal Study of Life

Change and Illness Patterns." *Journal of Psychosomatic Research*, 1967, *10*, 355-366.

Rahe, R. H., Meyer, M., Smith, M., Kjaer, G., and Holmes, T. H. "Social Stress and Illness Onset." *Journal of Psychosomatic Research*, 1964, *8*, 35-44.

Rahe, R. H., O'Neil, T., Hagan, A., and Arthur, R. J. "Brief Group Therapy Following Myocardial Infarction: Eighteen-Month Follow-Up of a Controlled Trial." *International Journal of Psychiatry in Medicine*, 1975, *6*, 349-358.

Rahe, R. H., Rubin, R. T., and Arthur, R. J. "The Three Investigators Study: Serum Uric Acid, Cholesterol, and Cortisol Variability During Stresses of Everyday Life." *Psychosomatic Medicine*, 1974, *36*, 258-268.

Rahe, R. H., Rubin, R. T., Gunderson, E. K. E., and Arthur, R. J. "Psychologic Correlates of Serum Cholesterol in Man: A Longitudinal Study." *Psychosomatic Medicine*, 1971, *33*, 399-410.

Raiffa, H. *Decision Analysis: Introductory Lectures on Choices Under Uncertainty*. Reading, Mass.: Addison-Wesley, 1968.

Rangell, L. "Discussion of the Buffalo Creek Disaster: The Course of Psychic Trauma." *American Journal of Psychiatry*, 1976, *133*, 313-316.

Rapoport, A. "Toward a Redefinition of Density." *Environment and Behavior*, 1975, *7*, 133-158.

Raskin, M. "Psychiatric Crises of Medical Students and the Implications for Subsequent Adjustments." *Journal of Medical Education*, 1972, *47*, 210-215.

Ravitch, M. M. "Informed Consent—Descent to Absurdity." *Resident and Staff Physician*, 1974, *20* (4), 10s-12s, 16s, and 20s.

Reavley, W. "The Relation of Life Events to Several Aspects of Anxiety." *Journal of Psychosomatic Research*, 1974, *18*, 421-424.

Reed, H., and Janis, I. L. "Effects of Induced Awareness of Rationalizations on Smokers' Acceptance of Fear-Arousing Warnings About Health Hazards." *Journal of Consulting and Clinical Psychology*, 1974, *42*, 748.

Reeder, L. G., Schrama, P. G. M., and Dirken, J. M. "Stress and Cardiovascular Health: An International Cooperative Study—I." *Social Science and Medicine*, 1973, *7*, 573-584.

Rees, W. D., and Lutkins, S. "Mortality of Bereavement." *British Medical Journal*, 1967, *4*, 13-16.

Reiss, J., and Menashe, V. "Genetic Counseling and Congenital Heart Disease." *Journal of Pediatrics*, 1972, *80*, 655-656.

Reitan, R. M. "A Research Program on the Psychological Effects of Brain Lesions in Human Beings." In N. R. Ellis (Ed.), *International Review of Research in Mental Retardation*. Vol. 1. New York: Academic Press, 1966.

Reite, M., Kaufman, I. C., Pauley, J. D., and Stynes, A. J. "Depression in Infant Monkeys: Physiological Correlates." *Psychosomatic Medicine*, 1974, *36*, 363-367.

Renneker, R., and Cutler, M. "Psychological Problems of Adjustment to

Cancer of the Breast." *Journal of the American Medical Association,* 1952, *148,* 833-838.

Revans, R. "Human Relations, Management, and Size." In E. M. Hugh-Jones (Ed.), *Human Relations and Modern Management.* Amsterdam: North Holland, 1958.

Reynolds, A. G., and Flagg, P. W. *Cognitive Psychology.* Cambridge, Mass.: Winthrop, 1977.

Reynolds, B. D., Puck, M., and Robertson, A. "Genetic Counseling: An Appraisal." *Clinical Genetics,* 1974, *5,* 177-187.

Rezler, A. G. "Attitude Changes During Medical School: A Review of the Literature." *Journal of Medical Education,* 1974, *49,* 1023-1030.

Rhoades, W. "Group Training in Thought Control for Relieving Nervous Disorders." *Mental Hygiene,* 1935, *19,* 373-386.

Rice, H., McDaniel, M., and Denny, B. "Operant Conditioning Techniques for Use in the Physical Rehabilitation of the Multiply Handicapped Retarded Person." *Physical Therapy,* 1968, *48,* 342-346.

Richardson, W. "Measuring the Urban Poor's Use of Physicians' Services in Response to Illness Episodes." *Medical Care,* 1970, *8,* 132-142.

Richter, C. P. "On the Phenomenon of Sudden Death in Animals and Man." *Psychosomatic Medicine,* 1957, *19,* 191-198.

Riker, W. H. "The Future of a Science of Politics." *American Behavioral Scientist,* 1977, *21,* 11-29.

Ritson, B. "Involvement in Treatment and Its Relation to Outcome Amongst Alcoholics." *British Journal of the Addictions,* 1969, *64,* 23-29.

Robbins, L. C., and Hall, J. H. *How to Practice Prospective Medicine.* Indianapolis: Slaymakers Enterprises, 1970.

Robertson, L., Kelley, A. B., O'Neill, B., Wixon, C. W., Eiswirth, R. S., and Haddon, W., Jr. "A Controlled Study of the Effect of Television Messages on Safety Belt Use." *American Journal of Public Health,* 1974, *64,* 1071-1080.

Robertson, L. S., and Heagarty, M. C. *Medical Sociology: A General Systems Approach.* Chicago: Nelson Hall, 1975.

Robinson, D. *The Process of Becoming Ill.* London: Routledge and Kegan Paul, 1971.

Robinson, D., and Rhode, S. "Two Experiments with an Anti-Semitism Poll." *Journal of Abnormal and Social Psychology,* 1946, *41,* 136-144.

Robinson, W. S. "Ecological Correlations and the Behavior of Individuals." *American Sociological Review,* 1950, *15,* 351-357.

Rodin, J. "Density, Perceived Choice, and Response to Controllable and Uncontrollable Outcomes." *Journal of Experimental Social Psychology,* 1976a, *12,* 564-578.

Rodin, J. "Menstruation, Reattribution, and Competence." *Journal of Personality and Social Psychology,* 1976b, *33,* 345-353.

Rodin, J. "Obesity: Why the Losing Battle." In *Master Lecture Series on Brain-Behavior Relationships.* Washington, D.C.: American Psychological Association, 1977.

Rodin, J. "Somatopsychics and Attribution." *Personality and Social Psychology Bulletin,* 1978, *4,* 531-540.

Rodin, J., and Langer, E. "Long-Term Effects of a Control-Relevant Intervention with the Institutionalized Aged." *Journal of Personality and Social Psychology,* 1977, *35,* 897-902.

Rodin, J., and Langer, E. "Rehearsal and Attributional Focus as Techniques for Effective Use of Memory in the Elderly." Unpublished manuscript, Yale University, 1978.

Roe, B. B. "Are Postoperative Narcotics Necessary?" *Archives of Surgery,* 1963, *87,* 50-53.

Rogers, C. R. *Counseling and Psychotherapy.* Boston: Houghton Mifflin, 1942.

Rogers, C. R. *Client-Centered Therapy.* Boston: Houghton Mifflin, 1951.

Rogers, C. R. "The Necessary and Sufficient Conditions for Therapeutic Personality Change." *Journal of Consulting Psychology,* 1957, *21,* 95-101.

Rogers, R. W., and Mewborn, C. R. "Fear Appeals and Attitude Change: Effects of a Threat's Noxiousness, Probability of Occurrence, and the Efficacy of Coping Responses." *Journal of Personality and Social Psychology,* 1976, *34,* 54-61.

Rogers, R. W., and Thistlethwaite, D. L. "Effects of Fear Arousal and Reassurance upon Attitude Change." *Journal of Personality and Social Psychology,* 1970, *15,* 227-233.

Roghmann, K., and Haggerty, R. "The Diary as a Research Instrument in the Study of Health and Illness Behavior." *Medical Care,* 1972, *10,* 143-163.

Rokeach, M. "Attitude Change and Behavior Change." *Public Opinion Quarterly,* 1966-1967, *30,* 529-550.

Rokeach, M. "Long-Range Experimental Modification of Values, Attitudes, and Behavior." *American Psychologist,* 1971, *26,* 453-459.

Rokeach, M. *The Nature of Human Values.* New York: Free Press, 1973.

Rollin, B. *First, You Cry.* Philadelphia: Lippincott, 1976.

Roman, P., and Trice, H. "The Sick Role, Labeling Theory, and the Deviant Drinker." *International Journal of Social Psychiatry,* 1968, *14,* 245-251.

Rosch, E. "Cognitive Representations of Semantic Categories." *Journal of Experimental Psychology: General,* 1975, *104,* 192-233.

Rose, K. D., and Rosow, I. "Marital Stability Among Physicians." *California Medicine,* 1972, *116,* 95-99.

Rose, K. D., and Rosow, I. "Physicians Who Kill Themselves." *Archives of General Psychiatry,* 1973, *29,* 800-805.

Rosen, G. "The Evolution of Social Medicine." In H. E. Freeman, S. Levine, and L. G. Reeder (Eds.), *Handbook of Medical Sociology.* (2nd ed.) Englewood Cliffs, N.J.: Prentice-Hall, 1972.

Rosen, J. L., and Bibring, G. L. "Psychological Reactions of Hospitalized Male Patients to a Heart Attack: Age and Social-Class Differences." *Psychosomatic Medicine,* 1966, *28,* 808-821.

Rosenbaum, E. H. *Living with Cancer.* New York: Praeger, 1975.

Rosenberg, M. "Cognitive Structure and Attitudinal Affect." *Journal of Abnormal and Social Psychology,* 1956, *53,* 367-373.

Rosenberg, P. P. "Students' Perceptions and Concerns During Their First Year in Medical School." *Journal of Medical Education,* 1971, *46,* 211-218.

Rosenberg, P. P., and Chilgren, R. "Sex Education Discussion Groups in a Medical Setting." *International Journal of Group Psychotherapy,* 1973, *23,* 23-41.

Rosenberg, S. "Patient Education—An Educator's View." In D. Sackett and R. Haynes (Eds.), *Compliance with Therapeutic Regimens.* Baltimore: Johns Hopkins University Press, 1976.

Rosenblatt, S. M., Gross, M. M., Malenowski, B., Broman, M., and Lewis, E. "Marital Status and Multiple Psychiatric Admissions for Alcoholism." *Quarterly Journal of Studies on Alcohol,* 1971, *32,* 1092-1096.

Rosenman, R. H. "Behavior Pattern Type A: Its Causal Relationship to Coronary Heart Disease." Paper presented at conference on "Stress: The Impact of Life Events and Life Styles," University of California School of Medicine, San Francisco, September 22, 1973.

Rosenman, R. H., Brand, R. J., Jenkins, C. D., Friedman, M., Straus, R., and Wurm, M. "Coronary Heart Disease in the Western Collaborative Group Study: Final Follow-Up Experience of 8.5 Years." *Journal of the American Medical Association,* 1975, *233,* 872-877.

Rosenman, R. H., Brand, R. J., Sholtz, R. I., and Friedman, M. "Multivariate Prediction of Coronary Heart Disease During 8.5 Year Follow-Up in the Western Collaborative Group Study." *American Journal of Cardiology,* 1976, *37,* 903-910.

Rosenman, R. H., Friedman, M., Straus, R., Jenkins, C. D., Zyzanski, S. H., and Wurm, M. "Coronary Heart Disease in the Western Collaborative Group Study." *Journal of Chronic Diseases,* 1970, *23,* 173-190.

Rosenman, R. H., Friedman, M., Straus, R., Wurm, M., Jenkins, C. D., and Messinger, H. B. "Coronary Heart Disease in the Western Collaborative Group Study: A Follow-up Experience of Two Years." *Journal of the American Medical Association,* 1966, *195,* 86-92.

Rosenman, R. H., Friedman, M., Straus, R., Wurm, M., Kositchek, R., Hahn, W., and Werthessen, N. T. "A Predictive Study of Coronary Heart Disease: The Western Collaborative Group Study." *Journal of the American Medical Association,* 1964, *189,* 15-22.

Rosenstock, I. M. "Cultural Anthropology, Social Psychology, and Sociology in Public Health." *American Journal of Public Health,* 1961, *51* (12), 1820-1827.

Rosenstock, I. M. "Why People Use Health Services." *Milbank Memorial Fund Quarterly,* 1966, *44,* 94-124.

Rosenstock, I. M. "The Health Belief Model and Preventive Health Behavior." *Health Education Monographs,* 1974, *2* (4), 354-386.

Rosenstock, I. M., Derryberry, M., and Carriger, B. "Why People Fail to Seek Poliomyelitis Vaccination." *Public Health Reports,* 1959, *74,* 98-103.

Rosenthal, G. "Planning in the Health Care System." In A. Sheldon, F. Baker, and C. McLaughlin (Eds.), *Systems and Medical Care*. Cambridge, Mass.: M.I.T. Press, 1970.

Rosenthal, R., and Rosnow, R. *Artifact in Behavioral Research*. New York: Academic Press, 1969.

Rosenthal, R., and Rosnow, R. *The Volunteer Subject*. New York: Wiley, 1975.

Ross, L., Lepper, M., and Hubbard, M. "Perseverance in Self-Perception and Social Perception: Biased Attributional Processes in the Debriefing Paradigm." *Journal of Personality and Social Psychology*, 1975, *32*, 880-892.

Ross, L., Rodin, J., and Zimbardo, P. "Toward an Attribution Therapy: The Reduction of Fear Through Induced Cognitive-Emotional Misattribution." *Journal of Personality and Social Psychology*, 1969, *12*, 279-288.

Rossi, J. J., Stach, A., and Bradley, N. J. "Effects of Treatment of Male Alcoholics in a Mental Hospital." *Quarterly Journal of Studies on Alcohol*, 1963, *34*, 91-108.

Roth, H., and Berger, D. "Studies on Patient Cooperation in Ulcer Treatment: Observation of Actual as Compared to Prescribed Antacid Intake on a Hospital Ward." *Gastroenterology*, 1960, *38*, 630-633.

Roth, H., Caron, H., and Hsi, B. "Estimating a Patient's Cooperation with His Regimen." *American Journal of Medical Science*, 1971, *262*, 269-273.

Rothberg, J. S. "Dependence and Anxiety in Male Patients Following Surgery: An Investigation of the Relationship Between Dependence, Anxiety, and Physical Manifestations of Recovery Following Surgery in Male Patients." Unpublished doctoral dissertation, New York University, 1965.

Rotter, J. B. *Social Learning and Clinical Psychology*. Englewood Cliffs, N.J.: Prentice-Hall, 1954.

Rotter, J. B. "Generalized Expectancies for Internal Versus External Control of Reinforcement." *Psychological Monographs*, 1966, *80* (1), No. 609.

Rotter, J. B., Chance, J. E., and Phares, E. J. *Applications of a Social Learning Theory of Personality*. New York: Holt, Rinehart and Winston, 1972.

Rousselot, L. M. "Federal Efforts to Influence Physicians' Education, Specialization Distribution, Projections, and Options." *American Journal of Medicine*, 1973, *55*, 123-130.

Routh, D. K. "Postdoctoral Training in Pediatric Psychology." *Professional Psychology*, 1977, *8*, 245-250.

Rowland, K. F. "Environmental Events Predicting Death for the Elderly." *Psychological Bulletin*, 1977, *84*, 349-372.

Rundall, T. G. "Life Change and Recovery from Surgery." Unpublished doctoral dissertation, Stanford University, 1976.

Ruphuy, R. S. "Psychology and Medicine: A New Approach for Community Health Development." *American Psychologist*, 1977, *32*, 910-913.

Rushner, R. F. *Humanizing Health Care: Alternative Future for Medicine*. Cambridge, Mass.: M.I.T. Press, 1975.

Rusk, T. N. "Opportunity and Technique in Crisis Psychiatry." *Comprehensive Psychiatry*, 1971, *12*, 249-263.

Russek, H. I. "Emotional Stress and Coronary Heart Disease in American Physicians, Dentists, and Lawyers." *American Journal of the Medical Sciences*, 1962, *243*, 716-726.

Russek, H. I. "Stress, Tobacco, and Coronary Heart Disease." *Journal of the American Medical Association*, 1965, *192*, 89-94.

Russek, H. I. "Role of Emotional Stress in the Etiology of Clinical Coronary Heart Disease." *Diseases of the Chest*, 1967, *52*, 1-9.

Russek, H. I., and Russek, L. G. "Is Emotional Stress an Etiological Factor in Coronary Heart Disease?" *Psychosomatics*, 1976, *17* (2), 63-67.

Russell, L. B., and Burke, C. S. "Political Economy of Federal Health Programs in the United States: Historical Review." *International Journal of Health Services*, 1978, *8*, 55-77.

Ryan, W. *Blaming the Victim*. New York: Pantheon Books, 1971.

Sachs, D. L., Hall, R. G., and Hall, S. M. "Rapid Smoking: Physiological Evaluation of a Smoking Cessation Therapy." *Annals of Internal Medicine*, 1978, *88*, 639-641.

Sachs, J. D. S. "Recognition Memory for Syntactic and Semantic Aspects of Connected Discourse." *Perception and Psychophysics*, 1967, *2*, 437-442.

Sackett, D. L. "The Magnitude of Compliance and Noncompliance." In D. L. Sackett and R. B. Haynes (Eds.), *Compliance with Therapeutic Regimens*. Baltimore: Johns Hopkins University Press, 1976.

Sackett, D. L., and Haynes, R. B. *Compliance with Therapeutic Regimens*. Baltimore: Johns Hopkins University Press, 1976.

Sackett, D. L., Haynes, R. B., Gibson, E. S., Hackett, B. C., Taylor, D. W., Roberts, R. S., and Johnson, A. L. "Randomized Clinical Trial of Strategies for Improving Medication Compliance in Primary Hypertension." *Lancet*, 1975, *1*, 1205-1207.

Sadler, M. M., Sadler, B. L., and Bliss, A. A. *The Physician's Assistant Today and Tomorrow*. Trauma Program of the Department of Surgery, School of Medicine, Yale University, 1972.

Saegert, S. "High-Density Environments: Their Personal and Social Consequences." In A. Baum and W. Epstein (Eds.), *Human Responses to Crowding*. Hillsdale, N.J.: Lawrence Erlbaum, 1977.

Safer, M. A., Tharps, Q. J., Jackson, T. C., and Leventhal, H. "Determinants of Three Stages of Delay in Seeking Care at a Medical Clinic." *Medical Care*, in press.

Salk, J. "Immunological Paradoxes: Theoretical Considerations in the Rejection or Retention of Grafts, Tumors, and Normal Tissue." *Annals of the New York Academy of Sciences*, 1969a, *164* (Art. 2), 365-380.

Salk, J. "Panel Discussion 2: The Immunologic Approach." *Annals of the New York Academy of Sciences*, 1969b, *164* (Art. 2), 620-627.

Saltzman, B. N. "Health Care for the Disadvantaged in the Rural Area." *Journal of the Arkansas Medical Society*, 1971, *67*, 319-321.

Sanderson, R. E., Campbell, D., and Laverty, S. G. "An Investigation of a New Oversize Conditioning Treatment for Alcoholism." *Quarterly Journal of Studies on Alcohol*, 1963, *24*, 261-275.

Sarason, I. G., de Monchaux, C., and Hunt, T. "Methodological Issues in the Assessment of Life Stress." In L. Levi (Ed.), *Emotions—Their Parameters and Measurement.* New York: Raven Press, 1975.

Sarnoff, I., and Zimbardo, P. "Anxiety, Fear, and Social Affiliation." *Journal of Abnormal and Social Psychology,* 1961, *62,* 356-363.

Savage, L. J. "The Theory of Statistical Decision." *Journal of the American Statistical Association,* 1951, *46,* 55-67.

Sawyer, J. "Measurement and Prediction: Clinical and Statistical." *Psychological Bulletin,* 1966, *66,* 178-200.

Schachter, S. *The Psychology of Affiliation.* Stanford, Calif.: Stanford University Press, 1959.

Schachter, S., and Singer, J. E. "Cognitive, Social, and Physiological Determinants and Emotional State." *Psychological Review,* 1962, *69,* 379-399.

Schaie, K., and Gribbin, K. "Adult Development and Aging." *Annual Review of Psychology,* 1975, *26,* 65-96.

Schiffenbauer, A. I., Brown, J. E., Perry, P. L., Shulack, L. K., and Zanzola, A. M. "The Relationship Between Density and Crowding: Some Architectural Modifiers." *Environment and Behavior,* 1977, *9,* 3-14.

Schmale, A. H., Jr. "Giving Up as a Final Common Pathway to Changes in Health." *Advances in Psychosomatic Medicine,* 1972, *8,* 20-40.

Schmale, A. H., Jr., and Engel, G. L. "The Giving Up-Given Up Complex Illustrated on Film." *Archives of General Psychiatry,* 1967, *17,* 135-145.

Schmale, A. H., Jr., and Iker, H. P. "The Affect of Hopelessness and the Development of Cancer: I. Identification of Uterine Cervical Cancer in Women with Atypical Cytology." *Psychosomatic Medicine,* 1966, *28,* 714-721.

Schmale, A. H., Jr., and Iker, H. P. "Hopelessness as a Predictor of Cervical Cancer." *Social Science and Medicine,* 1971, *5,* 95-100.

Schmidt, F. L. "The Relevant Efficiency of Regression in Simple Unit Predictor Weights in Applied Differential Psychology." *Educational and Psychological Measurement,* 1971, *31,* 699-714.

Schmidt, R. L. "An Exploratory Study of Nursing and Patient Readiness for Surgery." Unpublished master's thesis, School of Nursing, Yale University, 1966.

Schmitt, F. E., and Wooldridge, P. J. "Psychological Preparation of Surgical Patients." *Nursing Research,* 1973, *22,* 108-116.

Schmitt, N., and Levine, R. L. "Statistical and Subjective Weights: Some Problems and Proposals." *Organizational Behavior and Human Performance,* 1977, *20,* 15-30.

Schneider, J. M., Werner, D., and Kagan, N. "The Development of a Measure of Empathy: The Affective Sensitivity Scale." Paper presented at annual meeting of the American Psychological Association Convention, San Francisco, August 1977.

Schneider, W., and Shiffrin, R. M. "Controlled and Automatic Human Information Processing: I. Detection, Search, and Attention." *Psychological Review,* 1977, *84,* 1-66.

Schoenberg, B., and Carr, A. C. "Loss of External Organs: Limb Amputation, Mastectomy and Disfiguration." In B. Schoenberg, A. C. Carr, D. Peretz, and A. H. Kutscher (Eds.), *Loss and Grief: Psychological Management in Medical Practice.* New York: Columbia University Press, 1970.

Schoenberg, B., Carr, A. C., Peretz, D., and Kutscher, A. H. (Eds.). *Loss and Grief: Psychological Management in Medical Practice.* New York: Columbia University Press, 1970.

Schoenfield, J. "Psychological Factors Related to Delayed Return to an Earlier Life-Style in Successfully Treated Cancer Patients." *Journal of Psychosomatic Research,* 1972, *16,* 41-46.

Schofield, W. "Standards for Clinical Psychology: Origins and Evaluation." In L. Blank and H. P. David (Eds.), *Sourcebook for Training in Clinical Psychology.* New York: Springer, 1964.

Schofield, W. "The Role of Psychology in the Delivery of Health Services." *American Psychologist,* 1969, *24,* 565-584.

Schofield, W. "The Psychologist as a Health Care Professional." *Intellect,* January 1975, pp. 255-258.

Schofield, W. "The Psychologist as a Health Professional." *Professional Psychology,* 1976, *7,* 5-8.

Schoolman, H. M., and Bernstein, L. M. "Computer Use in Diagnosis, Prognosis and Therapy." *Science,* 1978, *200,* 926-931.

Schottenfeld, D., and Robbins, G. F. "Quality of Survival Among Patients Who Have Had Radical Mastectomy." *Cancer,* 1970, *26,* 650-654.

Schowalter, J. E. "The Child's Reaction to His Own Terminal Illness." In B. Schoenberg, A. C Carr, D. Peretz, and A. H. Kutscher (Eds.), *Loss and Grief: Psychological Management in Medical Practice.* New York: Columbia University Press, 1970.

Schulman, B. "Patient Participation in Treatment for Hypertension." Unpublished doctoral dissertation, University of Michigan, 1977.

Schulz, R. "Effects of Control and Predictability on the Physical and Psychological Well Being of the Institutionalized Aged." *Journal of Personality and Social Psychology,* 1976, *33,* 563-573.

Schulz, R., and Hanusa, B. M. "Long-Term Effects of Control and Predictability Enhancing Interventions: Findings and Ethical Issues." *Journal of Personality and Social Psychology,* 1978, *36,* 1194-1201.

Schumacher, C. F. "Personal Characteristics of Students Choosing Different Types of Medical Careers." *Journal of Medical Education,* 1964, *39,* 278-288.

Schuman, S. "Patterns of Urban Heat-Wave Deaths and Implications for Prevention: Data from New York and St. Louis During July 1966." *Environmental Research,* 1972, *5,* 59-75.

Schwartz, G. E. "Toward a Theory of Voluntary Control of Response Patterns in the Cardiovascular System." In P. A. Obrist, A. H. Black, J. Brener, and L. V. DiCara (Eds.), *Cardiovascular Psychophysiology.* Chicago: Aldine, 1974.

Schwartz, G. E. "Biofeedback, Self-Regulation, and the Patterning of Physiological Processes." *American Scientist*, 1975, *63*, 314-324.

Schwartz, G. E. "Self-Regulation of Response Patterning: Implications for Psychophysiological Research and Therapy." *Biofeedback and Self-Regulation*, 1976, *1*, 7-30.

Schwartz, G. E. "Biofeedback and Physiological Patterning in Human Emotion and Consciousness." In J. Beatty and H. Legewie (Eds.), *Biofeedback and Behavior*. New York: Plenum Press, 1977a.

Schwartz, G. E. "Biofeedback and the Self-Management of Disregulation Disorders." In R. B. Stuart (Ed.), *Behavioral Self-Management: Strategies, Techniques, and Outcome*. New York: Brunner/Mazel, 1977b.

Schwartz, G. E. "Psychosomatic Disorders and Biofeedback: A Psychobiological Model of Disregulation." In J. D. Maser and M. E. Seligman (Eds.), *Psychopathology: Experimental Models*. San Francisco: W. H. Freeman, 1977c.

Schwartz, G. E. "Psychobiological Foundations of Psychotherapy and Behavior Change." In S. L. Garfield and A. E. Bergin (Eds.), *Handbook of Psychotherapy and Behavior Change*. (2nd ed.) New York: Wiley, 1978.

Schwartz, G. E. "Disregulation and Systems Theory: A Biobehavioral Framework for Biofeedback and Behavioral Medicine." In N. Birbaumer and H. D. Kimmel (Eds.), *Biofeedback and Self-Regulation*. Hillsdale, N.J.: Lawrence Erlbaum, 1979.

Schwartz, G. E., and Beatty, J. (Eds.). *Biofeedback: Theory and Research*. New York: Academic Press, 1977.

Schwartz, G. E., Davidson, R. J., and Maer, F. "Right Hemisphere Lateralization for Emotion in the Human Brain: Interaction with Cognition." *Science*, 1975, *190*, 286-288.

Schwartz, G. E., and Johnson, H. J. "Affective Visual Stimuli as Operant Reinforcers of the GSR." *Journal of Experimental Psychology*, 1969, *80*, 28-32.

Schwartz, G. E., Shapiro, A. P., Ferguson, D. C. E., Redmond, D. P., and Weiss, S. M. "Behavioral and Biological Approaches to Hypertension: An Integrative Analysis of Theory and Research." Submitted for publication, 1978.

Schwartz, G. E., and Weiss, S. M. "What Is Behavioral Medicine?" *Psychosomatic Medicine*, 1977, *39*, 377-381.

Schwartz, G. E., and Weiss, S. M. (Eds.). "Proceedings of the Yale Conference on Behavioral Medicine." *Journal of Behavioral Medicine*, 1978, *1*, 3-12.

Schwartz, M. "The Role of the Pharmacist in the Patient-Health Team Relationship." In L. Lasagna (Ed.), *Patient Compliance*. Mt. Kisco, N.Y.: Futura, 1976.

Schwartz, R. "Follow-Up by Phone or by Mail." *Evaluation*, 1973, *1*, 25-26.

Schwartz, R. S. "Another Look at Immunologic Surveillance." *New England Journal of Medicine*, 1975, *293*, 181-184.

Scotch, N. A. "Medical Anthropology." In *Biennial Review of Anthropology*. Stanford, Calif.: Stanford University Press, 1963.

Sears, R. R. *Survey of Objective Studies of Psychoanalytic Concepts*. New York: Social Science Research Council, 1943.

Sechrest, L. "The Psychologist as a Program Evaluator." In P. J. Woods (Ed.), *Career Opportunities for Psychologists: Expanding and Emerging Areas*. Washington, D.C.: American Psychological Association, 1976.

Sechrest, L. "Methodological Problems in the Use of Health Status Indicators." Paper presented at annual meeting of the American Psychological Association, San Francisco, August 1977.

Sechrest, L., and Sukstorf, S. "Parental Visitation of the Institutionalized Retarded." *Journal of Applied Social Psychology*, 1977, *7*, 286-294.

Second Conference on Psychophysiological Aspects of Cancer. *Annals of the New York Academy of Sciences*, 1969, *164* (Art. 2).

Seeman, M. "On the Meaning of Alienation." *American Sociological Review*, 1959, *24*, 783-791.

Seeman, M., and Evans, J. "Alienation and Learning in a Hospital Setting." *American Sociological Review*, 1962, *27*, 772-783.

Segal, A. "The Sick-Role Concept: Understanding Illness Behavior." *Journal of Health and Social Behavior*, 1976, *17*, 162-169.

Seligman, M. E. "On the Generality of the Laws of Learning." *Psychological Review*, 1970, *77*, 406-418.

Seligman, M. E. *Helplessness*. San Francisco: W. H. Freeman, 1975.

Selltiz, C., Wrightsman, L. S., and Cook, S. W. *Research Methods in Social Relations*. (3rd ed.) New York: Holt, Rinehart and Winston, 1976.

Selvidge, J. "A Three-Step Procedure for Assigning Probabilities to Rare Events." In D. Wendt and C. A. J. Vlek (Eds.), *Utility, Probability, and Human Decision Making*. Dordrecht, The Netherlands: Reidel, 1975.

Selvin, H. "Durkheim's *Suicide*: Further Thoughts on a Methodological Classic." In R. A. Nisbet (Ed.), *Emile Durkheim*. Englewood Cliffs, N.J.: Prentice-Hall, 1965.

Selye, H. *The Stress of Life*. New York: McGraw-Hill, 1956.

Selye, H. "The Evolution of the Stress Concept—Stress and Cardiovascular Disease." In L. Levi (Ed.), *Society, Stress, and Disease*. Vol. 1. London: Oxford University Press, 1971.

Selye, H. *Stress Without Distress*. Philadelphia: Lippincott, 1974.

Selye, H. "Confusion and Controversy in the Stress Field." *Journal of Human Stress*, 1975, *1* (2), 37-44.

Selye, H. *The Stress of Life*. (rev. ed.) New York: McGraw-Hill, 1976.

Sexton, D. L. "A Study of the Relation Between Adults' Health Beliefs, Knowledge of Illness, and Health Behaviors." *Dissertation Abstracts International*, 1974, *35* (1-A), 159.

Shands, H. C., Finesinger, J. E., Cobb, S., and Abrams, R. D. "Psychological Mechanisms in Patients with Cancer." *Cancer*, 1951, *4*, 1159-1170.

Shapiro, A. P., Schwartz, G. E., Ferguson, D. C. E., Redmond, D. P., and

Weiss, S. M. "Behavioral Methods in the Treatment of Hypertension." *Annals of Internal Medicine,* 1977, *86,* 626-636.

Shapiro, D. *Neurotic Styles.* New York: Basic Books, 1965.

Shapiro, D., and Surwit, R. S. "Operant Conditioning: A New Theoretical Approach in Psychosomatic Medicine." *International Journal of Psychiatry in Medicine,* 1974, *5* (4), 377-387.

Sharpe, T., and Mikeal, R. "Patient Compliance with Prescription Medication Regimens." *Journal of the American Pharmacy Association,* 1975, *15,* 191-197.

Shaver, K. G. *An Introduction to Attribution Processes.* Cambridge, Mass.: Winthrop, 1975.

Shaw, M. E. *Group Dynamics.* New York: McGraw-Hill, 1971.

Shaw, M. E., and Wright, J. M. *Scales for the Measurement of Attitudes.* New York: McGraw-Hill, 1967.

Shepard, D., and Moseley, T. "Mailed Versus Telephoned Appointment Reminders to Reduce Broken Appointments in a Hospital Outpatient Department." *Medical Care,* 1976, *14,* 268-273.

Sherman, M. A. "An Evaluation of the Effectiveness of Mobile Intensive Care Units in Reducing Deaths Due to Myocardial Infarction." Unpublished doctoral dissertation, Northwestern University, 1977.

Shiffrin, R. M., and Schneider, W. "Controlled and Automatic Human Information Processing: II. Perceptual Learning, Automatic Attending, and a General Theory." *Psychological Review,* 1977, *84,* 127-190.

Shore, M. "Psychological Issues in Counseling the Genetically Handicapped." In C. Birch and P. Abrecht (Eds.), *Genetics and the Quality of Life.* Oxford, England: Pergamon Press, 1975.

Short, M. J., and Wilson, W. P. "Roles of Denial in Chronic Hemodialysis." *Archives of General Psychiatry,* 1969, *20,* 433-437.

Shortliffe, E. H. *Computer-Based Medical Consultations: MYCIN.* New York: American Elsevier, 1976.

Shulman, L. S., and Elstein, A. S. "Studies of Problem Solving, Judgment, and Decision Making: Implications for Educational Research." In F. N. Kerlinger (Ed.), *Review of Research in Education.* Itasca, Ill.: Peacock, 1975.

Shuval, J. T. "Sex Role Differentiation in the Professions: The Case of Israeli Dentists." *Journal of Health and Social Behavior,* 1970, *11,* 236-244.

Sibinga, M. S., and Friedman, C. J. "Complexities of Parental Understanding of Phenlketonuria." *Pediatrics,* 1971, *48* (2), 216-224.

Siegel, E., Thomas, D., Coulter, E., Tuthill, R., and Chipman, S. "Continuation of Contraception by Low-Income Women: A One Year Follow-Up." *American Journal of Public Health,* 1971, *61,* 1886-1898.

Sigerist, H. E. *Medicine and Human Welfare.* New Haven, Conn.: Yale University Press, 1941.

Sigerist, H. E. *A History of Medicine.* New York: Oxford University Press, 1951 (Vol. 1), 1961 (Vol. 2).

Silverman, S. *Psychological Aspects of Physical Illness: A Dynamic Study of*

Forty-Five Hospitalized Medical Patients. New York: Appleton-Century-Crofts, 1968.

Sime, A. M. "Relationship of Preoperative Fear, Type of Coping, and Information Received About Surgery to Recovery from Surgery." *Journal of Personality and Social Psychology,* 1976, *34,* 716-724.

Simmons, A. J., and Gross, A. E. "Animistic Responses as a Function of Sentence Context and Instruction." *Journal of Genetic Psychology,* 1957, *91,* 181-189.

Simon, H. A. *Models of Man.* New York: Wiley, 1957.

Simon, H. J. "Mortality Among Medical Students. 1947-1967." *Journal of Medical Education,* 1968, *43,* 1175-1182.

Simon, R., and Paredes, H. *Understanding Human Behavior in Health and Disease.* Baltimore: Waverly, 1977.

Simonton, O. C., and Simonton, S. S. "Belief Systems and Management of the Emotional Aspects of Malignancy." *Journal of Transpersonal Psychology,* 1975, *7,* 29-47.

Simpson, M. A. "Medical Student Evaluation in the Absence of Examinations." *Medical Education,* 1976, *10,* 22-26.

Simpson, M. T., Olewine, D. A., Jenkins, C. D., Ramsey, F. H., Zyzanski, S. J., Thomas, G., and Hames, C. G. "Exercise-Induced Catecholamines and Platelet Aggregation in the Coronary-Prone Behavior Pattern." *Psychosomatic Medicine,* 1974, *36,* 476-487.

Sims, J. H., and Baumann, D. D. "The Tornado Threat: Coping Styles of the North and South." *Science,* 1972, *176,* 1386-1392.

Singer, M. T. "Engagement-Involvement: A Central Phenomenon in Psychophysiological Research." *Psychosomatic Medicine,* 1974, *36,* 1-17.

Sisson, J. C., Schoomaker, E. B., and Ross, J. C. "Clinical Decision Analyses —The Hazard of Using Additional Data." *Journal of the American Medical Association,* 1976, *236,* 1259-1263.

Sjöbäck, H. *The Psychoanalytic Theory of Defensive Processes.* New York: Wiley, 1973.

Slawson, P. F. "Group Psychotherapy with Obese Women." *Psychosomatics,* 1965, *6,* 206-209.

Slovic, P., Fischhoff, B., and Lichtenstein, S. "Behavioral Decision Theory." *Annual Review of Psychology,* 1977, *28,* 1-39.

Slovic, P., and Lichtenstein, S. "Comparison of Bayesian and Regression Approaches to the Study of Information-Processing Judgment." *Organizational Behavior and Human Performance,* 1971, *6,* 649-744.

Slovic, P., Rorer, L. G., and Hoffman, P. J. "Analyzing Use of Diagnostic Signs." *Investigative Radiology,* 1971, *6,* 18-26.

Smedslund, J. "The Concept of Correlation in Adults." *Scandinavian Journal of Psychology,* 1963, *4,* 165-173.

Smith, E. E., Shoben, E. J., and Rips, L. J. "Structure and Process in Semantic Memory: A Featural Model for Semantic Decisions." *Psychological Review,* 1974, *81,* 214-241.

Smith, L. S. "An Investigation of Pre- and Postsurgical Anxiety as a Function of Relaxation Training." Unpublished doctoral dissertation, University of Southern Mississippi, 1974.

Smith, T. "Factors Involving Sociocultural Incongruity and Change: A Review of Empirical Findings." In S. L. Syme and L. G. Reeder (Eds.), "Social Stress and Cardiovascular Disease." *Milbank Memorial Fund Quarterly,* 1967, *45* (2), 23-39.

Snyder, M. "Social Psychological Perspectives on the Physician's Feelings and Behavior." Paper presented at annual meeting of the American Psychological Association, San Francisco, August 1977.

Sobell, M. B., and Sobell, L. C. "Individualized Behavior Therapy for Alcoholics: Rationale, Procedures, Preliminary Results, and Appendix." In *California Mental Health Research Monograph No. 13.* Sacramento, Calif.: Department of Mental Hygiene, 1972.

Sobell, M. B., and Sobell, L. C. "Alcoholics Treated by Individualized Behavior Therapy: One-Year Treatment Outcome." *Behavior Research and Therapy,* 1973, *11,* 599-618.

Sogin, S., and Pallek, M. "Bad Decisions, Responsibility, and Attitude Change: Effects of Volition, Foreseeability, and Locus of Causality of Negative Consequences." *Journal of Personality and Social Psychology,* 1976, *33,* 300-306.

Solomon, A. J. "The Effect of a Psychotherapeutic Interview on the Physical Results of Thoracic Surgery." Unpublished doctoral dissertation, California School of Professional Psychology, San Francisco, 1973.

Solomon, G. F. "Discussion. Emotions and Immunity." *Annals of the New York Academy of Sciences,* 1969a, *164* (Art. 2), 461-462.

Solomon, G. F. "Emotions, Stress, the Central Nervous System, and Immunity." *Annals of the New York Academy of Sciences,* 1969b, *164* (Art. 2), 335-343.

Somers, H., and Somers, A. *Doctors, Patients, and Health Insurance: Organization and Financing of Medical Care.* Washington, D.C.: The Brookings Institution, 1961.

Sommer, R. *Design Awareness.* New York: Rinehart Press, 1972.

Sommers, A. R. (Ed.). *Promoting Health.* Germantown, Md.: Aspen Systems Corporation, 1976.

Sorenson, J. "Genetic Counseling: Some Psychological Considerations." In M. Lipkin and D. Duncombe (Eds.), *Genetic Responsibility.* New York: Plenum Press, 1972.

Sorkin, A. L. *Health Economics: An Introduction.* Lexington, Mass.: Lexington Books, 1975.

Southam, C. M. "Discussion. Emotions, Immunology, and Cancer: How Might the Psyche Influence Neoplasia?" *Annals of the New York Academy of Sciences,* 1969, *164* (Art. 2), 473-475.

Southard, E. E. "Psychopathology and Neuropathology: The Problems of Teaching and Research Contrasted." *Journal of the American Medical Association,* 1912, *53,* 914-916.

Spark, R. "The Case Against Regular Physicals." *New York Times Magazine,* July 25, 1976, pp. 10-11 and 38-41.

Speisman, J. C., Lazarus, R. S., Mordkoff, A., and Davison, L. "Experimental Reduction of Stress Based on Ego-Defense Theory." *Journal of Abnormal and Social Psychology,* 1964, *68,* 367-380.

Spilken, A. Z., and Jacobs, M. A. "Prediction of Illness Behavior from Measures of Life Crisis, Manifest Distress, and Maladaptive Coping." *Psychosomatic Medicine,* 1971, *33,* 251-264.

Spitz, R. A. "Hospitalism: An Inquiry into the Genesis of Psychiatric Conditions in Early Childhood." *Psychoanalytic Study of the Child,* 1945, *1,* 53-74.

Spitz, R. A. "Anaclitic Depression: An Inquiry into the Genesis of Psychiatric Conditions in Early Childhood, II." *Psychoanalytic Study of the Child,* 1946, *2,* 313-342.

Spivack, J. S., and Kagan, N. "Laboratory to Classroom—The Practical Application of IPR in a Master's Level Pre-Practicum Counselor Education Program." *Counselor Education and Supervision,* 1972, *12,* 3-15.

Spriesterbach, D. C., and Farrell, W. J. "Impact of Federal Regulations at a University." *Science,* 1977, *198,* 27-30.

Stahl, S. M., Lawrie, T., Neill, P., and Kelley, C. "Motivational Interventions in Community Hypertension Screening." *American Journal of Public Health,* 1977, *67,* 345-352.

Standard, S., and Nathan, H. *Should the Patient Know the Truth?* New York: Springer, 1955.

Statistical Abstracts of the United States. 97th Annual Edition. Washington, D.C.: Bureau of the Census, U.S. Department of Commerce, 1976.

Staub, E., and Kellett, D. "Increasing Pain Tolerance by Information About Aversive Stimuli." *Journal of Personality and Social Psychology,* 1972, *21,* 198-208.

Staub, E., Tursky, B., and Schwartz, G. E. "Self-Control and Predictability: Their Effects on Reactions to Aversive Stimulation." *Journal of Personality and Social Psychology,* 1971, *18,* 157-162.

Stavraky, K. M., and others. "Psychological Factors in the Outcome of Human Cancer." *Journal of Psychosomatic Research,* 1968, *12,* 251-259.

Steele, F. *Physical Settings and Organization Development.* Reading, Mass.: Addison-Wesley, 1973.

Stefflre, B. (Ed.). *Theories of Counseling.* New York: McGraw-Hill, 1965.

Stein, H. F. "Commentary on Kleinman's 'Lessons from a Clinical Approach to Medical Anthropological Research.'" *Medical Anthropology Newsletter,* 1977, *8* (4), 15-16.

Stein, M., Schiavi, R. C., and Camerino, M. "Influence of Brain and Behavior on the Immune System." *Science,* 1976, *191,* 435-440.

Steiner, I. D. *Group Process and Productivity.* New York: Academic Press, 1972.

Stekel, S., and Swain, M. "The Use of Written Contracts to Increase Adherence." *Hospitals,* 1977, *51,* 81-84.

Stephens, G. G. *National Task Force on Training Family Practice Physicians in Patient Education: Final Report.* Washington, D.C.: Bureau of Health Manpower, Health Resources Administration, and National High Blood Pressure Education Program, National Institutes of Health, 1978.

Stephenson, J. H., and Grace, W. J. "Life Stress and Cancer of the Cervix." *Psychosomatic Medicine,* 1954, *16,* 287-294.

Steppacher, R. C., and Mausner, J. S. "Suicide in Male and Female Physicians." *Journal of the American Medical Association,* 1974, *228* (3), 323-328.

Stern, M., Farquhar, J. M., Maccoby, N., and Russell, S. H. "Results of a Two-Year Health Education Campaign on Dietary Behavior." *Circulation,* 1976, *54,* 826-833.

Sternbach, R. A. *Pain: A Psychophysiological Analysis.* New York: Academic Press, 1968.

Steward, M., and Regalbuto, B. A. "Do Doctors Know What Children Know?" *American Journal of Orthopsychiatry,* 1975, *45,* 146-149.

Stewart, A. L., Ware, J. E., Jr., and Brook, R. H. *A Study of the Reliability, Validity, and Precision of Scales to Measure Chronic Functional Limitations Due to Poor Health.* Rand Paper Series, P5660. Santa Monica, Calif.: Rand Corporation, 1977.

Stimson, G. "Obeying Doctors' Orders: A View from the Other Side." *Social Science and Medicine,* 1974, *8,* 97-104.

Stimson, G. "Doctor-Patient Interaction and Some Problems for Prescribing." *Journal of the Royal College of General Practitioners,* 1976, *26,* 712-718.

Stokols, D. "The Experience of Crowding in Primary and Secondary Environments." *Environment and Behavior,* 1976, *8,* 49-86.

Stokols, D. (Ed.). *Perspectives on Environment and Behavior.* New York: Plenum Press, 1977.

Stone, G. C. "Patient Compliance and the Role of the Expert." *Journal of Social Issues,* in press.

Stone, G. C., Carlton, P. L., Gentry, W. D., Matarazzo, J. D., Pattishall, E. G., and Wakely, J. H. "Teaching Psychology to Medical Students." *Teaching Psychology,* 1977, *4,* 111-115.

Stone, R. A., and DeLeo, J. D. "Psychotherapeutic Control of Hypertension." *New England Journal of Medicine,* 1976, *294,* 80-84.

Storms, M., and Nisbett, R. "Insomnia and the Attributional Process." *Journal of Personality and Social Psychology,* 1970, *16,* 319-328.

Stoyva, J. "Why Should Muscular Relaxation Be Clinically Useful? Some Data and 2-1/2 Models." In J. Beatty and H. Legewie (Eds.), *Biofeedback and Behavior.* New York: Plenum Press, 1977.

Straus, R. "The Nature and Status of Medical Sociology." *American Sociological Review,* 1957, *22,* 200-204.

Strauss, A. *Chronic Illness and the Quality of Life.* St. Louis, Mo.: Mosby, 1975.

Strickland, S. *Politics, Science, and Dread Disease.* Cambridge, Mass.: Harvard University Press, 1972.

Stuart, R. B. "Behavioral Control of Overeating." *Behavior Research and Therapy,* 1967, *5,* 357-365.

Stuart, R. B. (Ed.). *Behavioral Self-Management: Strategies, Techniques, and Outcome.* New York: Brunner/Mazel, 1977.

Stuart, R. B., and Davis, B. *Slim Chance in a Fat World: Behavioral Control of Obesity.* Champaign, Ill.: Research Press, 1972.

Stunkard, A. J. "New Therapies for the Eating Disorders: Behavior Modification of Obesity and Anorexia Nervosa." *Archives of General Psychiatry,* 1972, *26,* 391-398.

Stunkard, A. J. "Behavioral Treatment of Obesity: Failure to Maintain Weight Loss." In R. B. Stuart (Ed.), *Behavioral Self-Management: Strategies, Techniques, and Outcome.* New York: Brunner/Mazel, 1977a.

Stunkard, A. J. "Testimony Before Select Committee on Nutrition and Human Needs: Part II. Obesity." Washington, D.C.: U.S. Government Printing Office, 1977b.

Stunkard, A. J., and McClaren-Hume, M. "The Results of Treatment of Obesity: A Review of the Literature and Report of a Series." *Archives of Internal Medicine,* 1959, *103,* 79-85.

Stunkard, A. J., and Rush, J. "Dieting and Depression Reexamined." *Annals of Internal Medicine,* 1974, *81,* 526-533.

Suchman, E. "Sociomedical Variations Among Ethnic Groups." *American Journal of Sociology,* 1964, *70,* 319-331.

Suchman, E. "Social Patterns of Illness and Medical Care." *Journal of Health and Social Behavior,* 1965, *6,* 2-16.

Suchman, E. "Health Orientation and Medical Care." *American Journal of Public Health,* 1966, *56,* 97-105.

Suchman, E. "Preventive Health Behavior: A Model for Research on Community Health Campaigns." *Journal of Health and Social Behavior,* 1967, *8,* 197-209.

Sundberg, N. D. *Assessment of Persons.* Englewood Cliffs, N.J.: Prentice-Hall, 1977.

Sundberg, N. D., and Tyler, L. E. *Clinical Psychology: An Introduction to Theory and Practice.* New York: Appleton-Century-Crofts, 1962.

Sundstrom, E. "An Experimental Study of Crowding: Effects of Room Size, Intrusion, and Goal Blocking on Non-Verbal Behavior, Self-Disclosure, and Self-Reported Stress." *Journal of Personality and Social Psychology,* 1975, *32,* 645-654.

Super, D. E. "The Dimensions and Measurement of Vocational Maturity." *Teachers College Record,* 1955a, *57,* 151-163.

Super, D. E. "Transition: From Vocational Guidance to Counseling Psychology." *Journal of Counseling Psychology,* 1955b, *2,* 3-9.

Surman, O. S., Hackett, T. P., Silverberg, E. L., and Behrendt, D. M. "Usefulness of Psychiatric Intervention in Patients Undergoing Cardiac Surgery."
Archives of General Psychiatry, 1974, *30,* 830-835.

Susser, M. "Epidemiological Models." In E. L. Struening and M. Guttentag
(Eds.), *Handbook of Evaluation Research.* Beverly Hills, Calif.: Sage,
1975.

Sutherland, A. M. "Psychological Observations in Cancer Patients." *International Psychiatry Clinics,* 1967, *4,* 75-92.

Sutherland, A. M., Orbach, C. E., Dyk, R. B., and Bard, M. "The Psychological Impact of Cancer and Cancer Surgery: I. Adaptation to Dry Colostomy; Preliminary Report and Summary of Findings." *Cancer,* 1952, *5,*
857-872.

Svarstad, B. "Physician-Patient Communication and Patient Conformity with
Medical Advice." In D. Mechanic, *The Growth of Bureaucratic Medicine.*
New York: Wiley, 1976.

Swigar, M. E. "Interview Follow-Up of Abortion Applicant Dropouts." *Social Psychiatry,* 1976, *11,* 135-143.

Swinehart, J. "Voluntary Exposure to Health Communications." *American
Journal of Public Health,* 1968, *58,* 1265-1275.

Syme, S. L. "Implications and Future Prospects." In S. L. Syme and L. G.
Reeder (Eds.), "Social Stress and Cardiovascular Disease." *Milbank
Memorial Fund Quarterly,* 1967, *45* (2), 175-180.

Syme, S. L. "Social and Psychological Risk Factors in Coronary Heart Disease." *Modern Concepts of Cardiovascular Diseases,* 1975, *14,* 17-21.

Szasz, T. S. "The Role of the Counterphobic Mechanism in Addiction."
American Psychoanalytic Association Journal, 1958, *6,* 309-325.

Szasz, T. S., and Hollender, M. H. "A Contribution to the Philosophy of
Medicine: The Basic Models of the Doctor-Patient Relationship." *Archives
of Internal Medicine,* 1956, *97,* 585-592.

Szklo, M., Tonascia, J., and Gordis, L. "Psychosocial Factors and the Risk of
Myocardial Infarctions in White Women." *American Journal of Epidemiology,* 1976, *103,* 312-320.

Tagliacozzo, D., and Ima, K. "Knowledge of Illness as a Predictor of Patient
Behavior." *Journal of Chronic Diseases,* 1970, *22,* 765-775.

Tagliacozzo, D., Ima, K., and Lashof, J. C. "Influencing the Chronically Ill:
The Role of Prescriptions in Premature Separations of Outpatient Care."
Medical Care, 1973, *11,* 21-29.

Tagliacozzo, D., Luskin, D. B., Lashof, J. C., and Ima, K. "Nurse Intervention and Patient Behavior: An Experimental Study." *American Journal of
Public Health,* 1974, *64,* 596-603.

Taylor, C. *In Horizontal Orbit: Hospitals and the Cult of Efficiency.* New
York: Holt, Rinehart and Winston, 1970.

Taylor, D. W. "Health Beliefs and Compliance with Antihypertensive Regimens." In R. B. Haynes, D. W. Taylor, and D. L. Sackett (Eds.), *Compliance with Preventive and Therapeutic Regimens.* Baltimore: Johns Hopkins University Press, in press.

Taylor, D. W., Berry, P. C., and Block, C. H. "Does Group Participation When Using Brainstorming Facilitate or Inhibit Creative Thinking?" *Administrative Science Quarterly,* 1958, *3,* 23-47.

Taylor, S., and Levin, S. "The Psychological Impact of Breast Cancer: Theory and Practice." In A. J. Enelow and D. M. Panagis (Eds.), *Psychological Aspects of Breast Cancer.* Technical Bulletin No. 1. San Francisco: West Coast Cancer Foundation, 1977.

Tedeschi, J. T. "Attributions, Liking, and Power." In T. Huston (Eds.), *Foundations of Interpersonal Attraction.* New York: Academic Press, 1974.

Tesser, A., and Rosen, S. "The Reluctance to Transmit Bad News." In L. Berkowitz (Ed.), *Advances in Experimental Social Psychology.* New York: Academic Press, 1975.

Tessler, R., Mechanic, D., and Dimond, M. "The Effect of Psychological Distress on Physician Utilization: A Prospective Study." *Journal of Health and Social Behavior,* 1976, *17,* 353-364.

Theorell, T. "Life Events Before and After the Onset of a Premature Myocardial Infarction." In B. S. Dohrenwend and B. P. Dohrenwend (Eds.), *Stressful Life Events: Their Nature and Effects.* New York: Wiley, 1974.

Theorell, T., Lind, E., and Flodérus, B. "The Relationship of Disturbing Life Changes and Emotions to the Early Development of Myocardial Infarction and Other Serious Illnesses." *International Journal of Epidemiology,* 1975, *4,* 281-293.

Theorell, T., and Rahe, R. H. "Behavior and Life Satisfactions Characteristics of Swedish Subjects with Myocardial Infarction." *Journal of Chronic Diseases,* 1972, *25,* 139-147.

Thomas, C. B. "What Becomes of Medical Students: The Dark Side." *Johns Hopkins Medical Journal,* 1976, *136,* 185-195.

Thomas, C. B., and Greenstreet, R. L. "Psychobiological Characteristics in Youth as Predictors of Five Disease States: Suicide, Mental Illness, Hypertension, Coronary Heart Disease, and Tumor." *Johns Hopkins Medical Journal,* 1973, *132,* 16-43.

Thomas, C. B., and Murphy, E. A. "Further Studies on Cholesterol Levels in the Johns Hopkins Medical Students: The Effect of Stress at Examinations." *Journal of Chronic Diseases,* 1958, *8,* 661-668.

Thoresen, C. E., and Mahoney, M. J. *Behavioral Self-Control.* New York: Holt, Rinehart and Winston, 1974.

Thornbury, J. R., Fryback, D. G., and Edwards, W. "Likelihood Ratios as a Measure of the Diagnostic Usefulness of Excretory Urogram Information." *Radiology,* 1975, *114,* 561-565.

Thoroughman, J. C., Pascal, G. R., Jenkins, W. O., Crutcher, J. C., and Peoples, L. C. "Psychological Factors Predictive of Surgical Success in Patients with Intractable Duodenal Ulcer." *Psychosomatic Medicine,* 1964, *26,* 618-624.

Thurlow, H. J. "General Susceptibility to Illness: A Selective Review." *Canadian Medical Association Journal,* 1967, *97,* 1397-1404.

Titchener, J. L., and Kapp, F. T. "Family and Character Change at Buffalo Creek." *American Journal of Psychiatry,* 1976, *133,* 295-299.

Titchener, J. L., and Levine, M. *Surgery as a Human Experience.* New York: Oxford University Press, 1960.

Toomey, M. "Conflict Theory Approach to Decision Making Applied to Alcoholics." *Journal of Personality and Social Psychology,* 1972, *24,* 199-206.

Tornstam, L. "Health and Self-Perception: A Systems Theoretical Approach." *The Gerontologist,* 1975, *15,* 264-270.

Trice, H. M., and Roman, P. M. "Sociopsychological Predictors of Affiliation with Alcoholics Anonymous: A Longitudinal Study of Treatment Success." *Social Psychiatry,* 1970, *5,* 51-59.

Trice, H. M., Roman, P. M., and Belasco, J. A. "Selection for Treatment: A Predictive Evaluation of an Alcoholism Treatment Regimen." *International Journal of the Addictions,* 1969, *4,* 303-317.

Truax, C. B., and Mitchell, K. M. "Research on Certain Therapist Interpersonal Skills in Relation to Process and Outcome." In A. E. Bergin and S. L. Harfield (Eds.), *Handbook of Psychotherapy and Behavior Change.* New York: Wiley, 1971.

Tsushima, W. T. "Relationship Between the Mini-Mult and the MMPI with Medical Patients." *Journal of Clinical Psychology,* 1975, *31,* 673-675.

Tuch, R. H. "The Relationship Between a Mother's Menstrual Status and Her Response to Illness in Her Child." *Psychosomatic Medicine,* 1975, *37,* 388-394.

Tufo, H. M., and Ostfeld, A. M. "A Prospective Study of Open-Heart Surgery." *Psychosomatic Medicine,* 1968, *30,* 552-553.

Tulving, E., and Thomson, D. M. "Encoding Specificity and Retrieval Processes in Episodic Memory." *Psychological Review,* 1973, *80,* 352-373.

Turiel, E. "An Experimental Test of the Sequentiality of Developmental Stages in the Child's Moral Judgments." *Journal of Personality and Social Psychology,* 1966, *3,* 611-618.

Turk, D. C. "Cognitive Control of Pain: A Skills-Training Approach." Unpublished master's thesis, University of Waterloo, Ontario, 1975.

Tversky, A., and Kahneman, D. "Availability: A Heuristic for Judging Frequency and Probability." *Cognitive Psychology,* 1973, *5,* 207-232.

Tversky, A., and Kahneman, D. "Judgment Under Uncertainty: Heuristics and Biases." *Science,* 1974, *185,* 1124-1131.

Twaddle, A. C. "Health Decisions and Sick Role Variations: An Exploration." *Journal of Health and Social Behavior,* 1969, *10,* 105-114.

Twaddle, A. C., and Hessler, R. M. *A Sociology of Health.* St. Louis, Mo.: Mosby, 1977.

Tyler, V. D., and Straughan, J. H. "Coverant Control and Breath Holding as Techniques for the Treatment of Obesity." *Psychological Record,* 1970, *20,* 473-478.

Udry, J. R., Clark, L. T., Chase, C. L., and Levy, M. "Can Mass Media Advertising Increase Contraceptive Use?" *Family Planning Perspectives*, 1972, *4* (3), 37-44.

U.S. Department of Agriculture. *Health Services in Rural America*. Agricultural Information Bulletin No. 362. Washington, D.C.: U.S. Department of Agriculture, Rural Development Service, 1974.

U.S. Department of Health, Education, and Welfare, Public Health Service. *Health Statistics from the U.S. National Health Survey: Dental Care, Interval and Frequency of Visits, United States, July 1947-June 1959*. PHS Publication No. 584-B14. Washington, D.C.: U.S. Government Printing Office, 1960a.

U.S. Department of Health, Education, and Welfare, Public Health Service. *Health Statistics from the U.S. National Health Survey: Volume of Physician Visits, United States, July 1957-June 1959*. PHS Publication No. 584-B19. Washington, D.C.: U.S. Government Printing Office, 1960b.

U.S. Department of Health, Education, and Welfare, Public Health Service. *Health Statistics from the U.S. National Health Survey: Hospital Discharges and Length of Stay, Short-Stay Hospitals, United States, 1958-1960*. PHS Publication No. 584-B32, Washington, D.C.: U.S. Government Printing Office, 1962.

U.S. Department of Health, Education, and Welfare, Public Health Service. *Forward Plan for Health. FY 1977-1981*. DHEW Publication No. (OS) 76-50046. Washington, D.C.: U.S. Government Printing Office, 1976.

U.S. Department of Health, Education, and Welfare, Public Health Service, Health Resources Administration. *Health of the Disadvantaged: Chart Book*. DHEW Publication No. 77-628. Hyattsville, Md.: U.S. Government Printing Office, 1977.

U.S. Office of the Federal Register. "Health Maintenance Organizations: Designation of Medically Underserved Areas and Population Groups." *Federal Register*, 1975, *40*, 40315-40320.

University of Minnesota, Division of Health Care Psychology. "Proposal for a Professional Degree Program Leading to the Doctor of Psychology Degree in Health Care Psychology." Health Sciences Center, University of Minnesota, 1975.

Vaillant, G. E. "Natural History of Male Psychological Health: V. The Relation of Choice of Ego Mechanisms of Defense to Adult Adjustment." *Archives of General Psychiatry*, 1976, *33*, 535-545.

Vaillant, G. E., Sobowale, N. C., and McArthur, C. "Some Psychologic Vulnerabilities of Physicians." *New England Journal of Medicine*, 1972, *287*, 372-375.

Venzmer, G. *Five Thousand Years of Medicine*. (Marion Koenig, trans.) New York: Taplinger, 1972.

Verbrugge, L. "Females and Illness: Recent Trends in Sex Differences in the United States." *Journal of Health and Social Behavior*, 1976, *17*, 387-403.

Vernier, C. M., Barrell, R. P., Cummings, J. W., Dickerson, J. H., and

Hooper, H. E. "Psychosocial Study of the Patient with Pulmonary Tuberculosis: A Cooperative Research Approach." *Psychological Monographs,* 1961, *75* (6), 1-32.

Vernon, D. T. A., and Bigelow, D. A. "Effect of Information About a Potentially Stressful Situation on Responses to Stress Impact." *Journal of Personality and Social Psychology,* 1974, *29,* 50-59.

Vetter, N. J., Cay, E. L., Philip, A. E., and Strange, R. C. "Anxiety on Admission to a Coronary Care Unit." *Journal of Psychosomatic Research,* 1977, *21,* 73-78.

Vincent, P. "Factors Influencing Patient Noncompliance: A Theoretical Approach." *Nursing Research,* 1971, *20,* 509-516.

Vinokur, A., and Selzer, M. L. "Desirable Versus Undesirable Life Events: Their Relationship to Stress and Mental Distress." *Journal of Personality and Social Psychology,* 1975, *32,* 329-337.

Vinsonhaler, J., Wagner, C., and Elstein, A. S. "The Inquiry Theory: An Information-Processing Approach to Clinical Problem Solving." In D. B. Shires and H. K. Wolf (Eds.), *MEDINFO, 1977: Proceedings of the Second World Conference on Medical Informatics.* Amsterdam: North-Holland, 1977.

Virgilio, J. V. "Occupational Hazards of Dentistry." *Dental Student,* 1971, *49,* 77-78.

Visotsky, H. M., Hamburg, D. A., Goss, M. E., and Lebovitz, B. A. "Coping Under Extreme Stress: Observations of Patients with Severe Poliomyelitis." *Archives of General Psychiatry,* 1961, *5,* 423-448.

Vladeck, B. C. "Discussion." In C. Lee Jones (Ed.), *National Health Planning Act: Potential for Information Service Activities: Proceedings of a Seminar.* New York: Columbia University, 1976.

Vladeck, B. C. "Interest Group Representation and the HSAs: Health Planning and Political Theory." *American Journal of Public Health,* 1977, *67,* 23-29.

Voegtlin, W. L., and Lemere, F. "The Treatment of Alcohol Addiction: A Review of the Literature." *Quarterly Journal of Studies on Alcohol,* 1942, *2,* 717-803.

Voeks, V. "Sources of Apparent Animism in Studies." *Scientific Monthly,* 1954, *79,* 406-407.

von Bertalanffy, L. *General Systems Theory.* New York: Braziller, 1968.

von Brauchitsch, H. "Physicians' Suicide." *Journal of Nervous and Mental Disease,* 1976, *162,* 40-45.

von Kugelgen, E. R. "Psychological Determinants of the Delay in Decision to Seek Aid in Cases of Myocardial Infarction." Unpublished doctoral dissertation, University of California, Berkeley, 1975.

von Mehring, O., and Kasdan, L. (Eds.). *Unity Amid Diversity: Anthropology and the Behavioral and Health Sciences.* Pittsburgh: University of Pittsburgh Press, 1970.

von Neumann, J., and Morgenstern, O. *Theory of Games and Economic Behavior.* Princeton, N.J.: Princeton University Press, 1947.

Wagner, N. N., and Stegeman, K. L. "Psychologists in Medical Education: 1964." *American Psychologist*, 1964, *19*, 689-690.

Wagner, R. *Probleme und Beispiele Biologischer Regulung*. Stuttgart: Thieme, 1954.

Wagner, S. *Cigarette Country: Tobacco in American History and Politics*. New York: Praeger, 1971.

Waitzkin, H. B., and Waterman, B. *The Exploitation of Illness in Capitalist Society*. New York: Bobbs-Merrill, 1974.

Wallgren, H., and Barry, H. *Actions of Alcohol*. Vol. 2. Amsterdam: Elsevier, 1970.

Wallsten, T. S. "Three Biases in the Cognitive Processing of Diagnostic Information." Unpublished paper, Psychometric Laboratory, University of North Carolina, Chapel Hill, 1978.

Wallston, B., Wallston, K. A., and Maides, S. "Development and Validation of the Health Locus of Control (HLC) Scale." *Journal of Consulting and Clinical Psychology*, 1976, *44*, 580-585.

Wallston, K. A., Maides, S., and Wallston, B. "Health-Related Information Seeking as a Function of Health-Related Locus of Control and Health Value." *Journal of Research in Personality*, 1976, *10*, 215-222.

Walseth, H. K. "Repression-Sensitization and Reactions to Surgery." Unpublished doctoral dissertation, University of Minnesota, 1968.

Walster, E. "Assignment of Responsibility for an Accident." *Journal of Personality and Social Psychology*, 1966, *3*, 73-79.

Walton, H. O., Ritson, E. B., and Kennedy, R. I. "Response of Alcoholics to Clinic Treatment." *British Medical Journal*, 1966, *2*, 1171-1174.

Wapner, S. "Organismic-Developmental Theory: Some Applications to Cognition." In J. Langer, P. Mussen, and M. Covington (Eds.), *Trends and Issues in Developmental Psychology*. New York: Holt, Rinehart and Winston, 1969.

Ward, R. A. *The Economics of Health Resources*. Reading, Mass.: Addison-Wesley, 1975.

Ware, J. E., Jr., Snyder, M. K., and Wright, W. R. *Development and Validation of Scales to Measure Patient Satisfaction with Health Care Services: Volume I of a Final Report*. Part A: Review of Literature, Overview of Methods, and Results Regarding Construction of Scales. Carbondale, Ill.: School of Medicine, Southern Illinois University, 1976a.

Ware, J. E., Jr., Snyder, M. K., and Wright, W. R. *Development and Validation of Scales to Measure Patient Satisfaction with Health Care Services: Volume I of a Final Report*. Part B: Results Regarding Scales Constructed from the Patient Satisfaction Questionnaire and Measures of Other Health Care Perceptions. Carbondale, Ill.: School of Medicine, Southern Illinois University, 1976b.

Ware, J. E., Jr., Young J., Snyder, M. K., and Wright, W. R. "The Measurement of Health as a Value: Preliminary Findings Regarding Scale Reliability, Validity, and Administration Procedures." U.S. National Technical Information Service, Department of Commerce, 1974.

Warfield, F. *Cotton in My Ears.* New York: Viking Press, 1948.

Warheit, G. J. "The Use of the Field Survey to Estimate Health Needs in the General Population." In R. A. Bell, M. Sundel, J. F. Aponte, and S. A. Murrel (Eds.), *Need Assessment in Health and Human Services: Proceedings of the Louisville National Conference,* University of Louisville, Louisville, Ky., March 9-12, 1976. (Expanded version to be published by Human Sciences Press, 1979.)

Waring, E. M. "Psychiatric Illness in Physicians: A Review." *Comprehensive Psychiatry,* 1974, *15,* 519-530.

Wason, P., and Johnson-Laird, P. *Psychology of Reasoning.* Cambridge, Mass.: Harvard University Press, 1972.

Waters, J. "Using the Family Environment Scale as an Instructional Aid for Studying the Family." Social Science Division, Gordon Junior College, Barnesville, Ga., 1976.

Watson, J. B. "Content of a Course in Psychology for Medical Students." *Journal of the American Medical Association,* 1912, *58,* 916-918.

Watson, J. B. "Psychology as the Behaviorist Views It." *Psychological Review,* 1913, *20,* 158-177.

Watson, R. I. "A Brief History of Clinical Psychology." *Psychological Bulletin,* 1953, *50,* 321-346.

Wayne, A. L., Montgomery, R. L., and Pettit, W. W. "A Cigarette Information Program." *Journal of the American Medical Association,* 1964, *188,* 872-874.

Webb, E., Campbell, D., Schwartz, R., and Sechrest, L. *Unobtrusive Measures: Nonreactive Research in the Social Sciences.* Chicago: Rand McNally, 1969.

Webster, T. G. "The Behavioral Sciences in Medical Education and Practice." In R. H. Coombs and E. V. Clark (Eds.), *Psychosocial Aspects of Medical Training.* Springfield, Ill.: Thomas, 1971.

Weidman, H. "Trained Manpower and Medical Anthropology: Conceptual Organizational and Educational Priorities." *Social Science and Medicine,* 1971, *5,* 15-36.

Weidman, H. "On Mitchell's 'Changing Others.'" *Medical Anthropology Newsletter,* 1977, *8* (3), 25-26.

Weinberg, G. M. *An Introduction to General Systems Thinking.* New York: Wiley, 1975.

Weiner, H. *Psychobiology and Human Disease.* New York: American Elsevier, 1977.

Weiner, I. W. "Psychological Factors Related to Results of Subtotal Gastrectomy." *Psychosomatic Medicine,* 1956, *18,* 486-491.

Weinstein, P., and Gipple, C. "Some Determinants of Career Choice in the Second Year of Medical School." *Journal of Medical Education,* 1975, *50,* 194-198.

Weisbrod, B. A. *Economics of Public Health.* Philadelphia: University of Pennsylvania Press, 1961.

Weisenberg, M. "The Role of Psychology in the Delivery of Health Services." *American Psychologist,* 1970, *25,* 472.

Weisenberg, M. (Ed.). *Pain: Clinical and Experimental Perspectives.* St. Louis, Mo.: Mosby, 1975.

Weisenberg, M. "Pain and Pain Control." *Psychological Bulletin,* 1977, *84,* 1008-1044.

Weisman, A. D. *On Dying and Denying: A Psychiatric Study of Terminality.* New York: Behavioral Publications, 1972.

Weisman, A. D. "Early Diagnosis of Vulnerability in Cancer Patients." *American Journal of the Medical Sciences,* 1976, *27,* 187-196.

Weisman, A. D., and Hackett, T. P. "Denial as a Social Act." In S. Levin and R. Kahana (Eds.), *Psychodynamic Studies of Aging: Creativity, Reminiscing, and Dying.* New York: International Universities Press, 1967.

Weisman, A. D., and Worden, J. W. "The Existential Plight in Cancer: Significance of the First 100 Days." *International Journal of Psychiatry in Medicine,* 1976-1977, *7,* 1-15.

Weisman, A. D., and Worden, J. W. "Coping and Vulnerability in Cancer Patients." Unpublished research report, Project Omega, Department of Psychiatry, Harvard Medical School, Massachusetts General Hospital, 1977.

Weiss, A. R. "A Behavioral Approach to the Treatment of Adolescent Obesity." *Behavior Therapy,* 1977, *8,* 720-726.

Weiss, D. W. "Discussion." *Annals of the New York Academy of Sciences,* 1969, *164* (Art. 2), 427-429.

Weiss, J. M. "Somatic Effects of Predictable and Unpredictable Shock." *Psychosomatic Medicine,* 1970, *32,* 397-409.

Weiss, R. S. *Marital Separation.* New York: Basic Books, 1975.

Weiss, S. A., Fishman, S., and Krause, F. "Symbolic Impulsivity, the Bender-Gestalt Test, and Prosthetic Adjustment in Amputees." *Archives of Physical Medicine,* 1970, *51,* 152-158.

Weiss, S. M. (Ed.). *Proceedings of the National Heart and Lung Institute Working Conference of Health Behavior.* DHEW Publication No. (NIH) 76-868. Washington, D.C.: U.S. Government Printing Office, 1975.

Weizenbaum, J. "ELIZA: A Computer Program for the Study of Natural Language Communication Between Man and Machine." *Communications of the Association for Computing Machinery,* 1965, *9,* 36-45.

Weizenbaum, J. *Computer Power and Human Reasoning.* San Francisco: W. H. Freeman, 1976.

Weller, G. R. "From 'Pressure Group Politics' to 'Medical-Industrial Complex': The Development of Approaches to the Politics of Health." *Journal of Health Politics, Policy, and Law,* 1976-1977, *1,* 444-470.

Wells, F. L., and Ruesch, J. *Mental Examiners' Handbook.* New York: Psychological Corporation, 1969.

Werner, A., and Schneider, J. M. "Teaching Medical Students Interactional Skills: Research-Based Course in the Doctor-Patient Relationship." *New England Journal of Medicine,* 1974, *290,* 1232-1237.

Werner, H. *Comparative Psychology of Mental Development.* New York: Science Editions, 1948.

Werner, H., and Kaplan, B. *Symbol Formation.* New York: Wiley, 1963.

Wershow, H. J., and Reinhart, G. "Life Changes and Hospitalization—A Heretical View." *Journal of Psychosomatic Research,* 1974, *18,* 393-401.

Wertlake, P. T., Wilcox, A. A., Haley, M. I., and Peterson, J. E. "Relation of Mental and Emotional Stress to Serum Cholesterol Levels." *Proceedings of the Society for Experimental Biology and Medicine,* 1958, *97,* 163-165.

Wexler, M. "The Behavioral Sciences in Medical Education. A View from Psychology." *American Psychologist,* 1976, *31,* 275-283.

Whalen, R. R. "Health Care Begins with I's." *New York Times,* April 17, 1977, Section 4, p. 21.

Wheelis, A. *The Quest for Identity.* New York: Norton, 1958.

White, K. L., Williams, T. F., and Greenberg, B. G. "The Ecology of Medical Care." *New England Journal of Medicine,* 1961, *265,* 885-892.

White, M. S. "Career Satisfaction and the Nurse Practitioner." Paper presented at symposium on "Women's Careers in the Health Sciences," University of California, San Francisco, May 1977.

White, R. W. "Motivation Reconsidered: The Concept of Competence." *Psychological Review,* 1959, *66,* 297-333.

White, R. W. "Strategies of Adaptation: An Attempt at Systematic Description." In G. V. Coelho, D. A. Hamburg, and J. E. Adams (Eds.), *Coping and Adaptation.* New York: Basic Books, 1974.

Whiteman, M. "Children's Conceptions of Psychological Causality." *Child Development,* 1967, *38,* 143-156.

Wiener, M., Carpenter, B., and Carpenter, J. T. "Determination of Defense Mechanisms for Conflict Areas from Verbal Material." *Journal of Consulting Psychology,* 1956, *20,* 215-219.

Wiener, N. *Cybernetics: Control and Communication in the Animal and Machine.* Cambridge, Mass.: M.I.T. Press, 1948.

Wiggins, J. G. "The Psychologist as a Health Professional in the Health Maintenance Organization." *Professional Psychology,* 1976, *7,* 9-13.

Wiggins, N., and Hoffman, P. J. "Three Models of Clinical Judgment." *Journal of Abnormal Psychology,* 1968, *73,* 70-77.

Wilber, J., and Barrow, J. "Hypertension—A Community Problem." *American Journal of Medicine,* 1972, *52,* 653-663.

Wilcocks, C. *Medical Advance, Public Health, and Social Evolution.* Elmsford, N.Y.: Pergamon Press, 1965.

Wilcox, B., and Holahan, C. "Social Ecology of the Megadorm in University Student Housing." *Journal of Educational Psychology,* 1976, *68,* 453-458.

Willems, E. "Behavioral Ecology, Health Status, and Health Care: Applications to the Rehabilitation Setting." In I. Altman and J. Wohlwill (Eds.), *Human Behavior and Environment: Advances in Theory and Research.* Vol. 1. New York: Plenum Press, 1976.

Willems, E. "Behavioral Ecology." In D. Stokols (Ed.), *Perspectives on Envi-*

ronment and Behavior. New York: Plenum Press, 1977.

Willems, E., and Halstead, L. "An Eco-Behavioral Approach to Health Status and Health Care." In R. G. Barker and Associates, *Habitats, Environments, and Human Behavior: Studies in Ecological Psychology and Eco-Behavioral Science*. San Francisco: Jossey-Bass, 1978.

Williams, A., and Wechsler, H. "Interrelationship of Preventive Actions in Health and Other Areas." *Health Services Reports*, 1972, *87*, 969-976.

Williams, P. A. "Women in Medicine: Some Themes and Variations." *Journal of Medical Education*, 1971, *46*, 584-591.

Williamson, E. G. "Vocational Counseling: Trait-Factor Theory." In B. Stefflre (Ed.), *Theories of Counseling*. New York: McGraw Hill, 1965.

Williamson, J. W., Aronovitch, S., Simonson, L., Ramirez, C., and Kelly, D. "Health Accounting: An Outcome-Based System of Quality Assurance: Illustrative Application to Hypertension." *Bulletin of the New York Academy of Medicine* (2nd Series), 1975, *51*, 727-738.

Wilmer, H. "The Relationship of the Physician to the Self-Discharge Behavior of Tuberculosis Patients." In P. Sparer (Ed.), *Personality, Stress, and Tuberculosis*. New York: International Universities Press, 1956.

Wilner, D. M., Walkley, R. P., Pinkerton, T. C., and Tayback, M. *The Housing Environment and Family Life*. Baltimore: Johns Hopkins University Press, 1962.

Wilson, J. "Drug Compliance Problems for Hospitalized Children." In L. Lasagna (Ed.), *Patient Compliance*. Mt. Kisco, N.Y.: Futura, 1976.

Wilson, J. F. "Determinants of Recovery from Surgery: Preoperative Instruction, Relaxation Training, and Defensive Structure." Unpublished doctoral dissertation, University of Michigan, 1977.

Wirsching, M., Druner, H. V., and Herrmann, G. "Results of Psychosocial Adjustment to Long-Term Colostomy." *Psychotherapy and Psychosomatics*, 1975, *26*, 245-256.

Wishner, J. "Neurosis and Tension: An Exploratory Study of Physiological and Rorschach Measures." *Journal of Abnormal and Social Psychology*, 1953, *48*, 253-260.

Wishnie, H. A., Hackett, T. P., and Cassem, N. H. "Psychological Hazards of Convalescence Following Myocardial Infarction." *Journal of the American Medical Association*, 1971, *215*, 1292-1296.

Witkin, H. A., Mensh, I. N., and Cates, J. "Psychologists in Medical Schools." *American Psychologist*, 1972, *27*, 434-440.

Wittkower, E. D. "Historical Perspective on Contemporary Psychosomatic Medicine." *International Journal of Psychiatry in Medicine*, 1974, *5*, 309-319.

Wolf, S. "The End of the Rope: The Role of the Brain in Cardiac Death." *Canadian Medical Association Journal*, 1967, *97*, 1022-1025.

Wolfer, J. A. "Definition and Assessment of Surgical Patients' Welfare and Recovery." *Nursing Research*, 1973, *22*, 394-401.

Wolfer, J. A., and Davis, C. E. "Assessment of Surgery Patients' Preoperative Emotional Condition and Postoperative Welfare." *Nursing Research*, 1970, *19*, 402-414.

Wolfer, J. A., and Visintainer, M. A. "Pediatric Surgical Patients' and Parents' Stress Responses and Adjustment as a Function of Psychologic Preparation and Stress-Point Nursing Care." *Nursing Research,* 1975, *24,* 244-255.

Wolff, C. T., Friedman, S. G., Hofer, M. A., and Mason, J. W. "Relationship Between Psychological Defenses and Mean Urinary 17-Hydroxycorticosteroid Excretion Rates: I. A Predictive Study of Parents of Fatally Ill Children." *Psychosomatic Medicine,* 1964, *26,* 576-591.

Wolff, H., and Goodell, H. *Stress and Disease.* (2nd ed.) Springfield, Ill.: Thomas, 1968.

Wolff, K. "Hospitalized Alcoholic Patients: III. Motivating Alcoholics Through Group Psychotherapy." *Hospital and Community Psychiatry,* 1968, *19,* 206-209.

Wollersheim, J. P. "Effectiveness of Group Therapy Based upon Learning Principles in the Treatment of Overweight Women." *Journal of Abnormal Psychology,* 1970, *76,* 462-474.

Wolpe, J., and Lazarus, A. *Behavior Therapy Techniques.* Elmsford, N.Y.: Pergamon Press, 1966.

Woods, D. J. "The Repression-Sensitization of Variable and Self-Reported Emotional Arousal: Effects of Stress and Instructional Set." *Journal of Consulting and Clinical Psychology,* 1977, *45,* 173-183.

Woods, S. M., and Natterson, J. "Sexual Attitudes of Medical Students: Some Implications for Medical Education." *American Journal of Psychiatry,* 1967, *124,* 323-332.

Worchel, S., and Teddlie, C. "The Experience of Crowding: A Two-Factor Theory." *Journal of Personality and Social Psychology,* 1976, *34,* 30-40.

World Conference on Smoking and Health. *Summary of the Proceedings.* New York: National Interagency Council on Smoking and Health, 1967.

Wortman, C. G., and Brehm, J. W. "Responses to Uncontrollable Outcomes: An Integration of Reactance Theory and the Learned Helplessness Model." In C. Berkowitz (Ed.), *Advances in Experimental Social Psychology.* Vol. 8. New York: Academic Press, 1975.

Wright, B. A. *Physical Disability—A Psychological Approach.* New York: Harper & Row, 1960.

Wright, L. "Psychology as a Health Profession." *Clinical Psychologist,* 1976, *29,* 16-19.

Wright, L. "Conceptualizing and Defining Psychosomatic Disorders." *American Psychologist,* 1977, *32,* 625-628.

Wright, R. G., and Holmes, T. H. "Psychological Aspects of Hospitalization." In H. I. Lief, V. F. Lief, and N. R. Lief (Eds.), *The Psychological Basis of Medical Practice.* New York: Harper & Row, 1963.

Wülf, F. "Über die Veränderung von Vorstellungen (Gedächtnis und Gestalt)." *Psychologische Forschung,* 1922, *1,* 333-373. Translated and condensed in W. D. Ellis (Ed.), *A Source Book of Gestalt Psychology.* New York: Harcourt Brace Jovanovich, 1938.

Young, M., Benjamin, B., and Wallis, C. "The Mortality of Widowers." *Lancet,* 1963, *2,* 454-456.

Yufit, R. I., Pollack, G. H., and Wasserman, E. "Medical Specialty Choice and Personality." *Archives of General Psychiatry,* 1969, *20,* 89-99.

Zammuner, V. L. "Attitudes Toward Abortion: A Pilot Cross-Cultural Comparison." *Giornule Italiano de Psicologia,* 1976, *3,* 75-116.

Zborowski, M. "Cultural Components in Responses to Pain." *Journal of Social Issues,* 1952, *8,* 16-30.

Zedeck, S., and Kafry, D. "Capturing Rater Policies for Processing Evaluation Data." *Organizational Behavior and Human Performance,* 1977, *18,* 269-294.

Zieve, L. "Misinterpretation and Abuse of Laboratory Tests by Clinicians." *Annals of the New York Academy of Sciences,* 1966, *134,* 563-572.

Zimbardo, P. G. "The Human Choice." In W. Arnold and D. Levine (Eds.), *Nebraska Symposium on Motivation 1969.* Vol. 17. Lincoln: University of Nebraska Press, 1970.

Zimpfer, D. G. *Group Work in the Helping Professions: A Bibliography.* Washington, D.C.: American Personnel and Guidance Association, 1976.

Zinsser, O. *Rats, Lice, and History.* Boston: Little, Brown, 1935.

Zola, I. K. "Culture and Symptoms—An Analysis of Patients' Presenting Complaints." *American Sociological Review,* 1966, *31,* 615-630.

Zola, I. K. "Studying the Decision to See a Doctor: Review, Critique, Corrective." *Advances in Psychosomatic Medicine,* 1972, *8,* 216-236.

Zola, I. K. "Pathways to the Doctor—From Person to Patient." *Social Science and Medicine,* 1973, *7,* 677-689.

Zyzanski, S. J., Hulka, B. S., and Cassel, J. C. "Scale for the Measurement of Satisfaction with Medical Care: Modifications in Content, Format, and Scoring." *Medical Care,* 1974, *12,* 611-620.

Name Index

Subject Index